W9-BMA-059

Step 1: Learn

"A journey of a thousand miles begins with a single step."

— Lao-tzu

Congratulations! You are embarking on an exciting and rewarding career, and you have taken a great first step. Coding is a career that gives you a chance to pursue excellence at a variety of levels, and I am happy that you have chosen to start with my *Step* line of products. As a lifelong coder and educator, I am dedicated to giving you the tools you need to succeed. *So, get out there and code!*

— Carol J. Buck, MS, CPC-I, CPC, CPC-H, CCS-P

Track your progress!

See the checklist in the back of this book
to learn more about your next step toward coding success!

The tools for your
total coding success are here!

Build a **strong foundation** for career success
with the proven leader in coding education.

Workbook

Enhance your understanding with real-world documents and additional exercises!

ISBN: 978-1-4377-0218-7

Sold separately.

Medical Coding Online

Get extra practice and strengthen your understanding with this **interactive online course**!

ISBN: 978-1-4377-0369-6

Sold separately.

evolve
learning system

Evolve Resources

Stay up to date and **practice what you've learned** with the **Evolve** companion website, included with your textbook. Go to **http://evolve.elsevier.com**!

Included with this textbook!

Get the resources you need now!

- Visit your **local bookstore**
- Order securely at **www.elsevierhealth.com**
- Call toll-free **1-800-545-2522**

Virtual Medical Office

An interactive software program designed to work with your book, **Virtual Medical Office** lets you practice **critical thinking skills** in a simulated office setting.

ISBN: 978-1-4377-1505-7

Sold separately.

See the checklist in the back of this book for more information!

Need more ICD-9-CM study resources?

This clear, easy-to-use textbook is **your key to ICD-9-CM coding success,** offering **everything you need to understand and apply the official codes of the ICD-9-CM, while giving you a preview of ICD-10.** You'll find **detailed background information** on the evolution and importance of medical coding, as well as **reliable, straightforward guidelines** for each of the coding classifications you'll use in practice.

Master the ICD-9-CM and ICD-10-CM/PCS concepts needed to ensure proper reimbursement with features like...

- **Dual Codes** that let you practice finding ICD-10-CM/PCS codes in addition to learning ICD-9-CM

- **ICD-9-CM guidelines** that open each coding chapter with examples that clearly demonstrate their real-world applications.

- A **full-color design** that makes anatomy and physiology stand out and provides visual reinforcement of key content.

- **Illustrations and overviews of anatomy, physiology, and related disease conditions** in each coding chapter that help you better visualize and understand what the codes represent.

- **Problem-solving exercises** throughout each chapter that provide valuable practice using key coding principles as you learn them.

Foreword by
Carol J. Buck

2010

ICD-9-CM CODING
THEORY AND PRACTICE

Karla R. Lovaasen, RHIA, CCS, CCS-P
Jennifer Schwerdtfeger, BS, RHIT, CCS, CPC, CPC-H

SAUNDERS
ELSEVIER

evolve
learning system

ICD-9-CM Coding: Theory and Practice, 2010 Edition
Karla R. Lovaasen, RHIA, CCS, CCS-P, and
Jennifer Schwerdtfeger, BS, RHIT, CCS, CPC, CPC-H
2010 • 832 pp., 400 illus. • ISBN: 978-1-4377-0600-0

LOV-10

learning system

REGISTER TODAY!

To access your Student Resources, visit:

http://evolve.elsevier.com/Buck/step/

Evolve® Student Resources for **_Buck: Step-by-Step Medical Coding, 2010 Edition_** offer the following features:

Student Resources

- **Content Updates**
  Keep your textbook current with updates straight from the author.

- **Activities**
  Provides a variety of activity styles for added practice with each chapter (contact instructor for answers).

- **_SpeedECoder_**
  30-day access to _SpeedECoder_ online code editor, to be used at the end of your training course.

- **Coding Updates, Tips, and Links**
  Easy access to the latest ICD-9-CM Official Guidelines for Coding and Reporting; 1995 and 1997 Guidelines for E/M Services; CPT, ICD-9-CM, and HCPCS code updates; Study Tips; and WebLinks.

- **AAPC Salary Survey**
  Review the latest salary study published by the AAPC.

- **Extra Coding Cases**
  Realistic medical reports allow you to practice your coding skills and check your answers.

ELSEVIER

2010

STEP-BY-STEP

MEDICAL CODING

2010

STEP-BY-STEP

MEDICAL CODING

Carol J. Buck
MS, CPC-I, CPC, CPC-H, CCS-P
Program Director, Retired
Medical Secretary Programs
Northwest Technical College
East Grand Forks, Minnesota

Susan Thurston
MA, CHCA, CPC, CPC-I, CPC-H,
CPC-P, CCS-P, MCS-P, CHCO, CMM, RMC
CEO
Coder's Connection, Inc.
Executive Director of Education
Association of Health Care Auditors and Educators
Rifle, Colorado

learning system

SAUNDERS
ELSEVIER

3251 Riverport Lane
Maryland Heights, Missouri 63043

STEP-BY-STEP MEDICAL CODING, 2010 EDITION ISBN: 978-1-4160-6836-5

Copyright © 2010, 2009, 2008, 2007, 2006, 2005, 2004, 2002, 2000, 1998, 1996 by Saunders, an imprint of Elsevier Inc.

NOTE: *Current Procedural Terminology, 2010,* was used in updating this text.

Current Procedural Terminology (CPT) is copyright 2009 American Medical Association. All Rights Reserved. No fee schedules, basic units, relative values, or related listings are included in CPT. The AMA assumes no liability for the data contained herein. Applicable FARS/DFARS restrictions apply to government use.

All rights reserved. No part of this publication may be reproduced or transmitted in any form or by any means, electronic or mechanical, including photocopying, recording, or any information storage and retrieval system, without permission in writing from the publisher. Permissions may be sought directly from Elsevier's Rights Department: phone: (+1) 215 239 3804 (US) or (+44) 1865 843830 (UK); fax: (+44) 1865 853333; e-mail: healthpermissions@ elsevier.com. You may also complete your request on-line via the Elsevier website at http://www.elsevier.com/permissions.

NOTICE

Knowledge and best practice in this field are constantly changing. As new research and experience broaden our knowledge, changes in practice, treatment, and drug therapy may become necessary or appropriate. Readers are advised to check the most current information provided (i) on procedures featured or (ii) by the manufacturer of each product to be administered, to verify the recommended dose or formula, the method and duration of administration, and contraindications. It is the responsibility of the practitioner, relying on his or her own experience and knowledge of the patient, to make diagnoses, to determine dosages and the best treatment for each individual patient, and to take all appropriate safety precautions. To the fullest extent of the law, neither the Publisher nor the Author assumes any liability for any injury and/or damage to persons or property arising out of or related to any use of the material contained in this book.

The Publisher

Library of Congress Cataloging-in-Publication Data

Buck, Carol J.
  Step-by-step medical coding / Carol J. Buck. -- 2010 ed.
    p. ; cm.
  Includes bibliographical references and indexes.
  ISBN 978-1-4160-6836-5 (pbk. : alk. paper) 1. Nosology--Code numbers. I. Title. II. Title: Medical coding. III. Title: 2010 step-by-step medical coding.
  [DNLM: 1. Disease--classification. 2. Terminology as Topic. 3. Forms and Records Control--methods. 4. Insurance, Health, Reimbursement. WB 15 B922s 2010]
  RB115.B83 2010
  616.001'48--dc22

                                                                    2009033572

Publisher: Michael S. Ledbetter
Developmental Editor: Joshua S. Rapplean
Publishing Services Manager: Pat Joiner-Myers
Senior Designer: Amy Buxton

Working together to grow
libraries in developing countries

www.elsevier.com | www.bookaid.org | www.sabre.org

ELSEVIER   BOOK AID International   Sabre Foundation

Printed in Canada

Last digit is the print number: 9 8 7 6 5 4 3 2 1

To the students, whose drive and determination to learn serve as my endless source of inspiration and enrichment.

To teachers, whose contributions are immense and workloads daunting. May this work make your preparation for class a little easier.

Carol J. Buck

ACKNOWLEDGMENTS

This book was developed in collaboration with educators and employers in an attempt to meet the needs of students preparing for careers in the medical coding allied health profession. Obtaining employers' input about the knowledge, skills, and abilities desired of entry-level coding employees benefits educators tremendously. This text is an endeavor to use this information to better prepare our students.

There are several other people who deserve special thanks for their efforts in making this text possible.

Joan E. Wolfgang, who joined the effort and has lent her expertise and unending patience to this project and many others. She is a highly regarded member of our team.

Jacqueline Grass, Research Assistant, for her technical knowledge, interest in student learning, and long hours of dedicated service to developing education materials. Her gentle and quiet demeanor is a gift beyond measure.

Jody Klitz, Research Assistant, for her meticulous approach to a myriad of complex assignments. Her professionalism is beyond compare.

Nancy Maguire, for her dedication to superior education and a lifetime of devotion to the coding career.

Susan Thurston, Team Leader, who has joined the Village with enthusiasm and lends her expertise to this work.

Michael Ledbetter, Publisher, who managed to maintain an excellent sense of humor while jumping into the fray and who is a valued member of the team. **Josh Rapplean,** Developmental Editor, who manages the developmental duties of this text with calm, confidence, and tremendous efficiency. **Laura Slown Sullivan** and **Rhoda Bontrager,** Production Editors, Graphic World, who assumed responsibility for many projects while maintaining a high degree of professionalism.

The publisher would also like to acknowledge and thank the following people for their enthusiasm and dedication to the coding profession and tremendous contributions to this work:

Patricia Champion	Lynda Kross	Lynne Padilla
Beverly Comsa	Stephanie A. Lewis	Christine A. Patterson
Maria Coslett	Karla R. Lovaasen	Letitia Patterson
Ellen Dooley	Nancy Maguire	Damaris Ramirez
Robert H. Ekvall	Debbi Miller	Keith Russell
Christopher P. Galeziewski	Tom Mobley	Patricia Sommerfeld
Patricia Cordy Henricksen	Genieve R. Nottage	Cynthia Stahl
	John R. Nuemann III	Martha Tracy
Melony M. Jones	Sharon J. Oliver	Jane A. Tuttle
	Barbara Oviatt	Joan E. Wolfgang

Skip Stowers of Photography by Skip Stowers and Dan Kaufman of Las Vegas Photo and Video, for their talent, patience, and photographs.

Thank you for purchasing *Step-by-Step Medical Coding*, the leading textbook for medical coding education. This 2010 edition has been carefully reviewed and updated with the latest content, making it the most current textbook for your class. The author and publisher have made every effort to equip you with skills and tools you will need to succeed on the job. To this end, *Step-by-Step Medical Coding* presents essential information for all health care coding systems and covers the skills needed to be a successful medical coder. No other text on the market brings together such thorough coverage of all coding systems in one source.

ORGANIZATION OF THIS TEXTBOOK

Developed in collaboration with employers and educators, *Step-by-Step Medical Coding, 2010 Edition* takes a practical approach to training for a successful career in medical coding. The text is divided into four units covering Reimbursement, ICD-9-CM and ICD-10-CM, CPT and HCPCS, and Inpatient Coding.

Unit I, Reimbursement, is a chapter that introduces the reimbursement, HIPAA, and compliance processes, noting the connections between coding and reimbursement.

Unit II, ICD-9-CM and ICD-10-CM, provides an overview of both the ICD-9-CM and ICD-10-CM codes and their use in medical coding. A highlight of this unit is the inclusion of the *ICD-9-CM Official Guidelines for Coding and Reporting* within the chapter text, as they apply to the content.

Unit III, CPT and HCPCS, begins with an introduction to the CPT manual, followed by in-depth explanation of the sections found in the code set. Organized by body systems to follow the CPT codes, the chapters include important information about anatomy, terminology, and various procedures, as well as demonstration and examples of how to code each service.

Unit IV, Inpatient Coding, provides an overview of reporting facility services provided to patients in acute inpatient facilities and the reporting of these services with ICD-9-CM, Volume 3, Procedures codes.

DISTINCTIVE FEATURES OF OUR APPROACH

This book was designed to be the first step in your coding career, and it has many unique features to help you along the way.

- The repetition of skills in each chapter reinforces the material and creates a logical progression for learning and applying each skill—a truly "step-by-step" approach!
- In-text exercises further reinforce important concepts and allow you to check your comprehension as you read.

■ The format for exercise and review answers guides you in the development of your coding ability by including three response variations:

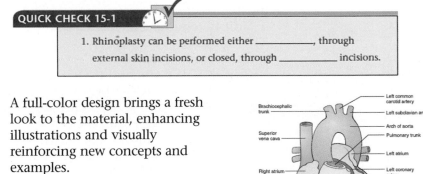

- ■ **One** answer blank for coding questions that require a one-code answer
- ■ **Multiple** answer blanks for coding questions that require a multiple-code answer
- ■ Answer blanks with a preceding symbol (⊛) indicate that **you must decide** the number of codes necessary to correctly answer the question

■ *Quick Checks* are located throughout the chapters, providing short follow-up questions after a key concept has been covered to immediately assess learning. Answers to the *Quick Checks* are located at the end of each chapter.

QUICK CHECK 15-1

1. Rhinoplasty can be performed either _____, through external skin incisions, or closed, through _____ incisions.

■ A full-color design brings a fresh look to the material, enhancing illustrations and visually reinforcing new concepts and examples.

■ Medical procedures or conditions are illustrated and discussed in the text to help you understand the services being coded.

FIGURE 16-3   External view of heart.

■ Using the login information on the bind-in card, access to *SpeedECoder* online code editor is available with this edition. *SpeedECoder* can be used with the exercises in Appendix C as a capstone experience after completing work with the textbook.

APPENDIX **C**

SpeedECoder
Exercises

Note: It is recommended that you wait to access this feature until you've finished working through the main text.
    As an additional bonus feature, we have included 30-day access to *SpeedECoder* online code editor.

CASES 1 THROUGH 15
Your supervisor has asked you to use the *SpeedECoder* to check the accuracy of several cases that were coded by another coder.

CASES 16 THROUGH 20
For Cases 16 through 20, you are to assign the correct CPT and ICD-9-CM codes. Be sure to check the codes you assign with the *SpeedECoder*. Once you have finished, your instructor will provide you with answers for Cases 16-20 so you can check your work.

CHAPTER 10

"I think having a goal of being a lifelong learner is important. One also has to have a great degree of integrity. It takes knowledge and character to adhere to the correct way to do things, and not be swayed by other factors, such as how to 'get it paid.'"

Joan E. Wolfgang, BA, CPC, CPC-H
Consultant, Educator,
PMCC Certified Instructor
Milwaukee, Wisconsin

Evaluation and Management (E/M) Section

Chapter Topics	Learning Objectives
Contents of the E/M Section	*After completing this chapter you should be able to*
Three Factors of E/M Codes	1 Identify and explain the three factors of E/M code assignment.
Various Levels of E/M Service	2 Differentiate between a new and an established patient.
An E/M Code Example	3 Differentiate between an inpatient and an outpatient.
Using the E/M Codes	4 Explain the levels of E/M service.
Documentation Guidelines	5 Review the key components.
Chapter Review	6 Analyze the key component history.
Quick Check Answers	7 Analyze the key component examination.
	8 Analyze the key component medical decision making.
	9 List contributory factors.
	10 Analyze code information.
	11 Analyze the types of E/M codes.
	12 Identify CMS Documentation Guidelines.
	13 Demonstrate the ability to code E/M services.

- Chapter learning objectives and end of chapter review questions help readers focus on essential chapter content.

CHAPTER 10 ■ Evaluation and Management (E/M) Section

CHAPTER REVIEW

CHAPTER 10, PART I, THEORY
Without using the CPT manual, complete the following:

1 Is examination of the back an organ system or body area examination?

2 The four types of patient status are
_____,
_____, and
_____.

3 The first outpatient visit is called the _____ visit, and the second visit is called the _____ visit.

4 The first three factors a coder must consider when coding are patient _____, _____, and _____.

5 How many types of histories are there?

6 Which history is more complex: the problem focused history or the expanded problem focused history? _____

7 The four types of examinations, in order of difficulty (from least difficult to most difficult), are as follows:

a _____
b _____
c _____
d _____

8 The examination that is limited to the affected body area is the _____.

9 What does VLBW stand for?

10 What medical decision making involves a situation in which the diagnosis and management options are minimal, data amount and complexity that must be reviewed are minimal/none, and there is a minimal risk to the patient of complications or death?

11 What term is used to describe a patient who has been formally admitted to a hospital?

- Concrete "real-life" examples illustrate the application of important coding principles and practices.

Example
During a cardiac catheterization procedure, contrast medium is injected into a bypass graft and into the coronary arteries. CPT codes would be used to identify each of the areas of injection as follows:
93540   injection into the bypass graft
93545   injection into selective coronary arteries

ICD-9-CM OFFICIAL GUIDELINES FOR CODING AND REPORTING

SECTION I.B.11.
11. Combination Code

A combination code is a single code used to classify:
Two diagnoses, or
A diagnosis with an associated secondary process (manifestation)
A diagnosis with an associated complication

Combination codes are identified by referring to subterm entries in the Alphabetic Index and by reading the inclusion and exclusion notes in the Tabular List.

Assign only the combination code when that code fully identifies the diagnostic conditions involved or when the Alphabetic Index so directs. Multiple coding should not be used when the classification provides a combination code that clearly identifies all of the elements documented in the diagnosis. When the combination code lacks necessary specificity in describing the manifestation or complication, an additional code should be used as a secondary code.

- *ICD-9-CM Official Guidelines for Coding and Reporting* boxes in Chapters 2-7 contain excerpts of the actual guidelines, presenting the official wording alongside in-text discussions.

- *From the Trenches* boxes highlight a different real-life medical coding practitioner in each chapter, with photographs throughout the chapter alongside quotes that offer practical advice or motivational comments.

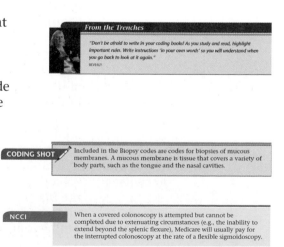

From the Trenches

"Don't be afraid to write in your coding books! As you study and read, highlight important rules. Write instructions 'in your own words' so you will understand when you go back to look at it again."
BEVERLY

- *Coding Shots* contain tips for the new coder.

CODING SHOT Included in the Biopsy codes are codes for biopsies of mucous membranes. A mucous membrane is tissue that covers a variety of body parts, such as the tongue and the nasal cavities.

- *NCCI* boxes highlight correct coding methods as recognized by the CPT in their National Correct Coding Initiative.

NCCI When a covered colonoscopy is attempted but cannot be completed due to extenuating circumstances (e.g., the inability to extend beyond the splenic flexure), Medicare will usually pay for the interrupted colonoscopy at the rate of a flexible sigmoidoscopy.

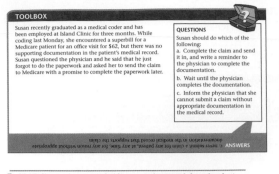

TOOLBOX

Susan recently graduated as a medical coder and has been employed at Island Clinic for three months. While coding last Monday, she encountered a superbill for a Medicare patient for an office visit for $62, but there was no supporting documentation in the patient's medical record. Susan questioned the physician and he said that he just forgot to do the paperwork and asked her to send the claim to Medicare with a promise to complete the paperwork later.

QUESTIONS

Susan should do which of the following:

a. Complete the claim and send it in, and write a reminder to the physician to complete the documentation.

b. Wait until the physician completes the documentation.

c. Inform the physician that she cannot submit a claim without appropriate documentation in the medical record.

ANSWERS: c. never submit a claim for any patient, at any time, for any reason without appropriate documentation in the medical record that supports the claim

- *Toolbox* features are located throughout the chapters, providing scenarios and questions to help apply chapter content to realistic scenarios.

STOP *You were just presented with some very important information about the use of certain codes in the CPT manual. The plus (+) symbol next to any CPT code—not just next to Qualifying Circumstances codes—indicates that that code cannot be used alone. Throughout the remaining sections of the CPT manual, the plus symbol will appear to caution you to use the code only as an adjunct code (with other codes).*

- *Stop!* notes halt you for a reality check, offering a brief summary of material that was just covered and providing a transition into the next topic.

CAUTION *Some CPT codes are for bilateral procedures and do not require a bilateral modifier. For example, 27395 is for a bilateral lengthening of the hamstring tendon, and it would be incorrect to place a bilateral modifier on the code.*

- *Caution!* notes warn you about common coding mistakes and reinforce the concept of coding as an exact science.

CHECK THIS OUT! The American Medical Association (AMA) has a Website located at http://www.ama-assn.org

- *Check This Out!* boxes offer notes about accessing reference information related to coding, primarily via the Internet.

CURRENT PROCEDURAL TERMINOLOGY (CPT) CODES

00100-01999: 218, 252
00142: 358
00400: 360
00740: 364
00810: 364
00901: 372
01916-01936: 350
01922: 350

- A *Coder's Index* can be found in the back of the book, providing easy reference when looking for specific codes.

EXTENSIVE SUPPLEMENTAL RESOURCES

Considering the broad range of students, programs, and institutions in which this textbook is used, we have developed an extensive package of supplements designed to complement *Step-by-Step Medical Coding.* Each of these comprehensive supplements has been developed with the needs of both students and instructors in mind.

STEP-BY-STEP   SAUNDERS

Activity 15-2, Match the Terms

Directions: Match the term with the correct definition by dragging the term to the definition.

A. lavage   B. pleurectomy   C. cordectomy

D. intramural   E. thoracotomy

[ ] 1. within the organ wall

[ ] 2. surgical incision into the chest wall

[ ] 3. surgical excision of the pleura

[ ] 4. surgical removal of the vocal cord(s)

[ ] 5. washing out of an organ

Exit   Main Menu   Print Activity   Reset Activity   Back   Next

Student Online Activities

The online activities supplement the text with 46 chapter activities and 25 coding cases. The variety of activity styles include multiple choice, fill in the blank, matching, and coding exercises. These activities will reinforce material learned in the text and offer students another study tool. Answers can be found in the TEACH Instructor Resources.

Student Workbook

The fully updated workbook supplements the text with more than 1000 questions and terminology exercises, as well as over 80 original source documents to familiarize the user with documents he or she will encounter in practice. Reports are included in a variety of areas, including arthroscopy, muscle repair, thoracentesis, tubal ligation, and endoarterectomy. The workbook questions also follow the same answer format of the main text, improving coding skills and promoting critical thinking.

TEACH Instructor Resources on Evolve

No matter what your level of teaching experience, this total-teaching solution will help you plan your lessons with ease, and the author has developed all the curriculum materials necessary to use *Step-by-Step Medical Coding* in the classroom. Included in the printed material are all answers to the textbook, online activities, and workbook exercises; extra coding cases with answers; a course calendar and syllabus; curriculum with TEACH Lesson Plans and Lecture Outlines; and ready-made tests for easy assessment. The instructor Evolve site includes all printed content, a comprehensive PowerPoint collection of the entire text, interactive PowerPoint slides, and a test bank in ExamView. The slides can be easily customized to support your lectures or formatted with PowerPoint as overhead transparencies or handouts for student note-taking. The ExamView test generator will help you quickly and easily prepare quizzes and exams, and the test banks can be customized to your specific teaching methods.

Evolve Learning Resources

The Evolve Learning Resources offer helpful material that will extend your studies beyond the classroom. Official Coding Guidelines, Code Updates, and Chapter WebLinks offer you the opportunity to expand your knowledge base and stay current with this ever-changing field, while extra Coding Cases and Coding Tips are available online to check your understanding. Instructors can also download all materials available from the Instructor's Resource Manual, as well as content updates and industry news.

A Course Management System is also available free to instructors who adopt this textbook. This web-based platform gives instructors yet another resource to facilitate learning and to make medical coding content accessible to students. In addition to the Evolve Learning Resources available to both faculty and students, there is an entire suite of tools available that allows for communication between instructors and students. Students can log on through the Evolve portal to take online quizzes, participate in threaded discussions, post assignments to instructors, or chat with other classmates, while instructors can use the online grade book to follow class progress.

To access this comprehensive online resource, simply go to the Evolve home page at http://evolve.elsevier.com and enter the user name and password provided by your instructor. If your instructor has not set up a Course Management System, you can still access the free Evolve Learning Resources at http://evolve.elsevier.com/Buck/step/.

Step-by-Step Medical Coding Online

Designed to accommodate diverse learning styles and environments, *Step-by-Step Medical Coding Online* is an online course supplement that works in conjunction with the textbook to provide you with a wide range of visual, auditory, and interactive learning materials. The course amplifies course content, synthesizes concepts, reinforces learning, and demonstrates practical applications in a dynamic and exciting way. As you move through the course, interactive exercises, quizzes, and activities allow you to check your comprehension and learn from immediate feedback, while still allowing you to use your textbook as a resource. Because of its design, this course offers students a unique and innovative learning experience.

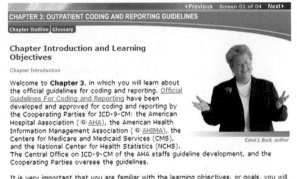

evolve|ebooks

Spend less time searching and more time learning with electronic access to *Step-by-Step Medical Coding, 2010 Edition.* With easy access from any computer or internet browser, you can search across all of your Elsevier e-textbooks, paste important text and images from multiple sources into a focused, custom document, make notes, highlights, and more. Please contact an Elsevier customer service representative for more information, or visit http://evolve.elsevier.com/ebooks.

DEVELOPMENT OF THIS EDITION

This book would not have been possible without a team of educators and professionals, including practicing coders and technical consultants. The combined efforts of the team members have made this text an incredible learning tool.

TEAM LEADER

Susan Thurston, MA, CHCA, CPC, CPC-I, CPC-H, CPC-P, CCS-P, MCS-P, CHCO, CMM, RMC
CEO
Coder's Connection, Inc.
Executive Director of Education
Association of Health Care Auditors and Educators
Rifle, Colorado

SENIOR ICD-9-CM AND ICD-10-CM CODING SPECIALIST

Karla R. Lovaasen, RHIA, CCS, CCS-P
Coding and Consulting Services
Abingdon, Maryland

—Co-author of *ICD-9-CM Coding: Theory and Practice, 2010 Edition*, St. Louis, 2010, Saunders.

SENIOR COLLABORATOR AND SPECIAL ICD-10-CM CONSULTANT

Nancy Maguire, ACS, CRT, PCS, FCS, CPC, CPC-H, HCS-D, APC, AFC
Physician Consultant for Auditing and Education
Universal City, Texas

SPECIAL ICD-10-CM CONSULTANT

Joan E. Wolfgang, BA, CPC, CPC-H, CPC-I
Coding QI & Provider Education Director
Lakeshore Medical Clinics
South Milwaukee, Wisconsin

CODING SPECIALISTS

Jacqueline Klitz Grass, MA, CPC
Coding Specialist
Grand Forks, North Dakota

Jody Klitz, CPC
Coding Reimbursement Specialist
Cancer Center of North Dakota
Grand Forks, North Dakota

Lindsay-Anne Jenkins, CRNA, CPC, CPC-H, CPC-I
Coding and Auditing Specialist
Healthcare Strategic Initiatives
St. Louis, Missouri

QUERY MANAGER

Patricia Cordy Henricksen, CPC, CCP
Approved PMCC Instructor
President, Lexington Local Chapter of AAPC
Bluegrass Medical Managers Association
Lexington, Kentucky

QUERY TEAM

Debra Kroll, RHIT
Altru Health System
Grand Forks, North Dakota

To ensure the accuracy of the material presented in this textbook, many reviewers have provided feedback over several editions of this text. We are deeply grateful to the numerous people who have shared their suggestions and comments. Reviewing a book or supplement takes an incredible amount of energy and attention, and we are glad so many colleagues were able to take the time to give us their feedback on the material.

EDITORIAL REVIEW BOARD

Kelly M. Anastasio, CPC, CPC-H, CPC-P, CPC-I
Billing Supervisor
Yale University, Department of Orthopaedics and Rehabilitation
PMCC Instructor
Medical Coding Academy
New Haven, Connecticut

Elaine Benton, CPC
Reimbursement Manager
University of Texas Southwestern Medical Center at Dallas
Dallas, Texas

Judy B. Breuker, CPC, CCS-P, CHBME, ACS, PCS
Certified E/M Auditor
President
Medical Education Services, LLC
Hudsonville, Michigan

Virginia Bryant, CPC-a
Interim Director of Medical Reimbursement Program
Career Learning Center of the Black Hills
Rapid City, South Dakota

Patrice A. Bush, CPC, PCS
Coding Consultant
Coding Reimbursement Consultants (CRC)
Canton, Ohio

Brenda J. Dombkowski, CPC
Compliance Auditor
New Haven, Connecticut

Karen Drummond, CPC-I, CPC-H, ACS-RA, ACS-OB/GYN, PCS, FCS, CMC, CMBS-I
Instructor and Consultant
Lexington, North Carolina

Patricia Cordy Henricksen, CPC, CCP
Approved PMCC Instructor
President, Lexington Local Chapter of AAPC
Bluegrass Medical Managers Association
Lexington, Kentucky

Miriam F. Hernandez, MD, NCICS
Physician Coding/Compliance Auditor
Miami Children's Hospital
Miami, Florida

Carolyn M. Hutt, CMA(AAMA), CPC, CPC-I, CCS-P, CCP, CMC, CPHT, BCS-M, RMC
Associate Director of Reimbursement
US Oncology
Houston, Texas

Linda D. Jackson, CPC, CMIS, CGCS, CCP, PCS
Reimbursement/Coding Coordinator
Washington Hospital Center, Department of Medicine
Washington, District of Columbia

Debra Kroll, RHIT
Altru Health System
Grand Forks, North Dakota

Maria N. Lesly, MEd, RHIT, CCS-P, CPC, CPC-I
Coding Knowledge Solutions
Lubbock, Texas

Jenny Mann-Francis, CCS-P, CPC, PMCC, CAPPM
Revenue Manager
University of California, Davis
Davis, California

Donna M. Martin, MBA, CPC-I, CPC, CPC-H, MCS-P
Owner/Chief Academic Officer
Codes Unlimited Healthcare Academy
Memphis, Tennessee

Allysen L. Martinez, RCC, CPC
Medical Coding and Billing Instructor
Purdue University, Calumet
Condensed Curriculum International College
Hammond, Indiana
Coding Supervisor
Medical Management and Data Services, Inc.
Munster, Indiana

Lois E. Mazza, CPC
Certified Professional Coder
Lahey Clinic
Burlington, Massachusetts

Denae M. Merrill, CPC-E/M
HCC Coding Specialist
The Coding Source
Owner
Merrill Medical Management
Los Angeles, California

Genieve R. Nottage, MBA, BSHA, CPC, CPC-I, CMBS
Healthcare Administration Consultant
Locust Grove, Georgia

Sharon J. Oliver, CPC, CPC-I, CPMA
Senior Inpatient Biller
Jonesborough, Tennessee

Eva R. Oltman, MEd, BS, CPC, EMT, CMA
Allied Health Division Chair
Jefferson Community and Technical College
Louisville, Kentucky

Lynn L. Pascoe, CPC, CPC-I, CPC-EMS, CCP
President
AAPC—Charm City Chapter (Baltimore East)
Baltimore, Maryland

Letitia Patterson, MPA, CPC, CCS-P
Senior Medical Coding Specialist
Wellcare
Chicago, Illinois

Sharon R. Peddycord, AAS, CPC
Medical Biller/Coder, Coding Consultant
Glenwood, Illinois

Susie Perryman, CPC
Coding Team Leader
Cardiovascular Associates of East Texas
Tyler, Texas

Amy Petry, CPC
Coding and Compliance Specialist
Bothell, Washington

Damaris Ramirez, CPC, CPC-I
Director of Education
CPC Exam Prep, LLC
Edgewater, New Jersey

Janet Schmitt, CPC, PCS
Financial Quality Team Lead
AAPC
Augusta, Georgia

Patricia Harrison Skibbe
Welcoming Officer
AAPC Richardson, Texas, Chapter
Richardson, Texas

Kathleen M. Skolnick, CPC, CPC-I, CCP-P
AAPC PMCC Approved Instructor
Consultant
Medical Coding for Professionals, LLC
Colonia, New Jersey

Geraldine Slawek, CPC, CPC-I, CPC-ED, RHIT
Medical Coding Manager
Florida Health Information Management Association
Tampa, Florida

Cynthia Stahl, CPC, CCS-P, CPC-H
Reimbursement and Coding Specialist
Lebanon, Indiana

Rebecca Stewart, CPC, CCS
Project Manager
Cleveland Clinic
Cleveland, Ohio

Mary Lynn Taylor, CMA, CPC, PMCCI
President/CEO
Professional Coding Services
Fairbanks, Alaska

Martha Tracy, CPC, CPC-I
Coding and Compliance Manager
Mid-America Cardiology
PMCC Instructor
Kansas City Coding Institute, LLC
Kansas City, Kansas

Linda M. Tunis, RHIT, CPC
Certified Professional Coder
Massachusetts General Hospital, Professional Billing Office
Charlestown, Massachusetts

Kathy Wittman, RHIT
Coding Specialist
North Valley Health Center
Warren, Minnesota

Jim Wright, CPC
Billing/Collections Manager
Cunningham Pathology, LLC
Birmingham, Alabama

The number of people seeking health care services has increased as a result of an aging population, technologic advances, and better access to health care. At the same time, there is an increase in the use of outpatient facilities. This increase is due in part to the government's introduction of tighter controls over patient services. The government continues to increase its involvement in and control over health care through reimbursement of services for Medicare and Medicaid patients. Other insurance companies are following the government's lead and adopting reimbursement systems that have proved effective in reducing third-party payer costs but place further pressure on the health care system.

Health care in America has undergone tremendous change in the recent past, and more changes are promised for the future. These changes have resulted in an ever-increasing demand for qualified medical coders. The Bureau of Labor Statistics states that medical records and health information technicians job growth will be "faster than average" with three out of five of these jobs being in the physician/outpatient setting.[1] The national shortage has increased the salary for the coding occupation, and salaries in general show a solid upward trend.

There is also a greater demand for coders because of the increase in the number of medical tests, treatments, and procedures and the increase in the claims review by third-party payers. Certified coders are on average paid more than the noncertified coder. According to the 2008 Salary Survey,* the certified coder earns an average of $43,100![2] Figure 1 illustrates the earnings by state; Figure 2 shows the average salary by experience; and Figure 3 lists the salary by workplace. The CPC-H®, the hospital outpatient certification, pays significantly more than the CPC®, the physician outpatient certification. Dual certification as a CPC and CPC-H is also gaining popularity. Further information can be obtained about the AAPC and the certifications offered by the organization at www.aapc.com.

---

*Check your Evolve resources for the latest AAPC Salary Survey information.

From the Trenches

"Coding can really open doors to a variety of things. You're not tied into one job—there are many roads you can take and many things you can do with a coding background."

MARIA

This map details the regions and their average salaries:

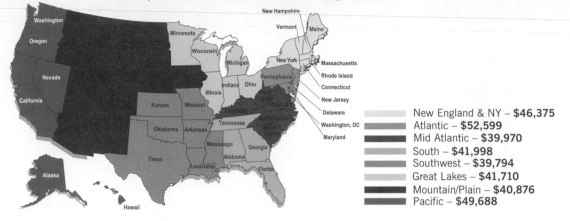

New England & NY – **$46,375**
Atlantic – **$52,599**
Mid Atlantic – **$39,970**
South – **$41,998**
Southwest – **$39,794**
Great Lakes – **$41,710**
Mountain/Plain – **$40,876**
Pacific – **$49,688**

FIGURE 1 Earnings by State. (From American Academy of Professional Coders: *2008 Salary Survey: Sunlight on Coders' Compensation* [website]: www.aapc.com/documents/OctCE_Salary%20Survey.pdf. Accessed March 3, 2009.)

How Hot is Your Specialty?

Experience in our field also matters with almost a steady increase as years of experience are gained, as shown in the table below:

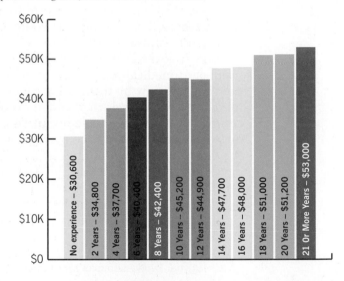

FIGURE 2 Average Salary by Experience. (From American Academy of Professional Coders: *2008 Salary Survey: Sunlight on Coders' Compensation* [website]: www.aapc.com/documents/OctCE_Salary%20Survey.pdf. Accessed March 3, 2009.)

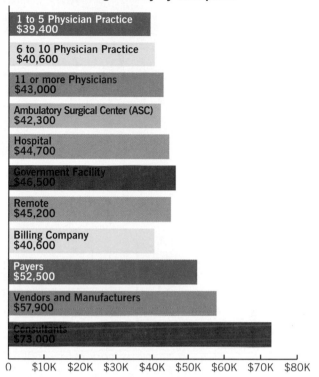

Average Salary by Workplace

Workplace	Salary
1 to 5 Physician Practice	$39,400
6 to 10 Physician Practice	$40,600
11 or more Physicians	$43,000
Ambulatory Surgical Center (ASC)	$42,300
Hospital	$44,700
Government Facility	$46,500
Remote	$45,200
Billing Company	$40,600
Payers	$52,500
Vendors and Manufacturers	$57,900
Consultants	$73,000

FIGURE 3 Average Salary by Workplace. (From American Academy of Professional Coders: *2008 Salary Survey: Sunlight on Coders' Compensation* [website]: www.aapc.com/documents/OctCE_Salary%20Survey.pdf. Accessed March 3, 2009.)

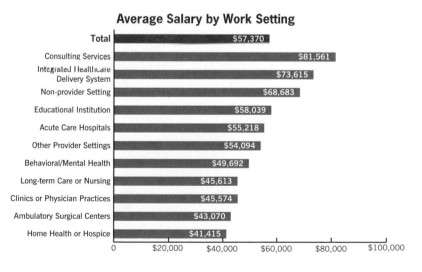

Average Salary by Work Setting

Work Setting	Salary
Total	$57,370
Consulting Services	$81,561
Integrated Healthcare Delivery System	$73,615
Non-provider Setting	$68,683
Educational Institution	$58,039
Acute Care Hospitals	$55,218
Other Provider Settings	$54,094
Behavioral/Mental Health	$49,692
Long-term Care or Nursing	$45,613
Clinics or Physician Practices	$45,574
Ambulatory Surgical Centers	$43,070
Home Health or Hospice	$41,415

FIGURE 4 Average Salaries by Work Setting. (From American Health Information Management Association: *2008 Salary Study Delves Deeper into Factors Driving Pay* [website]: www.ahima.org/salarystudy. Accessed March 3, 2009.)

Average Salary by Setting and Level

Average Salary by Setting and Level	Director	Manager	Supervisor	Coding Professional
Ambulatory Surgical Center	$59,386	$48,369	$35,276	$41,818
Behavioral/Mental Health	$56,532	$51,502	$41,833	$36,700
Consulting Services	$97,067	$86,214	$57,083	$57,700
Educational Institution	$62,698	$51,721	$50,500	NA
Integrated Healthcare Delivery System	$102,129	$75,809	$59,374	$46,813
Acute Care Hospital	$77,603	$65,068	$51,488	$43,673
Long-term Care or Nursing Facility	$47,134	$44,361	$39,998	$40,829
Clinic or Physician Practice	$68,481	$53,542	$45,304	$37,589
Home Health or Hospice	$55,389	$56,107	$42,758	$36,502
Other Provider Setting (e.g., rehab)	$72,653	$59,551	$48,329	$41,248
Non-provider Setting (government, vendor, assoc., etc.)	$94,435	$75,057	$53,799	$48,115
Total	$76,570	$64,225	$50,362	$43,359

FIGURE 5 Average Salary by Setting and Level. (From American Health Information Management Association: *2008 Salary Study Delves Deeper into Factors Driving Pay* [website]: www.ahima. org/salarystudy. Accessed March 3, 2009.)

The American Health Information Management Association (AHIMA) is a health care organization that offers the Certified Coding Specialist—Physician-based (CCS-P) certification. The AHIMA 2008 Salary Study indicated, ". . . the overall average annual salary of survey respondents being $57,370."[3] Figure 4 illustrates the average salary by the work setting. Figure 5 illustrates the average salary by job setting. Figure 6 illustrates the average salary for coders by credential. Further information about AHIMA and the certifications offered can be accessed at the organization's website, www.ahima.org.

Medical coding is far more than assigning numbers to services and diagnoses. Coders abstract information from the patient record and combine that information with their knowledge of reimbursement and coding guidelines to optimize physician payment. Coders have been called the "fraud squad" because they optimize but never maximize and code only for services provided to the patient that are documented in the medical record.

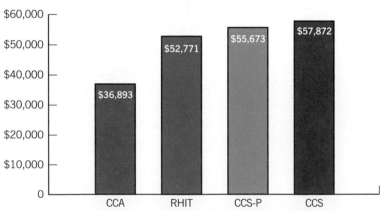

FIGURE 6 Average Coder Salaries by Credential. (From American Health Information Management Association: *2008 Salary Study Delves Deeper into Factors Driving Pay* [website]: www.ahima. org/salarystudy. Accessed March 3, 2009.)

From the Trenches

"You need to be committed . . . . Be prepared to spend some time and effort to study and work hard. Do whatever you have to do to get your foot in the door."

BARBARA

There is a demand for skilled coders, and you can be one of those in demand. Put your best efforts into building the foundation of your career, and you will be rewarded for a lifetime.

References

1. U.S. Department of Labor, Bureau of Labor Statistics, Employment Projections. www.bls.gov/oco/ocos103.htm#emply
2. 2008 Salary Survey, *AAPC Coding Edge,* Salt Lake City, UT. www.aapc.com/documents/OctCE_Salary%20Survey.pdf
3. American Health Information Management Association. www.ahima.org/salarystudy

CONTENTS

UNIT I
Reimbursement

CHAPTER 1
Reimbursement, HIPAA, and Compliance   1
Introduction   2
Basic Structure of the Medicare Program   2
Health Insurance Portability and Accountability Act   7
Federal Register   9
Outpatient Resource-Based Relative Value Scale (RBRVS)   11
Medicare Fraud and Abuse   17
Managed Health Care   21
Chapter Review   24
Quick Check Answers   25

UNIT II
ICD-9-CM and ICD-10-CM

CHAPTER 2
An Overview of ICD-9-CM   26
The ICD-9-CM   27
ICD-9-CM Format   28
Tabular List, Volume 1   29
Appendices in the Tabular List, Volume 1   38
Alphabetic Index, Volume 2   40
Procedures, Volume 3   60
Chapter Review   72
Quick Check Answers   74

CHAPTER 3
Outpatient Coding and Reporting Guidelines   75
First-Listed Diagnosis   76
Additional Diagnoses   80
V Codes   81
Specificity   87
Uncertain Diagnosis   88
Chronic Diseases   89
Diagnostic Services   90
Therapeutic Services   91
Surgery   92
Prenatal Visits   93
Chapter Review   95

CHAPTER 4
Using ICD-9-CM 97
Organization of the Guidelines 98
Level of Specificity 100
Integral Conditions 102
Multiple Coding 104
Acute and Chronic 107
Combination Codes 109
Late Effects 110
Impending or Threatened Condition 113
Chapter Review 115
Quick Check Answers 116

CHAPTER 5
Chapter-Specific Guidelines (ICD-9-CM Chapters 1-8) 117
Infectious and Parasitic Diseases 118
Neoplasms 120
Endocrine, Nutritional, and Metabolic Diseases and Immunity Disorders 128
Diseases of the Blood and Blood-Forming Organs 130
Mental Disorders 131
Diseases of the Nervous System and Sense Organs 133
Diseases of the Circulatory System 134
Diseases of the Respiratory System 140
Chapter Review 143
Quick Check Answers 146

CHAPTER 6
Chapter-Specific Guidelines (ICD-9-CM Chapters 9-17) 147
Diseases of the Digestive System 148
Diseases of the Genitourinary System 150
Complications of Pregnancy, Childbirth, and the Puerperium 151
Diseases of the Skin and Subcutaneous Tissue 157
Diseases of the Musculoskeletal System and Connective Tissue 159
Congenital Anomalies and Certain Conditions Originating in the Perinatal Period 161
Signs, Symptoms, and Ill-Defined Conditions 165
Injury and Poisoning 166
Chapter Review 189
Quick Check Answers 191

CHAPTER 7
ICD-10-CM 192
Development of the ICD-10-CM 193
Development of the ICD-10-PCS 197
Chapter Review 209

UNIT III
CPT and HCPCS

CHAPTER 8
Introduction to the CPT and Level II National Codes (HCPCS)   211

The Purpose of the CPT Manual   212
Updating the CPT Manual   212
CPT Manual Format   214
Starting with the Index   229
History of National Level Codes   233
Chapter Review   246
Quick Check Answers   248

CHAPTER 9
Modifiers   249

CPT Modifiers   250
Modifier -22   251
Modifier -23   252
Modifier -24   253
Modifier -25   254
Modifier -26   254
Modifier -32   256
Modifier -47   256
Modifier -50   256
Modifier -51   257
Modifier -52   261
Modifier -53   264
Modifier -54   264
Modifier -55   265
Modifier -56   265
Modifier -57   266
Modifier -58   267
Modifier -59   268
Modifier -62   269
Modifier -63   270
Modifier -66   270
Modifier -76   271
Modifier -77   271
Modifier -78   272
Modifier -79   273
Modifier -80   273
Modifier -81   273
Modifier -82   274
Modifier -90   275
Modifier -91   276
Modifier -92   276
Modifier -99   276
Chapter Review   277
Quick Check Answers   278

Contents

CHAPTER 10
Evaluation and Management (E/M) Services 279
Contents of the E/M Section 280
Three Factors of E/M Codes 280
Various Levels of E/M Service 283
An E/M Code Example 304
Using the E/M Codes 305
Documentation Guidelines 338
Chapter Review 341
Quick Check Answers 344

CHAPTER 11
Anesthesia 345
Types of Anesthesia 346
Anesthesia Section Format 349
Formula for Anesthesia Payment 351
Concurrent Modifiers 361
Unlisted Anesthesia Code 363
Other Reporting 364
Chapter Review 365
Quick Check Answers 366

CHAPTER 12
Surgery Guidelines and General Surgery 367
Introduction to the Surgery Section 368
Notes and Guidelines 368
Unlisted Procedures 371
Special Reports 372
Separate Procedure 372
Surgical Package 374
General Subsection 378
Chapter Review 379
Quick Check Answers 380

CHAPTER 13
Integumentary System 381
Integumentary System 382
Format 382
Skin, Subcutaneous, and Accessory Structures 383
Nails 394
Repair (Closure) 398
Burns 411
Destruction 415
Breast Procedures 417
Chapter Review 421
Quick Check Answers 422

CHAPTER 14
Musculoskeletal System 423
Format 424
Fractures and Dislocations 425
General 431
Application of Casts and Strapping 440

Endoscopy/Arthroscopy   443
Chapter Review   445
Quick Check Answers   446

CHAPTER 15
Respiratory System   447
Format   448
Endoscopy   449
Nose   451
Accessory Sinuses   457
Larynx   458
Trachea/Bronchi   460
Lungs and Pleura   463
Chapter Review   467
Quick Check Answers   469

CHAPTER 16
Cardiovascular System   470
Coding Highlights   471
Cardiovascular Coding in the Surgery Section   473
Cardiovascular Coding in the Medicine Section   495
Cardiovascular Coding in the Radiology Section   509
Chapter Review   513
Quick Check Answers   515

CHAPTER 17
Hemic, Lymphatic, Mediastinum, and Diaphragm   516
Hemic and Lymphatic Systems   517
Mediastinum and Diaphragm   522
Chapter Review   524
Quick Check Answers   525

CHAPTER 18
Digestive System   526
Format   527
Lips   527
Vestibule of Mouth   529
Tongue and Floor of Mouth   530
Dentoalveolar Structures   531
Palate and Uvula   533
Salivary Gland and Ducts   533
Pharynx, Adenoids, and Tonsils   535
Esophagus   537
Stomach   541
Intestines (Except Rectum)   543
Meckel's Diverticulum and the Mesentery   545
Appendix   546
Rectum   546
Anus   553
Liver   556
Biliary Tract   556
Pancreas   557

Contents

Abdomen, Peritoneum, and Omentum   557
Chapter Review   560
Quick Check Answers   562

CHAPTER 19
Urinary and Male Genital Systems   563
Urinary System   564
Male Genital System   582
Chapter Review   596
Quick Check Answers   598

CHAPTER 20
Reproductive, Intersex Surgery, Female Genital System,
and Maternity Care and Delivery   599
Reproductive System Procedures   600
Intersex Surgery   600
Female Genital System   600
Maternity Care and Delivery   615
Chapter Review   622
Quick Check Answers   624

CHAPTER 21
Endocrine and Nervous Systems   625
Endocrine System   626
Nervous System   630
Chapter Review   641
Quick Check Answers   642

CHAPTER 22
Eye, Ocular Adnexa, Auditory, and Operating Microscope   643
Eye and Ocular Adnexa   644
Auditory System   651
Operating Microscope   651
Chapter Review   658
Quick Check Answers   659

CHAPTER 23
Radiology   660
Format   661
Radiology Terminology   661
Terms   662
Planes   662
Guidelines   668
Diagnostic Radiology   672
Breast, Mammography   674
Diagnostic Ultrasound   675
Radiation Oncology   679
Nuclear Medicine   684
Chapter Review   686
Quick Check Answers   688

CHAPTER 24
Pathology/Laboratory 689
Format 690
Organ or Disease Oriented Panels 690
Drug Testing 691
Therapeutic Drug Assays 692
Evocative/Suppression Testing 693
Consultations (Clinical Pathology) 694
Urinalysis and Chemistry 695
Hematology and Coagulation 696
Immunology 698
Transfusion Medicine 698
Microbiology 699
Anatomic Pathology 700
Cytopathology and Cytogenic Studies 701
Surgical Pathology 701
Other Procedures 703
Chapter Review 704
Quick Check Answers 706

CHAPTER 25
Medicine 707
Format 708
Introduction to Immunizations 709
Psychiatry 714
Biofeedback 716
Dialysis 717
Gastroenterology 720
Ophthalmology 721
Special Otorhinolaryngologic Services 724
Cardiovascular 724
Pulmonary 726
Allergy and Clinical Immunology 727
Endocrinology 728
Neurology and Neuromuscular Procedures 729
Central Nervous System Assessments/Tests 731
Health and Behavior Assessment/Intervention 732
Chemotherapy Administration 733
Photodynamic Therapy 737
Special Dermatological Procedures 737
Physical Medicine and Rehabilitation 738
Medical Nutrition Therapy 741
Osteopathic Manipulative Treatment (OMT) 741
Chiropractic Manipulative Treatment (CMT) 741
Non-Face-to-Face Nonphysician Services 742
Special Services, Procedures, and Reports 742
Other Services and Procedures 743
Home Health Procedures/Services 743
Medication Therapy Management Services 743
Chapter Review 744
Quick Check Answers 746

UNIT IV
Inpatient Coding

CHAPTER 26
Inpatient Coding   747
Karla R. Lovaasen, RHIA, CCS, CCS-P
Differences between Inpatient and Outpatient Coding   748
Selection of Principal Diagnosis   749
Reporting Additional Diagnoses   760
Present on Admission (POA)   763
Chapter Review   764

APPENDIX A
Online Resources   766
ICD-9-CM Official Guidelines for Coding and Reporting
1995 Guidelines for E/M Services
1997 Documentation Guidelines for Evaluation and Management Services
CPT Updates
ICD-9-CM Updates
HCPCS Updates
Study Tips
WebLinks

APPENDIX B
Exercise Answers   767

APPENDIX C
***SpeedECoder* Exercises   806**

Glossary   836

Coder's Index   853

Index   867

"You will probably feel a bit 'lost' in the beginning, but don't let that slow you down! You are learning to identify the little pieces to a big puzzle. Wait until the puzzle is completed before deciding if you like the 'big picture'; you will be greatly rewarded."

Beverly Comsa, CPC
HealthCare Training Manager
New Horizons Learning Center
Anaheim, California

Reimbursement, HIPAA, and Compliance

Chapter Topics

Introduction

Basic Structure of the Medicare Program

Health Insurance Portability and Accountability Act

Federal Register

Outpatient Resource-Based Relative Value Scale (RBRVS)

Medicare Fraud and Abuse

Managed Health Care

Chapter Review

Quick Check Answers

Learning Objectives

After completing this chapter you should be able to

1 Distinguish among Medicare Parts A, B, C, and D.

2 Define QIO.

3 Interpret rules of Health Insurance Portability and Accountability Act (HIPAA).

4 Locate information in the *Federal Register*.

5 Explain the RBRVS system.

6 Understand the framework of Medicare Fraud and Abuse.

7 Identify the major components of Managed Health Care.

Make sure to check
evolve
learning system
for the latest content updates

INTRODUCTION

Coding systems are used in the outpatient and inpatient health care settings. Each of the coding systems plays a key role in the reimbursement of providers of patient health care services. In your role as a medical coder, it is your responsibility to ensure that you code accurately and completely to optimize reimbursement for services provided. To accomplish this, you not only need to know the coding systems, but also the environment in which the modern medical office functions.

Today, the elderly compose the fastest growing segment of our population. Medical advances allow people to live longer and healthier lives than ever before. Consider that in 1949 there were four persons age 19 and younger for every one person age 65 and older; in 2030 there will be one person age 19 and younger for every one person 65 and older.[1]

RATIO OF CHILDREN 18 AND YOUNGER TO PERSONS 65 AND OLDER[1,2]

- 4 : 1   1949
- 2 : 1   1988
- 1 : 1   2030

Persons enrolled in Medicare coverage increased from 19 million in 1967 to 43 million in 2008.[3] Medicare is big business, with Medicare spending at $207.9 billion in 1997 and $373.7 billion in 2006.[4] The program is expected to grow to $862 billion in 2016 and provide for 77 million beneficiaries.[5]

Increasing numbers of elderly people, technologic advances, and improved access to health care have increased consumer use of health care services. As more people utilize health care services, coding becomes even more important to appropriate reimbursement and cost control.

As a coder, it is your responsibility to ensure that the data reported are as accurate as possible, not only for classification and study purposes but also to obtain appropriate reimbursement. On an ethical level, issues will arise and will require attention by coding personnel. Guidelines must always be followed in the assignment of codes. Instruction from internal and external sources (e.g., administration, review organizations, third-party payers) that may increase reimbursement but conflict with coding guidelines must be discussed and resolved.

Reimbursement usually comes from third-party payers. By far, the largest third-party payer is the government through the Medicare program. Because the Medicare program plays such an important role in reimbursement, the rules and regulations that govern Medicare reimbursement will be your first topic of study.

BASIC STRUCTURE OF THE MEDICARE PROGRAM

The Medicare program was established in 1965 with the passage of the Social Security Act. The Medicare program dramatically increased the involvement of the government in health care and consists of Part A (Hospital Insurance) and Part B (Supplemental Medical Insurance). Part A pays for the cost of hospital/facility care, and Part B pays for physician services and durable medical equipment not paid for under Part A, which covers services that are provided by hospitals, skilled nursing facilities (non-custodial or long-term care), and critical access hospitals. Part A insurance also helps to cover hospice care and some care services that are rendered in the home.

Medicare was originally designed for people 65 and over. Later on people who were eligible for disability benefits from Social Security were also covered under the Medicare program, along with those patients experiencing permanent renal failure. Individuals covered under Medicare are termed **beneficiaries**.

The Secretary of the Department of Health and Human Services (DHHS) is responsible for the administration of the Federal Medicare program.

Within the Department, the operation of Medicare is delegated to the Centers for Medicare and Medicaid Services (CMS), formerly the Health Care Financing Administration (HCFA). The funds to run Medicare are generated from payroll taxes paid by employers and employees. The Social Security Administration is responsible for collecting and handling the funds. CMS's function is to promote the general welfare of the public and its stated mission and vision are:

CMS's Mission:	To ensure effective, up-to-date health care coverage and to promote quality care for beneficiaries.
CMS's Vision:	To achieve a transformed and modernized health care system.
CMS will accomplish our mission by continuing to transform and modernize America's health care system.[6]	

CMS handles the daily operation of the Medicare program through the use of Medicare Administrative Contractors (MACs) (formerly Fiscal Intermediaries, FIs). The MACs do the paperwork for Medicare and are usually insurance companies that bid for a contract with CMS to handle the Medicare program in a specific area. The monies for Medicare flow from the Social Security Administration through the CMS to the MACs and, finally, are paid to beneficiaries and providers.

In 2003, the Medicare Prescription Drug Improvement and Modernization Act passed and allowed CMS to reduce the administrative structure from 48 FIs to 19 MACs. There are 15 Part A and B MACs (Fig. 1–1) and 4 Durable

Part A and B MAC Jurisdictions

Jurisdiction	States Included in Jurisdiction
1	American Samoa, California, Guam, Hawaii, Nevada, and Northern Mariana Islands
2	Alaska, Idaho, Oregon, and Washington
3	Arizona, Montana, North Dakota, South Dakota, Utah, and Wyoming
4	Colorado, New Mexico, Oklahoma, and Texas
5	Iowa, Kansas, Missouri, and Nebraska
6	Illinois, Minnesota, and Wisconsin
7	Arkansas, Louisiana, and Mississippi
8	Indiana and Michigan
9	Florida, Puerto Rico, and U.S. Virgin Islands
10	Alabama, Georgia, and Tennessee
11	North Carolina, South Carolina, Virginia, and West Virginia
12	Delaware, District of Columbia, Maryland, New Jersey, and Pennsylvania
13	Connecticut and New York
14	Maine, Massachusetts, New Hampshire, Rhode Island, and Vermont
15	Kentucky and Ohio

FIGURE 1–1 Part A and B MAC jurisdictions.[7]

Durable Medical Equipment (DME) MAC Jurisdictions

Jurisdiction	States Included in Jurisdiction
A	Connecticut, Delaware, District of Columbia, Maine, Maryland, Massachusetts, New Hampshire, New Jersey, New York, Pennsylvania, Rhode Island, and Vermont
B	Illinois, Indiana, Kentucky, Michigan, Minnesota, Ohio, and Wisconsin
C	Alabama, Arkansas, Colorado, Florida, Georgia, Louisiana, Mississippi, New Mexico, North Carolina, Oklahoma, Puerto Rico, South Carolina, Tennessee, Texas, U.S. Virgin Islands, Virginia, and West Virginia
D	Alaska, American Samoa, Arizona, California, Guam, Hawaii, Idaho, Iowa, Kansas, Missouri, Montana, Nebraska, Nevada, North Dakota, Northern Mariana Islands, Oregon, South Dakota, Utah, Washington, and Wyoming

FIGURE 1–2   Durable Medical Equipment jurisdictions.[7]

Medical Equipment (DME) MACs (Fig. 1–2). The full implementation will take place in approximately 2011; however, under this schedule, the full fee-for-service workload transitioned to the MACs in October of 2009.

Physicians, hospitals, and other suppliers that furnish care or supplies to Medicare patients are called **providers**. Providers must be licensed by local and state health agencies to be eligible to provide services or supplies to Medicare patients. Providers must also meet various additional Medicare requirements before payment can be made.

Medicare pays for 80% of allowable charges, and the beneficiary pays the remaining 20%. The beneficiary pays deductibles, premiums, and coinsurance payments. (The 2009 deductible for Part A is $1068[8] and for Part B, $135.[8]) The **coinsurance** is the 20% that Medicare does not pay. Often, beneficiaries have additional insurance to cover out-of-pocket expenses or non-covered services.

Beneficiary Pays: Deductible, premiums, coinsurance (20%), non-covered services

Medicare Pays: Covered services (80%)

The maximum out-of-pocket amounts are set each year according to formulas established by Congress and published in the *Federal Register*. New amounts usually take effect each January 1.

Quality Improvement Organization (QIO)

Claims sent in by the providers of services are processed by MACs according to Medicare guidelines. Providers can sign a Quality Improvement Organization (QIO) agreement with a MAC to accept assignment on all claims submitted to Medicare. QIO providers were previously termed PROs (Participating Provider Organizations). Under the direction of CMS, the Quality Improvement Organization program consists of a national network of QIOs, responsible for each U.S. state, territory, and the District of Columbia. QIOs work with consumers and physicians, hospitals, and other caregivers to refine care delivery systems to make sure patients get the right care at the right time, particularly patients from underserved populations.[9] When a provider accepts assignment, the provider agrees to accept the Medicare allowable for services provided. The provider also agrees not to bill the patient for the difference between what the service costs and what Medicare allows. For example, a QIO provider renders a service that costs $100 and bills Medicare for the service; Medicare allows $58, and the provider accepts the Medicare payment as payment in full. Now, you are probably asking yourself why anyone would

Not covered CPC

agree to this. The patient does not pay the $42 difference, nor does Medicare. The amount is written off by the provider as if the service really cost only $58. This is a good deal for Medicare and the patient, but what about the provider? Why would a provider agree to decreased payments?

Incentives have been established to encourage providers to become QIO providers. Congress has mandated the following incentives:

FOR QIO PROVIDERS:

- Direct payment is made to the provider on all claims.
- A 5% higher fee schedule than that for non-QIO providers.
- Faster processing of claims.
- The provider's name is listed in the QIO directory, which is made available to each Medicare patient, along with identification as a QIO provider who accepts assignment on all claims.
- Hospital referrals for outpatient care must provide the patient with the name and address of at least one QIO provider.

FOR NON-QIO PROVIDERS:

- Payment goes to the patient on all claims.
- A 5% lower fee schedule than that for QIO providers.
- Slower processing of claims is the norm.
- A statement on the Medicare Summary Notice (MSN) sent to the patient reminds the patient that the use of a participating physician will lower out-of-pocket expenses.

FOR QIO:

- A bonus is offered for each recruited and enrolled QIO provider.

There are incentives for providers to participate in the Medicare program! These incentives are backed by Congress. Currently, more than half of all physicians in the nation are participating providers.

Part A: Hospital Insurance

Hospitals report services for Part A services by using ICD-9-CM codes and Medical Severity-Diagnosis Related Groups (MS-DRG) assignment. You will be learning more about MS-DRGs in Chapter 26 of this text.

Beneficiaries are automatically eligible for Part A, hospital insurance, when they are eligible for Medicare benefits.

During a hospital inpatient stay, Part A pays for a semiprivate room (two to four beds), meals and special diet, plus all other medically necessary services except personal-convenience items and private-duty nurses. Also covered are general nursing, drugs as part of the inpatient treatment, and other hospital services and supplies. Part A can also help pay for inpatient care in a Medicare-certified skilled nursing facility if the patient's condition requires daily skilled nursing or rehabilitation services that can be provided only in a skilled nursing facility. Skilled nursing care means care that can be performed only by or under the supervision of licensed nursing personnel. Skilled rehabilitation services may include such services as physical therapy performed by or under the supervision of a professional therapist. The skilled nursing care and skilled rehabilitation services received must be based on a physician's orders. Part A pays for a semiprivate room in the skilled nursing facility, plus meals, nursing services, and drugs. Personal-convenience items, private-duty nurses, and custodial nursing home services are provided to covered beneficiaries who have chronic long-term illnesses or disabilities.

Part A can pay for covered home health care visits from a participating home health agency. The visits can include part-time skilled nursing care and physical therapy or speech therapy when the services are approved by a physician.

Hospice provides relief (palliative) care and support care to terminally ill patients. Part A also pays for hospice care for terminally ill patients when a physician has certified that the patient is terminally ill and is expected to live 6 months or less if the disease runs its normal course. Further, the patient has elected to receive care from a hospice rather than the standard Medicare benefits, and the hospice is Medicare-certified. Items covered include nursing services, physician services, and certain other medically necessary services.[8]

Part B: Supplementary Insurance

Part B is not automatically provided to beneficiaries when they become eligible for Medicare. Instead, beneficiaries must purchase the benefits with a monthly premium.[8] Part B helps pay for medically necessary professional services, outpatient hospital services, home health care, and a number of other medical services and supplies that are not covered by Part A. Beneficiaries pay a premium each month. There are circumstances in which the premium may vary. If eligible Medicare recipients do not sign up for Medicare when they become eligible they will be penalized. The cost will inflate by 10% each year that they could have obtained coverage, unless they qualify under a special case. The penalty will be in effect as long as they obtain coverage. These Part B services are reported using ICD-9-CM codes for the diagnosis, CPT codes for the procedure (service), and HCPCS codes (National Level II codes) for the additional supplies and services.

Part C: Medicare Advantage

Medicare Part C is also known as Medicare Advantage (formerly Medicare + Choice) and is a set of health care options from which Medicare beneficiaries can choose their health care providers. The options available under Part C are:

- Health Maintenance Organization (HMO)
- Point of Service (POS)
- Provider-Sponsored Organizations (PSO)
- Preferred Provider Organization (PPO)
- Medical Savings Account (MSA)
- Private plans (fee-for-service)
- Religious fraternal benefit society plans

Medicare Advantage Plans may offer the option to purchase additional benefits, such as vision, hearing, dental, and/or health and wellness programs, and prescription drug coverage that the original Medicare does not offer. The managed plan, such as an HMO, has a contract to deliver Medicare services under the plan and provides the same services to all beneficiaries enrolled under Part C. The beneficiary is still under the coverage of Medicare, but has opted to utilize a different way of receiving services.

Part D: Prescription Drugs

The Medicare Prescription Drug, Improvement, and Modernization Act of 2003 (MMA) (Pub. L. 108–173, enacted December 8, 2003) established a prescription drug benefit under Part D of the Medicare program. On January 1, 2006, Medicare beneficiaries could enroll in the Medicare prescription drug plan (Part D) and choose between several plans that offered drug coverage. Medicare beneficiaries are charged a premium each month to be a member of these plans and receive the Medicare Part D drug benefit, pay a deductible, and a copayment.

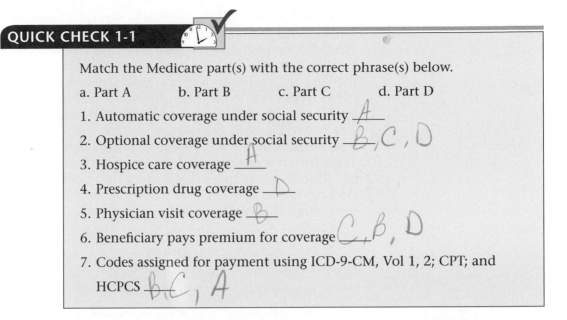

QUICK CHECK 1-1

Match the Medicare part(s) with the correct phrase(s) below.

a. Part A   b. Part B   c. Part C   d. Part D

1. Automatic coverage under social security _A_

2. Optional coverage under social security _B, C, D_

3. Hospice care coverage _A_

4. Prescription drug coverage _D_

5. Physician visit coverage _B_

6. Beneficiary pays premium for coverage _C, B, D_

7. Codes assigned for payment using ICD-9-CM, Vol 1, 2; CPT; and HCPCS _B, C, A_

EXERCISE 1-1 *Medicare*

Using the information presented in this chapter, complete the following:

1 The major third-party payer in the United States is the _federal gov_.

2 The Medicare program was established in what year? _1965_

3 Hospital Insurance is Medicare, Part _A_.

4 Supplemental Medical Insurance is Medicare, Part _B_.

CHECK THIS OUT 👉 The CMS website is located at www.cms.hhs.gov. It contains information about the Medicare program, and through it, you can link to useful information concerning Medicare providers.

HEALTH INSURANCE PORTABILITY AND ACCOUNTABILITY ACT[10]

HIPAA stands for the Health Insurance Portability and Accountability Act of 1996 and includes provisions for governing:

- Health coverage portability
- Health information privacy
- Administrative simplification
- Medical savings accounts
- Long-term care insurance

The section of the Act that has resulted in the most major change to the health care industry is the administrative simplification portion of which there are four parts:

- Electronic transactions and code sets standard requirements
- Privacy requirements
- Security requirements
- National identifier requirements

Electronic Transactions

Uniformity is one goal of the change that took place by adopting transaction standards for several types of electronic health information transactions. Third-party payers (insurers) can no longer have unique requirements for processing claims. Everyone covered by HIPAA is required to provide the same information using standard formats for processing claims and payments; as well as for the maintenance and transmission of electronic health care information and data. With the implementation of HIPAA there is now only one way to process electronic claims.

Transactions are activities involving the transfer of health care information. **Transmission** means the movement of electronic data between two entities and the technology that supports the transfer. For example, if you send claims electronically to a payer you are using Electronic Data Interchange **(EDI)** technology. HIPAA identified 10 standard transactions for EDI transmission:

1. Claims or equivalent encounter information
2. Payment and remittance advice
3. Claim status inquiry and response
4. Eligibility inquiry and response
5. Referral certification and authorization inquiry and response
6. Enrollment and disenrollment in a health plan
7. Health plan premium payments
8. Coordination of benefits
9. Claims attachments
10. First report of injury

Code Sets

Code sets are the codes that identify specific diagnosis and clinical procedures on claims and encounter forms. The CPT and ICD-9-CM codes are examples of code sets for procedure and diagnosis coding. Other code sets adopted under the administrative simplification provisions of HIPAA include codes sets used for claims involving:

Groups	Code Sets
1. Physician services/other health services	HCPCS and CPT
2. Medical supplies, orthotics, and DME (durable medical equipment) (A-V codes)	HCPCS
3. Diagnosis codes	ICD-9-CM, Vols 1, 2
4. Inpatient hospital procedures	ICD-9-CM, Vol 3
5. Dental services	Dental codes (HCPCS, D codes)
6. Drugs/biologics	National Drug Classifications (NDC)

Privacy Requirements

HIPAA also has privacy requirements that govern disclosure of patient protected health information (PHI). Protected health information is placed in the medical record by physicians, nurses, and other health care providers. This can include conversations about the patient's health care or treatment with nurses and other staff. All PHI is included in the privacy requirements.

Security Requirements

The security regulation adopted administrative, technical, and physical safeguards required to prevent unauthorized access to protected health care information. There are significant penalties for those that breach the security of the medical record. Always be certain not to access any medical record you are not authorized to access and always have a work-related reason to access those you do.

Facilities must train their employees in their privacy procedures and designate an individual to be responsible for ensuring the procedures are followed. If an employee fails to follow the established procedures, the facility is required by law to take appropriate disciplinary action.

Security has become a significant concern with the advent of computers to store patient information. The two major terms used to describe the format of the electronic health record are:

- Electronic medical record **(EMR)**—a computerized health record limited to one practice
- Electronic health record **(EHR)**—the entire health record including multiple practices

National Provider Identification

HIPAA also requires health care providers, health plans, and employers to have standard National Provider Identification (NPI) numbers that are unique identification on standard transactions. The NPI is entered onto the claim forms to identify the provider(s) of the services.

Further information about HIPAA is located on the CMS website: www.cms.hhs.gov/HIPAAGenInfo/.

FEDERAL REGISTER

The *Federal Register* is the official publication for all "Presidential Documents," "Rules and Regulations," "Proposed Rules," and "Notices." When the government institutes national changes, those changes are published in the *Federal Register*. You must be aware of the changes listed in the *Federal Register* that relate to reimbursement of Medicare so as to submit Medicare charges correctly.

Most of the information in this chapter is about rules that the government has developed and introduced through the *Federal Register*. You might wonder why so much time is to be spent on learning how to follow the guidelines set by the government for reimbursement when it is only one third-party payer. The answer is simple: Because the government is the largest third-party payer in the nation, even a slight change in the rules governing reimbursement to providers can have major consequences. For example, there was a 45% decrease in the number of inpatient hospital beds between 1975 and 1996,[2] directly related to a government-implemented inpatient reimbursement system that you will learn about in Chapter 26—MS-DRGs. Often, more than 33% of the patients in a hospital are Medicare patients. Because the government is such an important payer in the health care system, you must know how to interpret the government's directives published in the *Federal Register*. In addition, many commercial insurers have adopted Medicare payment philosophies for their own reimbursement policies. The government has changed health care reimbursement through the Medicare program, and even more changes are promised for the future.

From the Trenches

"Don't be afraid to write in your coding books! As you study and read, highlight important rules. Write instructions 'in your own words' so you will understand when you go back to look at it again."
BEVERLY

If you have the *Federal Register* available to you through a library or via the internet, locating and reviewing some of the issues would be an excellent educational activity for you.

CHECK THIS OUT 👉 You can access the *Federal Register* on the website for the National Archives and Records Administration at www.gpoaccess. gov/fr/index.html. This site houses issues of the *Federal Register* from 1994 to the present.

The October editions of the *Federal Register* are of special interest to **hospital** facilities because the hospital updates are released in that edition. **Outpatient** facilities are especially interested in the November or December edition of the *Federal Register* because Medicare reimbursements for outpatient services are usually published in one of those editions. Each year, when changes to the various payment systems are proposed, those proposed changes are published early in the year, and a period of several months is offered to interested parties to comment and make suggestions on the proposed changes. The final rules are usually published in the fall editions and implemented in the following calendar year. Some addendums are particularly helpful to the coder because they list the active codes, non-covered codes, bundled codes, etc.

Fig. 1–3 shows a copy of a portion of a *Federal Register;* it is marked to indicate the location of the following details[11]:

1. The regulation's issuing office
2. The subject of the notice
3. The agency
4. The action
5. A summary
6. The dates
7. The address
8. Contacts for further information
9. Supplementary information

Items 1 through 9 are always placed before the Final Rule, which is the official statement of the entire rule.

EXERCISE 1-2 *Federal Register*

Answer the following questions:

1 Which edition of the *Federal Register* is of special interest to hospital facilities? *October*

2 Which edition of the *Federal Register* is of special interest to outpatient facilities? *Nov or Dec*

Using Fig. 1–3, answer the following questions:

3 What is the issuing office? *Dept. Health Human Serv. HHS*

4 What is the date the provisions of this rule are effective? *1-26-2009*

5 According to the Summary section in Fig. 1–3, what does ASC mean? *Amb Surg Center*

6 According to the "For Further Information Contact" section in Fig. 1–3, who could give you further information related to the issue addressed in this *Federal Register*? *Alberta Dwivedi*

6. Dates   7. Further information

4343

Rules and Regulations

Federal Register
Vol. 74, No. 15
Monday, January 26, 2009

This section of the FEDERAL REGISTER contains regulatory documents having general applicability and legal effect, most of which are keyed to and codified in the Code of Federal Regulations, which is published under 50 titles pursuant to 44 U.S.C. 1510.

The Code of Federal Regulations is sold by the Superintendent of Documents. Prices of new books are listed in the first FEDERAL REGISTER issue of each week.

1. Issuing Office

DEPARTMENT OF HEALTH AND HUMAN SERVICES

Centers for Medicare & Medicaid Services

42 CFR Parts 410, 416, and 419

[CMS–1404–CN]

RIN 0938–AP17; RIN 0938–AL80; RIN 0938–AH17

2. Subject

Medicare Program; Changes to the Hospital Outpatient Prospective Payment System and CY 2009 Payment Rates; Changes to the Ambulatory Surgical Center Payment System and CY 2009 Payment Rates; Hospital Conditions of Participation: Requirements for Approval and Re-Approval of Transplant Centers To Perform Organ Transplants—Clarification of Provider and Supplier Termination Policy Medicare and Medicaid Programs: Changes to the Ambulatory Surgical Center Conditions for Coverage

3. Agency

AGENCY: Centers for Medicare & Medicaid Services (CMS), HHS.

4. Action

ACTION: Correction of final rule with comment period.

5. Summary

SUMMARY: This document corrects technical errors that appeared in the final rule with comment period published in the **Federal Register** on November 18, 2008, entitled "Medicare Program; Changes to the Hospital Outpatient Prospective Payment System and CY 2009 Payment Rates; Changes to the Ambulatory Surgical Center

Payment System and CY 2009 Payment Rates; Hospital Conditions of Participation: Requirements for Approval and Re-Approval of Transplant Centers To Perform Organ Transplants—Clarification of Provider and Supplier Termination Policy Medicare and Medicaid Programs: Changes to the Ambulatory Surgical Center Conditions for Coverage" (hereinafter referred to as the CY 2009 OPPS/ASC final rule with comment period).

DATES: *Effective Date:* this document is effective on January 26, 2009.
Applicability Date: The corrections in this document are applicable on and after January 1, 2009.

FOR FURTHER INFORMATION CONTACT: Alberta Dwivedi, (410) 786–0378.

SUPPLEMENTARY INFORMATION:

I. Background

In FR Doc. E8–20212 of November 18, 2008 (73 FR 68502), there were a few technical errors that are identified in the "Summary of Errors" section and corrected in the "Correction of Errors" section below.

II. Summary of Errors

We incorrectly determined the CY 2009 status indicator for new CY 2009 Healthcare Common Procedure Coding System (HCPCS) code J3300 (Injection, triamcinolone acetonide, preservative free, 1 mg) and, as a result, incorrectly assigned HCPCS code J3300 status indicator "N." Status indicator "N" indicates that items and services are packaged into ambulatory payment classification (APC) rates. Payment for those items and services assigned status indicator "N" is packaged into payment for other services, including, for example, outliers, and, therefore, there is no separate APC payment. The CY 2009 OPPS/ASC final rule with comment period included several Addenda. The erroneous assignment of status indicator "N" to HCPCS code J3300 appears in Addendum B on page 69228. On that page, we are changing

the status indicator of HCPCS code J3300 from "N" to "K" (Nonpass-Through Drugs and Biologicals; Paid under OPPS; separate APC payment) to correctly reflect its separately payable status for CY 2009. As a result of our error in determining the status indicator of HCPCS code J3300, and the corresponding incorrect indication of status indicator "N" in Addendum B, we need to make two additional conforming changes.

Because we incorrectly packaged HCPCS code J3300 in the CY 2009 OPPS/ASC final rule with comment period, we provided no APC assignment for the HCPCS code in that rule. With the correct assignment of status indicator "K" to HCPCS code J3300, an APC must be established for payment, because each separately payable drug or biological is assigned to its own unique APC under the OPPS. Therefore, in Addendum A, on page 68831, we are adding APC 1253 (Triamcinolone A inj PRS-free) with status indicator "K." Also, in Addendum BB, on page 69301, a similar change to that made in Addendum B needs to be made to correspond to the Ambulatory Surgical Center (ASC) payment system. Accordingly, we are changing the ASC payment indicator for HCPCS code J3300 from "N1" to "K2" (Drugs and biologicals paid separately when provided integral to a surgical procedure on ASC list; payment based on OPPS rate) to correctly reflect separate payment of HCPCS code J3300 under the ASC payment system.

III. Correction of Errors

In FR Doc. E8-26212 of November 10, 2008 (73 FR 68502), make the following corrections:

Addendum A.—Final OPPS APCs for CY 2009

1. On page 68831, in column 1, insert between APC 1251 and APC 1280, lines 24 and 25, the final OPPS CY 2009 entry for APC 1253 to read as follows:

APC	Group title	SI	Relative weight	Payment rate	National unadjusted copayment	Minimum unadjusted copayment
1253	Triamcinolone A inj PRS-free	K	....	$3.18	....	$0.64

8. Supplementary information

FIGURE 1–3 Example of page from *Federal Register*. (From *Federal Register*, January 26, 2009, Vol 74, No 15, Rules and Regulations.)

OUTPATIENT RESOURCE-BASED RELATIVE VALUE SCALE (RBRVS)

Physician payment reform was implemented to:

1. Decrease Medicare expenditures
2. Redistribute physicians' payments more equitably
3. Ensure quality health care at a reasonable rate

Before January 1, 1992, payment under Medicare Part B for physicians' services was based on a reasonable charge that, under the Social Security Act, could not exceed the lowest of (1) the physician's actual charge for the service, (2) the physician's customary charge for the service, or (3) the prevailing charges of physicians for similar services in the locality.

The act also required that the local prevailing charge for a physician's service not exceed the level in effect for that service in the locality for the fiscal year ending on June 30, 1973. Some provision was made for changes in the level on the basis of economic changes. When there were economic changes in the country, the Medicare Economic Index (MEI) reflected these changes. Until 1992, the MEI tied increases in the Medicare prevailing charges to increases in the costs of physicians' practice and general wage rates throughout the economy as compared with the index base year. The MEI was first published in the *Federal Register* on June 16, 1975, and has been recalculated annually since then.

Congress mandated the MEI as part of the 1972 Amendment to the Social Security Act. The 1972 Amendment to the Act did not specify the particular type of index to be used; however, the present form of the MEI follows the recommendations outlined by the Senate Finance Committee in its report accompanying the legislation. The MEI attempts to present an equitable measure for changes in the costs of physicians' time and operating expenses.

A major change took place in Medicare in 1989 with the enactment of the Omnibus Budget Reconciliation Act of 1989 (OBRA), Public Law 101-239. Section 6102 of PL 101-239 amended Title XVIII of the Social Security Act by adding Section 1848, Payment for Physician Services. The new section contained three major elements:

1. Establishment of standard rates of increase of expenditures for physicians' services
2. Replacement of the reasonable charge payment mechanism by a fee schedule for physicians' services
3. Replacement of the maximum actual allowable charge (MAAC), which limits the total amount non-QIO physicians could charge

Revisions were made and a new Omnibus Budget Reconciliation Act of 1990 was passed. OBRA 1990 contained several modifications and clarifications of the provisions establishing the physician fee schedule. This final rule required that before January 1 of each year, beginning with 1992, the Secretary establish, by regulation, fee schedules that determine payment amounts for all physicians' services furnished in all fee schedule areas for the year.

The physician fee schedule is updated each April 15 and is composed of three basic elements:

1. The relative value units (RVUs) for each service
2. A geographic adjustment factor to adjust for regional variations in the cost of operating a health care facility
3. A national conversion factor

CHECK THIS OUT ☞ The CMS Physician Fee Schedule Search can be accessed at www.cms.hhs.gov/pfslookup/02_PFSsearch.asp

Medicare volume performance standards have been developed to be used as a tool to monitor annual increases in Part B expenditures for physicians' services and, when appropriate, to adjust payment levels to reflect the success or failure in meeting the performance standards. Various financial protections have been designed and instituted on behalf of the Medicare beneficiary.

Relative Value Unit   Nationally, unit values are assigned for each service and are determined on the basis of the resources necessary to the physician's performance of the service. By analyzing a service, a Harvard team was able to identify its separate parts and assign each part a relative value unit (RVU). These parts or components are as follows:

1. **Work.** The work component is identified as the amount of time, the intensity of effort, and the technical expertise required for the physician to provide the service.

2. **Overhead.** The overhead component or **practice expense** is identified as the allocation of costs associated with the physician's practice (e.g., rent, staffing, supplies) that must be expended in order to provide a service.

3. **Malpractice.** The malpractice component is identified as the cost of the medical malpractice insurance coverage/risk associated with providing service.

The sum of the units established for each component of the service equals the total RVUs of a service.

A relative value was established for a midlevel, established-patient office visit (99213) and all other services are valued at, above, or below this service relative to the work, overhead, and malpractice expenses associated with the service.

Geographic Practice Cost Index

The Urban Institute developed scales that measure cost differences in various areas. The Geographic Practice Cost Indices (GPCIs) have been established for each of the prevailing charge localities. An entire state may be considered a locality for purposes of physician payment reform. The GPCIs reflect the relative costs of practice in a given locality compared with the national average. A separate GPCI has been established and is applied to each component of a service.

Conversion Factor

The conversion factor (CF) is a national dollar amount that is applied to all services paid on the basis of the Medicare Fee Schedule. Congress provided a CF to be used to convert RVUs to dollars. Updated annually on the basis of the data sources, the CF indicates:

- Percent changes to the Medicare Economic Index (MEI)
- Percent changes in physician expenditures
- The relationship of expenditures to volume performance standards
- Change in access and quality

The CF varies according to the type of service provided (e.g., medical, surgical, nonsurgical).

CHECK THIS OUT 👉 The Physician Fee Schedule (PFS) is located at www.cms.hhs.gov/PhysicianFeeSched/PFSRVF/list.asp#TopOfPage

Medicare Volume Performance Standards

The Medicare Volume Performance Standards (MVPS) are best thought of as an object. "It" represents the government's estimate of how much growth is appropriate for nationwide physician expenditures paid by the Part B Medicare program. The purpose of MVPS is to guide Congress in its consideration of the appropriate annual payment update.

The Secretary of Health and Human Services must make MVPS recommendations to Congress by April 15 for the upcoming fiscal year, and by May 15, the Physician Payment Review Commission (PPRC) must make its recommendations for the fiscal year. Congress has until October 15 to establish the MVPS by either accepting or modifying the two proposed MVPS recommendations.

If Congress does not react by October 15, the MVPS rate is established by using a default mechanism. If the default mechanism is used, the Secretary is then required to publish a notice in the *Federal Register* that provides the formula for deriving the MVPS.

Variations in health care usage by Medicare patients occur every year. Because Medicare strives for a balanced budget, if CMS agrees to pay for additional services not previously paid for or increases the weights of CPT codes, thus increasing reimbursement, then discounts are taken across the board so that more money than authorized is not spent and the budget remains balanced.

Beneficiary Protection

Several provisions in the Physician Payment Reform were designed to protect Medicare beneficiaries.

1. As of September 1, 1990, all providers must file claims for their Medicare patients (free of charge). In addition, claims must be submitted according to timely filing guidelines. The Social Security Act requires physicians and suppliers to submit claims within 12 months of the service date. Based on the date of service, there is an additional grace period of up to 26 months. Assigned claims submitted more than 12 months after the date of service will be subject to a 10% reduction of the allowable amount.

2. The Omnibus Budget Reconciliation Act of 1989 requires participating physicians to accept the amount paid for eligible Medicaid services (mandatory assignment) as payment in full.

3. Effective January 1, 1991, the Maximum Actual Allowable Charge (MAAC) limitations that applied to nonparticipating physician charges were replaced by new limits called limiting charges. The provisions of the new limitations state that nonparticipating physicians and suppliers cannot charge more than the stated limiting charge.

Limiting Charge

In 1991 and 1992, the limiting charge was specific to each physician. Beginning in 1993, the limiting charge for a service has been the same for all physicians within a locality, regardless of specialty. The limiting charge for each service also appears on the Advance Beneficiary Notice (ABN).

CODING SHOT The provider may receive a transmission in an electronic format, called the Electronic Remittance Advice (ERA), or in a paper format, called the Standard Paper Remittance Advice (SPR). Although the information featured on the ERA and SPR is similar, the two formats are arranged differently.

The limiting charge applies to every service listed in the Medicare Physicians' Fee Schedule that is performed by a nonparticipating physician. This includes global, professional, and technical services performed by a physician. When a nonphysician provider (e.g., portable x-ray supplier, laboratory technician) provides the technical component of a service that is on the fee schedule, the limiting charge does not apply. CPT codes are assigned many different prices. The amount is determined by multiplying the RVU weight by the geographic index. The conversion factor is called the fee schedule amount. If a physician is participating, he or she receives the fee schedule amount. If the physician is not participating, the fee schedule amount or the allowable payment is slightly less than the participating physician's payment. The limiting amount is a percentage over the allowable (e.g., 115% times the allowable amount). The limiting charge is important because that is the maximum amount a Medicare patient can be billed for a service. For covered services, Medicare usually pays 80% of the allowable amount. The beneficiary is then balance-billed, which means that the patient is billed the difference between what Medicare pays and the limiting charge.

Example

Limiting charge is	$115	(Maximum charge)
Allowable is	$100	
Medicare pays	$80	(Medicare pays 80%)
Patient is billed	$35	($20, 20% of $100, and $15, the remainder of the limiting charge maximum)

Physicians may round the limiting charge to the nearest dollar if they do this consistently for all services.

Uniformity Provision

Equitable use of the Medicare fee schedule requires a payment system with uniform policies and procedures. Because the relative value of the work component of a service is the same nationwide (except for a geographic practice cost adjustment), it is important that when physicians across the country are paid for a service they be paid for the same amount, or "package." For example, the preoperative and postoperative periods included in the payment must be the same. To prevent variation in interpretation, standard definitions of services are required.

Adjustments

Whenever an adjustment of the full fee schedule amount is made to a service, the limiting charge for that service must also be adjusted. These adjustments are identified on the physician disclosure, which is provided to all physicians during the participating enrollment period each year.

Adjustments to the limiting charge must be manually calculated before submitting claims for all services in which a fee schedule limitation applies.

Payments to nonparticipating physicians do not exceed 95% of the physician fee schedule for a service.

Site-of-Service Limitations

Services that are performed primarily in office settings are subject to a payment discount if they are performed in an outpatient hospital department. There is a national list of procedures that are performed 50% of the time in the office setting. These procedures are subject to site-of-service limitations, which means that a discount is taken on any service that is performed in a setting other than a clinic setting. For instance, an arthrocentesis is normally performed in the office. If a physician provides this service in a hospital outpatient setting, the limiting charge will be less than that for the office setting. This is because the hospital will also be billing Medicare for the use of the room and the supplies. Medicare has a built-in practice expense, or overhead, for the clinic setting (the RVU weight for practice expense), and Medicare doesn't want to pay twice for the overhead. So part of the overhead is reduced from the physician's payment to make up for the hospital payment. For these procedures, the practice expense RVU is reduced by 50%. Payment is the lower of the actual charge or the reduced fee schedule amount.

Surgical Modifier Circumstances

Multiple Surgeries

General. If a surgeon performs more than one procedure on the same patient on the same day, discounts are made on all subsequent procedures, excluding add-on codes. Medicare will pay 100% of the fee for the highest value procedure, 50% for the second most expensive procedure, and 25% for the third, fourth, and fifth procedures. Each procedure after the fifth procedure requires documentation and special review to determine the payment amount. Discounting is why the order of the codes and the use of modifiers are so important! These discount amounts are subject to review every year by the CMS.

Third-party payers often follow discount limits different from those of Medicare. It is necessary to keep abreast of payer discounting rules.

Endoscopic Procedures. In the case of multiple endoscopic procedures, in the same indented category of the CPT, Medicare allows the full value of the highest valued endoscopy, plus the difference between the next highest endoscopy and the highest valued endoscopy. As in all other reimbursement issues, some non-Medicare carriers follow this pricing method, whereas others follow their own multiple-procedure discounting policies.

Dermatologic Surgery. For certain dermatology services, there are CPT codes that indicate that multiple surgical procedures have been performed. When a CPT code description states "additional," the general multiple-procedure rules do not apply. For example, code 11001 which is an indented code under 11000 and states "each additional" in the code description and the general multiple-procedure rules do not apply because of this statement in the code description.

Providers Furnishing Part of the Global Fee Package. Under the fee schedule, Medicare pays the same amount for surgical services furnished by several physicians as it pays if only one physician furnished all of the services in the global package.

Medicare pays each physician for his or her part of the global surgical services. The policy is written with the assumption that the surgeon always furnishes the usual and necessary preoperative and intraoperative services and also, with a few exceptions, in-hospital postoperative services. In most cases, the surgeon also furnishes the postoperative office services necessary to ensure normal recovery from the surgery. Recognizing that there are cases in which the surgeon turns over the out-of-hospital recovery care to another physician, Medicare has determined percentages of payment if the postoperative care is furnished by someone other than the surgeon. These are weighted percentages based on the percentage of total global surgical work.
For example:

- Preoperative care   15%
- Intraoperative service   70%
- Postoperative care   15%

Again, become familiar with individual third-party payer policies, because some may not split their global payments in this manner.

Physicians Who Assist at Surgery. Physicians assisting the primary physician in a procedure receive a set percentage of the total fee for the service. Medicare sets the payment level for assistants-at-surgery at 16% of the fee schedule amount for the global surgical service. Non-Medicare payers may set this percentage at 20% or more. CPT modifiers -80 (Assistant Surgeon), -81 (Minimum Assistant Surgeon), and -82 (Assistant Surgeon, when qualified resident surgeon not available) and HCPCS modifier -AS (Assistant at Surgery) would be appended to the code to indicate the type of assistant.

Two Surgeons and Surgical Team. When two surgeons of different specialties perform a procedure, each is paid an equal percentage of the global fee. For co-surgeons, Medicare pays 125% of the global fee, dividing the payment equally between the two surgeons (each will receive 62.5% of the global fee). No payment is made for an assistant-at-surgery when co-surgeons perform the procedure.

For team surgery, a medical director determines the payment amounts on an individual basis. Modifiers -62 (Two Surgeons) or -66 (Surgical Team) would be appended to the procedure code.

Purchased Diagnostic Services. For physicians who bill for a diagnostic test performed by an outside supplier, the fee schedule amount is limited to the lower of the billing physician's fee schedule amount or the price paid for the service.

Reoperations. The amount paid by Medicare for a return to the operating room for treatment of a complication is limited to the intraoperative portion of the code that best describes the treatment of the complications.

When an unlisted procedure is reported because no other code exists to describe the treatment, payment is usually based on a maximum of 50% of the value of the intraoperative services originally performed.

Modifiers -78 (Return to Operating Procedure Room for a Related Procedure During the Postoperative Period) or -79 (Unrelated Procedure or Service by the Same Physician During the Postoperative Period) would be appended to the code to more specifically identify that the service was a reoperation.

Third-party payers have their own guidelines. Many do not apply discounts for these subsequent surgical procedures.

CHECK THIS OUT 🖝 CMS publishes the RVUs on their website (www.cms. hhs.gov/PhysicianFeeSched/PFSRVF/list.asp#TopOfPage). On your job in the medical office, you may be responsible for downloading the new RVUs when they are posted, usually in October of each year. So, it is good idea to know where to locate this information!

EXERCISE 1-3 *RBRVS*

Fill in the blanks with the correct words:

1 What does RBRVS stand for?
   Resource Based Relative Value Scale

2 The Medicare Economic Index is published in what publication?
   Federal Register

3 In 1989, a major change took place in Medicare with the enactment of
   OBRA Omnibus Budget Reconciliation Act

MEDICARE FRAUD AND ABUSE

Fraud and Abuse Defined

The Medicare program is subject to fraud and abuse, as is any third-party payer program. But because Medicare is the largest third-party payer, it has the most comprehensive anti-fraud and -abuse program. You must understand the specifics of this program because you will be submitting Medicare claims. CMS is responsible for establishing the regulations that monitor the Medicare program for fraud and abuse. CMS publishes fraud and abuse guidelines for professionals (www.cms.hhs.gov/FraudAbuseforProfs/) that contain links to the latest fraud and abuse alerts and bulletins.

Fraud is the intentional deception or misrepresentation that an individual knows to be false or does not believe to be true and makes it knowing that the deception could result in some unauthorized benefit to himself/herself or some other person. Fraud involves both deliberate intention to deceive and an expectation of an unauthorized benefit. By this definition, it is fraud if a claim is filed for a service rendered to a Medicare patient when that service was not actually provided. How could this type of fraud happen? The fact is that most Medicare patients sign a standing approval, which is kept on file in the medical office. Having a standing approval is convenient for the patient and for the coding staff. After the patient has received a service, the Medicare claim is filed automatically, without the patient's actual signature. But a standing approval also makes it easy for unscrupulous persons to submit charges for services never provided. This circumstance also makes it possible for extra services to be submitted in addition to services that were provided (up coding). Suppose, for example, a patient came in for an office visit and a claim was submitted for an in-office surgical procedure. That's also fraud.

> ✋ **CAUTION** *The most common kind of fraud arises from a false statement or misrepresentation made, or caused to be made, that results in additional payment by the Medicare program.*

Who Are the Violators? The violator may be a physician or other practitioner, a hospital or other institutional provider, a clinical laboratory or other supplier, an employee of any provider, a billing service, a beneficiary, a Medicare carrier employee, or any person in a position to file a claim for Medicare benefits. You will be the person filing Medicare claims so you have to be careful about the claims you submit. It is important to validate that the service was provided by consulting the medical record or the physician.

Medlearn, the CMS educational Center on the Web, contains publications and computer-based training (CBT) modules on fraud and abuse (www.cms.hhs.gov/MLNGenInfo/). The heading labeled "Related Links Inside CMS" has a link to "Web Based Training (WBT) Modules" that directs you to a list of courses and one of them is "Medicare Fraud and Abuse."

Fraud schemes range from those committed by individuals acting alone to broad-based activities perpetrated by institutions or groups of individuals, sometimes employing sophisticated telemarketing and other promotional techniques to lure consumers into serving as unwitting tools in the schemes. Seldom do such perpetrators target just one insurer; nor do they focus exclusively on either the public or the private sector. Rather, most are found to be defrauding several private- and public-sector victims such as Medicare simultaneously.

What Forms Does Fraud Take? The most common forms of Medicare fraud are:

- Billing for services not furnished
- Misrepresenting a diagnosis to justify a payment
- Soliciting, offering, or receiving a kickback
- Unbundling, or "exploding," charges
- Falsifying certificates of medical necessity, plans of treatment, and medical records to justify payment
- Billing for additional services not furnished as billed—up coding
- Routine waiver of copayment

Who Says What Is Fraudulent? CMS administers the Medicare program. CMS's responsibilities include managing claims payment, overseeing fiscal audit and/or overpayment prevention and recovery, and developing and monitoring the payment safeguards necessary to detect and respond to payment errors or abusive patterns of service delivery. Within CMS's Bureau of Program Operations is the Office of Benefits Integrity (OBI), which oversees Medicare's payment safeguard program related to fraud, audit, medical review, the collection of overpayments, and the imposition of civil monetary penalties (CMPs) for certain violations of Medicare law.

The Office of the Inspector General (OIG), Department of Health and Human Services, is responsible for developing an annual work plan that outlines the ways in which the Medicare program is monitored to identify fraud and abuse. The plan is a published public document that provides the evaluation methods and approaches that will be taken the following year to monitor the Medicare program. For example, in the 2009 Work Plan, the following is listed as the review of services provided by nonphysicians.

PHYSICIANS' MEDICARE SERVICES PERFORMED BY NONPHYSICIANS

We will review services physicians bill to Medicare but do not perform personally. Such services, called "incident to," are typically performed by nonphysician staff members in physicians' offices. The Social Security Act, § 18610(s)(2)(A), provides for Medicare coverage of services and supplies performed "incident to" the professional services of a physician. However, these services may be vulnerable to overutilization or put beneficiaries at risk of receiving services that do not meet professionally recognized standards of care. We will examine the qualifications of nonphysician staff that perform "incident to" services and assess whether these qualifications are consistent with professionally recognized standards of care.[12]

This excerpt from the OIG Work Plan identifies a specific area that was monitored in 2009. The OIG charges the MACs with doing the actual monitoring. The OIG Work Plan sets the broad boundaries for monitoring the Medicare program for fraud and abuse.

CHECK THIS OUT ☞ The site http://oig.hhs.gov/publications/docs/workplan/2009/WorkPlanFY2009.pdf contains the OIG work plan for the current year and previous years.

TOOLBOX

Susan recently graduated as a medical coder and has been employed at Island Clinic for three months. While coding last Monday, she encountered a superbill for a Medicare patient for an office visit for $62, but there was no supporting documentation in the patient's medical record. Susan questioned the physician and he said that he just forgot to do the paperwork and asked her to send the claim to Medicare with a promise to complete the paperwork later.

QUESTIONS

Susan should do which of the following:

a. Complete the claim and send it in, and write a reminder to the physician to complete the documentation.

b. Wait until the physician completes the documentation.

c. Inform the physician that she cannot submit a claim without appropriate documentation in the medical record.

ANSWERS c. never submit a claim for any patient, at any time, for any reason without appropriate documentation in the medical record that supports the claim

Specific Regulations Are in the IOMs

CMS establishes the specific regulations in the *Internet-Only Manuals (IOMs)* for the providers and carriers to follow. You will deal with regulations as you report Medicare services in order to know what is allowable and what fraud and abuse are.

CHECK THIS OUT ☞ The IOMs are located at www.cms.hhs.gov/Manuals/IOM/list.asp and publication 100-08, Medicare Program Integrity Manual with many directions on fraud and abuse.

Attempts to defraud the Medicare program may take a variety of forms. The following are some more examples of how fraud may be perpetrated:

- Billing for services or supplies not provided;
- Deliberately applying for duplicate payment (e.g., billing both Medicare and the beneficiary for the same service or billing both Medicare and another insurer in an attempt to get paid twice);
- Soliciting, offering, or receiving a kickback, bribe, or rebate (e.g., paying for a referral of patients in exchange for the ordering of diagnostic tests and other services or medical equipment);
- Unbundling or "exploding" charges (e.g., the billing of a multichannel set of lab tests to appear as if the individual tests had been performed);
- Completing Certificates of Medical Necessity (CMN) for patients not personally and professionally known by the provider;
- Misrepresenting the services rendered (up coding or the use of procedure codes not appropriate for the item or service actually furnished), amounts charged for services rendered, identity of the person receiving the services, dates of services, etc.;
- Billing for noncovered services (e.g., routine foot care billed as a more involved form of foot care to obtain payment);
- Participating in schemes that involve collusion between a provider and a beneficiary, or between a supplier and a provider, and result in higher costs or charges to the Medicare program;
- Using another person's Medicare card to obtain medical care;
- Utilizing split billing schemes (e.g., billing procedures over a period of days when all treatment occurred during one visit);
- Participating in schemes that involve collusion between a provider and a carrier employee where the claim is assigned (e.g., the provider deliberately overbills for services, and the carrier employee then generates adjustments with little or no awareness on the part of the beneficiary);
- Billing based on "gang visits" (e.g., a physician visits a nursing home and bills for 20 nursing home visits without furnishing any specific service to, or on behalf of, individual patients).

How to Protect Yourself. As you can see from the preceding information about Medicare fraud and abuse, CMS is very serious about identifying those who try to take advantage of the program. As the person submitting the Medicare claims, you are one of those whom the CMS holds responsible for submitting truthful and accurate claims. If you are unsure about a charge or a request, check with the physician or other supervisory personnel to ensure that you are submitting the correct charges for each patient. In this way, you protect the Medicare program, your facility, and yourself.

CHECK THIS OUT ☞ CMS Fraud and Abuse guidelines at www.medicare.gov/FraudAbuse/Overview.asp

MANAGED HEALTH CARE

People come from all over the world to the United States of America to access the health care that U.S. residents take for granted. Physicians and health care have traditionally been held in high esteem by U.S. citizens. Whatever it took to provide access to high-quality health care is what these citizens demanded. Historically, the government responded to these demands by funding the research, facilities, and services necessary to keep the U.S. health system on the cutting edge of medical advances. But the research, facilities, and services are extremely expensive, and many U.S. citizens are also demanding a balanced federal budget.

Health care services in the United States are undergoing rapid change. The U.S. health care system has been financed through traditional health insurance systems, which paid providers on a fee-for-service basis and allowed beneficiaries relative freedom in their selection of health care providers. Health insurance has become an important benefit of employment. Employers became the primary purchasers of health insurance, and the rising cost of health care is reflected in the premiums employers pay and the subsequent decrease in employer-sponsored coverage. Private purchasers of health insurance have also seen a steady increase in their health insurance premiums, until many are forced to go "bare," forgoing health insurance due to the high costs. Fewer people now have health insurance coverage as a benefit of their employment. The number of uninsured people was 45.7 million in 2007,[13] and the number of uninsured continues to rise as employers and individuals find health care insurance out of their reach. One way of containing health care costs that has widespread popularity is managed health care.

The term "managed health care" refers to the concept of establishing networks of health care providers that offer an array of health care services under the umbrella of a single organization. A managed health care organization may be a group of physicians, hospitals, and health plans responsible for the health services for an enrolled individual or group. The organization coordinates the total health care services required by its enrollees. The purpose of managed health care is to provide cost-effectiveness of services and theoretically to improve the health care services provided to the enrollee by ensuring access to all required health services.

Many models are used to deliver managed health care: Health Maintenance Organizations (HMOs), Individual Practice Associations (IPAs), Group Practice, Multiple Option Plan, Medicare Risk HMOs, Preferred Provider Organizations (PPOs), and the Staff model. Each of these models delivers managed health care using a different structure.

The use of the managed health care approach varies widely with geography. There continues to be a rise in the percentage of employers opting for a managed care health plan for their employees; this indicates the employers' search for cost containment while offering the benefit of health coverage to employees.

The pressure on the government to cut expenses and balance the budget guarantees the continued increases in market share for managed care. The government mandated the use of managed care within the Medicaid program, and the number of Medicaid beneficiaries enrolled in managed care continues to increase.

The managed care industry has evolved from small, regional nonprofit plans to large, national, for-profit companies. In the early stages of development, the managed care market included networks that allowed the enrollees a broad choice of providers. As the market segments for managed care expanded, choice for the enrollees decreased.

Types of HMOs

A **Managed Care Organization (MCO)** is a group that is responsible for the health care services offered to an enrolled group or person. The organization coordinates or manages the care of the enrollee. The MCO contains costs by negotiating with various health care entities—hospitals, clinics, laboratories, and so forth—for a discounted rate for services provided to its enrollees. Providers of the health care services must receive prior approval from the MCO before services are rendered. For example, a physician may want to conduct a certain high-cost diagnostic test, but before the test can be conducted, the MCO must give the physician approval. The MCO uses a gatekeeper, usually the primary care physician of the patient, who can authorize the patient's need to seek health care services outside of the established organization. For example, a certain specialist may not be available within the MCO, and the primary care physician may recommend that the enrollee be referred to such a specialist. If the enrollee were to see the specialist without the recommendation of the primary care physician and the approval of the MCO, the enrollee would be responsible for charges incurred. MCOs develop practice guidelines that evaluate the appropriateness and medical necessity of medical care provided to the enrollee by the physicians, which gives the MCO control over what care is provided to the enrollee.

A **Preferred Provider Organization (PPO)** is a group of providers who form a network and who have agreed to provide services to enrollees at a discounted rate. Enrollees are usually responsible for paying a portion of the costs (cost sharing) when using a PPO provider. Enrollees who seek health care outside of the PPO providers pay an additional out-of-pocket cost. The out-of-pocket costs are established by the PPO to discourage the use of outside providers. The PPOs do not use a gatekeeper, but they do have strict guidelines that denote approved expenses and how much the enrollee will pay.

A **Health Maintenance Organization (HMO)** is a delivery system that allows the enrollee access to all health care services. The HMO is the "total package" approach to health care organizations, and the out-of-pocket expenses are minimal. However, the enrollee is assigned a primary care physician who manages all the health care needs of the enrollee and acts as the gatekeeper for the enrollee. Services are prepaid by the HMO. For example, the HMO pays a laboratory to provide services at a negotiated price and the services are prepaid by the HMO. The gatekeeper has authority to allow the enrollee access to the services available or authorize services outside of those the HMO has available.

The gatekeeper has strong incentives to contain costs for the HMO by controlling and managing the health care services provided to the enrollee. The HMO can directly employ the physician in the Staff Model HMO or contract the physician through the **Individual Practice Associations (IPA)** model in which the physician provides services for a set fee. Either way, the physician has an incentive to service the cost containment needs of the HMO.

An **Exclusive Provider Organization (EPO)** has many of the same features as an HMO except that the providers of the services are not prepaid. Instead, the providers are paid on a fee-for-service basis. The **Group Practice Model (GPM)** is a form of HMO in which an organization of physicians contracts with the HMO to provide services to the enrollees of the HMO. A payment is negotiated, the HMO pays the group, and then the group pays the individual physicians.

Medicare Advantage (formerly Medicare + Choice) is a Medicare-funded alternative to the standard Medicare supplemental coverage. Medicare Advantage is an HMO; however, it is provided to Medicare beneficiaries rather than the traditional fee-for-service model historically used by Medicare. The enrollees pay out of pocket if they choose to go outside the network of providers. **Point-of-Service (POS)** benefits allow enrollees to receive services outside of the HMO's health care network, but at increased cost in copayments, in coinsurance, or in a deductible. The POS benefit is one that the HMO may choose to offer, but it is not required, and CMS does not provide any additional funding for this benefit. However, the HMO that offers this option is more attractive to a potential enrollee, because the lack of access to providers outside of a predefined network is the one reason people do not join a managed health care organization. The POS benefit option is also referred to as an **open-ended HMO** or a **self-referral option**. The POS benefit is attractive not only to Medicare enrollees who wish to be treated by providers not available in their plan's network but also to those who travel and would like access to routine medical care while temporarily (fewer than 90 days) out of their plan's service area.

Program for All-Inclusive Care for the Elderly (PACE) is a program developed to address the needs of long-term care clients, providers, and payers. The program provides a comprehensive package of services that permits the clients to continue to live in their homes while receiving services rather than being placed in an institution.

Managed health care is now part of the fabric of the U.S. health care system. The "richer" plans of traditional insurance companies are often no longer an option to a great segment of the population.

Drawbacks of the HMO. There are some significant drawbacks to the HMO concept in terms of access to health care. Consider that providers (physicians in particular) have an incentive to keep treatment costs to a minimum. Traditionally, a physician's primary concern was what was in the best interest of the patient, not what was in the best interest of cost containment. This fundamental change transformed physicians into gatekeepers for third-party payers and transformed third-party payers into developers of guidelines that ultimately control the services patients can and do receive. The patient-physician relationship has shifted to include a physician/third-party-payer relationship, which leaves the patient at the mercy of the third-party payer. Many lawsuits have been brought by patients who allege that lack of treatment caused harm and sometimes death. Cost-containment issues, and hence HMOs, raise many ethical and legal issues that will continue to involve patients, providers, and third-party payers.

EXERCISE 1-4 *Medicare Fraud/Abuse and Managed Care*

Fill in the blanks for the following questions:

1 This term is the intentional deception or misrepresentation that an individual knows to be false or does not believe to be true and makes knowing that the deception could result in some unauthorized benefit. ___fraud___

2 This organization develops a work plan to identify areas of the Medicare program that will be monitored. ___OIG___

3 The physician that is responsible to control and manage the health care of an HMO enrollee is the ___PCP = Gate Keeper___.

4 What does the abbreviation PACE stand for? ___Program for All Inclusive Care for the Elderly___

CHAPTER REVIEW

CHAPTER 1, PART I, THEORY

Complete the following:

1 Two insurance programs were established in 1965 by amendments to the Social Security Act known as Part _A_ and Part _B_.

2 The Secretary of DHHS has delegated responsibility for Medicare to which department? _CMS_

3 Who administers funds for Medicare? _SSA_

4 Who is eligible for Medicare? _65+, ESRD, disabled_

5 List the three components of the relative value unit:
Work
Overhead
Malpractice

6 What does RBRVS stand for? _Res. Based Relative Value Scale_

7 What is the fastest growing segment of our population today? _elderly_

8 What is the name given to the groups that handle the daily operations of the Medicare program? _MACs_

CHAPTER 1, PART II, PRACTICAL

Referencing the CPT manual, Appendix A, match the modifier or modifiers with the correct definition.

9 Multiple Surgery ___-51___

10 Part of Global Fee Package ___-54___, ___-55___, ___-56___

11 Assistant Physicians ___-80___, ___81___, ___82___

12 Two Surgeons ___-62___

13 Surgical Team ___66___

Modifiers

a. -56

b. -80

c. -54

d. -51

e. -55

f. -62

g. -82

h. -66

i. -81

j. -AS

QUICK CHECK ANSWERS

QUICK CHECK 1-1
1. a
2. b, c, d
3. a
4. d
5. b
6. b, c, d
7. a, b, c

REFERENCES

1. Resident Population of the United States: Middle Series Projections, by Age and Sex, US Bureau of the Census, March 1996, p. 2015-2030.
2. 1996 HCFA Statistics. Bureau of Data Management, HCFA Pub. No. 03394, Sept. 1996.
3. Medicare 2000, 35 Years of Improving Americans' Health and Security, www.cms.hhs.gov/TheChartSeries/downloads/35chartbk.pdf
4. www.cbo.gov/ftpdocs/77xx/doc7731/01-24-BudgetOutlook.pdf
5. www.nchc.org/facts/Economy/effects_on_the_federal_budget.pdf
6. www.cms.hhs.gov/MissionVisionGoals/downloads/CMSStrategicActionPlan06-09_061023a.pdf
7. www.cms.hhs.gov/MedicareContractingReform/Downloads/MACJurisdictionFactSheet.pdf
8. www.cms.hhs.gov/apps/media/press/factsheet.asp?Counter=2488&intNumPerPage=10&checkDate=&checkKey=&srchType=1&numDays=3500&srchOpt=0&srchData=&srchOpt=0&srchData=&keywordType=All&chkNewsType=6&intPage=&showAll=&pYear=&year=&desc=&cboOrder=date
9. www.cms.hhs.gov/QualityImprovementOrgs/01_overview.asp
10. www.cms.hhs.gov/EducationMaterials/Downloads/HIPAA101-1.pdf
11. *Federal Register,* 74(15), January 26, 2009, p. 4343.
12. http://oig.hhs.gov/publications/docs/workplan/2009/WorkPlanFY2009.pdf
13. www.census.gov/prod/2008pubs/p60-235.pdf

"Take some baby steps and figure out where you want to be—then as time progresses, you'll fall into your niche."

John R. Neumann III, RN, CPC
Account Executive
Durham, North Carolina

An Overview of ICD-9-CM

Chapter Topics

The ICD-9-CM

ICD-9-CM Format

Tabular List, Volume 1

Appendices in the Tabular List, Volume 1

Alphabetic Index, Volume 2

Procedures, Volume 3

Chapter Review

Quick Check Answers

Learning Objectives

After completing this chapter you should be able to

1 List the uses of ICD-9-CM.

2 Identify the characteristics of the Tabular List, Volume 1.

3 Identify the characteristics of the Alphabetic Index, Volume 2.

4 Explain the uses of coding conventions when assigning codes.

5 Identify the characteristics of the Procedures Index and Tabular List, Volume 3.

6 Demonstrate use of ICD-9-CM.

Make sure to check
evolve
learning system
for the latest
content updates

The ICD-9-CM

The International Classification of Diseases, 9th Revision, Clinical Modification (ICD-9-CM) is designed for the classification of patient morbidity (sickness) and mortality (death) information for statistical purposes and for the indexing of health records by disease and operation for data storage and retrieval.

The ICD-9-CM is based on the ICD-9, the ninth revision of the official version of the International Classification of Diseases compiled by the World Health Organization (WHO). In February 1977, a committee was convened by the National Center for Health Statistics (NCHS) to provide advice and counsel concerning the development of a clinical modification of the ICD-9. The ICD-9-CM is the resulting clinical modification (CM). The term "clinical" was used to emphasize the intent of the modification to serve as a tool in the area of classification of morbidity data for indexing of diseases, medical care review, ambulatory care, other medical care programs, and basic health statistics.

Through the years, the use of the ICD-9-CM (often called the ICD-9 or I-9) has grown. The Medicare Catastrophic Coverage Act of 1988 (P.L. 100-360) required the submission of the appropriate ICD-9-CM diagnosis codes, with charges submitted to Medicare Part B (outpatient services). The law was later repealed, but the coding requirement still stands.

Although coding was originally designed to provide access to medical records through retrieval for medical research, education, and administration, today codes are used to:

1. Facilitate payment of health services
2. Evaluate patients' use of health care facilities (utilization patterns)
3. Study health care costs
4. Research the quality of health care
5. Predict health care trends
6. Plan for future health care needs

The use and results of coding are widespread and evident in our everyday lives. Many people hear the results of coding on a regular basis and don't even know it. Anytime you listen to the news and hear the newscaster refer to a specific number of AIDS cases in the United States or read a newspaper article about an epidemic of measles, you are seeing the results of ICD-9-CM coding. The ICD-9-CM classification system is totally compatible with its parent system, ICD-9, thus meeting the need for comparability of morbidity and mortality statistics at the international level. This classification system is used to track morbidity and mortality. A classification system means that each condition or disease can be coded to only one code as much as possible to ensure the validity and reliability of data.

Coding must be performed correctly and consistently to produce meaningful statistics. (Refer to Fig. 2–1 for the AAPC's Medical Coding Code of Ethics.) To code accurately, it is necessary to have an in-depth knowledge of medical terminology, anatomy, and physiology, disease conditions, and pharmacology along with an understanding of the ICD-9-CM coding guidelines, format, and conventions.

Transforming verbal or narrative descriptions of diseases, injuries, conditions, and procedures into numeric designations is a complex activity and should not be undertaken without proper training. Learning to use the ICD-9-CM codes will be a valuable tool to you in any health care career.

Medical Coding Code of Ethics

Members of the American Academy of Professional Coders shall be dedicated to providing the highest standard of professional coding and billing services to employers, clients and patients. Professional and personal behavior of AAPC members must be exemplary.

AAPC members shall maintain the highest standard of personal and professional conduct. Members shall respect the rights of patients, clients, employers and all other colleagues.

Members shall use only legal and ethical means in all professional dealings and shall refuse to cooperate with, or condone by silence, the actions of those who engage in fraudulent, deceptive or illegal acts.

Members shall respect and adhere to the laws and regulations of the land and uphold the mission statement of the AAPC.

Members shall pursue excellence through continuing education in all areas applicable to their profession.

Members shall strive to maintain and enhance the dignity, status, competence and standards of coding for professional services.

Members shall not exploit professional relationships with patients, employees, clients or employers for personal gain.

Above all else we will commit to recognizing the intrinsic worth of each member.

This code of ethical standards for members of the AAPC strives to promote and maintain the highest standard of professional service and conduct among its members. Adherence to these standards assures public confidence in the integrity and service of professional coders who are members of the AAPC.

Failure to adhere to these standards, as determined by AAPC, will result in the loss of credentials and membership with the American Academy of Professional Coders.

FIGURE 2-1 AAPC's Medical Coding Code of Ethics. (From American Academy of Professional Coders: Medical Coding Code of Ethics [website]: www.aapc.com/aboutus/code-of-ethics.aspx. Accessed July 1, 2009.)

EXERCISE 2-1 *What Is ICD-9-CM?*

Using the information presented in this text, complete the following:

1 The ICD-9-CM is designed for the classification of patient _____

   or _____.

2 The ICD-9-CM manual is based on what text developed by the World Health Organization?

   _____

3 The CM in ICD-9-CM stands for _____.

4 List four of the six reasons why the ICD-9-CM codes are used today.

   _____

   _____

   _____

   _____

5 The ICD-9-CM is used to translate what descriptive information into numeric codes?

   _____ or _____

ICD-9-CM FORMAT Volume 1 contains the disease and condition codes and the code descriptions (nomenclature) as well as the Supplementary Classification of Factors Influencing Health Status and Contact with Health Services (V codes) and External Causes of Injury and Poisoning (E codes).

Volume 2 is the Alphabetic Index for Volume 1. Volumes 1 and 2 are used in inpatient and outpatient settings to substantiate the reason for receiving medical services (medical necessity) by assigning diagnosis codes. Volume 3 is used for coding surgical, therapeutic, and diagnostic procedures and is used primarily by hospitals. ICD-9-CM codes are reported on the CMS-1500 insurance claim form (Fig. 2–2) used in physician's offices and on the CMS-1450 form or UB-04 used in hospitals (Fig. 2–3). Private insurance carriers also require ICD-9-CM codes on forms submitted for payment for services. Most private insurance companies accept the CMS-1500 and the UB-04. Individual insurance companies may have different requirements as to what fields on the form need to be completed.

Depending on the publisher, Volume 2 may be in the front of the ICD-9-CM manual or in the middle of the book. Some publishers have the order as Volume 2, Volume 1, and Volume 3, and other publishers have the order as Volume 1, Volume 2, Volume 3.

To begin the study of ICD-9-CM codes, you will be introduced to the format and content of the volumes. When the review has been completed, you will begin to practice locating codes for various diseases and illnesses using the ICD-9-CM manual. The only way to learn to code is to practice.

Several publishing companies produce versions of the ICD-9-CM manual. All versions are based on the official government version of the ICD-9-CM.

There are four groups whose function it is to deal with in-depth coding principles and practices: Centers for Medicare and Medicaid Services (CMS), which was formerly known as the Health Care Financing Administration (HCFA); National Center for Health Statistics (NCHS); American Health Information Management Association (AHIMA); and American Hospital Association (AHA).

Format

The ICD-9-CM manual is published in three volumes:

Volume 1   Diseases: Tabular List
Volume 2   Diseases: Alphabetic Index
Volume 3   Procedures: Tabular List and Alphabetic Index

TABULAR LIST, VOLUME 1

The Tabular List is Volume 1 of the ICD-9-CM. After referencing the Index (Volume 2), you will locate the code(s) identified in the Tabular. **You can never code directly from the Index.** Rather, you must always reference the Index and then verify the code number in the Tabular. Let's begin by learning about the divisions in the Tabular.

Divisions

Volume 1: Tabular List is the listing of all the codes available for assignment, including their descriptions. When the exact word is not found in the code description in the Tabular List but the descriptive word is found in the Alphabetic Index, you must trust the code provided in the Alphabetic Index to be correct because the Index contains descriptive words that the Tabular List **does not.** Not listing all possible descriptive terms in the Tabular List saves space.

Anything that can happen, in the way of injury or disease, to a human body has a code in Volume 1. Although there are certainly many things that can happen to us, the people who developed the ICD-9-CM not only included them all but organized them in a systematic way.

1500

HEALTH INSURANCE CLAIM FORM

APPROVED BY NATIONAL UNIFORM CLAIM COMMITTEE 08/05

☐☐ PICA   PICA ☐☐

| 1. MEDICARE ☐ (Medicare #) | MEDICAID ☐ (Medicaid #) | TRICARE CHAMPUS ☐ (Sponsor's SSN) | CHAMPVA ☐ (Member ID#) | GROUP HEALTH PLAN ☐ (SSN or ID) | FECA BLK LUNG ☐ (SSN) | OTHER ☐ (ID) | 1a. INSURED'S I.D. NUMBER (For Program in Item 1) |

2. PATIENT'S NAME (Last Name, First Name, Middle Initial)

3. PATIENT'S BIRTH DATE MM DD YY   SEX M☐ F☐

4. INSURED'S NAME (Last Name, First Name, Middle Initial)

5. PATIENT'S ADDRESS (No., Street)

6. PATIENT RELATIONSHIP TO INSURED   Self☐ Spouse☐ Child☐ Other☐

7. INSURED'S ADDRESS (No., Street)

CITY   STATE

8. PATIENT STATUS   Single☐ Married☐ Other☐   Employed☐ Full-Time Student☐ Part-Time Student☐

CITY   STATE

ZIP CODE   TELEPHONE (Include Area Code) (   )

ZIP CODE   TELEPHONE (Include Area Code) (   )

9. OTHER INSURED'S NAME (Last Name, First Name, Middle Initial)

10. IS PATIENT'S CONDITION RELATED TO:

11. INSURED'S POLICY GROUP OR FECA NUMBER

a. OTHER INSURED'S POLICY OR GROUP NUMBER

a. EMPLOYMENT? (Current or Previous) YES☐ NO☐

a. INSURED'S DATE OF BIRTH MM DD YY   SEX M☐ F☐

b. OTHER INSURED'S DATE OF BIRTH MM DD YY   SEX M☐ F☐

b. AUTO ACCIDENT?   PLACE (State) YES☐ NO☐

b. EMPLOYER'S NAME OR SCHOOL NAME

c. EMPLOYER'S NAME OR SCHOOL NAME

c. OTHER ACCIDENT? YES☐ NO☐

c. INSURANCE PLAN NAME OR PROGRAM NAME

d. INSURANCE PLAN NAME OR PROGRAM NAME

10d. RESERVED FOR LOCAL USE

d. IS THERE ANOTHER HEALTH BENEFIT PLAN? YES☐ NO☐ *If yes*, return to and complete item 9 a-d.

READ BACK OF FORM BEFORE COMPLETING & SIGNING THIS FORM.

12. PATIENT'S OR AUTHORIZED PERSON'S SIGNATURE I authorize the release of any medical or other information necessary to process this claim. I also request payment of government benefits either to myself or to the party who accepts assignment below.

SIGNED _____ DATE _____

13. INSURED'S OR AUTHORIZED PERSON'S SIGNATURE I authorize payment of medical benefits to the undersigned physician or supplier for services described below.

SIGNED _____

14. DATE OF CURRENT: MM DD YY   ILLNESS (First symptom) OR INJURY (Accident) OR PREGNANCY(LMP)

15. IF PATIENT HAS HAD SAME OR SIMILAR ILLNESS. GIVE FIRST DATE MM DD YY

16. DATES PATIENT UNABLE TO WORK IN CURRENT OCCUPATION FROM MM DD YY TO MM DD YY

17. NAME OF REFERRING PROVIDER OR OTHER SOURCE   17a. / 17b.

18. HOSPITALIZATION DATES RELATED TO CURRENT SERVICES FROM MM DD YY TO MM DD YY

19. RESERVED FOR LOCAL USE

20. OUTSIDE LAB? YES☐ NO☐ $ CHARGES

21. DIAGNOSIS OR NATURE OF ILLNESS OR INJURY (Relate Items 1, 2, 3 or 4 to Item 24E by Line)

1. L___.___   3. L___.___
2. L___.___   4. L___.___

22. MEDICAID RESUBMISSION CODE   ORIGINAL REF. NO.

23. PRIOR AUTHORIZATION NUMBER

24. A. DATE(S) OF SERVICE From MM DD YY To MM DD YY	B. PLACE OF SERVICE	C. EMG	D. PROCEDURES, SERVICES, OR SUPPLIES (Explain Unusual Circumstances) CPT/HCPCS MODIFIER	E. DIAGNOSIS POINTER	F. $ CHARGES	G. DAYS OR UNITS	H. EPSDT Family Plan	I. ID. QUAL.	J. RENDERING PROVIDER ID. #
1									
2									
3									
4									
5									
6									

25. FEDERAL TAX I.D. NUMBER   SSN☐ EIN☐

26. PATIENT'S ACCOUNT NO.

27. ACCEPT ASSIGNMENT? (For govt. claims, see back) YES☐ NO☐

28. TOTAL CHARGE $

29. AMOUNT PAID $

30. BALANCE DUE $

31. SIGNATURE OF PHYSICIAN OR SUPPLIER INCLUDING DEGREES OR CREDENTIALS (I certify that the statements on the reverse apply to this bill and are made a part thereof.)

SIGNED _____ DATE _____

32. SERVICE FACILITY LOCATION INFORMATION
a.   b.

33. BILLING PROVIDER INFO & PH # (   )
a.   b.

NUCC Instruction Manual available at: www.nucc.org   **PLEASE PRINT OR TYPE**   APPROVED OMB-0938-0999 FORM CMS-1500 (08-05)

CARRIER

PATIENT AND INSURED INFORMATION

PHYSICIAN OR SUPPLIER INFORMATION

FIGURE 2–2 CMS-1500 Health Insurance Claim Form. (Courtesy U.S. Department of Health and Human Services, Centers for Medicare and Medicaid Services.)

FIGURE 2-3 CMS-1450 was updated to the UB-04 paper form effective May 23, 2007. (Courtesy U.S. Department of Health and Human Services, Public Health Service, Centers for Medicare and Medicaid Services.)

Volume 1 is separated into two major divisions:

1. Classification of Diseases and Injuries
2. Supplementary Classifications
   - Supplementary Classification of Factors Influencing Health Status and Contact with Health Services (V codes) (V01-V89)
   - Supplementary Classification of External Causes of Injury and Poisoning (E codes) (E800-E999)

The Supplementary Classifications will be covered in detail in Chapter 3.

Classification of Diseases and Injuries. The Classification of Diseases and Injuries is the main part of the ICD-9-CM, Volume 1, Tabular List;

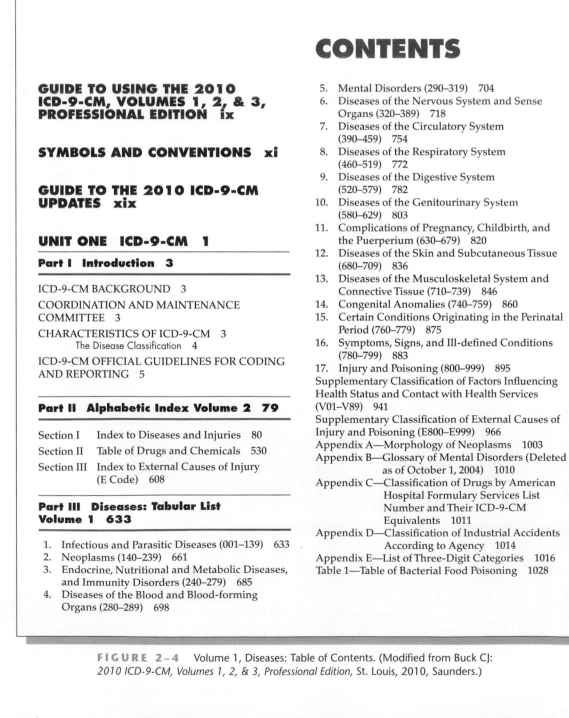

CONTENTS

GUIDE TO USING THE 2010 ICD-9-CM, VOLUMES 1, 2, & 3, PROFESSIONAL EDITION ix

SYMBOLS AND CONVENTIONS xi

GUIDE TO THE 2010 ICD-9-CM UPDATES xix

UNIT ONE ICD-9-CM 1

Part I Introduction 3

ICD-9-CM BACKGROUND 3
COORDINATION AND MAINTENANCE COMMITTEE 3
CHARACTERISTICS OF ICD-9-CM 3
  The Disease Classification 4
ICD-9-CM OFFICIAL GUIDELINES FOR CODING AND REPORTING 5

Part II Alphabetic Index Volume 2 79

Section I Index to Diseases and Injuries 80
Section II Table of Drugs and Chemicals 530
Section III Index to External Causes of Injury (E Code) 608

Part III Diseases: Tabular List Volume 1 633

1. Infectious and Parasitic Diseases (001–139) 633
2. Neoplasms (140–239) 661
3. Endocrine, Nutritional and Metabolic Diseases, and Immunity Disorders (240–279) 685
4. Diseases of the Blood and Blood-forming Organs (280–289) 698

5. Mental Disorders (290–319) 704
6. Diseases of the Nervous System and Sense Organs (320–389) 718
7. Diseases of the Circulatory System (390–459) 754
8. Diseases of the Respiratory System (460–519) 772
9. Diseases of the Digestive System (520–579) 782
10. Diseases of the Genitourinary System (580–629) 803
11. Complications of Pregnancy, Childbirth, and the Puerperium (630–679) 820
12. Diseases of the Skin and Subcutaneous Tissue (680–709) 836
13. Diseases of the Musculoskeletal System and Connective Tissue (710–739) 846
14. Congenital Anomalies (740–759) 860
15. Certain Conditions Originating in the Perinatal Period (760–779) 875
16. Symptoms, Signs, and Ill-defined Conditions (780–799) 883
17. Injury and Poisoning (800–999) 895
Supplementary Classification of Factors Influencing Health Status and Contact with Health Services (V01–V89) 941
Supplementary Classification of External Causes of Injury and Poisoning (E800–E999) 966
Appendix A—Morphology of Neoplasms 1003
Appendix B—Glossary of Mental Disorders (Deleted as of October 1, 2004) 1010
Appendix C—Classification of Drugs by American Hospital Formulary Services List Number and Their ICD-9-CM Equivalents 1011
Appendix D—Classification of Industrial Accidents According to Agency 1014
Appendix E—List of Three-Digit Categories 1016
Table 1—Table of Bacterial Food Poisoning 1028

FIGURE 2–4 Volume 1, Diseases: Table of Contents. (Modified from Buck CJ: *2010 ICD-9-CM, Volumes 1, 2, & 3, Professional Edition,* St. Louis, 2010, Saunders.)

it consists of 17 chapters with codes ranging from 001 to 999. Fig. 2–4 illustrates that most chapters are based on body system (e.g., nervous system [Chapter 6], respiratory system [Chapter 8], or digestive system [Chapter 9]). Some chapters are based on the cause or type of disease (e.g., infectious and parasitic diseases [Chapter 1] or neoplasms [Chapter 2]). Fig. 2–5 indicates the format of each chapter.

Chapter.   A chapter is the main division in the ICD-9-CM manual.

Section.   A section is a group of three-digit categories that represent a group of conditions or related conditions.

Category.   A three-digit category is a code that represents a single condition or disease. There are approximately 100 codes at the category level; most others require a fourth or fifth digit. If you look at the footnote area of your ICD-9-CM manual, you will see there is a symbol that is used to direct the coder to assign further digits.

Subcategory.   A four-digit subcategory code provides more information or specificity as compared to the three-digit code in terms of the cause, site, or manifestation of the condition. You must assign the fourth digit if it is available. Always code to the highest level of specificity based on the documentation in the medical record.

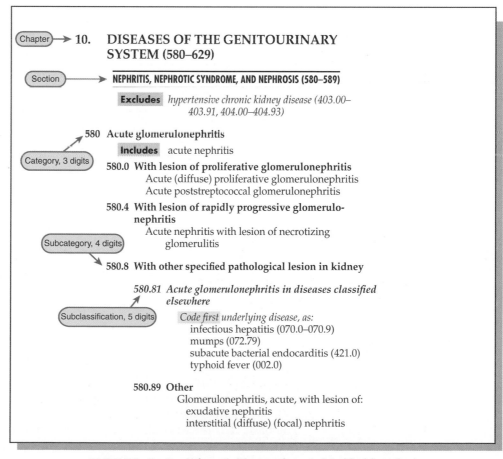

FIGURE 2–5   Volume 1, Diseases: format. (Modified from Buck CJ: *2010 ICD-9-CM, Volumes 1, 2, & 3, Professional Edition,* St. Louis, 2010, Saunders.)

Subclassification. A five-digit subclassification code adds even more information and specificity to a condition's description. You must assign the fifth digit if it is available. Instructions on the use of fifth digits may appear at the beginning of a chapter, a section or third/fourth digit category.

Bold Type   Bold type is used for all codes and titles in the Tabular List in Volume 1.

Example
244.8   Other specified acquired hypothyroidism
      Secondary hypothyroidism NEC

Italicized Type   Italicized type is used for all exclusion notes and to identify those codes that are not usually sequenced as the first-listed diagnosis. Italicized type codes cannot be assigned as a first-listed diagnosis because they always follow another code. Italicized codes are to be sequenced in the order specified in the Alphabetic Index, Volume 2, or according to specific coding instructions in the Tabular List, Volume 1, such as "Code first..."

Example
420.0   Acute pericarditis in diseases classified elsewhere
      Code first underlying disease, as:
         actinomycosis (039.8)
         amebiasis (006.8)
         chronic uremia (585.9)
         nocardiosis (039.8)
         tuberculosis (017.9)
         uremia NOS (586)

EXERCISE 2-2   *ICD-9-CM Chapter Format*

Using ICD-9-CM, Volume 1, Tabular List, locate the first page of Chapter 3 and answer the following questions about the chapter:

1 The name of the chapter: _____

2 The name of the first section: _____

3 The description of the first category: _____

4 The description of the first subcategory: _____

The information in this activity was important to your learning because it will enable you to communicate effectively about information in the ICD-9-CM manual using common terminology.

The basic ICD-9-CM code is a three-digit code, as shown in Fig. 2–6. Each code is a rubric (something under which something else is classed). Both the code number and the entry are in bold type. Diagnosis codes always contain at least three digits before the decimal point. If the diagnosis code is "1," it is written 001. Procedure codes from Volume 3 always consist of two digits, both

| Basic three-digit category code | ⟶ | 730 | Osteomyelitis, periostitis, and other infections involving bone |

FIGURE 2–6   ICD-9-CM three-digit category code. (Modified from Buck CJ: *2010 ICD-9-CM, Volumes 1, 2, & 3, Professional Edition*, St. Louis, 2010, Saunders.)

placed before the decimal point. You can always tell a procedure code from a diagnosis code by noting the number of digits before the decimal point.

Example

496	Diagnosis code
27.54	Procedure code
461.9	Diagnosis code
21.1	Procedure code

Fourth and Fifth-Digit Specificity.   The addition of the fourth and fifth digits to the basic three-digit code provides greater specificity to the numeric designation of the patient's condition and reduces third-party payer (insurance company) returns of claims for further clarification of the diagnosis code(s). When four digits (one digit after the decimal point) are used, they are called **subcategory** codes. If five digits are used (two digits after the decimal point), they are called **subclassification** codes. Fig. 2–7 shows the first three digits of the code used to identify the disease "Osteomyelitis, periostitis, and other infections involving bone"; the fourth digit provides further specificity by distinguishing between acute and chronic osteomyelitis. Pay special attention to the symbols that indicate fourth and fifth digits are to be assigned to the code.

Not all codes have fourth or fifth digits, but when a fourth or fifth digit is available, it must be used. Most ICD-9-CM manuals have a symbol to remind the coder to assign a fourth or fifth digit as shown in Fig. 2–8. As an example of the fifth digit: Code 730.0 appears with a list of fifth digits that are used to identify the location of acute osteomyelitis as:

- 0 site unspecified
- 1 shoulder region
- 2 upper arm
- 3 forearm
- 4 hand
- 5 pelvic region and thigh
- 6 lower leg
- 7 ankle and foot
- 8 other specified sites
- 9 multiple sites

You indicate that the acute osteomyelitis is located in the patient's shoulder by adding the fifth digit 1 to the 730.0; code 730.01.

CODING SHOT   Remember that the goal is to be as accurate, as complete, and as specific as possible. The code(s) selected must be supported by physician documentation.

Use of fourth subcategory digit ⟶ 730.0 **Acute osteomyelitis**
730.1 **Chronic osteomyelitis**

FIGURE 2–7 ICD-9-CM four-digit subcategory code. (Modified from Buck CJ: *2010 ICD-9-CM, Volumes 1, 2, & 3, Professional Edition,* St. Louis, 2010, Saunders.)

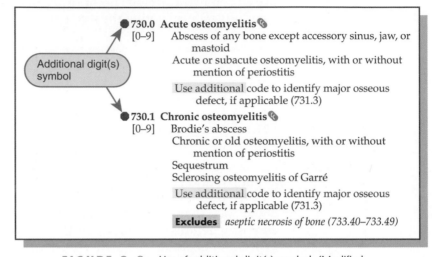

● **730.0 Acute osteomyelitis** 🦴
[0–9]   Abscess of any bone except accessory sinus, jaw, or mastoid
Acute or subacute osteomyelitis, with or without mention of periostitis

Use additional code to identify major osseous defect, if applicable (731.3)

● **730.1 Chronic osteomyelitis** 🦴
[0–9]   Brodie's abscess
Chronic or old osteomyelitis, with or without mention of periostitis
Sequestrum
Sclerosing osteomyelitis of Garré

Use additional code to identify major osseous defect, if applicable (731.3)

Excludes *aseptic necrosis of bone (733.40–733.49)*

Additional digit(s) symbol

FIGURE 2–8 Use of additional digit(s) symbol. (Modified from Buck CJ: *2010 ICD-9-CM, Volumes 1, 2, & 3, Professional Edition,* St. Louis, 2010, Saunders.)

Fig. 2–9 illustrates how adding the fourth and fifth digits adds specificity to the information about the patient's condition.

The addition of a fourth or fifth digit to a three-digit code provides greater specificity to the diagnosis. Greater specificity decreases the number of third-party-payer returns for further clarification of the diagnosis code(s). Delayed claims result in delayed payment to a physician practice or hospital.

Three-digit code + Fourth digit + Fifth digit

730   +   .0   +   .01   = 730.01 = acute ostemyelitis of the shoulder

Osteomyelitis + Acute + Shoulder

FIGURE 2–9 Specificity in ICD-9-CM codes.

EXERCISE 2-3   *Fifth-Digit Specificity*

Locate the first page of Chapter 13, Diseases of the Musculoskeletal System and Connective Tissues, in the ICD-9-CM manual. Notes immediately following the chapter title indicate the fifth-digit subclassifications and the specific categories with which these fifth digits are used. Read the notes for Chapter 13.

The following is a part of the fifth-digit subclassifications used with categories 711-712, 715-716, 718-719, and 730:

0 site unspecified

1 shoulder region

　　Acromioclavicular joint(s)

　　Clavicle

　　Glenohumeral joint(s)

　　Scapula joint(s)

　　Sternoclavicular

2 upper arm

　　Elbow joint

　　Humerus

The various joints of the shoulder region or the elbow joint and humerus of the upper arm are the specific anatomic terms to which the main term refers. The use of the 2 indicates the elbow joint, the humerus, and so forth. These anatomic terms serve to provide further specificity to the code selection.

Locate code 711 in the ICD-9-CM manual, then answer the following:

The patient record states: Pyogenic arthritis in lower leg.

1 What would the correct five-digit code be?

　　Code: _____

2 Is the use of the fifth digit optional? _____

3 How is specificity added to ICD-9-CM codes? _____

CODING SHOT   Sometimes you will have to go back two or three pages to locate the additional digit that is to be added.

QUICK CHECK 2-1

1. Locate code 719 in the Tabular. Read the notes there. The code for effusion of the knee would be 719.0_. You choose the fifth digit.

   a. 6
   b. 7
   c. 8
   d. 9

2. By reading the notes, how did you identify which of the fifth digits represented "knee"?

   _____

APPENDICES IN THE TABULAR LIST, VOLUME 1

Volume 1, Tabular List, contains five appendices:

Appendix A	Morphology of Neoplasms
Appendix B	Glossary of Mental Disorders (Deleted in 2004)
Appendix C	Classification of Drugs by American Hospital Formulary Service List Number and Their ICD-9-CM Equivalents
Appendix D	Classification of Industrial Accidents According to Agency
Appendix E	List of Three-Digit Categories

Appendices are included as a reference for the coder so it is possible to:

1. Provide further information about the patient's clinical picture

2. Further define a diagnostic statement

3. Aid in classifying new drugs

4. Reference three-digit categories

The appendices are titled Appendix A, B, C, D, and E to indicate their positions in the back of Volume 1 of the ICD-9-CM manual.

Appendix A: Morphology of Neoplasms

The World Health Organization has published an adaptation of the International Classification of Diseases for Oncology (ICD-O). The ICD-O contains codes for the **location (topography)** and morphology of tumors. **Morphology** is the study of neoplasms. The morphology codes consist of five digits: the first four identify the histologic type of the neoplasm and the fifth indicates the behavior of the neoplasm.

Examples of **types** of neoplasm are epithelial, papillary, basal cell, and adenoma. Refer to a medical dictionary if you are not familiar with the types of neoplasms presented in Appendix A of the ICD-9-CM.

Examples of the **behaviors** of neoplasms are the terms "benign," "malignant," and "carcinoma in situ." "In situ" means the neoplasm has not spread from another site and is located in its original place without invasion into neighboring tissue. ICD-O codes are used to gather data about the behavior, type, and location of tumors. For example, the coder would assign an ICD-9-CM code from Chapter 2, Neoplasms (140-239); the Certified Tumor Registrar (CTR) would receive a listing of coded data for all neoplasm codes. The CTR would then assign an M code for the morphology (histological type) along with an ICD-O code to indicate the location of the tumor. For example, the coder indicates a breast tumor (basal cell) of the upper-outer quadrant as the diagnosis, using ICD-9-CM code 174.4. The CTR then researches the patient's medical record and assigns an M code to indicate infiltrating ductal (M8500/3) and an ICD-O code to indicate the location of the tumor as C50.4 (upper-outer quadrant of the breast).

The one-digit morphology behavior code is as follows:

/0	Benign
/1	Uncertain whether benign or malignant Borderline malignancy
/2	Carcinoma in situ Intraepithelial (within the epithelial cells, those cells that cover the internal organs and vessels of the body) Noninfiltrating (cancer that has not spread to other, adjacent areas) Noninvasive (cancer that has not spread outside the original area)
/3	Malignant, primary site
/6	Malignant, metastatic site (secondary site, or site spread to) Secondary site
/9	Malignant, uncertain whether primary or metastatic site (secondary site, or site spread to)

A primary site is the originating site of the tumor, and a secondary site is the metastatic site (a spread from the primary to the secondary site).

Appendix B: Glossary of Mental Disorders

The psychiatric terms that appear in ICD-9-CM, Chapter 5, Mental Disorders, used to be listed in alphabetic order in Appendix B. Appendix B was deleted in 2004. Most psychiatric disorders are classified using the Diagnostic and Statistical Manual of Mental Disorders (DSM-IV).

Appendix C: Drugs

This alphabetized subsection is entitled Classification of Drugs by American Hospital Formulary Services List Number and Their ICD-9-CM Equivalents. (Have you noticed how few short titles there are in the ICD-9-CM!) A division of the American Hospital Formulary Service (AHFS) regularly publishes a coded listing of drugs. These AHFS codes have as many as five digits. Each has a number, then a colon, and then up to four additional digits to provide specificity.

Example

AHFS		ICD-9-CM
8:12.04	Antifungal Antibiotics	960.1

Note that the ICD-9-CM code and the AHFS poisoning codes mean the same thing. For example, both AHFS 8:12.04 and ICD-9-CM 960.1 are poisoning by Antifungal Antibiotics. AHFS codes are assigned primarily by pharmacists and are not placed on the insurance forms that you will be responsible to complete.

From the Trenches

"Coding is like solving a mystery . . . . I think It Is lIke detectIve work. There are some easy codes that you'll find very quickly, but there are others that take a great deal of intellect and research to determine whether or not you are actually getting it right."

JOHN

Appendix D: Industrial Accidents

The subsection Classification of Industrial Accidents According to Agency contains three-digit codes to identify occupational hazards. The subsection is divided into the following categories:

1. Machines
2. Means of Transport and Lifting Equipment
3. Other Equipment
4. Materials, Substances, and Radiations
5. Working Environment
6. Other Agencies, Not Elsewhere Classified (NEC)
7. Agencies Not Classified for Lack of Sufficient Data

The identification of occupational hazards is especially important in coding injury or death that is job-related. Statisticians analyze the data and make statements about the risks involved in various occupations based on the data collected from the forms completed by health care workers. Occupational hazard codes are not placed on the insurance or billing forms. Instead, these specialized codes are used by state and federal organizations to summarize data concerning industrial accidents.

Appendix E: Three-Digit Categories

Appendix E is a list of all the three-digit categories in the ICD-9-CM, presented by chapter. The categories are labeled 1 through 17, V01-V89, and E800-E999.

Example

1. **INFECTIOUS AND PARASITIC DISEASES**
    Intestinal infectious diseases (001-009)
    001   Cholera
    002   Typhoid and paratyphoid fevers
    003   Other salmonella infections
    004   Shigellosis
    005   Other food poisoning (bacterial)
    006   Amebiasis
    007   Other protozoal intestinal diseases
    008   Intestinal infections due to other organisms
    009   Ill-defined intestinal infections

Reviewing Appendix E is a good way to get a quick overview of all of the codes in the ICD-9-CM manual.

EXERCISE 2-4 *The Five Appendices in Volume 1*

Fill in the following:

1 In which appendix of the ICD-9-CM manual would you find the following information?

a. Glossary of Mental Disorders _____

b. Classification of Industrial Accidents According to Agency _____

c. Morphology of Neoplasms _____

d. List of Three-Digit Categories _____

e. Classification of Drugs by American Hospital Formulary Service List _____

2 In which appendix of the ICD-9-CM manual would you find the code to identify an injury

resulting from a job-related accident involving a machine? _____

ALPHABETIC INDEX, VOLUME 2

The Alphabetic Index is Volume 2 of the ICD-9-CM. As a coder, you will reference the Index first and then locate the code identified in the Index in the Tabular List, Volume 1. Everything in the Index is listed by condition—meaning diagnosis, signs, symptoms, and conditions such as pregnancy, admission, encounter, or complication. Some types of codes may be a little difficult to find, such as those dealing with complications, late effects, and V codes.

> ✋ **CAUTION** *There are terms in the Index that do not appear in the Tabular. For example, "Anton syndrome," 307.9, is listed in the Index but not in the Tabular. Even though the term is not listed in the Tabular description for the code, the code is correct because of the term "Anton syndrome" in the Index.*

The Alphabetic Index consists of three sections:

- Index to Diseases
- Table of Drugs and Chemicals
- Index to External Causes of Injury (E codes)

There are two tables located within the Index to Diseases. These tables are used to better list the subterms under the main term entries of hypertension and neoplasm.

**Please refer to the companion Evolve website for the most current guidelines.

ICD-9-CM OFFICIAL GUIDELINES FOR CODING AND REPORTING

SECTION I. Conventions, general coding guidelines and chapter specific guidelines

The conventions, general guidelines and chapter-specific guidelines are applicable to all health care settings unless otherwise indicated. The conventions and instructions of the classification take precedence over guidelines.

A. Conventions for the ICD-9-CM

The conventions for the ICD-9-CM are the general rules for use of the classification independent of the guidelines. These conventions are incorporated within the index and tabular of the ICD-9-CM as instructional notes. The conventions are as follows:

1. Format:

The ICD-9-CM uses an indented format for ease in reference

The ICD-9-CM Index utilizes three levels of indentation in the Alphabetic Index. They are the:

- Main terms
- Subterms
- Carryover lines

The main terms are identified by **bold** print and are flush with the left margin of each column. Alphabetization rules apply in locating main terms and subterms in the Alphabetic Index. Numerical entries appear first under the main term or subterm. Each term is followed by the code or codes that apply to the term (Fig. 2–10).

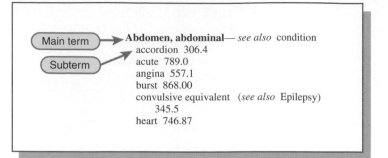

FIGURE 2–10 Main terms are capitalized and in bold print. Subterms are indented two spaces to the right under the term above. (Modified from Buck CJ: *2010 ICD-9-CM, Volumes 1, 2, & 3, Professional Edition,* St. Louis, 2010, Saunders.)

EXERCISE 2-5   *Main Terms*

Underline the main terms to be located in the Alphabetic Index in the following diagnostic statements:

1 Normocytic anemia

2 Acute prostatitis

3 Severe protein calorie malnutrition

4 Granuloma lung

5 Pain in neck

The subterms under the main terms are indented to the right. They begin with a lowercase letter and are not bolded. These subterms modify the main term and are called **essential modifiers.** These subterms provide greater specificity for proper code assignment. It is possible for a subterm to be followed by an additional subterm(s). These additional subterms are indented even further to the right.

Example
Incoordination
  esophageal-pharyngeal (newborn) 787.24

  muscular 781.3

  papillary muscle 429.81

The term in parentheses (newborn) is nonessential and merely supplementary. The indented subterms are essential modifiers, such as muscular or papillary muscle.

General adjectives such as "acute," "chronic," "epidemic," or "hereditary" and references to anatomic site, such as "arm," "stomach," and "uterus," will appear as main terms, but they will have a *"see"* or *"see also* condition" reference.

> *Example*
> **Hereditary**—*see* condition
> **Uterus**—*see* condition

Certain subterms are called **connecting words.** These define a relationship between a main term or a subterm and an associated condition or etiology. The connecting words "with" or "without" are located immediately after the main term and before any other subterms. Some additional connecting words are "associated with," "due to," "with mention of" or "in" (see Fig. 2–10).

Carryover lines are used when there is not enough space on a single line for an entry. They are indented to the right even further than a subterm to avoid confusion as illustrated in Fig. 2–11.

Conventions   The ICD-9-CM manual contains symbols, abbreviations, punctuation, and notations called conventions. Some conventions are used in all three volumes of the ICD-9-CM manual, and others are used in only one or two of the volumes. The ICD-9-CM manual contains a list of the conventions and definitions to be used when assigning codes, usually in the front matter of the manual. It is important that you be familiar with the conventions as you prepare to assign ICD-9-CM codes.

Although the maintenance of the ICD-9-CM is the responsibility of the NCHS (National Center for Health Statistics) and CMS (Centers for Medicare and Medicaid Services), many private companies publish editions of the ICD-9-CM, and each publisher has its own conventions in addition to the standard conventions. For example, some publishers indicate that a fifth digit is required by placing a special symbol next to the code in the index. These additional symbols are helpful to coders but are not a recognized convention.

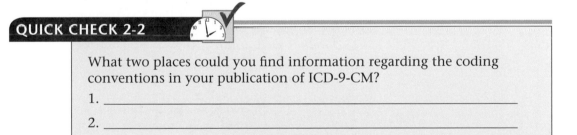

QUICK CHECK 2-2

What two places could you find information regarding the coding conventions in your publication of ICD-9-CM?

1. _____

2. _____

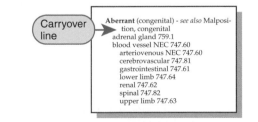

FIGURE 2–11   Carryover lines are indented five spaces to the right. (Modified from Buck CJ: *2010 ICD-9-CM, Volumes 1, 2, & 3, Professional Edition,* St. Louis, 2010, Saunders.)

NEC and NOS

ICD-9-CM OFFICIAL GUIDELINES FOR CODING AND REPORTING

SECTION I.A.

2. Abbreviations

   a. **Index abbreviations**

      NEC "Not elsewhere classifiable"

         This abbreviation in the index represents "other specified" when a specific code is not available for a condition, the index directs the coder to the "other specified" code in the tabular.

   b. **Tabular abbreviations**

      NEC "Not elsewhere classifiable"

         This abbreviation in the tabular represents "other specified". When a specific code is not available for a condition the tabular includes an NEC entry under a code to identify the code as the "other specified" code.

         (See Section I.A.5.a. "Other" codes").

      NOS "Not otherwise specified"

         This abbreviation is the equivalent of unspecified.

         (See Section I.A.5.b., "Unspecified" codes).

The two main abbreviations NEC (not elsewhere classifiable) and NOS (not otherwise specified) are often used and very important.

NEC.   NEC is used in both the Alphabetic Index and the Tabular List. In the Alphabetic Index, NEC represents "other specified." When a specific disease or condition is documented and there is not a specific code available, the Index will direct the coder by using the abbreviation NEC to an "other specified" code.

The NEC abbreviation in the Tabular List also means "other specified" and it often is classified to the final digit 8. The code may not fully describe the disease process or medical condition.

Example from Tabular List

244 Acquired hypothyroidism

      Includes: athyroidism (acquired)

                 hypothyroidism (acquired)

                 myxedema (adult) (juvenile)

                 thyroid (gland) insufficiency (acquired)

    244.8 Other specified acquired hypothyroidism

         Secondary hypothyroidism NEC

NOS.   NOS (not otherwise specified) is the equivalent of "unspecified." It is used when the information at hand does not permit a more specific code assignment. The coder should query the physician for more specific information so that a more specific code assignment can be made.

Example

159 Malignant neoplasm of other and ill-defined sites within the digestive organs and peritoneum

    159.0 Intestinal tract, part unspecified

         Intestine NOS

From the Trenches

"I try to always keep people aware that we're not just translating an ICD-9 narrative into a code—that's a patient we're dealing with. It's not just a piece of paper, it's not just words we're handling—it's still a patient."

JOHN

Example

NEC

Diagnosis: Pneumonia due to gram-negative bacteria

Index: **Pneumonia**
gram-negative bacteria NEC 482.83

Tabular: **482.8 Pneumonia due to other specified bacteria**
482.83 Other gram-negative bacteria

Code: 482.83 Pneumonia due to gram-negative bacteria

Code 482.83 identifies gram-negative bacterial pneumonia that cannot be classified more specifically. The other subclassifications within 482.8 are for anaerobes (482.81), Escherichia coli [E. coli] (482.82), other than gram-negative bacteria (482.83), Legionnaire's disease (482.84), and other specified bacteria (482.89). None of these other subclassifications can be assigned to the diagnostic statement; therefore, 482.83 is the most appropriate code assignment.

NEC can be used in two ways:

1. NEC directs the coder to other classifications, if appropriate. Other subterms or Excludes notes may provide hints as to what the other classifications may be.
2. NEC is used when the ICD-9-CM does not have any codes that provide greater specificity.

Example

NOS

Diagnosis: Bronchitis

Index: **Bronchitis 490**

Tabular: **490 Bronchitis, not specified as acute or chronic**
Bronchitis NOS

Assign: 490 Bronchitis

The diagnosis was not specified by the physician as acute or chronic; therefore, the "not otherwise specified" code 490 must be assigned. In this situation, it would be appropriate for the coder to query the physician for more specific information.

CODING SHOT Third-party payers prefer specific codes and do not appreciate a coder's dependence on NOS codes. If the NOS code is the only correct code, you must assign it, but only after a thorough review of all available documentation.

ICD-9-CM OFFICIAL GUIDELINES FOR CODING AND REPORTING

SECTION I.A.

3. Punctuation

[ ] Brackets are used in the tabular list to enclose synonyms, alternative wording or explanatory phrases. Brackets are used in the index to identify manifestation codes.
(See Section I.A.6. "Etiology/manifestations")

( ) Parentheses are used in both the index and tabular to enclose supplementary words that may be present or absent in the statement of a disease or procedure without affecting the code number to which it is assigned. The terms within the parentheses are referred to as nonessential modifiers.

: Colons are used in the Tabular list after an incomplete term which needs one or more of the modifiers following the colon to make it assignable to a given category.

Brackets [ ] Brackets enclose synonyms, alternative wording, or explanatory phrases and are found in the Tabular List.

Example

426.8   Other specified conduction disorders
    426.89   Other
            Dissociation:
                atrioventricular [AV]

Slanted Brackets *[ ]* Slanted brackets used in the Alphabetic Index, Volume 2, are used to enclose the manifestation of the underlying condition. You sequence the code inside the slanted brackets after the underlying condition code.

Example

Diabetic retinal hemorrhage

    Hemorrhage, hemorrhagic (nontraumatic) 459.0
        retina, retinal (deep) (superficial) (vessels) 362.81
            diabetic 250.5 *[362.01]*

You sequence the 250.5X (X means the appropriate fifth digit would have to be added) and then 362.01 to indicate that the retinal hemorrhage (the manifestation) was due to diabetes (the underlying disease or etiology).

Parentheses ( ) Parentheses enclose supplementary words (nonessential modifiers) that may be present or absent in the statement of a disease or procedure without affecting code assignment. Parentheses are located in both the Alphabetic Index and the Tabular List.

Example from Tabular List

158   **Malignant neoplasm of retroperitoneum and peritoneum**

    158.8   **Specified parts of peritoneum**
        Cul-de-sac (of Douglas)
        Mesentery

The nonessential modifier is "of Douglas." A cul-de-sac is a pouch that is closed at one end. A pouch of Douglas specifically refers to a type of cul-de-sac pouch that is located in the peritoneal cavity between the rectum and the back wall of the uterus (rectouterine pouch).

Example from Alphabetic Index

Ileus (adynamic) (bowel) (colon) (inhibitory) (intestine) (neurogenic) (paralytic) 560.1

The nonessential modifiers are the words "(adynamic) (bowel) (colon) (inhibitory) (intestine) (neurogenic) (paralytic)." Nonessential modifiers are words that may be used to clarify the diagnosis but do not affect code assignment. The code for ileus is 560.1, and the code for adynamic ileus is also 560.1. The addition of the modifier "adynamic" does not affect the code assignment.

EXERCISE 2-6   *Essential/Nonessential Modifier*

Using ICD-9-CM, Volume 2, Alphabetic Index, locate the following main terms and identify if the bolded subterm is an essential or nonessential modifier:

1 Otitis **externa** _____

2 **Acute** otitis externa _____

3 **Streptococcal** nasopharyngitis _____

4 **Suppurative** mastitis _____

5 **Congenital** spondylolisthesis _____

Colon : Colons are located in the Tabular List after an incomplete term that needs one or more of the modifiers that follow in order to make the condition assignable to a given category.

Example

628 **Infertility, female**
     628.4 **Of cervical or vaginal origin**
          Infertility associated with:
            anomaly of cervical mucus
            congenital structural anomaly
            dysmucorrhea

Brace } A brace is used in some publications to enclose a series of terms, each of which is modified by the statement appearing at the right of the brace.

Example

473 **Chronic sinusitis**
       Includes: abscess

               empyema

                            } (chronic) of sinus (accessory) (nasal)

               infection

               suppuration

ICD-9-CM OFFICIAL GUIDELINES FOR CODING AND REPORTING

SECTION I.A.

4. Includes and Excludes Notes and Inclusion terms

Includes: This note appears immediately under a three-digit code title to further define, or give examples of, the content of the category.

Excludes: An excludes note under a code indicates that the terms excluded from the code are to be coded elsewhere. In some cases the codes for the excluded terms should not be used in conjunction with the code from which it is excluded. An example of this is a congenital condition excluded from an acquired form of the same condition. The congenital and acquired codes should not be used together. In other cases, the excluded terms may be used together with an excluded code. An example of this is when fractures of different bones are coded to different codes. Both codes may be used together if both types of fractures are present.

Inclusion terms: List of terms is included under certain four and five digit codes. These terms are the conditions for which that code number is to be used. The terms may be synonyms of the code title, or, in the case of "other specified" codes, the terms are a list of the various conditions assigned to that code. The inclusion terms are not necessarily exhaustive. Additional terms found only in the index may also be assigned to a code.

Includes. Includes notes appear in the Tabular List, Volume 1 and they further define or provide examples and may apply to the chapter, section, or category. The notes at the beginning of a **chapter** apply to that entire chapter; the notes at the beginning of the **section** apply to that entire section; and the notes at the beginning of the **category** apply to that entire category. You have to refer to the beginning of the chapter or section for any Includes notes that refer to an entire chapter or section because the Includes notes are not repeated within the chapter or section. Includes notes may also be located before or after category codes.

Includes and Excludes notes that apply to codes 001-139 at the beginning of a chapter:

Example

1. **INFECTIOUS AND PARASITIC DISEASES (001-139)**
   Note: Categories for "late effects" of infectious and parasitic diseases are to be found at 137-139.

   INCLUDES   diseases generally recognized as communicable or transmissible as well as a few diseases of unknown but possibly infectious origin

   EXCLUDES   *acute respiratory infections (460-466)*
   carrier or suspected carrier of infectious organism (V02.0-V02.9)
   certain localized infections
   influenza (487.0-487.8, 488.0-488.1)

Includes notes that apply to codes 010-018 at the beginning of a section:

Example

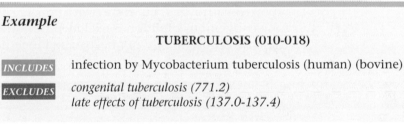

TUBERCULOSIS (010-018)

INCLUDES   infection by Mycobacterium tuberculosis (human) (bovine)

EXCLUDES   *congenital tuberculosis (771.2)*
late effects of tuberculosis (137.0-137.4)

Includes notes that apply to code 006 at the beginning of a category:

Example

006   Amebiasis

   INCLUDES   infection due to Entamoeba histolytica

   EXCLUDES   *amebiasis due to organisms other than Entamoeba histolytica (007.8)*

Excludes.   *Excludes* notes appear in the Tabular List, Volume 1, and indicate terms that are to be coded elsewhere. Excludes notes can be located at the beginning of a chapter or section or below a category or subcategory.

Excludes notes alert the coder to circumstances as in the following three examples:

Example 1

861   **Injury to heart and lung**

   EXCLUDES   *injury to blood vessels of thorax (901.0-901.9)*

This *Excludes* note indicates that injuries to the blood vessels of the thorax are assigned within the codes 901.0-901.9 and are not included within the codes in 861. If a patient had an injury to the thorax along with injury to blood vessels of the thorax, two codes would be assigned.

The code cannot be assigned if an associated condition is present and noted in the Excludes note.

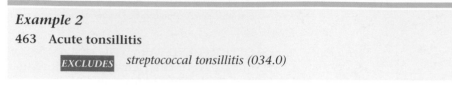

Example 2

463   **Acute tonsillitis**

EXCLUDES   *streptococcal tonsillitis (034.0)*

This *Excludes* note indicates that if the tonsillitis is documented as being caused by a streptococcal organism, it would be coded 034.0, not 463.

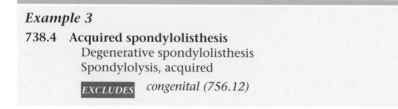

Example 3

738.4   **Acquired spondylolisthesis**
Degenerative spondylolisthesis
Spondylolysis, acquired

EXCLUDES   *congenital (756.12)*

This *Excludes* note instructs the coder that congenital spondylolisthesis is not reported with 738.4, but rather with 756.12. As the guidelines state, a code for a congenital condition is excluded from the acquired condition code and these two codes should not be assigned together.

EXERCISE 2-7 *Excludes*

Using the Tabular List, answer the following questions:

1 Is acute exacerbation of chronic myeloid leukemia assigned code 205.00? _____

   If not, what code is assigned? _____

2 Is rupture of the esophagus assigned code 530.4? _____

   If not, what code is assigned? _____

3 Is congenital clubfoot assigned code 736.71? _____

   If not, what code is assigned? _____

4 Is Shy-Drager syndrome assigned code 333.0? _____

   If not, what code is assigned? _____

5 Is duodenal ulcer included in code category 533? _____

   If not, what code category is assigned? _____

ICD-9-CM OFFICIAL GUIDELINES FOR CODING AND REPORTING

SECTION I.A.

5. Other and Unspecified codes

    a. **"Other" codes**

        Codes titled "other" or "other specified" (usually a code with a 4th digit 8 or fifth-digit 9 for diagnosis codes) are for use when the information in the medical record provides detail for which a specific code does not exist. Index entries with NEC in the line designate "other" codes in the tabular. These index entries represent specific disease entities for which no specific code exists so the term is included within an "other" code.

    b. **"Unspecified" codes**

        Codes (usually a code with a 4th digit 9 or 5th digit 0 for diagnosis codes) titled "unspecified" are for use when the information in the medical record is insufficient to assign a more specific code.

Subcategories.   Subcategories consist of fourth-digit codes that provide more information or specificity. The specificity may provide insight to the etiology of the disease as well as to the location of the disease or to the manifestation. A manifestation is a symptom or condition that is the result of a disease. A fourth digit of .8 is usually assigned for other specified conditions for that category. A .9 is usually assigned for unspecified conditions of that category as illustrated in Fig. 2–12.

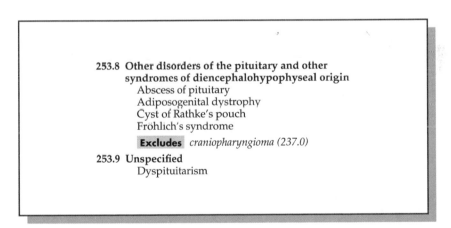

253.8 Other disorders of the pituitary and other syndromes of diencephalohypophyseal origin
    Abscess of pituitary
    Adiposogenital dystrophy
    Cyst of Rathke's pouch
    Frohlich's syndrome
      Excludes *craniopharyngioma (237.0)*

253.9 Unspecified
    Dyspituitarism

FIGURE 2–12   Other specified conditions and unspecified conditions. (From Buck CJ: *2010 ICD-9-CM, Volumes 1, 2, & 3, Professional Edition*, St. Louis, 2010, Saunders.)

Codes in Brackets

ICD-9-CM OFFICIAL GUIDELINES FOR CODING AND REPORTING

SECTION I.A.

6. Etiology/manifestation convention ("code first", "use additional code" and "in diseases classified elsewhere" notes)

Certain conditions have both an underlying etiology and multiple body system manifestations due to the underlying etiology. For such conditions, the ICD-9-CM has a coding convention that requires that the underlying condition be sequenced first followed by the manifestation. Wherever such a combination exists there is a "use additional code" note at the etiology code, and a "code first" note at the manifestation code. These instructional notes indicate the proper sequencing order of the codes, etiology followed by manifestation.

In most cases the manifestation codes will have in the code title, "in diseases classified elsewhere." Codes with this title are a component of the etiology/manifestation convention. The code title indicates that it is a manifestation code. "In diseases classified elsewhere" codes are never permitted to be used as first listed or principal diagnosis codes. They must be used in conjunction with an underlying condition code and they must be listed following the underlying condition.

There are manifestation codes that do not have "in diseases classified elsewhere" in the title. For such codes a "use additional code" note will still be present and the rules for sequencing apply.

In addition to the notes in the tabular, these conditions also have a specific index entry structure. In the index both conditions are listed together with the etiology code first followed by the manifestation codes in brackets. The code in brackets is always to be sequenced second.

The most commonly used etiology/manifestation combinations are the codes for Diabetes mellitus, category 250. For each code under category 250 there is a use additional code note for the manifestation that is specific for that particular diabetic manifestation. Should a patient have more than one manifestation of diabetes, more than one code from category 250 may be used with as many manifestation codes as are needed to fully describe the patient's complete diabetic condition. The category 250 diabetes codes should be sequenced first, followed by the manifestation codes.

"Code first" and "Use additional code" notes are also used as sequencing rules in the classification for certain codes that are not part of an etiology/ manifestation combination.

See – Section I.B.9. "Multiple coding for a single condition".

EXERCISE 2-8 *Etiology/Manifestation*

1 A patient is admitted with a diagnosis of malarial hepatitis.

a You might not be sure whether the first-listed diagnosis is hepatitis or malaria.

b Locate the term "Malaria" in the Index. Under the subterm "any type, with," locate "hepatitis 084.9 *[573.2].*" The slanted brackets alert you that *[573.2]* cannot be sequenced as the first-listed diagnosis.

c Locate the term "Hepatitis" and then the subterm "malarial." Again the entry states 084.9 *[573.2].*

d Both Index entries direct you to the first-listed diagnosis of malaria. Hepatitis can be a manifestation of malaria. The slanted brackets in 084.9 *[573.2]* indicate that this hepatitis is a manifestation of the condition malaria. "Hepatitis" is the condition and "malarial" describes the type of hepatitis.

e In the Tabular locate 084.9. Next locate "malarial" under "Use additional . . ." and then "hepatitis." 084.9 Malaria is the first-listed diagnosis and *[573.2]* hepatitis is the complication, and you would report both (084.9, 573.2) after checking 573.2 in the Tabular, which states *"Hepatitis in other infectious diseases classified elsewhere."*

You do the next one.

2 The patient's record states: endocarditis due to disseminated lupus erythematosus.

a When you locate the term "Endocarditis, due to, disseminated lupus erythematosus" in the Index, what do you find? _____

b In the Index, locate the main term (condition) "Lupus," the subterm "erythematosus," and the second subterm "systemic." What code are you directed to?

   ICD-9-CM Code: _____

c What is the title of 710 in the Tabular? _____

d According to the Includes notes in the Tabular following 710, what does 710 include?

   _____

e Under the four-digit code 710.0, you are directed to "Use additional code to identify manifestation," which is endocarditis in this case. What code are you directed to?

   ICD-9-CM Code: _____

That "Use additional code..." under 710.0 directs you to assign endocarditis (424.91) if the first-listed diagnosis is 710.0 and specified as "with endocarditis."

Again, the importance of verification in the Tabular is critical. This is where you receive instruction regarding the coding of endocarditis.

f What four-digit code designates the first-listed diagnosis of "systemic lupus erythematosus"?

   ICD-9-CM Code: _____

g What are the two codes to be reported for this case?

   ICD-9-CM Codes: _____, _____

ICD-9-CM OFFICIAL GUIDELINES FOR CODING AND REPORTING

SECTION I.A.
7. "And"

The word "and" should be interpreted to mean either "and" or "or" when it appears in a title.

SECTION I.A.
8. "With"

The word "with" in the alphabetic index is sequenced immediately following the main term, not in alphabetical order.

And and With. Although the two words "and" and "with" have similar meanings in everyday language, in ICD-9-CM terminology they have special significance and meanings. "And" means and/or, whereas "with" indicates that two conditions are included in the code and both conditions must be present to report the code.

And

Example

474   Chronic disease of tonsils and adenoids

Code 474 is assigned to identify the disease as one of tonsils and/or adenoids.

With

Example

Diabetes, diabetic (brittle) (congenital) (familial) (mellitus) (poorly controlled) (severe) (slight) (without complication) 250.0
   with
      coma (with ketoacidosis) 250.3
         due to secondary diabetes 249.3
         hyperosmolar (nonketotic) 250.2
            due to secondary diabetes 249.2
      complication NEC 250.9
         due to secondary diabetes 249.9
         specified NEC 250.8
            due to secondary diabetes 249.8
      gangrene 250.7 *[785.4]*
         due to secondary diabetes 249.7 *[785.4]*
      hyperglycemia - *code to Diabetes, by type, with 5th digit for not stated as uncontrolled*
      hyperosmolarity 250.2
         due to secondary diabetes 249.2
      ketosis, ketoacidosis 250.1
         due to secondary diabetes 249.1
      osteomyelitis 250.8 *[731.8]*

The "Diabetes" entry in the Index of the ICD-9-CM illustrates the use of "with" to direct the coder to the correct codes and the sequence of codes for conditions that may be present with the diabetes.

ICD-9-CM OFFICIAL GUIDELINES FOR CODING AND REPORTING

SECTION I.A.
9. "See" and "See Also"

The "see" instruction following a main term in the index indicates that another term should be referenced. It is necessary to go to the main term referenced with the "see" note to locate the correct code.

A "see also" instruction following a main term in the index instructs that there is another main term that may also be referenced that may provide additional index entries that may be useful. It is not necessary to follow the "see also" note when the original main term provides the necessary code.

Cross References

Cross references provide the coder with possible alternatives or synonyms for a term. There are three types of cross references:

1. *see*
2. *see* also
3. *see* category

The *"see"* cross reference is an explicit direction to look elsewhere. It is used for anatomic sites and many modifiers not normally used in the Alphabetic Index. The *"see"* cross reference is also used to reference the appropriate main term under which all the information concerning a specific disease will be located.

Example

Encephalomeningitis—*see* Meningoencephalitis
Endamebiasis—*see* Amebiasis
Kidney—*see* condition
Leukosis—*see* Leukemia
Lipofibroma (M8851/0)—*see* Lipoma, by site

The *"see also"* cross reference directs the coder to reference another main term if all the information being searched for cannot be located under the first main term entry.

Example

Laryngoplegia—(*see also* Paralysis, vocal cord) 478.30

The *"see category"* cross reference directs you to Volume 1, Tabular List, for important information governing the use of the specific code.

Example

Late—*see also* condition
    effect(s) (of)—*see also* condition
        abscess
            intracranial or intraspinal (conditions classifiable to 324)—*see* category
                326

EXERCISE 2-9   *See, See Also, See Category*

Using the Alphabetic Index, answer the following questions:

1 Locate the main term "Acquired immunodeficiency syndrome" in the Index. Is there another term for acquired immune deficiency syndrome that may be located in the Index and if so what is the term?

_____

2 Locate the main term "Malaria" in the Index. Is there a cross reference located there?

_____

3 Locate the main term "Itch" in the Index. Is there another term for itch that may be located in the Index and if so what is the term?

_____

4 Locate the main term "Polyadenitis" in the Index. Is there another term for polyadenitis that may be located in the Index and if so what is the term?

_____

5 Locate the main term "Polypoid" in the Index and what cross reference is given?

_____

Use Additional Code.   You add information by assigning an additional code to provide a more complete picture of the diagnosis or procedure. The use of an additional code is mandatory when supporting physician documentation is located in the record.

For example, if you are reporting empyema due to pseudomonas, the codes would be empyema (510.9), due to pseudomonas (041.7). If the organism that is causing the pseudomonas is known, the organism should be reported as indicated in the "Use additional code...." located with 510. If no organism has been identified, no additional code is assigned.

Example

510   **Empyema**

        Use additional code to identify infectious organism (041.0-041.9)

Code First Underlying Disease.   The phrase "Code first underlying disease" is used in the categories in the Tabular List, Volume 1. In some cases, the code, title, and instructions appear in italics to indicate that the underlying disease (etiology) be sequenced first.

Example

366.4   **Cataract associated with other disorders**

        366.41   Diabetic cataract

                Code first diabetes (249.5, 250.5)

By following this convention, diabetes 249.5X or 250.5X is sequenced first to indicate that the diabetes is the etiology, followed by 366.41 to indicate that the diabetic cataract is the manifestation.

Code, If Applicable, Any Causal Condition.   This is an instructional note that appears in the Tabular List. This note instructs the coder to sequence the causal condition (etiology) first. Unlike the instructional note "Code first underlying disease," if no causal condition is present or documented then the code may be sequenced first.

Example

707   **Chronic ulcer of skin**

    707.1   **Ulcer of lower limbs, except pressure ulcer**
        Ulcer, chronic, of lower limb:
          neurogenic of lower limb
          trophic of lower limb
        Code, if applicable, any causal condition first:
          atherosclerosis of the extremities with ulceration (440.23)
          chronic venous hypertension with ulcer (459.31)
          chronic venous hypertension with ulcer and inflammation (459.33)
          diabetes mellitus (249.80-249.81, 250.80-250.83)
          postphlebitic syndrome with ulcer (459.11)
          postphlebitic syndrome with ulcer and inflammation (459.13)

A postphlebitic syndrome with ulcer of the lower limb is the etiology and is reported with 459.11 (postphlebitic syndrome with ulcer) and 707.10 (ulcer of lower limb, unspecified) to report the manifestation.

Notes   Certain main terms are followed by notes that are used to define terms and give coding instructions.

Example

Amputation
  traumatic (complete) (partial)

  Note 06 "Complicated" includes traumatic amputation with delayed healing, delayed treatment, foreign body, or infection.

  arm 887.4
    at or above elbow 887.2
      complicated 887.3

EXERCISE 2-10 *Application of Sequencing Rules*

Using the Tabular and instructional notes, assign and sequence the following:

1 In the Tabular, see category 331 and assign code(s) for a patient who has Pick's disease with behavioral disturbances.

   Code(s): _____

2 In the Tabular, see code 484.6 and assign code(s) for a patient with pneumonia due to aspergillosis.

   Code(s): _____

3 In the Tabular, see code 707.1 and assign code(s) for a patient with atherosclerosis of the lower extremities with an ankle ulcer.

   Code(s): _____

4 In the Tabular, see code 600.01 and assign code(s) for a patient with benign hypertrophy of the prostate with urinary retention.

   Code(s): _____

5 In the Tabular, see code 713.3 and assign code(s) for a patient with arthropathy due to erythema multiforme.

   Code(s): _____

Notes in the Index list the fifth-digit subclassifications for subcategories—such as the entries "Tuberculosis" or "Diabetes." Only the four-digit code is given for the individual entry, and you must refer to the note following the main term to locate the appropriate fifth-digit subclassification. For example, Fig. 2–13 shows the fifth digits assigned when coding diabetes.

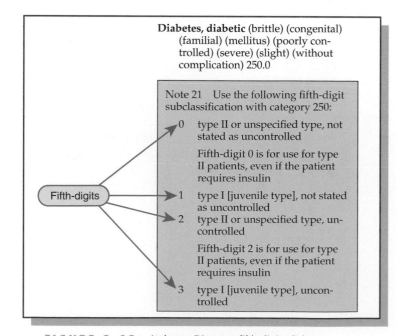

FIGURE 2–13 Index to Diseases, fifth digit, diabetes. (Modified from Buck CJ: *2010 ICD-9-CM, Volumes 1, 2, & 3, Professional Edition,* St. Louis, 2010, Saunders.)

Eponyms **Eponyms** (diseases, procedures, or syndromes named for persons) are listed both as main terms in their appropriate alphabetic sequence in the Index and under the main terms "Disease" or "Syndrome." A description of the disease or syndrome is usually included in parentheses following the eponym.

Example

Crigler-Najjar disease or syndrome
(congenital hyperbilirubinemia) 277.4

Disease
Crigler-Najjar (congenital hyperbilirubinemia) 277.4

Syndrome
Crigler-Najjar (congenital hyperbilirubinemia) 277.4

The cross-reference feature will be very helpful to you as you assign ICD-9-CM codes.

EXERCISE 2-11 *Conventions*

Match the convention to the definition:

1 *see* category _____

2 subterms _____

3 *see* _____

4 Notes _____

5 modifiers _____

6 *see also* _____

7 eponym _____

a. terms in parentheses or following main terms; they may or may not be essential

b. terms indented under main terms, considered essential modifiers

c. explicit direction to look elsewhere

d. defines and gives instructions

e. directs coder to look under another term if all information is not located under the first term

f. directs coder to use Volume 1, Tabular List, for additional information

g. disease, procedure, or syndrome named for a person

EXERCISE 2-12   *More Conventions*

Match the abbreviations, punctuation, symbols, and words to the correct descriptions:

1 [] _____

2 NOS _____

3 : _____

4 italics _____

5 *Excludes* _____

6 Includes _____

7 } _____

8 NEC _____

9 ( ) _____

10 *[ ]* _____

11 bold type _____

a. must be modified by an additional term to complete the code description

b. used in Volume 2 to enclose the disease manifestation codes that are sequenced after the underlying disease

c. typeface used for all codes and titles in Volume 1

d. indicates the use of code assignment for "other" when a more specific code does not exist

e. encloses a series of terms that modify the statement to the right

f. encloses synonyms, alternative words, or explanatory phrases

g. equals unspecified

h. typeface used for all exclusion notes or diagnosis codes not to be used for first-listed diagnosis

i. appears under a code to further define or explain the content

j. encloses supplementary words that do not affect the code assignment

k. indicates terms that are to be coded elsewhere

Answer the following questions about conventions:

12 Includes and *Excludes* notes have no bearing on the code selection.

   True   False

13 Brackets enclose synonyms, alternative wordings, or explanatory phrases.

   True   False

PROCEDURES, VOLUME 3

Procedure codes are located in Volume 3 of the ICD-9-CM. These codes are used only in the hospital setting. You can purchase the ICD-9-CM manual with or without Volume 3.

History

The World Health Organization (WHO) recognized the growing need for a classification of procedures used in medicine and in 1971 sponsored an international working party that was convened by the American Hospital Association to coordinate the recommendations for a classification of procedures, with the primary emphasis on surgery. The International Conference for the 9th Revision of the International Classification of Diseases was convened at WHO Headquarters in Geneva in 1975. From that gathering, a proposal for a classification of procedures was submitted. The recommendations of the working party were to publish the provisional procedures classification as a supplement to the ICD-9. When the ICD-9 manual was published, a series of separate sections called fascicles (supplements) were also published. Each fascicle provides a classification of a different mode (type) of therapy (e.g., surgery, radiology, and laboratory procedures).

Subsequently, the ICD-9-CM was published in a three-volume set, including Volume 3, Procedures. Volume 3 was drawn primarily from WHO's

Fascicle V, Surgical Procedures. At the same time, the codes in Volume 3 were expanded from three to four digits to allow for greater detail.

Volume 3 of the ICD-9-CM manual did not maintain compatibility with the ICD-9 as Volumes 1 and 2 had done. A different approach was taken in the development of Volume 3 that was deemed more appropriate to a classification system that would report surgical and therapeutic procedures.

Format   Volume 3 contains two parts—the Tabular List and the Alphabetic Index. Approximately 90% of the codes in Volume 3 refer to surgical procedures (Fig. 2–14). The remaining 10% of the codes are diagnostic (to diagnose) and therapeutic (to treat) procedures, as shown in Fig. 2–15. For the most part, nonsurgical procedures are segregated from surgical procedures and confined to the codes 87 to 99.

Volume 3 is **not** used in physicians' offices because procedures performed by physicians are reported using the CPT codes. Hospitals use Volume 3 extensively to report procedures provided to inpatients, including surgery, therapy, and diagnostic procedures. Hospitals use the ICD-9-CM codes to bill for inpatient charges (e.g., operating room, room and board, nurses, supplies). For example, a patient is admitted for a total abdominal hysterectomy. The physician would report his or her services and bill for the service of the total abdominal hysterectomy using the CPT code 58150. The hospital would report and bill for facility services for the hysterectomy procedure using the ICD-9-CM procedure code 68.49. The physician and the hospital would report the diagnosis using ICD-9-CM diagnosis codes. If the patient in this example had a diagnosis of chronic endometriosis, both the physician and the hospital would indicate the patient's diagnosis and the reason for their services due to endometriosis of the uterus with 617.0.

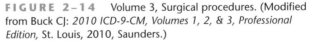

FIGURE 2–14   Volume 3, Surgical procedures. (Modified from Buck CJ: *2010 ICD-9-CM, Volumes 1, 2, & 3, Professional Edition*, St. Louis, 2010, Saunders.)

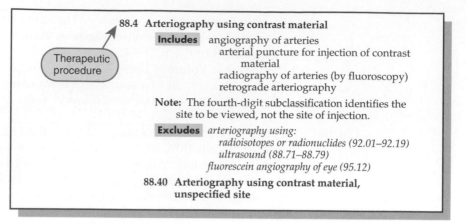

FIGURE 2-15 Volume 3, Therapeutic procedures. (Modified from Buck CJ: *2010 ICD-9-CM, Volumes 1, 2, & 3, Professional Edition,* St. Louis, 2010, Saunders.)

Example

Physician Codes
    Diagnosis: ICD-9-CM, Vols. 1 and 2
    Procedure: CPT

Inpatient Hospital Codes
    Diagnosis: ICD-9-CM, Vols. 1 and 2
    Procedure: ICD-9-CM, Vol. 3

Outpatient Hospital Codes
    Diagnosis: ICD-9-CM, Vols. 1 and 2
    Procedure: CPT

EXERCISE 2-13 *Table of Contents*

The Table of Contents, Volume 3 (Fig. 2–16) indicates the 16 chapters in Volume 3. Note that each chapter is based on a body system, except for Chapters 13 and 16.

1 What is Chapter 13?

_____

2 What is Chapter 16?

_____

3 What is Chapter 00?

_____

Part IV   Procedures Volume 3   1029

Index to Procedures   1030
Classification of Procedures   1140
  0. Procedures and Interventions, Not Elsewhere
     Classified (00)   1140
  1. Operations on the Nervous System
     (01–05)   1145
  2. Operations on the Endocrine System
     (06–07)   1149
  3. Operations on the Eye (08–16)   1151
  3A. Other Miscellaneous Diagnostic and
     Therapeutic Procedures   1157
  4. Operations on the Ear (18–20)   1158
  5. Operations on the Nose, Mouth, and Pharynx
     (21–29)   1160
  6. Operations on the Respiratory System
     (30–34)   1164
  7. Operations on the Cardiovascular System
     (35–39)   1168
  8. Operations on the Hemic and Lymphatic
     System (40–41)   1182
  9. Operations on the Digestive System
     (42–54)   1184
  10. Operations on the Urinary System
     (55–59)   1199
  11. Operations on the Male Genital Organs
     (60–64)   1204
  12. Operations on the Female Genital Organs
     (65–71)   1207
  13. Obstetrical Procedures (72–75)   1213
  14. Operations on the Musculoskeletal System
     (76–84)   1215
  15. Operations on the Integumentary System
     (85–86)   1227
  16. Miscellaneous Diagnostic and Therapeutic
     Procedures (87–99)   1231

FIGURE 2–16   Volume 3, Table of Contents. (Modified from Buck CJ: *2010 ICD-9-CM, Volumes 1, 2, & 3, Professional Edition,* St. Louis, 2010, Saunders.)

Tabular List, Volume 3

Volume 3 has abbreviations, punctuation, symbols, and terms similar to those used in Volumes 1 and 2. The following are the conventions, which are the same in all volumes:

1. Abbreviations of NEC and NOS
2. Punctuation symbols brackets, parentheses, colons, and braces
3. Bold type for all codes and titles
4. Italicized type for all exclusion notes
5. Instructional notations of Includes and Excludes

The term "Code also" has two purposes in Volume 3:

A. To allow the coding of each component of a procedure
B. To allow the coding of the use of special adjunctive (at the same time) procedures or equipment

These instructions are not mandatory, but they serve as a reminder to code these additional procedures if they were performed.

Using the following ICD-9-CM code as an example, let us take a closer look at the code to make sure you understand what the procedure is and how the term "Code also" is used.

Example

42.6 Antesternal anastomosis of esophagus
   Code also any synchronous:
      esophagectomy (42.40-42.42)
      gastrostomy (43.1)

The word "antesternal" will not be located in most medical dictionaries. It is at this time that your skill in medical terminology will help you out. The prefix "ante" means before, and "sternal" refers to sternum. Anastomosis is the joining together of two openings; in this case it is an opening into the esophagus. The location of the opening into the esophagus is above the sternum, which stated in medical terms is antesternal anastomosis of esophagus. The term **"synchronous"** means occurring at the same time; "esophagectomy" is the removal of a part of the esophagus, and "gastrostomy" is the creation of an opening into the stomach. The statement from code 42.6 is translated into "Code also any [esophagectomy or gastrostomy] occurring at the same time." The medical coder needs excellent skills in medical terminology, anatomy, and persistence in the search for accurate definitions of the words used in the medical records. The study of terminology is a lifelong endeavor. There are always new words to be discovered. Just remember to always look up any word you are not certain of and take the time to understand the word in the context in which it is used. If you make a practice of doing this, you will soon find that you have a very dependable medical terminology vocabulary. All coders need excellent medical terminology skills.

The second use of the instruction notation "Code also" is as a reminder to code the use of special adjunctive (accessory) procedures or equipment.

Example

39.21 Caval-pulmonary artery anastomosis
   Code also cardiopulmonary bypass (39.61)

The "Code also" note with code 39.21 directs you to report 39.61 [extracorporeal (outside the body) circulation]. Extracorporeal circulation is an auxiliary procedure performed during heart surgery.

If the procedure or equipment was not used, no additional code would be assigned.

EXERCISE 2-14 *Terminology*

State the definitions of the following terms:

1 cava(l) _____

2 pulmonary_____

3 anastomosis _____

4 cardiopulmonary_____

5 extracorporeal _____

6 What is a caval-pulmonary artery anastomosis? _____

_____

7 What does a heart-lung machine do for a patient who is having a caval-pulmonary artery

anastomosis? _____

Alphabetic Index, Volume 3

The Index of Procedures is an important complement to the Tabular List of Procedures because the Index contains many procedure terms that do not appear in the Tabular List of Procedures. The list of procedures included in the two-digit category code of the Tabular List of Procedures is not meant to be exhaustive; the terms serve as examples of the content of the category. The Index to Procedures, however, includes most procedure terms currently in use in North America. When the exact word is not located in the Tabular List of Procedures but is located in the Index to Procedures, you must trust that the code listed in the Index to Procedures is correct.

Example

In the Index to Procedures, there is an entry "Gastrostomy," subterm "Janeway," which is a type of gastrostomy. The entry directs you to code 43.19. When you then verify 43.19 in the Tabular List of Procedures, there is no mention of the term Janeway.

Never code directly from the Index to Procedures. After locating a code in the Index, refer to that code in the Tabular List of Procedures for important instructions. Instructions in the form of notes suggesting the use of additional codes and exclusion notes that indicate the circumstances under which a procedure would be coded elsewhere are found only in the Tabular List of Procedures.

The Index to Procedures is arranged primarily by procedure (Fig. 2–17). Procedure codes are numbers only, with no alphabetic characters. The classification is based on a two-digit structure with two additional digits when necessary for greater specificity.

Fig. 2–18 indicates the two-digit category codes, the three-digit subcategory codes, and the four-digit subclassification codes contained in the Tabular List of Procedures. All category codes in Volume 3, Procedures, are **two-digit codes,** whereas all category codes in Volume 1, Tabular List, Disease, are **three-digit codes.**

The sequence of the Index to Procedures is letter-by-letter alphabetic order. Letter-by-letter alphabetizing ignores single spaces and hyphens and produces sequences.

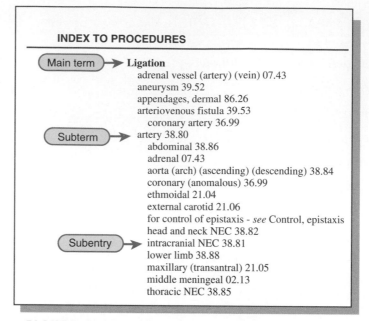

INDEX TO PROCEDURES

Main term → **Ligation**
adrenal vessel (artery) (vein) 07.43
aneurysm 39.52
appendages, dermal 86.26
arteriovenous fistula 39.53
coronary artery 36.99
Subterm → artery 38.80
abdominal 38.86
adrenal 07.43
aorta (arch) (ascending) (descending) 38.84
coronary (anomalous) 36.99
ethmoidal 21.04
external carotid 21.06
for control of epistaxis - *see* Control, epistaxis
head and neck NEC 38.82
Subentry → intracranial NEC 38.81
lower limb 38.88
maxillary (transantral) 21.05
middle meningeal 02.13
thoracic NEC 38.85

FIGURE 2–17 Index to procedures. (Modified from Buck CJ: *2010 ICD-9-CM, Volumes 1, 2, & 3, Professional Edition,* St. Louis, 2010, Saunders.)

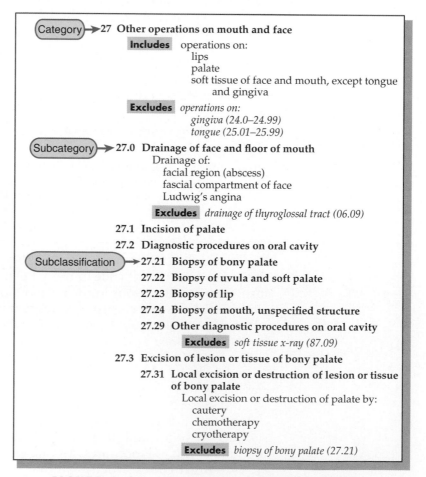

Category → **27 Other operations on mouth and face**
Includes operations on:
lips
palate
soft tissue of face and mouth, except tongue and gingiva
Excludes *operations on:*
gingiva (24.0–24.99)
tongue (25.01–25.99)
Subcategory → **27.0 Drainage of face and floor of mouth**
Drainage of:
facial region (abscess)
fascial compartment of face
Ludwig's angina
Excludes *drainage of thyroglossal tract (06.09)*
27.1 Incision of palate
27.2 Diagnostic procedures on oral cavity
Subclassification → **27.21 Biopsy of bony palate**
27.22 Biopsy of uvula and soft palate
27.23 Biopsy of lip
27.24 Biopsy of mouth, unspecified structure
27.29 Other diagnostic procedures on oral cavity
Excludes *soft tissue x-ray (87.09)*
27.3 Excision of lesion or tissue of bony palate
27.31 Local excision or destruction of lesion or tissue of bony palate
Local excision or destruction of palate by:
cautery
chemotherapy
cryotherapy
Excludes *biopsy of bony palate (27.21)*

FIGURE 2–18 Volume 3, format. (Modified from Buck CJ: *2010 ICD-9-CM, Volumes 1, 2, & 3, Professional Edition,* St. Louis, 2010, Saunders.)

> *Example*
>
> Opening
>
> open reduction
>
> Upon first consideration, you would think that these two words were not in correct alphabetical order; "open" should come before "opening." The old filer's rule of "nothing comes before something" does not apply here. To alphabetize "opening" and "open reduction," you consider the beginning of the two words as "o-p-e-n"; the fifth letter in "opening" is "i" and the fifth letter in "open reduction" is "r." For alphabetizing purposes, the terms are considered as
>
> opening
>
> openreduction

Numbers, whether Arabic (1, 2, 3), Roman (I, II, III), or ordinal (first, second, third), are all placed in numeric sequence *before* alphabetic characters. Simply stated, numbers come before letters (Fig. 2–19).

The **prepositions** as, by, and with immediately follow the main term to which they refer. When multiple prepositional references are present, they are listed in alphabetic sequence.

> *Example*
>
> Aneurysmorrhaphy NEC 39.52
>   by or with
>   anastomosis -- see Aneurysmectomy, with anastomosis, by site
>   clipping 39.51
>   coagulation 39.52
>   electrocoagulation 39.52
>   endovascular graft

The Index to Procedures is organized according to main terms, which are printed in bold type. Main terms usually identify the type of procedure performed, rather than the anatomic site involved.

A main term may be followed by a series of terms in parentheses. The presence or absence of these parenthetic terms in the procedure description has no effect on the selection of the code listed for the main term. These parenthetic terms are called **nonessential modifiers**. For example, all of the following words in parentheses are nonessential modifiers.

Operation
  Beck I (epicardial poudrage) 36.39
  Beck II (aorto-coronary sinus shunt) 36.39
  Beck-Jianu (permanent gastrostomy) 43.19

FIGURE 2–19 Numbers alphabetized in the Index. (Modified from Buck CJ: *2010 ICD-9-CM, Volumes 1, 2, & 3, Professional Edition,* St. Louis, 2010, Saunders.)

FIGURE 2–20 Essential and nonessential subterms. (Modified from Buck CJ: *2010 ICD-9-CM, Volumes 1, 2, & 3, Professional Edition,* St. Louis, 2010, Saunders.)

Example

Clipping
    aneurysm (basilar) (carotid) (cerebellar) (cerebellopontine) (communicating
       artery) (vertebral) 39.51

A main term may also be followed by a list of subterms (modifiers) that do have an effect on the selection of the appropriate code for a given procedure. These subterms form individual line entries and describe essential differences in site or surgical technique (Fig. 2–20).

Terms that identify incisions are listed as main terms in the Index to Procedures. If the incision was made only for the purpose of performing further surgery, the instruction "omit code" is given. The incision for the operative approach is bundled into (included in) the surgical code and would not be coded separately. Closure of a surgical wound is not coded separately unless the closure takes place during a separate operative procedure.

Example

Arthrotomy 80.10
    as operative approach—*omit* code with
        arthrography—*see* Arthrogram
        arthroscopy—*see* Arthroscopy
        injection of drug 81.92
        removal of prosthesis (*see also* Removal, prosthesis, joint structures) 80.00
    ankle 80.17
    elbow 80.12

For some operative procedures it is necessary to record the individual components of the procedure. In these instances the Index to Procedures lists both codes.

Example

Code 57.87 describes the reconstruction of a urinary bladder, and 45.51 indicates the intestinal resection (cutting out of a portion of the intestine) necessary to create an ileal bladder.

Ileal
    bladder
        closed 57.87 *[45.51]*

It is important to record these codes in the same sequence as that used in the Index to Procedures.

The cross references section provides you with possible modifiers for a term or its synonyms. There are three types of cross references used in the Index to Procedures:

1. The term *"see"* is an explicit direction to look elsewhere. It is used with terms that do not define the type of procedure performed.

> ### Example
>
> Bacterial smear—*see* Examination, microscopic

2. The term *"see also"* directs you to look under another main term because all of the information being searched for cannot be located under the first main term entry.

> ### Example
>
> Immunization—*see also* Vaccination

3. The term *"see* category" directs you to the Tabular List of Procedures for further information or specific site references.

> ### Example
>
> Osteolysis—*see* category 78.4

Notes are used in the Index to Procedures to list fourth-digit subclassifications for those categories that use the same fourth digit. In these cases, only the three-digit code is given for the individual entry; you must refer to the note following the main term to obtain the appropriate fourth digit. For an example of a note in the Index, see Fig. 2–21.

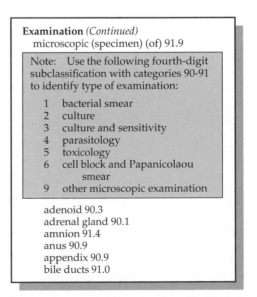

FIGURE 2–21 Note in the Index. (Modified from Buck CJ: *2010 ICD-9-CM, Volumes 1, 2, & 3, Professional Edition*, St. Louis, 2010, Saunders.)

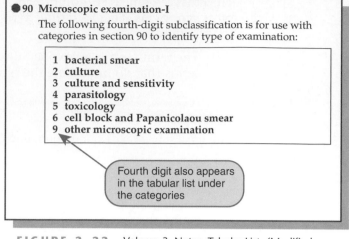

●90 **Microscopic examination-I**
The following fourth-digit subclassification is for use with categories in section 90 to identify type of examination:

1 **bacterial smear**
2 **culture**
3 **culture and sensitivity**
4 **parasitology**
5 **toxicology**
6 **cell block and Papanicolaou smear**
9 **other microscopic examination**

Fourth digit also appears in the tabular list under the categories

FIGURE 2–22   Volume 3, Notes, Tabular List. (Modified from Buck CJ: *2010 ICD-9-CM, Volumes 1, 2, & 3, Professional Edition*, St. Louis, 2010, Saunders.)

The fourth-digit subclassification codes also appear in the Tabular List of Procedures with the category codes 90 and 91. See Fig. 2–22 for an example of a note in the Tabular.

Operations named for persons **(eponyms)** are listed both as main terms in their appropriate alphabetic sequence and under the main term "Operation." A description of the procedure or anatomic site affected usually follows the eponym.

Example

Under O:

Operation

Thompson
cleft lip repair 27.54
correction of lymphedema 40.9
quadricepsplasty 83.86
thumb apposition with bone graft 82.69

Under T:

Thompson operation
cleft lip repair 27.54
correction of lymphedema 40.9
quadricepsplasty 83.86
thumb apposition with bone graft 82.69

EXERCISE 2-15   *Procedures, Volume 3*

Code the following using Volume 3 of the ICD-9-CM manual:

1 Flexible sigmoidoscopy

ICD-9-CM Code: _____

2 Vasectomy

ICD-9-CM Code: _____

3 Closed reduction of maxillary fracture

ICD-9-CM Code: _____

4 Transfusion of 2 units packed cells

ICD-9-CM Code: _____

5 Control of epistaxis by cauterization

ICD-9-CM Code: _____

 CONGRATULATIONS! You have now completed the study of the arrangement of the information in the ICD-9-CM manual. The knowledge you have gained will be used as the foundation that will be built upon in Chapters 3-6. In Chapters 3-6 you will begin further work with the correct assignment and sequencing of ICD-9-CM codes.

CHAPTER REVIEW

CHAPTER 2, PART I, THEORY

Match the appendix to the information contained in the appendix:

1 Appendix A _____
2 Appendix B _____
3 Appendix C _____
4 Appendix D _____
5 Appendix E _____

a. Industrial Accidents
b. Classification of Drugs
c. Morphology of Neoplasms
d. Three-Digit Categories
e. Deleted in 2004

Circle the correct answer in each of the following:

6 The ICD-9-CM is designed to classify what two things?

a. sickness and disease
b. symptoms and illness
c. causes of morbidity and mortality
d. diagnosis and disease

7 Which of the following is *not* a stated use for the ICD-9-CM?

a. facilitate payment of health services
b. study health care costs
c. plan for future health care needs
d. evaluate appropriateness of treatment

Match the ICD-9-CM volume number to the correct name of the volume:

8 Volume 1 _____
9 Volume 2 _____
10 Volume 3 _____

a. Tabular List of Procedures and Alphabetic Index to Procedures
b. Diseases: Alphabetic Index
c. Diseases: Tabular List

Identify the format of the chapters in the ICD-9-CM Volume 1, Tabular List, in the proper sequence, from first to last:

11 _____
12 _____
13 _____
14 _____
15 _____

a. subcategory
b. chapter
c. subclassification
d. section
e. category

CHAPTER 2, PART II, PRACTICAL

Using an ICD-9-CM manual, answer the following questions:

16 What does the *Excludes* note state under category code 175?

_____

17 What does the Includes note state under category 444?

_____

18 Under category 805, which codes use the subclassification 0-8?

_____

19 Would code 362.72 be sequenced as the first-listed diagnosis? _____

Using ICD-9-CM, Volume 1, Tabular List, locate the first pages of Chapter 8 and answer the following questions about the chapter:

20 The name of the chapter:

_____

21 The name of the first section:

_____

22 The description of the second category:

_____

23 The description of the first subcategory:

_____

24 The description of the first subclassification:

_____

25 What instructional note applies to the entire chapter?

_____

26 What excludes note applies to the first section?

_____

Underline the main terms to be located in the Alphabetic index in the following diagnostic statements:

27 Chronic pancreatitis

28 Paralytic ileus

29 Acute and chronic cholecystitis

30 Abdominal pain

31 Suppurative mastitis

Using ICD-9-CM, Volume 2, Alphabetic Index, locate the following main terms and identify if the bolded subterm is an essential or nonessential modifier:

32 **Chemical** esophagitis _____

33 **Reflux** esophagitis _____

34 **Primary** hyperparathyroidism

_____

35 **Uncontrolled** hypertension

_____

36 **Congenital** Schatzki's ring

_____

Using the Alphabetic Index, answer the following questions:

37 Locate the main term "Roseola infantum" in the index. The other term for infantum roseola located in the index is this term.

_____

38 Locate the main term "Emotional" in the index. The other term for emotional crisis located in the index is this term.

_____

Using the Tabular List, answer the following questions.

39 Is acute exacerbation of chronic lymphoid leukemia assigned code 204.00? _____

If not, what code is assigned? _____

40 Is congenital hydronephrosis assigned code 591? _____

If not, what code is assigned? _____

Using the Tabular and instructional notes, assign and sequence the following code(s):

41 See category 331 and assign code(s) for a patient who has Alzheimer's disease with behavioral disturbances.

_____

42 See code 484.5 and assign code(s) for a patient with pneumonia due to anthrax.

_____

QUICK CHECK ANSWERS

QUICK CHECK 2-1
1. a. 6
2. Notes instruct coder to "See listing at the beginning of the chapter for definitions" where a full list is included under each subclassification and "Knee joint" is listed under "6 lower leg."

QUICK CHECK 2-2
1. Official Guidelines for Coding and Reporting
2. Footer of each page

"Professional coding is a job that goes with you. You can work in any state, work in different types of companies, and do many different jobs."

Damaris Ramirez, CPC, CPC-I
National Director for
Documentation and Education
EmCare, Inc.—Inpatient Services
Dallas, Texas

Outpatient Coding and Reporting Guidelines

Chapter Topics

First-Listed Diagnosis

Additional Diagnoses

V Codes

Specificity

Uncertain Diagnosis

Chronic Diseases

Diagnostic Services

Therapeutic Services

Surgery

Prenatal Visits

Chapter Review

Learning Objectives

After completing this chapter you should be able to

1 Identify the first-listed diagnosis.

2 Demonstrate ability to assign diagnoses codes to unconfirmed conditions.

3 Assign the first-listed diagnosis in the outpatient surgery setting.

4 Report first-listed diagnoses in the observation setting.

5 Validate V code assignment.

6 Apply codes to suspected conditions.

7 Report uncertain diagnoses.

8 Demonstrate ability to report chronic conditions.

9 Examine guidelines for reporting therapeutic services.

10 Evaluate diagnoses reporting for surgical procedures.

11 Identify the guidelines for reporting prenatal visits.

Make sure to check
evolve
learning system
for the latest
content updates

FIRST-LISTED DIAGNOSIS

The majority of the services that a physician will provide are outpatient services. This chapter introduces you to assigning ICD-9-CM diagnosis codes for outpatient services in accordance with the ICD-9-CM Official Guidelines for Coding and Reporting.

Read the following guideline:

ICD-9-CM OFFICIAL GUIDELINES FOR CODING AND REPORTING

SECTION IV. Diagnostic Coding and Reporting Guidelines for Outpatient Services

These coding guidelines for outpatient diagnoses have been approved for use by hospitals/providers in coding and reporting hospital-based outpatient services and provider-based office visits.

Information about the use of certain abbreviations, punctuation, symbols, and other conventions used in the ICD-9-CM Tabular List (code numbers and titles), can be found in Section IA of these guidelines, under "Conventions Used in the Tabular List." Information about the correct sequence to use in finding a code is described in Section I.

The terms encounter and visit are often used interchangeably in describing outpatient service contacts and, therefore, appear together in these guidelines without distinguishing one from the other.

Though the conventions and general guidelines apply to all settings, coding guidelines for outpatient and provider reporting of diagnoses will vary in a number of instances from those for inpatient diagnoses, recognizing that:

> The Uniform Hospital Discharge Data Set (UHDDS) definition of principal diagnosis applies only to inpatients in acute, short-term, long-term care and psychiatric hospitals.

> Coding guidelines for inconclusive diagnoses (probable, suspected, rule out, etc.) were developed for inpatient reporting and do not apply to outpatients.

A. Selection of first-listed condition

> In the outpatient setting, the term first-listed diagnosis is used in lieu of principal diagnosis.

> In determining the first-listed diagnosis the coding conventions of ICD-9-CM, as well as the general and disease specific guidelines take precedence over the outpatient guidelines.

> Diagnoses often are not established at the time of the initial encounter/visit. It may take two or more visits before the diagnosis is confirmed.

> The most critical rule involves beginning the search for the correct code assignment through the Alphabetic Index. Never begin searching initially in the Tabular List as this will lead to coding errors.

SELECTING THE FIRST-LISTED DIAGNOSIS

Examples

1. Established 50-year-old patient was seen in the clinic for acute bronchitis. Patient also received a prescription for refill of medication for hypertension. The first-listed diagnosis is acute bronchitis.

2. Initial office visit for a 36-year-old female complaining of irregular menses. Review of systems identified unexplained weight loss. The first-listed diagnosis is irregular menses.

3. Established patient is a 75-year-old male complaining of substernal chest pain which is relieved with rest. Patient has a hypertension and blood pressure is above baseline on this visit. The first-listed diagnosis is substernal chest pain.

EXERCISE 3-1   *First-Listed Diagnosis*

Identify the term for first-listed diagnosis in the following encounters or visits:

1 Established patient complaining of painful urination and frequency. Patient is a type II diabetic. Lab work revealed a urinary tract infection and blood glucose was within normal limits.

   First-listed Diagnosis Term(s): _____

2 Established patient presented to clinic with exacerbation of Crohn's disease. Patient's rheumatoid arthritis is stable. No medication changes were made.

   First-listed Diagnosis Term(s): _____

3 Initial office visit for sprained left knee.

   First-listed Diagnosis Term(s): _____

4 Initial office visit for patient requiring management of COPD and CHF.

   First-listed Diagnosis Term(s): _____

5 Established patient seen for cough, fever, and shortness of breath. Chest x-ray confirmed physician's diagnosis of pneumonia and patient was sent home on antibiotics.

   First-listed Diagnosis Term(s): _____

Unconfirmed Diagnosis

TWO OR MORE VISITS BEFORE A DIAGNOSIS IS CONFIRMED

Examples

1. Initial office visit, 30-year-old woman complains of fatigue, weight gain, and constipation. Lab studies including thyroid function test were ordered. Patient will return in two weeks.

   In this case the only reportable diagnoses are symptom codes as no specific diagnosis have been confirmed during this visit.

   Codes: 780.79 fatigue, 783.1 weight gain, and 564.00 constipation.

2. Follow-up office visit, 30-year-old woman with continued complaints of fatigue, weight gain, and constipation. Lab results confirm that patient has hypothyroidism and she was started on Synthroid. She will have repeat thyroid function studies on her next visit.

   Code: 244.9 hypothyroidism. The patient was told that she has hypothyroidism and the fatigue, weight gain, and constipation are common symptoms and would likely improve with treatment of her hypothyroidism. No additional treatment was directed at the patient's symptoms.

3. Follow-up office visit, 30-year-old woman is seen following her repeat thyroid function studies and her hypothyroidism has responded to the Synthroid. She will be maintained on her current dose.

   Code: 244.9 hypothyroidism is the reason for the visit.

EXERCISE 3-2 *Two or More Visits Before a Diagnosis is Confirmed*

Identify the first-listed diagnosis for the following and assign the correct code(s):

1 Initial office visit for a 28-year-old male with persistent abdominal pain and bloody diarrhea. Patient was scheduled for small-bowel x-rays and colonoscopy. The patient will be seen in the office following the scheduled outpatient procedures.

    Codes: _____, _____

2 Follow-up office visit for a 28-year-old male with recent colonoscopy with biopsy and small bowel x-rays. The biopsy and small bowel x-rays confirmed that the patient had ulcerative colitis. The patient was started on Sulfasalazine.

    Code: _____

3 Initial office visit for 55-year-old male with fatigue and jaundice. Laboratory tests were ordered. He will return in 1 week for the results.

    Codes: _____, _____

4 Follow-up office visit for 55-year-old male with jaundice and fatigue. Diagnostic tests confirm that the patient has hepatitis C. He will be treated with interferon therapy.

    Code: _____

Outpatient Surgery

ICD-9-CM OFFICIAL GUIDELINES FOR CODING AND REPORTING

SECTION IV.A.

1. Outpatient Surgery

When a patient presents for outpatient surgery, code the reason for the surgery as the first-listed diagnosis (reason for the encounter), even if the surgery is not performed due to a contraindication.

Examples

OUTPATIENT SURGERY

Patient presents for an outpatient T&A due to chronic tonsillitis.

    First-listed diagnosis: 474.00 Chronic tonsillitis

OUTPATIENT SURGERY THAT HAS BEEN CANCELED

Patient presented for a right inguinal hernia repair. Following assessment of the patient by the nurse, it was discovered that the patient had breakfast and the surgery was canceled and will be rescheduled for next week.

    First-listed diagnosis: 550.90 Inguinal hernia (V64.3, surgery not carried out, would also be reported)

EXERCISE 3-3 *First-Listed Diagnosis for Outpatient Surgery*

Identify the term(s) that describe the first-listed diagnosis for the following:

1 A female patient was admitted as an outpatient for elective bilateral tubal ligation. The patient was noted to be wheezing during the nurse's assessment. She was seen by her physician and her surgery was cancelled because of an exacerbation of her asthma.

   First-listed Diagnosis Term(s): _____

2 A male patient was admitted as an outpatient for transurethral prostatic resection for symptomatic benign prostatic hypertrophy.

   First-listed Diagnosis Term(s): _____

3 A patient was admitted an outpatient for a cystoscopy for hematuria. The procedure was performed without complications. No abnormality or explanation for the hematuria was found.

   First-listed Diagnosis Term(s): _____

Observation Stay

ICD-9-CM OFFICIAL GUIDELINES FOR CODING AND REPORTING

SECTION IV.A.
2. Observation Stay

   When a patient is admitted for observation for a medical condition, assign a code for the medical condition as the first-listed diagnosis.

   When a patient presents for outpatient surgery and develops complications requiring admission to observation, code the reason for the surgery as the first reported diagnosis (reason for the encounter), followed by codes for the complications as secondary diagnoses.

OBSERVATION FOR A MEDICAL CONDITION

Example

Patient was admitted for observation due to chest pain. Patient has chronic obstructive pulmonary disease (COPD). After testing, no evidence of cardiac cause was found. Patient was discharged home. Discharge Diagnosis: Noncardiac chest pain.
   First-listed diagnosis: 786.59 Noncardiac chest pain.

OUTPATIENT SURGERY WITH COMPLICATION

Example

Patient had a right direct inguinal hernia repair with mesh in the ambulatory surgery center. While in the recovery room, the patient developed atrial fibrillation as a result of the procedure. The patient was admitted for observation and cardiac consult was obtained.
   First-listed diagnosis: 550.90 Right direct inguinal hernia.

EXERCISE 3-4 *Observation Stay*

Identify the term(s) that describe the first-listed diagnosis for the following:

1 A 35-year-old female patient was admitted to observation for severe nausea and vomiting (due to pelvic pain) following diagnostic laparoscopy for pelvic pain.

First-listed Diagnosis Term(s): _____

2 A male patient was admitted to observation following an endoscopic retrograde cholangiopancreatography (ERCP) for acute pancreatitis. Patient has a biliary duct stricture.

First-listed Diagnosis Term(s): _____

3 Patient was admitted for observation because of urinary retention following a dilation and curettage (D&C) for post-menopausal bleeding.

First-listed Diagnosis Term(s): _____

ADDITIONAL DIAGNOSES

In the preceding guidelines and exercises, we were concerned primarily with the identification of the first-listed diagnosis. In some cases, additional diagnoses would be reported to describe manifestations, complications, reasons for canceled procedures, and other coexisting conditions.

ICD-9-CM OFFICIAL GUIDELINES FOR CODING AND REPORTING

SECTION IV.
B. Codes from 001.0 through V89

The appropriate code or codes from 001.0 through V89 must be used to identify diagnoses, symptoms, conditions, problems, complaints, or other reason(s) for the encounter/visit.

The guidelines state that it is acceptable to use any of the codes throughout the entire Tabular List to identify the reason(s) for an outpatient visit including the use of V codes. V codes are used more frequently in the outpatient setting. This guideline is the same as General Coding Guidelines Section I.B.4.

ICD-9-CM OFFICIAL GUIDELINES FOR CODING AND REPORTING

SECTION IV.
C. Accurate reporting of ICD-9-CM diagnosis codes

For accurate reporting of ICD-9-CM diagnosis codes, the documentation should describe the patient's condition, using terminology which includes specific diagnoses as well as symptoms, problems, or reasons for the encounter. There are ICD-9-CM codes to describe all of these.

This guideline assures data integrity by promoting accurate ICD-9-CM diagnosis codes that are supported by documentation in the health record. It is important to code all the conditions or problems that are being managed during an encounter.

ICD-9-CM OFFICIAL GUIDELINES FOR CODING AND REPORTING

SECTION IV.

D. Selection of codes 001.0 through 999.9

The selection of codes 001.0 through 999.9 will frequently be used to describe the reason for the encounter. These codes are from the section of ICD-9-CM for the classification of diseases and injuries (e.g. infectious and parasitic diseases; neoplasms; symptoms, signs, and ill-defined conditions, etc.).

This guideline is the same as General Coding Guidelines Section I.B.5 and reaffirms that any code from the ICD-9-CM manual can be used to describe the reason for an encounter or visit.

ICD-9-CM OFFICIAL GUIDELINES FOR CODING AND REPORTING

SECTION IV.

E. Codes that describe symptoms and signs

Codes that describe symptoms and signs, as opposed to diagnoses, are acceptable for reporting purposes when a diagnosis has not been established (confirmed) by the provider. Chapter 16 of ICD-9-CM, Symptoms, Signs, and Ill-defined conditions (codes 780.0-799.9), contains many, but not all codes for symptoms.

This guideline is the same as General Coding Guidelines Section I.B.6. The examples and exercises used to illustrate the coding of two or more visits before a definite diagnosis can be confirmed shows the use of sign and symptom codes as the reason for the encounter. Remember that you can only code the condition(s) to the highest degree of certainty for a given encounter/visit. This may mean coding symptoms, signs, abnormal test results, or other reason for the encounter.

ICD-9-CM OFFICIAL GUIDELINES FOR CODING AND REPORTING

SECTION IV.

F. Encounters for circumstances other than a disease or injury

ICD-9-CM provides codes to deal with encounters for circumstances other than a disease or injury. The Supplementary Classification of factors Influencing Health Status and Contact with Health Services (V01.0-V89) is provided to deal with occasions when circumstances other than a disease or injury are recorded as diagnosis or problems. *See Section I.C.18 for information on V-codes.*

V CODES   There are 17 chapters in Volume 1, Tabular List, of the ICD-9-CM. Each of the chapters represents a different organ system or type of disease. You will review each of the ICD-9-CM chapters in this text, but first, there are some special codes that you need to know more about—V codes.

ICD-9-CM OFFICIAL GUIDELINES FOR CODING AND REPORTING

SECTION I.C.

18. Classification of Factors Influencing Health Status and Contact with Health Service (Supplemental V01-V89)

Note: The chapter specific guidelines provide additional information about the use of V codes for specified encounters.

a. Introduction

ICD-9-CM provides codes to deal with encounters for circumstances other than a disease or injury. The Supplementary Classification of Factors Influencing Health Status and Contact with Health Services (V01.0-V89.09) is provided to deal with occasions when circumstances other than a disease or injury (codes 001-999) are recorded as a diagnosis or problem.

There are four primary circumstances for the use of V codes:

1) A person who is not currently sick encounters the health services for some specific reason, such as to act as an organ donor, to receive prophylactic care, such as inoculations or health screenings, or to receive counseling on health related issues.

2) A person with a resolving disease or injury, or a chronic, long-term condition requiring continuous care, encounters the health care system for specific aftercare of that disease or injury (e.g., dialysis for renal disease; chemotherapy for malignancy; cast change). A diagnosis/symptom code should be used whenever a current, acute, diagnosis is being treated or a sign or symptom is being studied.

3) Circumstances or problems influence a person's health status but are not in themselves a current illness or injury.

4) Newborns, to indicate birth status

b. V codes use in any healthcare setting

V codes are for use in any healthcare setting. V codes may be used as either a first listed (principal diagnosis code in the inpatient setting) or secondary code, depending on the circumstances of the encounter. Certain V codes may only be used as first listed, others only as secondary codes.
See Section I.C.18.e, V codes that may only be Principal/First-Listed Diagnosis.

Index Locations

In the Tabular, the V codes follow code 999.9. If you have an ICD-9-CM manual available, locate the V codes now. Notice that V codes have only two digits before the decimal point, and a V precedes the number. V codes can be located in the Index like any other code. Often, the most difficult thing about the V code is locating the V code term in the Index. To help you become familiar with how to locate V codes in the Index, review the following, the most common Index terms for locating V codes:

Admission	Dialysis	Observation	Test
Aftercare	Donor	Problem	Transplant
Attention to	Examination	Procedure (surgical)	Unavailability of medical facilities
Boarder	Fitting of		
Care (of)	Follow-up	Prophylactic	Vaccination
Carrier	Health, Healthy	Replacement	
Checking	History	Screening	
Contraception	Maintenance	Status	
Counseling	Maladjustment	Supervision (of)	

Four Circumstances to Assign

V codes are most often used in outpatient settings, that is, ambulatory care centers, physicians' offices, and outpatient departments of hospitals. There are four circumstances in which V codes are used:

1. When a person who is currently not sick encounters the health services for some specific purpose, such as to act as donor of an organ or tissue, to receive a preventive vaccination, or to discuss a problem that is in itself not a disease or injury. Occurrences such as these are more common among outpatients at health clinics.

Example

The patient is donating a kidney.
Code: V59.4 indicates a donor of a kidney; the donor is not sick but encounters
         health care
V59   **Donors**
          V59.4 Kidney
V59 is the category and V59.4 is the subcategory. You would first locate Donor, kidney, in the Index (Volume 2), and then verify code V59.4 in the Tabular List.

Example

A well child receives a polio vaccination:
V04   **Need for prophylactic vaccination and inoculation against certain
          diseases**
          V04.0 Poliomyelitis
Code: V04.0 indicates a patient who is not ill but encounters health care for a
         polio vaccination.
V04 is the category and V04.0 is the subcategory.
   The Index (Volume 2) entry is "Vaccination, poliomyelitis." If you want to indicate that a child has been in contact with poliomyelitis, assign code V01.2, which has an Index location of "Contact, poliomyelitis."

Example

A student seeks health care to discuss a problem with school:
V62   **Other psychosocial circumstances**
          V62.3 Educational circumstances
                    Dissatisfaction with school environment
V62 is the category code and V62.3 is the subcategory code.
   Code V62.3 indicates a patient who is not ill but encounters health care for a psychosocial circumstance, specifically educational circumstances. The Index location is "Dissatisfaction with, education."

---

2. A patient with a known disease or injury receives health services for specific treatment of the disease or injury.

Example

A patient with breast cancer reports to the outpatient department of the hospital for a chemotherapy session. The patient is not currently ill but receives health care services for specific treatment of cancer.

Index:　　**Chemotherapy**, encounter (for) V58.11

Tabular:　**V58 Encounter for other and unspecified procedures and aftercare**

　　　　　　　　V58.11 Encounter for antineoplastic chemotherapy

Code:　　V58.11 Chemotherapy treatment

The breast cancer (174.9) would also be coded, but you will learn about the details of that later in Chapter 5; for now, concentrate on the use of the V codes. V codes should not be mistaken for procedure codes. There is an ICD-9-CM procedure code to identify chemotherapy (99.25). Facility policy and the health care setting will determine the assignment of the procedure code.

3. A circumstance or problem is present and influences a patient's health status but is not in itself a current illness or injury. In these situations the V code should be used only as a supplementary or secondary code.

Example

A patient who is allergic to penicillin is admitted to the hospital for treatment of pneumonia using intravenous antibiotic. The patient receives treatment for the pneumonia, but the patient's allergy to penicillin is a special consideration in the treatment received.

Index:　　**History** (personal) of, allergy to, antibiotic agent NEC V14.1, penicillin V14.0

Tabular:　**V14 Personal history of allergy to penicillin**

　　　　　　　　V14.0 Penicillin

Code:　　V14.0 History of allergy to penicillin

Additionally, the pneumonia (486) would be reported as the first-listed diagnosis, but you are focusing only on the use of V codes right now.

4. To indicate the birth status and outcome of the delivery of a newborn.

Example

A live, healthy newborn infant is the result of a vaginal delivery in the hospital.

Index:　　**Newborn**, single, born in hospital V30.00

Tabular:　**V30 Single live born**

Code:　　V30.00 Vaginal delivery of a single, live-born newborn

The third digit "0" means born in hospital, and the fourth digit "0" means delivery without mention of cesarean delivery.

EXERCISE 3-5   *V Codes*

Locate the V codes in the ICD-9-CM manual in Volume 2, Alphabetic Index, and then in Volume 1, Tabular List. Code the following:

1 A person who has been in contact with smallpox

     Index location: _____

     V Code: _____

2 Prophylactic vaccination against smallpox

     Index location: _____

     V Code: _____

3 Personal history of malignant neoplasm of the tongue

     Index location: _____

     V Code: _____

Assign the V code for the following:

4 Admission for cardiac pacemaker adjustment

     Code: _____

5 Insertion of subdermal implantable contraceptive

     Code: _____

6 Personal history of cancer of the prostate

     Code: _____

7 Baby in for MMR (measles, mumps, rubella) vaccination

     Code: _____

8 Screening mammogram

     Code: _____

9 Clinic visit for pre-employment physical examination

     Code: _____

CAUTION *Often, the patient record states that there is a "history of" a disease: for example, "history of diabetes mellitus." This does not mean that the patient no longer has diabetes mellitus, but that the patient's medical history includes diabetes mellitus. You would not assign a V code to indicate a previous history of diabetes mellitus, but instead would assign the code for the current disease of diabetes mellitus (250.0X). If there is any question regarding the current status of the disease, check with the physician. You may also want to offer some physician education regarding the documentation of past history of diseases.*

Observation

Codes from the V71.0-V71.9 series, Observation and evaluation for suspected conditions, are assigned as first-listed diagnoses for encounters or admissions to evaluate the patient's condition when there is some evidence to suggest the existence of an abnormal condition or following an accident or other incident that ordinarily results in a health problem, and where no supporting evidence for the suspected condition is found that requires no further treatment. The fact that the patient may be scheduled for continuing observation in the office/clinic setting following discharge does not limit the use of this series of codes.

EXERCISE 3-6 *Observation for Suspected Conditions*

Assign ICD-9-CM codes to the following as directed:

1 The patient fell off his motorcycle when turning too sharply and hit his head on the sidewalk. The patient was wearing a helmet. The examination reveals no outwardly apparent head injury. The only injury noted on examination is abrasion of the elbow. The patient is admitted overnight to the observation unit to rule out head injury.

There will be three codes on this case: one for the **observation** of the head injury (a V code), one for the **abrasion,** and one for the **cause** (falling from motorcycle reported with an E code).

   a Hospital observation is located in the Index under the main term "Observation." Listed under the main term are the reasons for observation. The subterm is "accident NEC." Check the code in the Tabular. What is the V code?

   Code: _____

   b The second code is for the abrasion to the elbow. When you locate the term "abrasion" in the Index, you are referred to "*see also* Injury, superficial, by site." Locate "Injury, superficial, arm." What is the code for the abrasion?

   Code: _____

   (See the cross reference in the Tabular, and discover whether a fourth digit is needed for specificity.)

   c The E code would be E816.2.

2 A patient is admitted for observation and further evaluation following an alleged rape.

   a There is only one code for this case. What is that V code?

   Code: _____

From the Trenches

"In a medical practice, teamwork is the glue that keeps the practice together. With physicians, the back and forth education is priceless. They cannot work without us coders, while we cannot do our job well without their support."

DAMARIS

SPECIFICITY

ICD-9-CM OFFICIAL GUIDELINES FOR CODING AND REPORTING

SECTION IV.

G. Level of Detail in Coding

1. **ICD-9-CM codes with 3, 4, or 5 digits**

   ICD-9-CM is composed of codes with either 3, 4, or 5 digits. Codes with three digits are included in ICD-9-CM as the heading of a category of codes that may be further subdivided by the use of fourth and/or fifth digits, which provide greater specificity.

2. **Use of full number of digits required for a code**

   A three-digit code is to be used only if it is not further subdivided. Where fourth-digit subcategories and/or fifth-digit subclassifications are provided, they must be assigned. A code is invalid if it has not been coded to the full number of digits required for that code.

   See also discussion under Section I.b.3., General Coding Guidelines, Level of Detail in Coding.

The addition of fourth and fifth digits to the basic three-digit code category was discussed in Chapter 2. Not all codes have fourth or fifth digits, but when a fourth or fifth digit is available it must be assigned. Most ICD-9-CM manuals have a symbol to remind the coder to assign the additional digits.

ICD-9-CM OFFICIAL GUIDELINES FOR CODING AND REPORTING

SECTION IV.

H. ICD-9-CM code for the diagnosis, condition, problem, or other reason for encounter/visit

List first the ICD-9-CM code for the diagnosis, condition, problem, or other reason for encounter/visit shown in the medical record to be chiefly responsible for the services provided. List additional codes that describe any coexisting conditions. In some cases the first-listed diagnosis may be a symptom when a diagnosis has not been established (confirmed) by the physician.

You have already had practice at selecting the first-listed diagnoses and you know that it is possible for the first-listed diagnosis to be a symptom. The important information in this guideline is that additional codes should be assigned for any coexisting conditions that are present or treated during that visit or encounter. Sometimes there is more than one symptom that is present.

Examples

1. An established patient was seen for dyspnea on exertion. The patient has hypertension and Graves disease. No etiology for the dyspnea was determined. Patient's medication prescriptions for hypertension and Graves' disease were refilled.

   Codes: 786.09 dyspnea, 401.9 hypertension, 242.00 Graves' disease.

2. Initial office visit for 55-year-old male with jaundice and fatigue. Laboratory tests were ordered and patient will return in 1 week for the results.

   Codes: 782.4 jaundice, 780.79 fatigue (either of these diagnoses could be the first-listed diagnosis).

EXERCISE 3-7 *First-Listed Diagnoses and Coexisting Conditions*

Identify the first-listed diagnosis and any coexisting conditions. Assign the ICD-9-CM codes:

1 Patient was seen in the office for a consultation of palpitations. Patient has rheumatoid arthritis. Medications that the patient takes for the arthritis were reviewed to see if they could be the cause of the palpitations.

First-listed Diagnosis Term(s): _____

Code: _____

Other Diagnoses Term(s): _____

Code(s): _____

2 Patient is an established patient with memory loss. Patient also takes medication for diabetes type II.

First-listed Diagnosis Term(s): _____

Code: _____

Other Diagnoses Term(s): _____

Code(s): _____

3 A new patient was seen for flank pain. He or she was diagnosed with a urinary tract infection and antibiotics were prescribed. Patient has psoriasis, which is stable at this time.

First-listed Diagnosis Term(s): _____

Code: _____

Other Diagnoses Term(s): _____

Code(s): _____

UNCERTAIN DIAGNOSIS

ICD-9-CM OFFICIAL GUIDELINES FOR CODING AND REPORTING

SECTION IV.
I. Uncertain diagnosis

Do not code diagnoses documented as "probable", "suspected," "questionable," "rule out," or "working diagnosis" or other similar terms indicating uncertainty. Rather, code the condition(s) to the highest degree of certainty for that encounter/visit, such as symptoms, signs, abnormal test results, or other reason for the visit.

Please note: This differs from the coding practices used by short-term, acute care, long-term care, and psychiatric hospitals.

This guideline states you can only code the condition(s) to the highest degree of certainty for a given encounter/visit in the outpatient setting. This may mean coding symptoms, signs, abnormal test results, or another reason for the encounter.

Examples

1. A chest x-ray is ordered to rule out pneumonia. Patient has cough and fever. The x-ray is normal.

   Codes: 786.2 cough, 780.60 fever. The pneumonia cannot be coded as it is documented as a rule out and has not been confirmed.

2. A 55-year-old male was seen with loss of appetite and jaundice. Further diagnostic studies are needed for suspected cancer of the pancreas.

   Codes: 782.4 jaundice, 783.0 loss of appetite. No code can be assigned for cancer of the pancreas because it is "suspected" and not yet confirmed.

EXERCISE 3-8 *Uncertain Diagnoses*

Identify the diagnoses and ICD-9-CM codes to be assigned.

1 Patient is seen in the office for pain and stiffness of the right knee. X-rays to rule out osteoarthritis were performed.

   Diagnoses Terms and Codes: _____

2 Office visit for established patient with wrist pain and numbness of fingertips. Studies ordered for probable carpal tunnel syndrome.

   Diagnoses Terms and Codes: _____

3 Office consultation for a new patient with amenorrhea and galactorrhea. Studies to rule out pituitary tumor were ordered.

   Diagnoses Terms and Codes: _____

4 Initial visit for a patient with a breast lump. Working diagnosis is breast cancer. Diagnostic workup has been scheduled.

   Diagnoses Terms and Code: _____

CHRONIC DISEASES

ICD-9-CM OFFICIAL GUIDELINES FOR CODING AND REPORTING

SECTION IV.
J. Chronic diseases
   Chronic diseases treated on an ongoing basis may be coded and reported as many times as the patient receives treatment and care for the condition(s)

Examples

1. Patient is an established patient who is seen in for management of asthma and diabetes.
   Codes: 493.90 Asthma, 250.00 Diabetes (either code could be the first-listed)
2. Established patient is seen for continued management of systemic lupus erythematosus.
   Code: 710.0 Systemic lupus erythematosus

ICD-9-CM OFFICIAL GUIDELINES FOR CODING AND REPORTING

SECTION IV.

K. Code all documented conditions that coexist

Code all documented conditions that coexist at the time of the encounter/visit, and require or affect patient care treatment or management. Do not code conditions that were previously treated and no longer exist. However, history codes (V10-V19) may be used as secondary codes if the historical condition or family history has an impact on current care or influences treatment.

Examples

1. An established patient is seen in follow-up for coronary artery disease. Patient is also a diabetic on oral medications. The patient had a coronary artery bypass graft 6 months ago. Labs were reviewed and prescriptions for diabetic medications were renewed.

   Codes: 414.00 coronary artery disease, 250.00 diabetes (chronic coexisting conditions that were managed during this visit), V45.81 history of CABG (acceptable to code as this is important in a patient with coronary artery disease).

2. An established patient is seen for management of hypertension and congestive heart failure. Patient has a family history of colonic polyps.

   Codes: 401.9 hypertension, 428.0 congestive heart failure (either could be first-listed diagnosis). No V code is necessary to identify the family history of colonic polyps as it has no bearing on the treatment of hypertension and congestive heart failure.

DIAGNOSTIC SERVICES

ICD-9-CM OFFICIAL GUIDELINES FOR CODING AND REPORTING

SECTION IV.

L. Patients receiving diagnostic services only

For patients receiving diagnostic services only during an encounter/visit, sequence first the diagnosis, condition, problem, or other reason for encounter/visit shown in the medical record to be chiefly responsible for the outpatient services provided during the encounter/visit. Codes for other diagnoses (e.g., chronic conditions) may be sequenced as additional diagnoses.

For encounters for routine laboratory/radiology testing in the absence of any signs, symptoms, or associated diagnosis, assign V72.5 **and a code from subcategory** V72.6. If routine testing is performed during the same encounter as a test to evaluate a sign, symptom, or diagnosis, it is appropriate to assign both the V code and the code describing the reason for the non-routine test.

For outpatient encounters for diagnostic tests that have been interpreted by a physician, and the final report is available at the time of coding, code any confirmed or definitive diagnosis(es) documented in the interpretation. Do not code related signs and symptoms as additional diagnoses.

Please note: This differs from the coding practice in the hospital inpatient setting regarding abnormal findings on test results.

Examples

DIAGNOSTIC SERVICES ONLY

1. Patient encounter for blood typing prior to outpatient surgery tomorrow.

    Code: V72.86 encounter for blood typing

2. Patient is having an MRI of the head to monitor the progression of brain tumor.

    Code: 239.6 brain tumor

3. Patient requested a CBC (complete blood count).

    Code: V72.60 laboratory examination without any sign or symptom documented

4. Patient was seen for shortness of breath and fever with negative x-ray. Patient returned the next day for a CT of chest, which confirmed the presence of pneumonia.

    Code: 486 pneumonia

THERAPEUTIC SERVICES

ICD-9-CM OFFICIAL GUIDELINES FOR CODING AND REPORTING

SECTION IV.

M. Patients receiving therapeutic services only

For patients receiving therapeutic services only during an encounter/visit, sequence first the diagnosis, condition, problem, or other reason for encounter/visit shown in the medical record to be chiefly responsible for the outpatient services provided during the encounter/visit. Codes for other diagnoses (e.g., chronic conditions) may be sequenced as additional diagnoses.

The only exception to this rule is that when the primary reason for the admission/encounter is chemotherapy, radiation therapy, or rehabilitation, the appropriate V code for the service is listed first, and the diagnosis or problem for which the service is being performed listed second.

A therapeutic service is one in which some type of treatment is performed to treat a specific disease. Therapeutic services can range from a medication to a surgical procedure.

Examples

THERAPEUTIC SERVICES ONLY

1. Patient had an outpatient phlebotomy performed for polycythemia vera.

    Code: 238.4 polycythemia vera

2. Patient received outpatient chemotherapy for breast cancer with metastasis to the axillary lymph nodes.

    Code: V58.11 encounter for chemotherapy, 174.9 breast cancer, and 196.3 metastasis to axillary lymph nodes

3. Patient had monthly B12 shot for pernicious anemia.

    Code: 281.0 pernicious anemia

SURGERY

ICD-9-CM OFFICIAL GUIDELINES FOR CODING AND REPORTING

SECTION IV.
N. Patients receiving preoperative evaluations only

For patients receiving preoperative evaluations only, sequence first a code from category V72.8, Other specified examinations, to describe the pre-op consultations. Assign a code for the condition to describe the reason for the surgery as an additional diagnosis. Code also any findings related to the pre-op evaluation.

Often a surgeon will want a preoperative clearance performed by the patient's primary care provider, often due to a chronic or pre-existing condition. When the primary care provider is reporting the diagnosis for the visit the first-listed diagnosis must be the appropriate V code to indicate the encounter is for preop clearance, followed by the reason for the upcoming surgery, and finally, the condition requiring the clearance. The V code will be one of the following:

V72.81 Preoperative cardiovascular examination

V72.82 Preoperative respiratory examination

V72.83 Other specified preoperative examination

V72.84 Preoperative examination, unspecified

Examples

PREOPERATIVE EVALUATIONS ONLY

1. Patient is seen by cardiologist for surgical clearance for upcoming cataract surgery. The patient has coronary artery disease (CAD) and has a cardiac stent. Patient's medical condition from a cardiac standpoint is stable. Patient can proceed with cataract removal.

   Code: V72.81 preoperative cardiovascular examination, 414.01 coronary artery disease, V45.82 history of cardiac angioplasty, 366.9 cataract

2. Patient is seen by internist for medical clearance for inguinal hernia repair. The patient has a number of chronic medical conditions including hypertension, diabetes type II, and atrial fibrillation.

   Code: V72.83 other specified preoperative examination, 401.9 hypertension, 250.00 diabetes type II, 472.31 atrial fibrillation, 550.90 inguinal hernia

ICD-9-CM OFFICIAL GUIDELINES FOR CODING AND REPORTING

SECTION IV.
O. Ambulatory surgery

For ambulatory surgery, code the diagnosis for which the surgery was performed. If the postoperative diagnosis is known to be different from the preoperative diagnosis at the time the diagnosis is confirmed, select the postoperative diagnosis for coding, since it is the most definitive.

Examples

1. **PRE AND POSTOPERATIVE DIAGNOSES ARE THE SAME**

   The patient has an EGD for upper gastrointestinal bleeding. The postoperative diagnosis is upper gastrointestinal bleeding, etiology undetermined.

   Code: 578.9

2. **PRE AND POSTOPERATIVE DIAGNOSES ARE DIFFERENT**

   The patient has an EGD for upper gastrointestinal bleeding. The postoperative diagnosis is gastrointestinal bleeding due to gastric ulcer.

   Code: 531.40

PRENATAL VISITS

ICD-9-CM OFFICIAL GUIDELINES FOR CODING AND REPORTING

SECTION IV.

P. Routine outpatient prenatal visits

For routine outpatient prenatal visits when no complications are present, codes V22.0, Supervision of normal first pregnancy, or V22.1, Supervision of other normal pregnancy, should be used as the principal diagnosis. These codes should not be used in conjunction with chapter 11 codes.

Examples

1. **FIRST PREGNANCY WITHOUT COMPLICATION**

   A 25-year-old female presents for initial prenatal visit. This is her first pregnancy. No problems were identified.

   Code: V22.0

2. **SECOND PREGNANCY WITHOUT COMPLICATION**

   A 25-year-old female presents for initial prenatal visit. Patient had an uncomplicated vaginal delivery of a term female infant 3 years ago. No problems were identified.

   Code: V22.1

3. **PRENATAL VISIT WITH COMPLICATION (CODE FROM CHAPTER 11)**

   A 25-year-old female is seen for a routine prenatal visit. Her laboratory results indicate that she has a urinary tract infection. She is given a prescription for antibiotics and will return in 1 week for repeat urinalysis.

   Codes: 646.63, 599.0

EXERCISE 3-9 *Chronic Disease, Diagnostic/Therapeutic Services, Surgery, and Prenatal Visits*

Match each code from the list of codes with the report to which it should be assigned and place the letters for the codes in the correct order:

a. 493.90	c. 710.0	e. 250.00	g. V88.01	i. 692.4	k. V72.0
b. V67.01	d. V45.81	f. 414.01	h. V10.41	j. V55.3	

1 A patient with chronic asthma and systemic lupus erythematosus presents to the clinic for an office visit during which the physician assesses the status of the asthma and lupus erythematosus.

   🔮 Code(s): _____

2 A patient with a history of coronary artery bypass graft of the native coronary artery 6 months earlier due to arteriosclerosis. The patient is also evaluated by his internal medicine physician for his longstanding diabetes for which the patient takes insulin. The physician revises the patient's diabetic medications and the Lipitor prescription based on review of laboratory results.

   🔮 Code(s): _____

3 A patient with a colostomy is evaluated by his internist for the patient's complaints of redness and itching at the skin level opening of his colostomy bag. The physician diagnosed dermatitis due to a new brand of skin level plastic seal. He prescribes a topical salve, replaced the seal, and requested the patient to return in 2 weeks if there is not significant improvement.

   🔮 Code(s): _____

4 The patient is examined by the ophthalmologist for an annual eye examination. The patient has no complaints and the physician indicates the patient's vision is excellent.

   🔮 Code(s): _____

5 A follow-up vaginal pap smear is performed for a patient who is status-post hysterectomy that included the removal of both the cervix and the uterus. The procedure was performed for a primary malignancy. The patient had a previous smear and both that smear and the current smear were negative for malignance.

   🔮 Code(s): _____

CHAPTER REVIEW

CHAPTER 3, PART I, THEORY

Answer the following questions about the Diagnostic Coding and Reporting Guidelines for Outpatient Services.

1 When a patient is to have outpatient surgery and the surgery is not performed due to contraindication, the reason that the surgery was not performed is the first-listed diagnosis.

True   False

2 It is appropriate to code the postoperative diagnosis as it is the most definitive diagnosis for ambulatory surgery.

True   False

3 Chronic diseases that are treated on an ongoing basis should be coded and reported as often as the patient receives treatment and care for the chronic conditions.

True   False

4 In the physician office it is acceptable to code V codes as a first-listed diagnosis.

True   False

5 In the outpatient setting it is unacceptable to have a sign or symptom as the first-listed diagnosis.

True   False

6 When coding an encounter for preoperative evaluation, the reason that the patient is having the surgery or procedure performed is the first-listed diagnosis.

True   False

7 In the outpatient setting, diagnoses that are documented as "probable," "suspected," "rule out," or "questionable" are coded only to the highest degree of certainty.

True   False

8 The first-listed diagnosis is defined as the diagnosis that is the most serious.

True   False

9 It is acceptable to use a code from the ICD-9-CM manual, Chapter 11 in conjunction with V22.0 or V22.1.

True   False

10 It is acceptable to code signs and symptoms even when a definitive diagnosis has been confirmed.

True   False

CHAPTER 3, PART II, PRACTICAL

Identify the first-listed diagnoses and assign the appropriate ICD-9-CM codes in the following encounters or visits.

11 Initial office visit for diaper rash

First-listed Diagnosis Term(s): _____

Code: _____

12 Established patient presents with dyspnea and lower extremity edema. The physician determined that the patient's symptoms were due to an exacerbation of congestive heart failure.

First-listed Diagnosis Term(s): _____

Code: _____

Other Diagnoses Term(s): _____

Code(s): _____

13 Established patient seen for management of vitamin B12 deficiency and hypertension

First-listed Diagnosis Term(s): _____

Code: _____

Other Diagnoses Term(s): _____

Code(s): _____

14 Patient was admitted as an outpatient for an arthroscopic knee procedure to repair old anterior cruciate ligament tear.

First-listed Diagnosis Term(s): _____

Code: _____

15 Patient is admitted to observation for syncope. Patient has diabetes mellitus.

After testing, no cardiac or other cause was found.

First-listed Diagnosis Term(s): _____

Code: _____

Other Diagnoses Term(s): _____

Code(s): _____

16 Patient was admitted for pain management following biopsy of the kidney for Stage IV chronic kidney disease.

First-listed Diagnosis Term(s): _____

Code: _____

Other Diagnoses Term(s): _____

Code(s): _____

17 Patient is seen by pulmonologist for surgical clearance for upcoming surgery. Patient has emphysema and is scheduled to have an endarterectomy for severe carotid stenosis on the right.

First-listed Diagnosis Term(s): _____

Code: _____

Other Diagnoses Term(s): _____

Code(s): _____

18 Patient had an outpatient cystoscopy. The preoperative diagnosis is hematuria. Postoperative diagnosis is hematuria due to bladder cancer.

First-listed Diagnosis Term(s): _____

Code: _____

Other Diagnoses Term(s): _____

Code(s): _____

Assign the appropriate V code for the following:

19 Exposure to asbestos _____

20 Personal history of colonic polyps

_____

21 Heart transplant status _____

"Coders should be patient, willing to research, detailed, not afraid to ask questions, and always looking to learn more so proper coding is done. Don't allow comfort to set in. Grow, grow, grow!"

Melony M. Jones, CPC
HCC Chart Specialist
Windsor Health Group
Little Rock, Arkansas

Using ICD-9-CM

Chapter Topics

Organization of the Guidelines

Level of Specificity

Integral Conditions

Multiple Coding

Acute and Chronic

Combination Codes

Late Effects

Impending or Threatened Condition

Chapter Review

Quick Check Answers

Learning Objectives

After completing this chapter you should be able to

1 Explain the organization of the Guidelines.

2 Determine the level of highest specificity.

3 Identify conditions integral to a disease process.

4 Assign multiple codes to a single condition.

5 Report acute and chronic conditions.

6 Demonstrate application of combination codes.

7 Differentiate between residual and late effects.

8 Abstract information that determines if a condition is impending or threatened.

Make sure to check
evolve learning system
for the latest
content updates

ORGANIZATION OF THE GUIDELINES

As was discussed in Chapter 3, Official Guidelines for Coding and Reporting have been developed and approved for coding and reporting by the Cooperating Parties for ICD-9-CM: the American Hospital Association (AHA), American Health Information Management Association (AHIMA), Centers for Medicare and Medicaid Services (CMS), and National Center for Health Statistics (NCHS).

The complete Official Guidelines for Coding and Reporting appears on the companion CD and is posted on the web at www.cdc.gov/nchs/icd.htm. The Guidelines are organized into sections. Section I of the Guidelines includes the structure and conventions of the classification and general guidelines that apply to the entire classification, and chapter-specific guidelines that correspond to the chapters as they are arranged in the classification. Section II includes guidelines for selection of principal diagnosis for non-outpatient (hospital) settings. Section III includes guidelines for reporting additional diagnoses in non-outpatient settings. Section IV is for outpatient coding and reporting. Outpatient coders, however, use guidance from throughout the Official Guidelines for Coding and Reporting because not all of the coding circumstances are fully explained in the Section IV of the Guidelines. Appendix I of the Guidelines includes Present on Admission Reporting Guidelines that are guidance for reporting certain conditions in the hospital setting.

QUICK CHECK 4-1

1. Examine your ICD-9-CM manual to determine if the Official Guidelines for Coding and Reporting are included in your publication. If so, where are they located? _____

The number that appears to the left of the guideline in this text is the number of the guideline as listed in the Official Guidelines for Coding and Reporting. For the purposes of this text, the Guidelines will sometimes appear out of order.

In the examples in this text, main terms and subterms are often noted for you after the term enclosed in parentheses to help you locate the terms in the Alphabetic Index. For example, Hodgkin's (main term) disease (subterm) directs you to the location of Hodgkin's disease in the Alphabetic Index like this: "(Hodgkin's, disease)." Remember, the extensive indexing system in the ICD-9-CM allows you many options for locating codes in the Alphabetic Index. The examples and subsequent identification of main terms and subterms represent only one way a term can be located.

You will be practicing coding using the ICD-9-CM throughout this chapter. You need to practice using the steps that are always necessary to assign an ICD-9-CM code. If you begin your ICD-9-CM coding using these steps, you will develop good coding habits that will last throughout your career.

Steps to Accurate Coding

1. Identify the main term(s) in the diagnostic statement.
2. Locate the main term(s) in the Alphabetic Index (Volume 2) (referred to in this text as the Index).
3. Review any subterms under the main term in the Index.
4. Follow any cross-reference instructions, such as *see also*.
5. Verify the code(s) selected from the Index (Volume 2) in the Tabular List (Volume 1) (referred to in this text as the Tabular).
6. Refer to any instructional notations in the Tabular.
7. Assign codes to the highest level of specificity. For example, if a fourth digit is available, you cannot assign only a three-digit code, and if a fifth digit is available, you cannot assign only a four-digit code.
8. Code the diagnosis until all elements are completely identified.

Guidelines are presented and followed by examples or exercises to illustrate the rule(s).

Let's get started with a general coding Guideline:

ICD-9-CM OFFICIAL GUIDELINES FOR CODING AND REPORTING

SECTION I.
B. General Coding Guidelines

1. **Use of Both Alphabetic Index and Tabular List**
   Use both the Alphabetic Index and the Tabular List when locating and assigning a code. Reliance on only the Alphabetic Index or the Tabular List leads to errors in code assignments and less specificity in code selection.

2. **Locate each term in the Alphabetic Index**
   Locate each term in the Alphabetic Index and verify the code selected in the Tabular List. Read and be guided by instructional notations that appear in both the Alphabetic Index and the Tabular List.

USE BOTH THE ALPHABETIC INDEX AND THE TABULAR LIST

Examples

1. Diagnosis: Hodgkin's Disease

   Index: **Hodgkin's** (main term)
                     disease (subterm) 201.9

   Tabular: **201 Hodgkin's disease** [category code]
                     201.9 Hodgkin's disease, unspecified [subcategory code]

   Code: 201.9X Hodgkin's Disease [subclassification code]

Verify 201.9 in the Tabular and note that the code requires a fifth-digit assignment of 0 to 8 to indicate the disease location. You would have missed the required fifth-digit subclassification (indicated by the X in the example) if you had referenced only the Index and not verified the code in the Tabular. You must also always go back to the beginning of the section in the Tabular and read any notes located there. In the case of 201, the section notes (above code 200) indicate the fifth digits to be used with codes 200-202. Code 201.90 is assigned because the type and location of the Hodgkin's disease were both unspecified.

Continued

2. Diagnosis: Stroke, due to vertebral artery occlusion

Index: **Stroke** (main term) 434.91

Tabular: **434.9 Cerebral artery occlusion, unspecified**

As the occlusion is specified as "due to vertebral artery occlusion," 434.9X, cerebral artery occlusion, unspecified, does not accurately describe the condition. Return to the Index and locate the term "occlusion" to see what other codes might more accurately describe this condition.

Index: **Occlusion**

artery (subterm), vertebral (subterm) 433.2

Tabular: **433 Occlusion and stenosis of precerebral arteries**

0 without mention of cerebral infarction

1 with cerebral infarction

433.2 Vertebral artery

Code: 433.21 Stroke, due to vertebral artery occlusion

The diagnosis statement "fits" or is classifiable to 433.21. You would have incorrectly reported the diagnosis as 434.91 if you had not verified the code in the Tabular. The fifth digit is "1, with cerebral infarction" because a stroke is an infarction. There are no shortcuts in this process: Always check the Tabular.

The level of specificity is the level of detail and detail is very important in diagnosis coding. Review the Guideline regarding specificity.

LEVEL OF SPECIFICITY

ICD-9-CM OFFICIAL GUIDELINES FOR CODING AND REPORTING

SECTION I.B.

3. Level of Detail in Coding

Diagnosis and procedure codes are to be used at their highest number of digits available.

ICD-9-CM diagnosis codes are composed of codes with 3, 4, or 5 digits. Codes with three digits are included in ICD-9-CM as the heading of a category of codes that may be further subdivided by the use of fourth and/or fifth digits, which provide greater detail.

A three-digit code is to be used only if it is not further subdivided. Where fourth-digit subcategories and/or fifth-digit subclassifications are provided, they must be assigned. A code is invalid if it has not been coded to the full number of digits required for that code. For example, Acute myocardial infarction, code 410, has fourth digits that describe the location of the infarction (e.g., 410.2, Of inferolateral wall), and fifth digits that identify the episode of care. It would be incorrect to report a code in category 410 without a fourth and fifth digit.

ICD-9-CM Volume 3 procedure codes are composed of codes with either 3 or 4 digits. Codes with two digits are included in ICD-9-CM as the heading of a category of codes that may be further subdivided by the use of third and/or fourth digits, which provide greater detail.

LEVEL OF SPECIFICITY

Examples

1. *Three-Digit Category*

Diagnosis:	Subarachnoid hemorrhage
Index:	**Hemorrhage**, subarachnoid, nontraumatic 430
Tabular:	**430 Subarachnoid hemorrhage** [category code]
Code:	430 Subarachnoid hemorrhage

Diagnosis:	AIDS
Index:	**AIDS 042**
Tabular:	**042 Human immunodeficiency virus (HIV) disease** [category code]
Code:	042 AIDS

Both of the preceding diagnostic statements are correctly assigned to three-digit category codes because there are no four-digit subcategory codes available within either code.

2. *Four-Digit Subcategory*

Diagnosis:	Crohn's disease of large intestine
Index:	**Crohn's disease** (see also Enteritis, regional) 555.9
Tabular:	**555 Regional enteritis (Includes: Crohn's disease)** [category code]
	555.1 Large intestine [subcategory code]
Code:	555.1 Crohn's disease of large intestine

Diagnosis:	Cellulitis of the upper right leg
Index:	**Cellulitis**, leg
Tabular:	**682 Other cellulitis and abscess** [category code]
	682.6 Leg, except foot [subcategory code]
Code:	682.6 Cellulitis of the upper right leg

Both of the preceding diagnostic statements are correctly assigned to four-digit subcategory codes because no five-digit subclassification codes are available.

3. *Five Digit Subclassification*

Diagnosis:	RUQ abdominal pain
Index:	**Pain**, abdominal
Tabular:	**789.0 Abdominal pain** [subcategory code]
	789.01 Right upper quadrant [subclassification code]
Code:	789.01 RUQ abdominal pain

Diagnosis:	Bilateral, congenital bowing of femur
Index:	**Bowing**
	femur 736.89
	congenital 754.42
Tabular:	**754 Certain congenital musculoskeletal deformities** [category code]
	754.4 Congenital genu recurvatum and bowing of long bones of leg [subcategory code]
	754.42 Congenital bowing of femur [subclassification code]
Code:	754.42 Bilateral, congenital bowing of femur

Both of the preceding diagnostic statements are correctly assigned to five-digit subclassification codes, having been carried out to the highest level of specificity available.

EXERCISE 4-1 *Level of Specificity in Coding*

Identify the category, subcategory, and subclassifications of the following codes:

1 Diagnosis: Recurrent right inguinal hernia, with obstruction

    Index: **Hernia**

                inguinal 550.9

    Tabular: **550 Inguinal hernia** _____

             550.1 Inguinal hernia, with obstruction, without mention of gangrene

             _____

             550.11 Inguinal hernia, with obstruction, without mention of gangrene, unilateral, recurrent _____

2 Diagnosis: Transient hypertension, 30 weeks' gestation, undelivered

    Index: **Hypertension**

                transient

                  of pregnancy (soubrette) 642.3

    Tabular: **642 Hypertension complicating pregnancy, childbirth, and the puerperium**

             _____

             642.3 Transient hypertension of pregnancy _____

             642.33 Antepartum condition or complication _____

INTEGRAL CONDITIONS

ICD-9-CM OFFICIAL GUIDELINES FOR CODING AND REPORTING

SECTION I.B.

7. Conditions that are an integral part of a disease process

Signs and symptoms that are associated routinely with a disease process should not be assigned as additional codes, unless otherwise instructed by the classification.

INTEGRAL PART OF A DISEASE PROCESS

Example 1

Diagnosis: Fever and shortness of breath due to pneumonia

Index: **Pneumonia 486**

Tabular: **486 Pneumonia, organism unspecified**

Code: 486 Pneumonia, organism unspecified

Fever and shortness of breath are common symptoms of pneumonia so additional codes would not be assigned.

INTEGRAL PART OF A DISEASE PROCESS

Example 2

Diagnosis:	Abdominal pain which is exacerbated by eating. The patient was found to have a gastric ulcer.
Index:	**Ulcer, stomach, 531.9**
Tabular:	**531 Gastric ulcer**
	531.90 Unspecified as acute or chronic, without mention of hemorrhage or perforation
Code:	531.90 Gastric ulcer

Abdominal pain that is exacerbated (made worse) by eating is a common symptom of a gastric ulcer.

ICD-9-CM OFFICIAL GUIDELINES FOR CODING AND REPORTING

SECTION I.B.

8. Conditions that are not an integral part of a disease process

Additional signs and symptoms that may not be associated routinely with a disease process should be coded when present.

NOT AN INTEGRAL PART OF A DISEASE PROCESS

Example 1

Diagnosis:	Dehydration due to pneumonia
Index:	**Pneumonia 486**
Tabular:	**486 Pneumonia, organism unspecified**
Code:	486 Pneumonia, organism unspecified
Index:	**Dehydration 276.51**
Tabular:	**276.5 Volume depletion**
	276.51 Dehydration
Code:	276.51 Dehydration
Codes:	486 (pneumonia) and 276.51 (dehydration)

Dehydration can result from a wide range of diseases, but not all patients who have pneumonia become dehydrated. Dehydration would be assigned as an additional code.

NOT AN INTEGRAL PART OF A DISEASE PROCESS

Example 2

Diagnosis:	Ascites due to cirrhosis of the liver
Index:	**Cirrhosis, cirrhotic**
	liver 571.5
Tabular:	**571.5 Cirrhosis of liver without mention of alcohol**
Code:	571.5 Cirrhosis of liver
Index:	**Ascites 789.59**
Tabular:	**789.59 Other ascites**
Code:	789.59 Ascites
Codes:	571.5 (cirrhosis) and 789.59 (ascites)

Ascites is not present in all patients with cirrhosis of the liver. The ascites should be coded in this case as the patient's treatment may be affected by the ascites.

It is necessary to have strong anatomy, terminology, and pathophysiology skills to know if a condition is an integral part of a disease process.

EXERCISE 4-2 *Integral and Not Integral Conditions*

Without the use of reference material, answer the following:

1 List two common symptoms of appendicitis.

_____

2 List the most common symptom associated with costochondritis.

_____

3 Patient has rheumatoid arthritis and anemia. The anemia is integral to the rheumatoid arthritis.

True   False

4 Patient has dyspnea due to congestive heart failure. Dyspnea should be assigned as an additional code.

True   False

Circle the diagnoses that should NOT be coded for the condition in bold typeface:

5 **Acute myocardial infarction**

Chest pain

Shortness of breath

Congestive heart failure

6 **Fractured hip**

Hip pain

Contusion of hip

MULTIPLE CODING

ICD-9-CM OFFICIAL GUIDELINES FOR CODING AND REPORTING

SECTION I.B.

9. Multiple coding for a single condition

In addition to the etiology/manifestation convention that requires two codes to fully describe a single condition that affects multiple body systems, there are other single conditions that also require more than one code. "Use additional code" notes are found in the tabular at codes that are not part of an etiology/manifestation pair where a secondary code is useful to fully describe a condition. The sequencing rule is the same as the etiology/manifestation pair- "use additional code" indicates that a secondary code should be added.

For example, for infections that are not included in chapter 1, a secondary code from category 041, Bacterial infection in conditions classified elsewhere and of unspecified site, may be required to identify the bacterial organism causing the infection. A "use additional code" note will normally be found at the infectious disease code, indicating a need for the organism code to be added as a secondary code.

"Code first" notes are also under certain codes that are not specifically manifestation codes but may be due to an underlying cause. When a "code first" note is present and an underlying condition is present the underlying condition should be sequenced first.

"Code, if applicable, any causal condition first", notes indicate that this code may be assigned as a principal diagnosis when the causal condition is unknown or not applicable. If a causal condition is known, then the code for that condition should be sequenced as the principal or first-listed diagnosis.

Multiple codes may be needed for late effects, complication codes and obstetric codes to more fully describe a condition. See the specific guidelines for these conditions for further instruction.

MULTIPLE CODING (ALSO KNOWN AS DUAL CODING)

Example 1

Diagnosis: Diabetic retinopathy with type I diabetes

(Note: Retinopathy is the manifestation and diabetes is the etiology (cause) of the retinopathy or retinal hemorrhage.)

Diagnosis: Index: **Retinopathy,** diabetic 250.5 *[362.01]*
diabetic 250.5 *[362.01]*

The Index subterm "diabetic" located under "Retinopathy" identifies the code for the etiology as 250.5 and directs you to the code for the manifestation of *[362.01]* retinopathy. The italicized code is never sequenced first as the first-listed diagnosis but is assigned to identify a manifestation.

Tabular: **250 Diabetes mellitus**

250.5 Diabetes with ophthalmic manifestations

Use additional code to identify manifestation

250.51 Type I, not stated as uncontrolled

Note that the diagnosis of diabetes mellitus will always be reported with a five-digit code because the fifth digit indicates the type of diabetes. See the fifth-digit codes listed after code 250 in the Tabular of your ICD-9-CM.

Code 250.51 is the correct code to describe the diabetes (etiology). The statement "Use additional code to identify manifestation..." in the Tabular at 250.5 directs you to assign a code that identifies the manifestation (retinopathy).

Tabular: **362 Other retinal disorders**

362.0 Diabetic retinopathy

Code first diabetes (250.5)

362.01 Background diabetic retinopathy

Note that the "*Code first diabetes 250.5*" directs you to the etiology code (diabetes).

Codes: 250.51, 362.01 Diabetic retinopathy with type I diabetes

The multiple codes fully describe the diagnostic statement. The Guideline directs you to place the etiology code first, followed by the manifestation code.

Let's review another example of multiple coding.

MULTIPLE CODING (ALSO KNOWN AS DUAL CODING)

Example 2

Diagnosis: Staphylococcal cellulitis of the face

(Staphylococcal infection is the etiology and cellulitis is the manifestation.)

Index: **Cellulitis,** face (any part, except eye) 682.0

Tabular: **682 Other cellulitis and abscess**

                   682.0 Face

Code: 682.0 Cellulitis of the face

You now must identify the code for the etiology (staphylococcal).

Index: **Infection,** staphylococcal NEC 041.10

Tabular: **041 Bacterial infection in conditions classified elsewhere and of unspecified site**

                   Note: This category is to be used as an additional code to identify the bacterial agent in diseases classified elsewhere. This category is also used to classify bacterial infections of unspecified nature or site.

                   041.1 Staphylococcus

                      041.10 Staphylococcus, unspecified

Codes: 682.0, 041.10 Staphylococcal cellulitis of the face

Note that it is acceptable to sequence the manifestation code first in this example because code 682.0 is not italicized in the Tabular, and the instructional notation listed under category 682 in the Tabular specifically states, "Use additional code to identify organism…"

QUICK CHECK 4-2

1. When verifying 682.0 in the Tabular, what note(s) pertaining to infections is stated?

   _____

2. In Question 1, is 041.1 a valid code (one that you would report)? Yes or No?

EXERCISE 4-3 *Multiple Coding*

Using multiple codes, fill in the codes for the following diagnoses:

1 Chronic prostatitis due to *Streptococcus*

    ICD-9-CM Codes: _____, _____

2 Acute bronchitis due to *Pseudomonas*

    ICD-9-CM Codes: _____, _____

3 Gangrene due to diabetes mellitus, type I, not stated as uncontrolled

    ICD-9-CM Codes: _____, _____

4 Urinary tract infection due to *Escherichia coli*

    ⊗ ICD-9-CM Code(s): _____

5 Amyloid cardiomyopathy

    ⊗ ICD-9-CM Code(s): _____

ACUTE AND CHRONIC

ICD-9-CM OFFICIAL GUIDELINES FOR CODING AND REPORTING

SECTION I.B.

10. Acute and Chronic Conditions

If the same condition is described as both acute (subacute) and chronic, and separate subentries exist in the Alphabetic Index at the same indentation level, code both and sequence the acute (subacute) code first.

See Fig. 4–1 for the format of acute pancreatitis and chronic pancreatitis. Both acute and chronic forms of pancreatitis are subcategorized under code 577. Acute pancreatitis is 577.0 and chronic pancreatitis is 577.1. If the same condition is described as acute and chronic pancreatitis, and occur at the same indentation level in the Alphabetic Index two codes are required and the acute code is listed first.

FIGURE 4–1 Indent level of acute and chronic. (Modified from Buck CJ: *2010 ICD-9-CM, Volumes 1, 2, & 3, Professional Edition,* St. Louis, 2010, Saunders.)

577.0 Acute pancreatitis
    Abscess of pancreas
    Necrosis of pancreas:
      acute
      infective
    Pancreatitis:
      NOS
      acute (recurrent)
      apoplectic
      hemorrhagic
      subacute
      suppurative
    Excludes *mumps pancreatitis (072.3)*

577.1 Chronic pancreatitis
    Chronic pancreatitis: Pancreatitis:
      NOS   painless
      infectious   recurrent
      interstitial   relapsing

ACUTE AND CHRONIC CONDITIONS

Example 1

Diagnosis: Acute and chronic thyroiditis

Index: **Thyroiditis**

        acute 245.0

        chronic 245.8

Note that acute and chronic are at the same indention level in the Index and Guideline Section I.B.10. directed the coder to sequence the acute code first, followed by the chronic code if both conditions were being reported.

Tabular: **245 Thyroiditis**

        245.0 Acute thyroiditis

        245.8 Other and unspecified chronic thyroiditis

Sequence: 245.0, 245.8 Acute and chronic thyroiditis

Note that the acute form of thyroiditis is sequenced before the chronic form, as directed by Section I.B.10. Guideline.

ACUTE AND CHRONIC CONDITIONS

Example 2

Diagnosis: Acute and chronic pericarditis

Index: **Pericarditis**

        acute 420.90

        chronic 423.8

Tabular: **420 Acute pericarditis**

        420.9 Other and unspecified acute pericarditis

          420.90 Acute pericarditis, unspecified

Tabular: **423 Other diseases of pericardium**

        423.8 Other specified diseases of the pericardium

Sequence: 420.90, 423.8 Acute and chronic pericarditis

Note that while the Index directs you to code 423.8 for chronic pericarditis, when the Tabular is verified, there is no mention of chronic pericarditis. This is an example of a common coding situation in which you must trust the Index to have more descriptive terms than the Tabular. When the condition is both acute and chronic, and both acute and chronic are listed in the Index as separate entries and at the same indentation level, both codes are assigned and the code for acute is sequenced *first*.

COMBINATION CODES

ICD-9-CM OFFICIAL GUIDELINES FOR CODING AND REPORTING

SECTION I.B.

11. Combination Code

A combination code is a single code used to classify:
Two diagnoses, or
A diagnosis with an associated secondary process (manifestation)
A diagnosis with an associated complication

Combination codes are identified by referring to subterm entries in the Alphabetic Index and by reading the inclusion and exclusion notes in the Tabular List.

Assign only the combination code when that code fully identifies the diagnostic conditions involved or when the Alphabetic Index so directs. Multiple coding should not be used when the classification provides a combination code that clearly identifies all of the elements documented in the diagnosis. When the combination code lacks necessary specificity in describing the manifestation or complication, an additional code should be used as a secondary code.

COMBINATION CODES

Example 1

Diagnosis: Acute cholecystitis with cholelithiasis

Index: **Cholecystitis** with calculus (stones in the gallbladder) directs you to *See* Cholelithiasis

Index: **Cholelithiasis** with, cholecystitis, acute 574.0

Tabular: **574 Cholelithiasis**

574.0 Calculus of gallbladder with acute cholecystitis

A fifth-digit subclassification is indicated as 0 for a case without mention of obstruction and as 1 when there is obstruction. There was no mention of obstruction in this case, so assign the fifth digit 0.

Code: 574.00 Acute cholecystitis with cholelithiasis

The single code 574.00 fully describes the diagnosis of acute cholecystitis with cholelithiasis.

COMBINATION CODES

Example 2

Another example of a diagnosis (streptococcal) and manifestation (pharyngitis or sore throat) reported with a combination code is as follows:

Diagnosis: Streptococcal pharyngitis

Index: **Pharyngitis**, streptococcal 034.0

Tabular: **034 Streptococcal sore throat and scarlet fever**

034.0 Streptococcal sore throat

Septic:	Streptococcal:
angina	angina
sore throat	laryngitis
	pharyngitis
	tonsillitis

The single code 034.0 fully describes the diagnosis of streptococcal pharyngitis.

Code: 034.0 Streptococcal pharyngitis

EXERCISE 4-4 *Combination Codes*

Assign combination codes to the following:

1 Pneumonia due to *Hemophilus influenzae*

ICD-9-CM Code: _____

2 Candidiasis of the mouth (thrush)

ICD-9-CM Code: _____

3 Enteritis due to *Clostridium difficile*

ICD-9-CM Code: _____

4 Gastroenteritis due to *Salmonella*

ICD-9-CM Code: _____

5 Closed fracture of the tibia and fibula

ICD-9-CM Code: _____

LATE EFFECTS Late effects codes are not assigned to a separate chapter in the Tabular. Instead, you must first identify a case as a late effect and then code it as such. You report late effects codes when the acute phase of the illness or injury has passed but a residual remains. Sometimes an acute illness or injury leaves a patient with a residual health problem that remains after the illness or injury has resolved. The **residual** is coded **first** and **then** the **late effects** code is assigned to indicate the cause of the residual. An example would be scars (residual) that remain after a severe burn (cause).

In most instances, two codes will be assigned—one code for the residual that is being treated and one code that indicates the late effect. There is no time limit for the development of a residual. It may be evident at the time of the acute illness or it may occur months after an injury. It is also possible that a patient may develop more than one residual. For example, a patient who has had a stroke may develop right-sided hemiparesis (paralysis of one side) and aphasia (loss of ability to communicate).

A person cannot have a current hip fracture (820.8) and a late effect of hip fracture (905.3) at the same time. The code is either a current injury or a condition caused by a prior injury. It cannot be both. The only exception to this rule is in category 438, Late effects of cerebrovascular disease; this is explained in the following Guideline.

ICD-9-CM OFFICIAL GUIDELINES FOR CODING AND REPORTING

SECTION I.B.
12. Late Effects

A late effect is the residual effect (condition produced) after the acute phase of an illness or injury has terminated. There is no time limit on when a late effect code can be used. The residual may be apparent early, such as in cerebrovascular accident cases, or it may occur months or years later, such as that due to a previous injury. Coding of late effects generally requires two codes sequenced in the following order: The condition or nature of the late effect is sequenced first. The late effect code is sequenced second.

An exception to the above guidelines are those instances where the code for late effect is followed by a manifestation code identified in the Tabular List and title, or the late effect code has been expanded (at the fourth and fifth-digit levels) to include the manifestation(s). The code for the acute phase of an illness or injury that led to the late effect is never used with a code for the late effect.

The late effects codes are accessed in the Index under the main term "Late."

ICD-9-CM OFFICIAL GUIDELINES FOR CODING AND REPORTING

SECTION I.C.7.
d. **Late Effects of Cerebrovascular Disease**

(1) **Category 438, Late Effects of Cerebrovascular disease**
Category 438 is used to indicate conditions classifiable to categories 430-437 as the causes of late effects (neurologic deficits), themselves classified elsewhere. These "late effects" include neurologic deficits that persist after initial onset of conditions classifiable to 430-437. The neurologic deficits caused by cerebrovascular disease may be present from the onset or may arise at any time after the onset of the condition classifiable to 430-437.

(2) **Codes from category 438 with codes from 430-437**
Codes from category 438 may be assigned on a health care record with codes from 430-437, if the patient has a current cerebrovascular accident (CVA) and deficits from an old CVA

(3) **Code V12.54**
Assign code V12.54, Transient ischemic attack (TIA), and cerebral infarction without residual deficits (and not a code from category 438) as an additional code for history of cerebrovascular disease when no neurologic deficits are present.

RESIDUAL AND CAUSE

Example

Diagnosis: Aphasia due to a previous cerebrovascular accident

Residual: Aphasia

The aphasia is a condition that remains following the acute illness of the cerebrovascular accident.

Cause: Cerebrovascular accident

This patient had a previous cerebrovascular accident.

Terms to code: Aphasia [residual]

Cerebrovascular accident [cause]

The late effect of cerebrovascular accident is reported with a combination code. Locate the terms "Late, effect, cerebrovascular disease, with aphasia" in the Index of the ICD-9-CM and you will be directed to 438.11, which reports both the residual and the cause in one combination code.

EXERCISE 4-5 *Residual and Cause*

Write the term(s) that represent the residual and the cause terms on the lines provided:

1 Scars of the face resulting from third-degree burns suffered 1 year ago

Residual: _____

Cause: _____

2 Constrictive pericarditis due to old tuberculosis infection

Residual: _____

Cause: _____

3 Residual foreign body in femur due to gunshot injury years ago

Residual: _____

Cause: _____

4 Mental retardation due to previous poliomyelitis

Residual: _____

Cause: _____

5 Leg pain resulting from old fracture of femur

Residual: _____

Cause: _____

To locate the late effects codes in the Index of the ICD-9-CM, use the entry "Late, effects." There are numerous subterms that describe the various late effects. Review and become familiar with the late effects subterms in the Index.

Assign the code for the acute injury or disease first; then refer to the Index "Late, effects" for that injury or disease. Next, reference the Tabular to ensure the codes are correct and assign any further digits indicated.

EXERCISE 4-6 *Residual and Cause Codes*

Identify the residual and cause terms and then code the following:

1 Traumatic arthritis following fracture of the left ankle 3 years ago

Residual: _____

Code: _____

Cause: _____

Code: _____

2 Dysphasia due to cerebrovascular accident 6 months ago (requires one combination code)

Residual: _____

Cause: _____

Code: _____

3 Sensorineural deafness due to previous meningitis

Residual: _____

Code: _____

Cause: _____

Code: _____

IMPENDING OR THREATENED CONDITION

ICD-9-CM OFFICIAL GUIDELINES FOR CODING AND REPORTING

SECTION I.B.

13. Impending or Threatened Condition

Code any condition described at the time of discharge as "impending" or "threatened" as follows:

If it did occur, code as confirmed diagnosis.

If it did not occur, reference the Alphabetic Index to determine if the condition has a subentry term for "impending" or "threatened" and also reference main term entries for "Impending" and for "Threatened."

If the subterms are listed, assign the given code.

If the subterms are not listed, code the existing underlying condition(s) and not the condition described as impending or threatened.

IMPENDING OR THREATENED CONDITION

Example 1

Diagnosis: Threatened abortion

Index: **Threatened**, abortion 640.0

Tabular: **640 Hemorrhage in early pregnancy**

               640.0 Threatened abortion

Code: 640.03 Threatened abortion

Fifth-digit 3 indicates an antepartum condition or complication

---

IMPENDING OR THREATENED CONDITION

Example 2

Diagnosis: Impending myocardial infarction

Index: **Impending**, myocardial infarction 411.1

Tabular: **411 Other acute and subacute forms of ischemic heart disease**

               411.1 Intermediate coronary syndrome

                        Impending infarction

                        Preinfarction angina

                        Preinfarction syndrome

                        Unstable angina

Code: 411.1 Impending myocardial infarction

If the infarction had occurred, you would have reported it as a confirmed diagnosis by coding myocardial infarction (with the appropriate fifth digit to denote the episode of care).

EXERCISE 4-7   *Uncertain and Impending/Threatened Condition*

Assign codes for the following:

1 Evolving stroke

    ICD-9-CM Code: _____

2 Impending delirium tremens

    ICD-9-CM Code: _____

3 Threatened miscarriage

    ICD-9-CM Code: _____

4 Threatened labor

    ICD-9-CM Code: _____

5 Impending coronary syndrome

    ICD-9-CM Code: _____

CHAPTER REVIEW

CHAPTER 4, PART I, THEORY

Without the use of reference material, answer the following:

1 List two of the four cooperating parties that agree on coding principles:

_____

_____

2 Fill in the missing words in the Steps to Accurate Coding:

1. Identify the main _____ in the diagnostic statement.

2. Locate the main term(s) in the Alphabetic Index (Volume _____).

3. Review any _____ under the main term in the index.

4. Follow any _____-_____ instructions, such as *see also.*

5. Verify the code(s) selected from the Index (Volume _____) in the Tabular List (Volume _____) (referred to in this text as the Tabular).

6. Refer to any instructional notations in the _____.

7. Assign codes to the highest level of _____. For example, if a fourth digit is available, you cannot assign only a three-digit code, and if a fifth digit is available, you cannot assign only a four-digit code.

8. Code the diagnosis until all _____ are completely identified.

3 A combination code is a single code used to classify:

a. two diagnoses
b. a diagnosis with an associated manifestation
c. a diagnosis with an associated complication
d. all of the above

4 Additional signs and symptoms that may not routinely be associated with the disease process being reported should be coded when present.

True   False

5 In the outpatient setting, an impending condition should be coded as if it actually exists.

True   False

6 When separate codes exist to identify acute and chronic conditions, the chronic code is sequenced first.

True   False

7 It is acceptable to use only the Alphabetic Index to assign ICD-9-CM codes.

True   False

8 When sequencing codes for residuals and late effects, the residual is sequenced first followed by a late effect code.

True   False

9 A code is invalid if it has not been coded to the full number of digits available for that code.

True   False

10 The Official Guidelines for Coding and Reporting are updated annually.

True   False

CHAPTER 4, PART II, PRACTICAL

List the following:

11 List two common symptoms associated with kidney stones.

_____

12 List two common symptoms associated with pneumonia.

_____

Assign ICD-9-CM codes to the following diagnoses:

13 Acute and chronic prostatitis

ICD-9-CM Code(s): _____,

_____

14 Headache, stiff neck, and fever due to viral meningitis

ICD-9-CM Code: _____

15 Acute and chronic pyelonephritis

ICD-9-CM Code(s): _____,

_____

16 Abdominal pain due to acute and chronic cholecystitis

ICD-9-CM Code: _____

17 Urinary tract infection due to *proteus mirabilis*

ICD-9-CM Code(s): _____

18 Impending cerebrovascular accident

ICD-9-CM Code(s): _____

19 Traumatic arthritis wrist due to fracture 5 years ago

ICD-9-CM Code(s): _____

20 Dysphagia due to previous cerebrovascular accident

ICD-9-CM Code(s): _____

21 What is the code for respiratory syncytial virus (RSV)?

ICD-9-CM Code: _____

QUICK CHECK ANSWERS

QUICK CHECK 4-1
1. The presence and location of the Official Guidelines for Coding and Reporting may vary depending on the publisher of the ICD-9-CM manual and some do not include them at all.

QUICK CHECK 4-2
1. There is an instructional note to use an additional code to identify organism, such as Staphylococcus (041.1).
2. No, the fifth digit is missing.

"It is necessary to set yourself apart, to demonstrate a level of professionalism, to ensure your employer that you see coding as a career, rather than just a job. It serves to prove your proficiency and makes you more marketable."

Debbi Miller, RNC, BSN, CPC
Manager, Revenue Integrity
LifePoint Hospitals, Inc.
Brentwood, Tennessee

Chapter-Specific Guidelines (ICD-9-CM Chapters 1-8)

Chapter Topics

Infectious and Parasitic Diseases

Neoplasms

Endocrine, Nutritional, and Metabolic Diseases and Immunity Disorders

Diseases of the Blood and Blood-Forming Organs

Mental Disorders

Diseases of the Nervous System and Sense Organs

Diseases of the Circulatory System

Diseases of the Respiratory System

Chapter Review

Quick Check Answers

Learning Objectives

After completing this chapter you should be able to

1   Review infectious and parasitic disease codes.

2   Analyze the neoplasms codes.

3   Examine the endocrine, nutritional, metabolic diseases, and immunity disorders codes.

4   Review the blood conditions, mental disorders, nervous system, and sense organs codes.

5   Review the circulatory system codes.

6   Review the respiratory system codes.

Make sure to check
evolve
learning system
for the latest content updates

INFECTIOUS AND PARASITIC DISEASES

Chapter 1 in the ICD-9-CM Tabular is Infectious and Parasitic Diseases that classifies diseases according to the etiology, or cause, of the disease. Because infectious and parasitic conditions can affect various parts of the body, the chapter contains a wide variety of codes.

In this chapter there are many instances of combination coding and multiple coding. Remember: **Combination coding** applies when one code fully describes the condition. **Multiple coding** applies when it takes more than one code to fully describe the condition and then sequencing of multiple codes may have to be considered.

From the Trenches

"Always follow the coding guidelines! 'If it's not documented, it wasn't done' is a familiar phrase among coding professionals."

DEBBI

Examples

COMBINATION CODING

Diagnosis:	Candidiasis infection of the mouth
Index:	**Candidiasis,** candidal, mouth 112.0
Tabular:	**112.0 Candidiasis of mouth**
Code:	112.0 Candidiasis infection of the mouth

Code 112.0 fully describes the diagnosis.

MULTIPLE CODING

Diagnosis:	Urinary tract infection due to *Escherichia coli (E. coli)*
Index:	**Infection,** infected, infective; urinary (tract) NEC 599.0
Tabular:	**599.0 Urinary tract infection, site not specified**
	Use additional code to identify organism, such as *Escherichia coli [E. coli]* (041.4)

Code 599.0 does not fully describe the condition. The instructions in the Tabular for code 599.0 state that you are to also code the organism causing the urinary tract infection. To locate a causative organism, you locate the main term "Infection" in the Index and then the subterm of the specific organism, which in the example is *Escherichia coli.* The urinary tract infection is sequenced first, followed by the bacterial organism.

Index:	**Infection,** infected, infective, Escherichia coli NEC 041.4
Tabular:	**041 Bacterial infection in conditions classified elsewhere and of unspecified site**
	041.4 Escherichia coli [E. coli]
Codes:	599.0, 041.4 Urinary tract infection due to *Escherichia coli (E. coli)*

Multiple coding is necessary to fully describe the infection of the urinary tract and the causative organism, *E. coli.*

Human Immunodeficiency

Another important category in Chapter 1 is 042 Human Immunodeficiency Virus (HIV) Disease. Review the guidelines for HIV codes.

ICD-9-CM OFFICIAL GUIDELINES FOR CODING AND REPORTING

SECTION I.C.1.

a. Human Immunodeficiency Virus (HIV) Infections

1) **Code only confirmed cases**

   Code only confirmed cases of HIV infection/illness. This is an exception to the hospital inpatient guideline Section II, H.

   In this context, "confirmation" does not require documentation of positive serology or culture for HIV; the provider's diagnostic statement that the patient is HIV positive, or has an HIV-related illness is sufficient.

2) **Selection and sequencing of HIV code**

   (a) **Patient admitted for HIV-related condition**

   If a patient is admitted for an HIV-related condition, the principal diagnosis should be 042, followed by additional diagnosis codes for all reported HIV-related conditions.

   (b) **Patient with HIV disease admitted for unrelated condition**

   If a patient with HIV disease is admitted for an unrelated condition (such as a traumatic injury), the code for the unrelated condition (e.g., the nature of injury code) should be the principal diagnosis. Other diagnoses would be 042 followed by additional diagnosis codes for all reported HIV-related conditions.

   (c) **Whether the patient is newly diagnosed**

   Whether the patient is newly diagnosed or has had previous admissions/encounters for HIV conditions is irrelevant to the sequencing decision.

   (d) **Asymptomatic human immunodeficiency virus**

   V08 Asymptomatic human immunodeficiency virus [HIV] infection, is to be applied when the patient without any documentation of symptoms is listed as being "HIV positive," "known HIV," "HIV test positive," or similar terminology. Do not use this code if the term "AIDS" is used or if the patient is treated for any HIV-related illness or is described as having any condition(s) resulting from his/her HIV positive status; use 042 in these cases.

   (e) **Patients with inconclusive HIV serology**

   Patients with inconclusive HIV serology, but no definitive diagnosis or manifestations of the illness, may be assigned code 795.71, Inconclusive serologic test for Human Immunodeficiency Virus [HIV].

   (f) **Previously diagnosed HIV-related illness**

   Patients with any known prior diagnosis of an HIV-related illness should be coded to 042. Once a patient has developed an HIV-related illness, the patient should always be assigned code 042 on every subsequent admission/encounter. Patients previously diagnosed with any HIV illness (042) should never be assigned to 795.71 or V08.

   (g) **HIV Infection in Pregnancy, Childbirth and the Puerperium**

   During pregnancy, childbirth or the puerperium, a patient admitted (or presenting for a health care encounter) because of an HIV-related illness should receive a principal diagnosis of 647.6X, Other specified infectious and parasitic diseases in the mother classifiable elsewhere, but complicating the pregnancy, childbirth or the puerperium, followed by 042 and the code(s) for the HIV-related illness(es). Codes from Chapter 15 always take sequencing priority.

Patients with asymptomatic HIV infection status admitted (or presenting for a health care encounter) during pregnancy, childbirth, or the puerperium should receive codes of 647.6X and V08.

(h) **Encounters for testing for HIV**

If a patient is being seen to determine his/her HIV status, use code V73.89, Screening for other specified viral disease. Use code V69.8, Other problems related to lifestyle, as a secondary code if an asymptomatic patient is in a known high risk group for HIV. Should a patient with signs or symptoms or illness, or a confirmed HIV related diagnosis be tested for HIV, code the signs and symptoms or the diagnosis. An additional counseling code V65.44 may be used if counseling is provided during the encounter for the test.

When a patient returns to be informed of his/her HIV test results use code V65.44, HIV counseling, if the results of the test are negative.

If the results are positive but the patient is asymptomatic use code V08, Asymptomatic HIV infection. If the results are positive and the patient is symptomatic use code 042, HIV infection, with codes for the HIV related symptoms or diagnosis. The HIV counseling code may also be used if counseling is provided for patients with positive test results.

As stated in Guideline Section I.C.1., you do not assign 042 to a patient's record or insurance claim unless the diagnosis of AIDS is a **confirmed** diagnosis. The assignment of the code prior to confirmation may cause the patient many unwarranted problems if the patient does not have HIV. Use extreme caution when assigning 042.

> ✋ **CAUTION** *This statement is **very** important. You are **never** to code HIV unless you are certain of the diagnosis. This diagnosis stays in the patient's record forever!*

EXERCISE 5-1 *Infectious and Parasitic Diseases*

Code the following infectious diseases:

1 Viral gastroenteritis

   ICD-9-CM Code: _____

2 Septicemia due to *Pseudomonas* with septic shock

   ICD-9-CM Codes: _____, _____, _____

3 Acute poliomyelitis

   ICD-9-CM Code: _____

4 Candidal vaginal infection

   ICD-9-CM Code: _____

NEOPLASMS   Chapter 2 in the Tabular of the ICD-9-CM is similar to Chapter 1, Infectious and Parasitic Diseases, in that it classifies diseases according to the etiology, or cause, of the disease. Neoplastic conditions can affect all parts of the body. Before you learn more about what is in Chapter 2, you will review some of the specific terminology by completing the following exercise.

EXERCISE 5-2 *Neoplasms Terminology*

Match the following terms to the correct definitions:

1 neoplasm _____

2 malignant _____

3 primary _____

4 secondary _____

5 benign _____

6 in situ _____

7 uncertain behavior _____

8 unspecified nature _____

9 morphology _____

a. not usually progressive

b. malignancy that is located within the original site of development

c. used to describe a cancerous tumor that grows worse over time

d. study of neoplasms

e. refers to the behavior of a neoplasm as neither malignant nor benign but having characteristics of both malignant and benign neoplasms

f. when the behavior or histology of a neoplasm is not known or not specified

g. site to which a malignant tumor has spread

h. site of origin or where the tumor originated

i. new tumor growth that can be benign or malignant

Neoplasm Codes

Neoplasms are **staged,** which means that they are evaluated for placement on a common grading scale based on the level of invasion. For example, staging for endometrial, cervical, and ovarian malignancies is staged based on if the malignancy (I) is confined to corpus, (II) involves corpus and cervix, (III) extends outside uterus but not outside true pelvis, (IV) extends outside true pelvis or involves rectum or bladder or staging for renal cancer staged on Stage I tumor of kidney capsule only, Stage II tumor invading renal capsule/vein but within fascia, Stage III tumor extending to regional lymph/vena cava, or Stage IV other organ metastasis. The pathology report and staging information will be documented in the medical record.

To assign a diagnosis code to a neoplasm is a two-step process:

1. First, locate the morphology or histologic type of the neoplasm in the Index of the ICD-9-CM. Examples of histology types are carcinoma, adenocarcinoma, sarcoma, melanoma, lymphoma, lipoma, adenoma.

2. Once you have located the morphology, review all modifiers and subterms, and then follow the instructions or verify the code listed. Most often you will be instructed to reference the Neoplasm Table in the Index to locate the code, as illustrated in Fig. 5–1.

Although M codes are not assigned in the outpatient setting, M Codes are still important because the information will assist you in learning about how neoplasms are classified. In addition, there are coding employees whose job it is to classify neoplasms based on the medical documentation. So a basic knowledge of M codes is important. Mostly, M codes are assigned by the tumor registrar (the person who records morphology information). M codes are not required on insurance forms, but you will see them throughout the Index.

M codes are alphanumeric codes and are listed in Appendix A of the ICD-9-CM manual. The alphanumeric structure of the morphology codes starts with the letter M (for morphology), followed by four digits that indicate the histologic type of neoplasm, and a slash, followed by a fifth digit that indicates the behavior.

| Neoplasm (Continued) | Malignant | | | | | |
	Primary	Secondary	Ca in situ	Benign	Uncertain Behavior	Unspecified
jaw (Continued)						
carcinoma (any type) (lower) (upper)	195.0	—	—	—	—	—
skin	173.3	198.2	232.3	216.3	238.2	239.2
soft tissues	143.9	198.89	230.0	210.4	235.1	239.0
lower	143.1	198.89	230.0	210.4	235.1	239.0
upper	143.0	198.89	230.0	210.4	235.1	239.0
jejunum	152.1	197.4	230.7	211.2	235.2	239.0
joint NEC (see also Neoplasm, bone)	170.9	198.5	—	213.9	238.0	239.2
acromioclavicular	170.4	198.5	—	213.4	238.0	239.2
bursa or synovial membrane - see Neoplasm, connective tissue						
costovertebral	170.3	198.5	—	213.3	238.0	239.2
sternocostal	170.3	198.5	—	213.3	238.0	239.2
temporomandibular	170.1	198.5	—	213.1	238.0	239.2
junction						
anorectal	154.8	197.5	230.7	211.4	235.5	239.0
cardioesophageal	151.0	197.8	230.2	211.1	235.2	239.0
esophagogastric	151.0	197.8	230.2	211.1	235.2	239.0
gastroesophageal	151.0	197.8	230.2	211.1	235.2	239.0
hard and soft palate	145.5	198.89	230.0	210.4	235.1	239.0
ileocecal	153.4	197.5	230.3	211.3	235.2	239.0
pelvirectal	154.0	197.5	230.4	211.4	235.2	239.0

FIGURE 5–1 Neoplasm Table. (Modified from Buck CJ: *2009 ICD-9-CM, Volumes 1, 2, & 3, Professional Edition*, St. Louis, 2009, Saunders.)

Behavior Indicated by Fifth Digit

/0 = Benign

/1 = Uncertain whether benign or malignant
Borderline malignancy

/2 = Carcinoma in situ
Intraepithelial
Noninfiltrating
Noninvasive

/3 = Malignant, primary site

/6 = Malignant, metastatic site
Secondary site

/9 = Malignant, uncertain whether primary or metastatic site

The following example shows how the morphology codes are assigned.

ICD-9-CM CODES AND MORPHOLOGY CODES

Example

Diagnosis: Adenocarcinoma of the upper-outer quadrant right breast with metastasis to the axillary lymph nodes

Index: **Adenocarcinoma** (M8140/3)—*see also* Neoplasm, by site, malignant

Neoplasm Table: Breast, upper-outer quadrant, 174.4 (Primary column)

Lymph-, lymphatic, gland (Secondary column), axilla, axillary, 196.3

Tabular: **174 Malignant neoplasm of female breast**

174.4 Upper-outer quadrant

196 Secondary and unspecified malignant neoplasm of lymph nodes

196.3 Lymph nodes of axilla and upper limb

Codes: 174.4, 196.3 Adenocarcinoma of the upper-outer quadrant right breast with metastasis to the axillary lymph nodes

But wait, you're not finished yet. You have two M codes to assign to this diagnosis before you are finished—one for the primary adenocarcinoma and one for a secondary adenocarcinoma. Both M codes will have the same histologic type of adenocarcinoma, but the fifth digit will be different to indicate the primary and secondary behaviors.

Index: **Adeno-carcinoma** (M8140/3)—*see also* Neoplasm, by site, malignant

M code: **Primary** adenocarcinoma of the breast, M8140/3 (3 indicates primary site)

M code: **Secondary** adenocarcinoma of the axillary lymph nodes, M8140/6 (6 indicates secondary site)

ICD-9-CM and M Codes: 174.4, M8140/3, 196.3, M8140/6 Adenocarcinoma of the upper-outer quadrant right breast with metastasis to the axillary lymph nodes

Note that the M codes are sequenced after the ICD-9-CM diagnosis code to which they refer.

The Guidelines provide the following information regarding reporting neoplasms:

ICD-9-CM OFFICIAL GUIDELINES FOR CODING AND REPORTING

SECTION I.C.

2. Chapter 2: Neoplasms (140-239)

General guidelines

Chapter 2 of the ICD-9-CM contains the codes for most benign and all malignant neoplasms. Certain benign neoplasms, such as prostatic adenomas, may be found in the specific body system chapters. To properly code a neoplasm it is necessary to determine from the record if the neoplasm is benign, in situ, malignant, or of uncertain histologic behavior. If malignant, any secondary (metastatic) sites should also be determined.

The neoplasm table in the Alphabetic Index should be referenced first. However, if the histological term is documented, that term should be referenced first, rather than going immediately to the Neoplasm Table, in order to determine which column in the Neoplasm Table is appropriate. For example, if the documentation indicates "adenoma," refer to the term in the Alphabetic Index to review the entries under this term and the instructional note to "see also neoplasm, by site, benign." The table provides the proper code based on the type of neoplasm and the site. It is important to select the proper column in the table that corresponds to the type of neoplasm. The tabular should then be referenced to verify that the correct code has been selected from the table and that a more specific site code does not exist.

See Section I.C.18.d.4. for information regarding V codes for genetic susceptibility to cancer.

a. Treatment directed at the malignancy

If the treatment is directed at the malignancy, designate the malignancy as the principal diagnosis.

The only exception to this guideline is if a patient admission/encounter is solely for the administration of chemotherapy, immunotherapy or radiation therapy, assign the appropriate V58.X code as the first-listed or principal diagnosis, and the diagnosis or problem for which the service is being performed as a secondary diagnosis.

b. **Treatment of secondary site**

When a patient is admitted because of a primary neoplasm with metastasis and treatment is directed toward the secondary site only, the secondary neoplasm is designated as the principal diagnosis even though the primary malignancy is still present

c. **Coding and sequencing of complications**

Coding and sequencing of complications associated with the malignancies or with the therapy thereof are subject to the following guidelines:

1) **Anemia associated with malignancy**

When admission/encounter is for management of an anemia associated with the malignancy, and the treatment is only for anemia, the appropriate anemia code (such as code 285.22, Anemia in neoplastic disease) is designated as the principal diagnosis and is followed by the appropriate code(s) for the malignancy.

Code 285.22 may also be used as a secondary code if the patient suffers from anemia and is being treated for the malignancy.

Code 285.22, Anemia in neoplastic disease, and code 285.3, Antineoplastic chemotherapy induced anemia, may both be assigned if anemia in neoplastic disease and anemia due to antineoplastic chemotherapy are both documented.

2) **Anemia associated with chemotherapy, immunotherapy and radiation therapy**

When the admission/encounter is for management of an anemia associated with chemotherapy, immunotherapy or radiotherapy and the only treatment is for the anemia, the anemia is sequenced first. The appropriate neoplasm code should be assigned as an additional code.

3) **Management of dehydration due to the malignancy**

When the admission/encounter is for management of dehydration due to the malignancy or the therapy, or a combination of both, and only the dehydration is being treated (intravenous rehydration), the dehydration is sequenced first, followed by the code(s) for the malignancy.

4) **Treatment of a complication resulting from a surgical procedure**

When the admission/encounter is for treatment of a complication resulting from a surgical procedure, designate the complication as the principal or first-listed diagnosis if treatment is directed at resolving the complication.

d. **Primary malignancy previously excised**

When a primary malignancy has been previously excised or eradicated from its site and there is no further treatment directed to that site and there is no evidence of any existing primary malignancy, a code from category V10, Personal history of malignant neoplasm, should be used to indicate the former site of the malignancy. Any mention of extension, invasion, or metastasis to another site is coded as a secondary malignant neoplasm to that site. The secondary site may be the principal or first-listed with the V10 code used as a secondary code.

e. **Admission/Encounters involving chemotherapy, immunotherapy and radiation therapy**

1) **Episode of care involves surgical removal of neoplasm**

When an episode of care involves the surgical removal of a neoplasm, primary or secondary site, followed by adjunct chemotherapy or radiation treatment during the same episode of care, the neoplasm code should be assigned as principal or first-listed diagnosis, using codes in the 140-198 series or where appropriate in the 200-203 series.

2) **Patient admission/encounter solely for administration of chemotherapy, immunotherapy and radiation therapy**

If a patient admission/encounter is solely for the administration of chemotherapy, immunotherapy or radiation therapy assign code V58.0, Encounter for radiation therapy, or V58.11, Encounter for antineoplastic chemotherapy, or V58.12, Encounter for antineoplastic immunotherapy as the first-listed or principal diagnosis. If a patient receives more than one of these therapies during the same admission more than one of these codes may be assigned, in any sequence.

The malignancy for which therapy is being administered should be assigned as a secondary diagnosis.

3) **Patient admitted for radiotherapy/chemotherapy and immunotherapy and develops complications**

When a patient is admitted for the purpose of radiotherapy, immunotherapy or chemotherapy and develops complications such as uncontrolled nausea and vomiting or dehydration, the principal or first-listed diagnosis is V58.0, Encounter for radiotherapy, or V58.11, Encounter for antineoplastic chemotherapy, or V58.12, Encounter for antineoplastic immunotherapy, followed by any codes for the complications.

f. **Admission/encounter to determine extent of malignancy**

When the reason for admission/encounter is to determine the extent of the malignancy, or for a procedure such as paracentesis or thoracentesis, the primary malignancy or appropriate metastatic site is designated as the principal or first-listed diagnosis, even though chemotherapy or radiotherapy is administered.

g. **Symptoms, signs, and ill-defined conditions listed in Chapter 16 associated with neoplasms**

Symptoms, signs, and ill-defined conditions listed in Chapter 16 characteristic of, or associated with, an existing primary or secondary site malignancy cannot be used to replace the malignancy as principal or first-listed diagnosis, regardless of the number of admissions or encounters for treatment and care of the neoplasm.

h. **Admission/encounter for pain control/management**

See Section I.C.6.a.5 for information on coding admission/encounter for pain control/management.

V codes are also frequently reported with neoplasms to indicate the history of a malignant neoplasm (V10.00-V10.9). These history codes are used to report a malignant neoplasm that is no longer present. Remember that in the V code section, you were presented with information about documenting a "history of" a disease. Be careful in determining whether the physician is indicating a past and current history of a condition or a true past history. With neoplasms there is often a true "history of" whereby the condition previously existed but is no longer present.

There are also encounter V codes for chemotherapy (V58.11), immunotherapy (V58.12), and radiotherapy (V58.0). When coding an encounter solely for chemotherapy, immunotherapy, or radiotherapy, place the V code first, followed by the active code for the malignant neoplasm, even if that neoplasm has already been removed. As long as the neoplasm is being treated with adjunctive therapy (another treatment used in conjunction with the primary treatment) following a surgical removal of the cancer (primary treatment), you code the neoplasm as if it still exists. You would **not** assign a "history of" V code because the neoplasm is the reason for the treatment. Instead, the neoplasm is coded as a current or active disease.

EXERCISE 5-3   *Neoplasm Codes*

Assign diagnosis codes to the following:

1 A patient is admitted for chemotherapy for ovarian cancer.

Two codes are needed for this case: one for the encounter for chemotherapy and the other for the malignant, primary, ovarian neoplasm.

> Locate the code in the Index and verify in the Tabular.
>
> ICD-9-CM Codes: _____, _____

2 A patient is admitted for radiation therapy for metastatic bone cancer. The patient had a mastectomy for breast cancer 3 years earlier.

There is a code for the admission for radiation management, which will be a V code; a code for the secondary, malignant, bone neoplasm; and a V code for the history of malignant neoplasm of the breast.

> ICD-9-CM Code(s): _____, _____, _____

3 A patient is admitted with chest pain, shortness of breath, and a history of bloody sputum. Diagnostic x-ray film shows a mass in the bronchial tube. A diagnostic bronchoscopy is performed and is positive for cancer. The pathology report states "metastatic carcinoma of bronchus, primary unknown." The patient chooses to undergo chemotherapy.

   a What is the description of the first-listed diagnosis? _____

   b What is the subsequent diagnosis description? _____

   c Is the metastatic carcinoma of the bronchus a primary or secondary malignant neoplasm?

   _____

   d What are the diagnosis codes for this case?

   > ICD-9-CM Codes: _____, _____

4 A patient is admitted with uncontrolled nausea and vomiting after chemotherapy treatment for lung cancer.

   a How many codes would be needed to accurately report this case? _____ (plus an E code)

   b What is the first-listed diagnosis? _____

   c What is the secondary diagnosis? _____

   d What is the code for the first-listed diagnosis?

   > ICD-9-CM Code: _____

   e What is the code for the secondary diagnosis and the E code?

   > ICD-9-CM Code(s): _____, _____

Unknown Site or Unspecified

There is an entry on the Neoplasm Table that states "unknown site or unspecified." This code, 199.1, is assigned to indicate either an unknown or an unspecified primary or secondary malignancy. If there is a **known** secondary site, a code must be assigned to the primary site or the history of a primary site. It is possible for the primary site to be unknown and the secondary site to be known.

QUICK CHECK 5-1

1. What entry in the Neoplasm Table reports a benign neoplasm of an unspecified site? _____

UNKNOWN PRIMARY SITE

Example

Diagnosis: Metastatic bone cancer

This statement indicates that the bone cancer is a secondary neoplasm, but there is no indication of the location of the primary site.

Index: **Cancer**—*see also* Neoplasm, by site, malignant

Neoplasm Table: Bone 198.5 (Secondary)

                 Unknown site or unspecified 199.1 (Primary)

Tabular: **198 Secondary malignant neoplasm of other specified site**

                 198.5 Bone and bone marrow

Tabular: **199 Malignant neoplasm without specification of site**

                 199.1 Other

Codes: 198.5, 199.1 Metastatic bone cancer (if the treatment is for the secondary site)

                 199.1, 198.5 Metastatic bone cancer (if the treatment or diagnostic workup is for the primary site)

The sequencing of the primary and secondary neoplasms is dependent on the treatment circumstances documented in the health record. If treatment was directed toward the secondary malignancy, the code for the secondary would be sequenced first. If treatment was focused on determining the site of the unknown primary malignancy, the code for the unknown site would be sequenced first.

EXERCISE 5-4 *More Neoplasms*

Assign ICD-9-CM codes for the following neoplasms:

1 Multiple myeloma

　　ICD-9-CM Code: _____

2 Carcinoma in situ, cervix

　　ICD-9-CM Code: _____

3 Cancer of the sigmoid colon with spread to the peritoneum

　　ICD-9-CM Codes: _____, _____

4 Adenocarcinoma of the prostate with metastasis to the bone

　　ICD-9-CM Codes: _____, _____

5 Metastatic cancer to the brain; primary unknown (treatment directed to metastatic site)

　　ICD-9-CM Codes: _____, _____

6 Metastatic carcinoma of the breast to the lungs; the breast carcinoma has been removed by mastectomy

　　ICD-9-CM Codes: _____, _____

ENDOCRINE, NUTRITIONAL, AND METABOLIC DISEASES AND IMMUNITY DISORDERS

Chapter 3 in the Tabular of the ICD-9-CM describes diseases or conditions affecting the endocrine system. The endocrine system involves glands that are located throughout the body and are responsible for secreting hormones into the bloodstream. Also included in Chapter 3 are diseases or conditions that affect nutritional and metabolic status as well as disorders of the immune system.

One of the frequently used category codes in Chapter 3 is 250, Diabetes Mellitus. When you locate diabetes in the Index, you will note that for many of the subterms, two codes are listed. The 250.XX code is followed by an italicized code in brackets. This is because multiple coding is common for diabetes because both the manifestation (symptom) and the etiology (cause—diabetes) are reported.

Example

Index:　　　　**Diabetes,** retinopathy, background, 250.5X *[362.01]*

There are four five-digit subclassifications for use with category 250. It is essential that you read these before assigning codes for diagnosis of diabetes mellitus (DM). The fifth digits identify the type of diabetes: 2 is type II or unspecified type, uncontrolled; and 3 is type I [juvenile type], uncontrolled. The health care providers usually document the type of diabetes mellitus. You should not assume that because a patient is receiving insulin that he or she is a type I diabetic because a type II diabetic may be receiving insulin. If there is any question regarding the type of diabetes, query the physician.

In order to appropriately assign the fifth digits 2 or 3, uncontrolled diabetes, the physician must document that the patient's DM is uncontrolled or out of control. If a complication is specified (250.1-250.8), assign the appropriate fourth and fifth digits; do not use the .9 (unspecified).

Example

Diagnosis: Diabetic iritis

Index: **Diabetes, diabetic, iritis 250.5 *[364.42]***

The first code (250.5) indicates the etiology (diabetes) and the second code *[364.42]* indicates the manifestation (iritis). You need two codes to describe the diagnoses. You will always list the etiology first and then the manifestation.

Tabular: **250.5 Diabetes with ophthalmic manifestations**

                Use additional code to identify manifestation, as...:

             364.4 Vascular disorders of iris and ciliary body

The Tabular also indicates that a fifth digit should be added for greater specificity.

Tabular: **364.4 Vascular disorders of iris and ciliary body**

             364.42 Rubeosis iridis

Even though the 364.42 entry does not specifically indicate iritis, you trust the code that is listed in the Index. You could also reference the main term "Iritis" in the Index and be directed to the same codes.

Index: **Iritis 364.3, diabetic 250.5 *[364.42]***

You are directed to the same codes.

Codes: 250.50, 364.42 Diabetic iritis

The codes must be sequenced in this order to indicate that the iritis is a manifestation of the diabetes.

To code a disease or condition as a manifestation of DM, it must be stated that the disease or condition is diabetic or due to the diabetes. A cause-and-effect relationship must be stated or evident. If you are unsure of the relationship, you must clarify this relationship with the physician.

If a cause-and-effect relationship is not evident or stated and no further indication of the relationship can be obtained, the following codes would be assigned.

Example

Diagnosis: Diabetes mellitus and iritis

Index: **Diabetes, diabetic 250.0**

             Note—Use the following fifth-digit subclassification with category 250:

The Note in the Index directs you to use a fifth digit for greater specificity.

Tabular: **250.0 Diabetes mellitus without mention of complication**

Index: **Iritis 364.3**

Tabular: **364.3 Unspecified iridocyclitis**

Codes: 250.00 Diabetes and 364.3 Iritis

Note that codes (250.00 and 364.3) are individual codes because a cause-and-effect relationship was not established—the iritis is not reported as a manifestation of the diabetes in this case.

EXERCISE 5-5 *Endocrine, Nutritional, and Metabolic Diseases and Immunity Disorders*

Fill in the codes for the following:

1 Addison's disease

ICD-9-CM Code: _____

2 Dehydration

ICD-9-CM Code: _____

3 Diabetes mellitus with hypoglycemic coma

ICD-9-CM Code: _____

4 Graves' disease with thyrotoxic crisis

ICD-9-CM Code: _____

DISEASES OF THE BLOOD AND BLOOD-FORMING ORGANS

Chapter 4, Diseases of the Blood and Blood-Forming Organs, in the ICD-9-CM is a short chapter with only 10 categories. The **anemia** category is often used because anemia is the most common blood disease. Anemia is the main term under which you will find the many subterms that relate to anemia. In addition to there being numerous subterms for anemia, many of those subterms have lengthy additional subterms listed under them.

There are two anemias that are easy to confuse—anemia of chronic disease and chronic simple anemia. These two diagnostic statements do not have the same meaning. In anemia of chronic disease, the word "chronic" describes the nature of the disease that is the cause of the anemia, for example, anemia due to neoplastic disease. The neoplasm is the chronic disease causing the anemia. Code anemia (285.22) and then assign the appropriate code to identify the neoplasm. In the diagnostic statement chronic, simple anemia, the word "chronic" describes simple anemia. Let's see what difference these diagnostic statements make in code assignment.

ANEMIA

Example 1

Diagnosis: Anemia of chronic disease

In this diagnosis statement, you do not know what the chronic disease is.

Index: **Anemia**

The Index has a subterm (in, chronic illness, 285.29) that further directs you in the choice of the correct code.

Tabular: **285.2 Anemia of chronic disease**

Code: 285.29 Anemia of other chronic disease

ANEMIA

Example 2

Diagnosis: Chronic simple anemia

Index: **Anemia 285.9, chronic simple 281.9**

In this example, the Index does indicate a subterm that further directs you to chronic simple 281.9.

Tabular: **281.9 Unspecified deficiency anemia**

Code: 281.9 Chronic simple anemia

If there is any question about the classification of the anemia, check with the physician.

EXERCISE 5-6   *Diseases of the Blood and Blood-Forming Organs*

Assign codes for the following:

1 Pernicious anemia

   ICD-9-CM Code: _____

2 Disseminated intravascular coagulation (DIC)

   ICD-9-CM Code: _____

3 Hemophilia

   ICD-9-CM Code: _____

4 Acute blood-loss anemia

   ICD-9-CM Code: _____

5 Familial polycythemia

   ICD-9-CM Code: _____

MENTAL DISORDERS

Chapter 5 in the Tabular of the ICD-9-CM is Mental Disorders. The chapter includes four sections: organic psychotic conditions; other psychoses; neurotic, personality, and other nonpsychotic mental disorders; and mental retardation.

Your understanding of the definitions of these mental disorders is necessary to enable you to code accurately. When assigning codes from Chapter 5, you need to take extra care to select the appropriate code(s) and report only diagnoses that are documented in the medical record. Mental disorders can be difficult to code because physicians are not always as specific in the diagnostic statements as might be required by the codes in the ICD-9-CM chapter. When in doubt, always check with the physician. Just one term in the medical record can make a big difference in the code(s) you use.

Five-Digit Subclassification

A five-digit subclassification is provided for categories 303-305 to indicate the patient's pattern of use of alcohol or drugs:

0	unspecified	
1	continuous:	Alcohol: refers to daily intake of large amounts of alcohol or regular heavy drinking on weekends or days off from work
		Drugs: daily or almost daily use of drugs
2	episodic:	Alcohol: refers to alcoholic binges lasting weeks or months, followed by long periods of sobriety
		Drugs: indicates short periods between drug use or use on weekends
3	in remission:	Refers either to a complete cessation of alcohol or drug intake or to the period during which decreasing intake leading toward cessation is taking place

CODING SHOT

You should be aware that there is a V code for history of alcoholism (V11.3). Instead of using that code you should use the **alcoholism** code (303.9x) with the fifth digit 3, which specifies in remission. It is rare to assign code V11.3 because the disease of alcoholism cannot be cured, only be in a state of remission.

Another commonly encountered instance is the instruction to "Use additional code to identify the associated neurological condition" or "Use additional code to identify cerebral atherosclerosis." Pay close attention to the instructions given in the Tabular when you see a "Use additional . . . " statement.

Example

Diagnosis: Arteriosclerotic dementia with delirium

Index: **Dementia** 294.8, arteriosclerotic (simple type) (uncomplicated) 290.40, with, delirium 290.41

Tabular: **290 Senile and presenile organic psychotic conditions**

　　　290.4 Vascular dementia

　　　　　Use additional code to identify cerebral atherosclerosis (437.0)

　　　290.41 Vascular dementia with delirium

Tabular: **437 Other and ill-defined cerebrovascular disease**

　　　437.0 Cerebral atherosclerosis

Codes: 290.41, 437.0 Arteriosclerotic dementia with delirium

According to the Guidelines, you are to sequence the etiology before the manifestation; however, if the Tabular directs the manifestation before the etiology, such as in 290, you must adhere to the Tabular direction. The "Use additional code to identify cerebral atherosclerosis (437.0)" is a direction to report the vascular dementia (290.4), which is the manifestation, before the cerebral atherosclerosis, which is the etiology.

EXERCISE 5-7 *Mental Disorders*

Now you have a chance to show your skill by coding the following:

1 Alzheimer's dementia with aggressive behavior

   ICD-9-CM Codes: _____, _____

2 Depression with anxiety

   ICD-9-CM Code: _____

3 Profound mental retardation

   🌐 ICD-9-CM Code(s): _____

4 Anorexia nervosa

   🌐 ICD-9-CM Code(s): _____

5 Delirium tremens due to chronic alcoholism, continuous

   🌐 ICD-9-CM Code(s): _____

DISEASES OF THE NERVOUS SYSTEM AND SENSE ORGANS

Chapter 6 of the Tabular ICD-9-CM is Diseases of the Nervous System and Sense Organs and describes diseases or conditions affecting the central nervous system and the peripheral nervous system. It also includes disorders and diseases of the eyes and ears.

The chapter contains some combination codes in which one code identifies both the manifestation and the etiology.

COMBINATION CODES

Example

Diagnosis: Pneumococcal meningitis

This diagnostic statement means the meningitis is due to pneumococcal bacteria.

Index: **Meningitis, pneumococcal 320.1**

Tabular: **320 Bacterial meningitis**

             320.1 Pneumococcal meningitis

Code: 320.1 Pneumococcal meningitis

Code 320.1 includes the manifestation of meningitis and also the etiology of pneumococcal organism. No separate code is required for the organism in this diagnostic statement.

In Chapter 6 of the ICD-9-CM, you will also locate conditions that are manifestations of other diseases. These categories appear in italics in the Tabular and provide instructions to code the underlying disease process first.

MANIFESTATIONS

Example

Diagnosis: Chronic iridocyclitis due to sarcoidosis

Index: **Iridocyclitis** NEC 364.3, chronic, in, sarcoidosis 135 *[364.11]*

Entries such as 135 *[364.11]* instruct you to code the sarcoidosis (135) first, followed by the chronic iridocyclitis (364.11). Both codes need to be verified in the Tabular.

Tabular: **135 Sarcoidosis**

Tabular: **364 Disorders of iris and ciliary body**

                364.11 Chronic iridocyclitis in diseases classified elsewhere

                     Code first underlying disease, as:

                            sarcoidosis (135)

                            tuberculosis (017.3)

Codes: 135, 364.11 Chronic iridocyclitis due to sarcoidosis

EXERCISE 5-8   *Diseases of the Nervous System and Sense Organs*

Assign codes for the following:

1 Meningitis due to *Proteus morganii*

    ICD-9-CM Code: _____

2 Multiple sclerosis

    ICD-9-CM Code: _____

3 Acute otitis media

    ICD-9-CM Code: _____

4 Primary open-angle glaucoma

    ICD-9-CM Code: _____

5 Bell's palsy

    ICD-9-CM Code: _____

DISEASES OF THE CIRCULATORY SYSTEM

Hypertension

Chapter 7 of the ICD-9-CM Tabular, Diseases of the Circulatory System, contains diseases of heart and blood vessels.

Hypertension is one of the most common conditions coded in this chapter. The Hypertension Table is located in the Index, as shown in Fig. 5–2. This table provides a complete listing of all conditions due to or associated with hypertension. The first column identifies the hypertensive condition, such as accelerated, antepartum, cardiovascular disease, cardiorenal, and cerebrovascular disease. The remaining three columns are Malignant, Benign, and Unspecified and constitute the subcategories of hypertensive disease.

Malignant hypertension is also known as accelerated hypertension and is a severe form of hypertension, manifested by headaches, blurred vision, dyspnea, and uremia. This type of hypertension usually causes permanent organ damage and has a poor prognosis. **Benign hypertension** is a continuous, mild blood pressure elevation that can usually be controlled

	Malignant	Benign	Unspecified
Hypertension, hypertensive (arterial) (arteriolar) (crisis) (degeneration) (disease) (essential) (fluctuating) (idiopathic) (intermittent) (labile) (low renin) (orthostatic) (paroxysmal) (primary) (systemic) (uncontrolled) (vascular)	401.0	(#1) 401.1	(#3) 401.9
with			
chronic kidney disease	—	—	—
stage I through stage IV, or unspecified	403.00	403.10	403.90
stage V or end stage renal disease	403.01	403.11	403.91
heart involvement (conditions classifiable to 429.0–429.3, 429.8, 429.9 due to hypertension) (*see also* Hypertension, heart)	402.00	402.10	402.90
with kidney involvement - *see* Hypertension, cardiorenal			
renal involvement (only conditions classifiable to 585, ~~586, 587~~) (excludes conditions classifiable to 584) (*see also* Hypertension, kidney)	403.00	403.10	403.90
with heart involvement - *see* Hypertension, cardiorenal failure (and sclerosis) (*see also* Hypertension, kidney)	403.01	403.11	(#4) 403.91
sclerosis without failure (*see also* Hypertension, kidney)	403.00	403.10	403.90
accelerated (*see also* Hypertension, by type, malignant)	401.0	—	
antepartum - *see* Hypertension, complicating pregnancy, childbirth, or the puerperium			
cardiorenal (disease)	404.00	404.10	404.90
with			
chronic kidney disease	—	—	—
stage I through stage IV, or unspecified	404.00	404.10	404.90
and heart failure	404.01	404.11	404.91
stage V or end stage renal disease	404.02	404.12	404.92
and heart failure	404.03	404.13	404.93
heart failure	404.01	404.11	404.91
and chronic kidney disease	404.01	404.11	404.91
stage I through stage IV or unspecified	404.01	404.11	404.91
stage V or end stage renal disease	404.03	404.13	404.93
cardiovascular disease (arteriosclerotic) (sclerotic)	(#2) 402.00	402.10	402.90
with			
heart failure	402.01	402.11	402.91
renal involvement (conditions classifiable to 403) (*see also* Hypertension, cardiorenal)	404.00	404.10	404.90
cardiovascular renal (disease) (sclerosis) (*see also* Hypertension, cardiorenal)	404.00	404.10	404.90

Condition

FIGURE 5–2 Hypertension Table, Index to Diseases. (Modified from Buck CJ: *2010 ICD-9-CM, Volumes 1, 2, & 3, Professional Edition,* St. Louis, 2010, Saunders.)

by medication. **Unspecified hypertension** has not been specified in the medical record as either benign or malignant.

There is no defined threshold of blood pressure above which an individual is considered hypertensive. Commonly, a sustained diastolic pressure of above 90 mm Hg and a sustained systolic pressure of above 140 mm Hg constitutes hypertension.

Benign hypertension remains fairly stable over the years and is compatible with a long life, but if untreated it is an important risk factor in coronary heart disease and cerebrovascular disease.

Malignant hypertension is commonly associated with abrupt onset and runs a course measured in months. It causes irreversible organ damage and often ends with renal failure or cerebral hemorrhage. Usually a person with malignant hypertension complains of headaches and vision difficulties and a blood pressure of 200/140 mm Hg is not uncommon.

Essential hypertension is high blood pressure for which the cause is not known.

Hypertensive heart disease refers to the secondary effects on the heart of prolonged, sustained, systemic hypertension. The heart has to work against greatly increased resistance, and that results in high blood pressure. The primary effect is the thickening of the left ventricle, which eventually may lead to heart failure.

There are two sections in this ICD-9-CM chapter that have instructions to "Use additional code to identify presence of hypertension (401-405)." The sections are Ischemic Heart Disease (410-414) and Cerebrovascular Disease (430-438). There are also a number of guidelines that pertain to hypertension or other hypertensive disease processes. Read the hypertension Guidelines that follow.

ICD-9-CM OFFICIAL GUIDELINES FOR CODING AND REPORTING

SECTION I.C.7.
a. Hypertension

Hypertension Table

The Hypertension Table, found under the main term, "Hypertension", in the Alphabetic Index, contains a complete listing of all conditions due to or associated with hypertension and classifies them according to malignant, benign, and unspecified.

1) Hypertension, Essential, or NOS

Assign hypertension (arterial) (essential) (primary) (systemic) (NOS) to category code 401 with the appropriate fourth digit to indicate malignant (.0), benign (.1), or unspecified (.9). Do not use either .0 malignant or .1 benign unless medical record documentation supports such a designation.

2) Hypertension with Heart Disease

Heart conditions (425.8, 429.0-429.3, 429.8, 429.9) are assigned to a code from category 402 when a causal relationship is stated (due to hypertension) or implied (hypertensive). Use an additional code from category 428 to identify the type of heart failure in those patients with heart failure. More than one code from category 428 may be assigned if the patient has systolic or diastolic failure and congestive heart failure.

The same heart conditions (425.8, 429.0-429.3, 429.8, 429.9) with hypertension, but without a stated causal relationship, are coded separately. Sequence according to the circumstances of the admission/encounter.

3) Hypertensive Chronic Kidney Disease

Assign codes from category 403, Hypertensive chronic kidney disease, when conditions classified to category 585 are present. Unlike hypertension with heart disease, ICD-9-CM presumes a cause-and-effect relationship and classifies chronic kidney disease (CKD) with hypertension as hypertensive chronic kidney disease.

Fifth digits for category 403 should be assigned as follows:

- 0 with CKD stage I through stage IV, or unspecified.
- 1 with CKD stage V or end stage renal disease.

The appropriate code from category 585, Chronic kidney disease, should be used as a secondary code with a code from category 403 to identify the stage of chronic kidney disease.

See Section I.C.10.a for information on the coding of chronic kidney disease.

4) Hypertensive Heart and Chronic Kidney Disease

Assign codes from combination category 404, Hypertensive heart and chronic kidney disease, when both hypertensive kidney disease and hypertensive heart disease are stated in the diagnosis. Assume a relationship between the hypertension and the chronic kidney disease, whether or not the condition is so designated. Assign an additional code from category 428, to identify the type of heart failure. More than one code from category 428 may be assigned if the patient has systolic or diastolic failure and congestive heart failure.

Fifth digits for category 404 should be assigned as follows:

- 0 without heart failure and with chronic kidney disease (CKD) stage I through stage IV, or unspecified
- 1 with heart failure and with CKD stage I through stage IV, or unspecified
- 2 without heart failure and with CKD stage V or end stage renal disease
- 3 with heart failure and with CKD stage V or end stage renal disease

The appropriate code from category 585, Chronic kidney disease, should be used as a secondary code with a code from category 404 to identify the stage of kidney disease. *See Section I.C.10.a for information on the coding of chronic kidney disease.*

5) Hypertensive Cerebrovascular Disease
First assign codes from 430-438, Cerebrovascular disease, then the appropriate hypertension code from categories 401-405.

6) Hypertensive Retinopathy
Two codes are necessary to identify the condition. First assign the code from subcategory 362.11, Hypertensive retinopathy, then the appropriate code from categories 401-405 to indicate the type of hypertension.

7) Hypertension, Secondary
Two codes are required: one to identify the underlying etiology and one from category 405 to identify the hypertension. Sequencing of codes is determined by the reason for admission/encounter.

8) Hypertension, Transient
Assign codes 796.2, Elevated blood pressure reading without diagnosis of hypertension, unless patient has an established diagnosis of hypertension. Assign code 642.3X for transient hypertension of pregnancy.

9) Hypertension, Controlled
Assign appropriate code from categories 401-405. This diagnostic statement usually refers to an existing state of hypertension under control by therapy.

10) Hypertension, Uncontrolled
Uncontrolled hypertension may refer to untreated hypertension or hypertension not responding to current therapeutic regimen. In either case, assign the appropriate code from categories 401-405 to designate the stage and type of hypertension. Code to the type of hypertension.

11) Elevated Blood Pressure
For a statement of elevated blood pressure without further specificity, assign code 796.2, Elevated blood pressure reading without diagnosis of hypertension, rather than a code from category 401.

Kidney Disease and Hypertension

The guidelines instruct you to assume that there is a cause-and-effect relationship between hypertension and chronic kidney disease reported with category 585. The physician might not indicate that the hypertension and chronic kidney disease are related, but the coder is to assume this relationship.

Chronic renal failure (CRF), chronic kidney disease (CKD), and chronic renal insufficiency (CRI) when reported with hypertension are reported as follows:

CRF/CKD/CRI + hypertension	403.90 + 585.9
CKD stage 1 + hypertension	403.90 + 585.1
CKD stage 2 + hypertension	403.90 + 585.2
CKD stage 3 + hypertension	403.90 + 585.3
CKD stage 4 + hypertension	403.90 + 585.4
CKD stage 5 + hypertension	403.91 + 585.5
ESRD or on dialysis + hypertension	403.91 + 585.6
Patient with CKD on any type of dialysis	403.91 + 585.6 + V45.1

Myocardial Infarction

Code 410, acute myocardial infarction (MI), requires a fifth digit assignment and includes specific instructions that must be carefully read.

A fifth digit of 1 indicates an initial episode of care for an MI and can be assigned to the same patient for a different encounter providing treatment for the initial episode of care for the MI. A patient could be diagnosed with acute MI and be transferred to a larger facility for further investigation and care. The diagnoses reported by both facilities would be the acute MI with the fifth-digit 1.

A fifth digit of 2 indicates subsequent care and is assigned when a patient is readmitted for testing or further care within 8 weeks of the initial episode. For example, a patient had an acute myocardial infarction and was discharged from the hospital. Four weeks later, that same patient was admitted for a cardiovascular procedure. The myocardial infarction would be coded 410.92 to indicate a subsequent episode of care with fifth digit 2. Note that code 412 is assigned for a healed (old) myocardial infarction that is not showing any symptoms (asymptomatic). You would not assign a V code history of MI in this situation.

As you review the following examples, refer to Fig. 5-2 for the codes highlighted in each example.

HYPERTENSION

Example 1

Diagnosis: Congestive heart failure **with** benign hypertension

Tabular: **428.0 Congestive heart failure**

401.1 Hypertension, benign (indicated as 1 in Fig. 5–2)

The key word in the above diagnosis statement is "with," which indicates two conditions. Both the congestive heart failure and the benign hypertension are coded because each is a separate condition.

HYPERTENSION

Example 2

Diagnosis: Dilated cardiomyopathy **due to** malignant hypertension

Index: **Hypertension**, cardiovascular disease, 402.00 (indicated as 2 in Fig. 5–2)

Tabular: **402 Hypertensive heart disease**

402.0 Malignant

402.00 Without heart failure

In this example, the hypertension caused the cardiomyopathy. The key words here are "due to," which indicates that one condition caused the other condition.

HYPERTENSION

Example 3

Diagnosis: Acute renal failure **with** hypertension

Tabular: **584.9 Acute renal failure**, unspecified

Tabular: **401.9 Hypertension**, unspecified (indicated as 3 in Fig. 5–2)

You would code the hypertension separately because the word "with" is included in the diagnostic statement. Under "Hypertension, renal involvement," in Fig. 5–2, you will see an *Excludes* note. The note indicates that conditions classifiable to 584 (acute renal failure) are excluded from the codes for hypertension with renal involvement. The condition in this example is acute renal failure (584); so, you cannot assign a renal involvement hypertension code. Thus, the code for the hypertension in this example is 401.9, Hypertension, unspecified, with no code for the acute renal failure. The key term included in this diagnosis is "acute" renal failure. See how the coding changes when the term chronic is stated within the diagnosis statement.

Fig. 5–3 shows the portion of the Hypertension Table that includes the secondary hypertension codes. **Secondary hypertension** means that the hypertension is caused by another condition.

	Malignant	Benign	Unspecified
pulmonary (artery)	—	—	416.8
with cor pulmonale (chronic)	—	—	416.8
acute	—	—	415.0
idiopathic	—	—	416.0
primary	—	—	416.0
of newborn	—	—	747.83
secondary	—	—	416.8
renal (disease) (*see also* Hypertension, kidney)	403.00	403.10	403.90
renovascular NEC	405.01	405.11	405.91
secondary NEC	405.09	405.19	405.99
due to			
aldosteronism, primary	405.09	405.19	405.99
brain tumor	405.09	405.19	405.99
bulbar poliomyelitis	405.09	405.19	405.99
calculus			
kidney	405.09	405.19	405.99
ureter	405.09	405.19	405.99
coarctation, aorta	405.09	405.19	405.99
Cushing's disease	405.09	405.19	405.99
glomerulosclerosis (*see also* Hypertension, kidney)	403.00	403.10	403.90
periarteritis nodosa	405.09	405.19	405.99
pheochromocytoma	405.09	405.19	405.99
polycystic kidney(s)	405.09	405.19	405.99
polycythemia	405.09	405.19	405.99
porphyria	405.09	405.19	405.99
pyelonephritis	405.09	405.19	405.99
renal (artery)			
aneurysm	405.01	405.11	405.91
anomaly	405.01	405.11	405.91
embolism	405.01	405.11	405.91
fibromuscular hyperplasia	405.01	405.11	405.91
occlusion	405.01	405.11 (#5)	405.91
stenosis	405.01	405.11	405.91
thrombosis	405.01	405.11	405.91
transient	—	—	796.2
of pregnancy	—	—	642.3
venous, chronic (asymptomatic) (idiopathic)	—	—	459.30
with			
complication, NEC	—	—	459.39
inflammation	—	—	459.32
with ulcer	—	—	459.33
ulcer	—	—	459.31
with inflammation	—	—	459.33
due to			
deep vein thrombosis (*see also* Syndrome, postphlebitic)	—	—	459.10

(Secondary hypertension label with arrow pointing to "secondary NEC" row)

FIGURE 5–3 Secondary hypertension. (Modified from Buck CJ: *2010 ICD-9-CM, Volumes 1, 2, & 3, Professional Edition,* St. Louis, 2010, Saunders.)

SECONDARY HYPERTENSION

Example

Diagnosis: Secondary, benign hypertension, due to renal artery occlusion

Tabular: **405.11 Hypertension,** secondary, due to renal (artery), occlusion, benign (indicated as 5 in Fig. 5–3)

In this example, the renal artery occlusion caused the hypertension and so is correctly coded to category 405. You would also assign a code to the renal artery occlusion (593.81) because the renal artery occlusion is causing the secondary hypertension.

Code: 593.81, 405.11 Secondary, benign hypertension, due to renal artery occlusion

According to Guideline Section I.C.7.a.7. the sequencing is determined by the reason for admission/encounter.

EXERCISE 5-9 *Diseases of the Circulatory System*

Assign codes for the following:

1 Congestive heart failure

ICD-9-CM Code: _____

2 Acute subendocardial infarction, initial episode

ICD-9-CM Code: _____

3 Secondary hypertension due to periarteritis nodosa

✤ ICD-9-CM Code(s): _____

4 Cerebral infarction due to thrombosis, brain

✤ ICD-9-CM Code(s): _____

5 Subarachnoid hemorrhage

✤ ICD-9-CM Code(s): _____

DISEASES OF THE RESPIRATORY SYSTEM

Chapter 8, Diseases of the Respiratory System, in the Tabular includes diseases and disorders of the respiratory tract, beginning with the nasal passages and following a path to the lungs. Note that at the beginning of ICD-9-CM Chapter 8 there is an instructional note that covers the entire chapter. The note states, "Use additional code to identify infectious organism." You should be aware that the organism is already identified in some codes, and in that case, you would not assign an additional code to identify the specific infectious organism.

IDENTIFYING INFECTIOUS ORGANISMS

Example 1

Diagnosis: Pneumonia due to *Klebsiella pneumoniae*

Index: **Pneumonia**, *Klebsiella pneumoniae*, 482.0

Tabular: **482 Other bacterial pneumonia**

482.0 Pneumonia due to Klebsiella pneumoniae

Code: 482.0 Pneumonia due to *Klebsiella pneumoniae*

Code 482.0 is a combination code that includes the disease process (pneumonia) with the causative organism *(Klebsiella pneumoniae)*. In this instance, you would not assign an additional code because the organism is identified in the code 482.0.

IDENTIFYING INFECTIOUS ORGANISMS

Example 2

In the following example, two codes are necessary, one to describe the disease process (manifestation) and one to indicate the causative organism (etiology).

Diagnosis: Acute maxillary sinusitis due to *Hemophilus influenzae*

Index: **Sinusitis** (accessory) (nasal) (hyperplastic) (nonpurulent) (purulent) (chronic) 473.9

   acute 461.9

   maxillary 461.0

Tabular: **461 Acute sinusitis**

   461.0 Maxillary

Index: **Infection, infected, infective** (opportunistic), *Hemophilus influenzae* NEC 041.5

Tabular: **041 Bacterial infection in conditions classified elsewhere and of unspecified site**

   041.5 Hemophilus influenzae [H. influenzae]

Codes: 461.0, 041.5 Acute maxillary sinusitis due to *Hemophilus influenzae*

The manifestation is listed first and the etiology is listed second.

Now, let's learn how to code the respiratory condition of chronic obstructive pulmonary disease (COPD), which falls within the category 496 Chronic airway obstruction NEC. The note in the Tabular under code 496 indicates that this code cannot be assigned with any code from categories 491-493 (491 is chronic bronchitis, 492 is emphysema, and 493 is asthma). The *Excludes* note under code 496 indicates that COPD specified "(as) (with) asthma (493.2)" cannot be assigned to code 496; rather, reference 493.2.

CHRONIC OBSTRUCTIVE PULMONARY DISEASE

Example

Diagnosis: COPD with asthma

Index: **Asthma, asthmatic** (bronchial) (catarrh) (spasmodic) 493.9, with, chronic obstructive pulmonary disease (COPD) 493.2

Tabular: **493 Asthma**

   493.2 Chronic obstructive asthma

This code is not complete yet because it requires a fifth digit. You have three fifth-digit choices:

   0 unspecified

   1 with status asthmaticus

   2 with (acute) exacerbation

Status asthmaticus is the most severe form of asthma attack and can last for days or weeks. To report the asthma with status asthmaticus, the physician provides specific documentation of the condition. If the clinical condition is severe enough that you suspect that the patient has status asthmaticus, clarification by the physician should be sought.

Code: 493.20 COPD with asthma

EXERCISE 5-10 *Diseases of the Respiratory System*

Assign codes for the following:

1 Croup

ICD-9-CM Code: _____

2 Respiratory failure due to congestive heart failure

ICD-9-CM Codes: _____, _____

3 COPD with chronic bronchitis (without exacerbation)

ICD-9-CM Code: _____

4 Influenza with acute bronchitis

ICD-9-CM Code: _____

5 Pneumonia due to *Hemophilus influenzae*

ICD-9-CM Code: _____

CHAPTER REVIEW

CHAPTER 5, PART I, THEORY

Without the use of reference material, answer the following:

1 ICD-9-CM assumes a relationship between hypertension and renal failure.

   True   False

2 If a patient is admitted for an HIV-related condition, the first-listed diagnosis is the related condition followed by the diagnosis code 042.

   True   False

3 A fifth digit of 1 should be assigned to 305.0X for someone who abuses alcohol by binge drinking.

   True   False

4 Another term to describe malignant hypertension is accelerated hypertension.

   True   False

5 Hypertension that is caused by another condition is called essential hypertension.

   True   False

6 A fifth digit of 1 to indicate status asthmaticus can be assigned if the physician documents an acute exacerbation.

   True   False

7 If a patient's diabetes is documented as poorly controlled, a fifth digit for out of control should be assigned.

   True   False

8 If a patient receives insulin for diabetes, type I diabetes should be reported.

   True   False

9 The site to which a malignant neoplasm has spread is the:

   a. metastatic site
   b. primary site
   c. benign site
   d. morphology

10 The site in which a malignant neoplasm originated is the:

   a. metastatic site
   b. primary site
   c. benign site
   d. morphology

CHAPTER 5, PART II, PRACTICAL

Using the ICD-9-CM and coding guidelines, assign codes for the following:

11 Combined spinal cord degeneration due to pernicious anemia

ICD-9-CM Codes: _____,

_____

12 Carcinoma, in situ, of skin of lip, vermilion border

ICD-9-CM Code: _____

13 Subacute bacterial endocarditis

ICD-9-CM Code: _____

14 Acute bronchitis with chronic obstructive bronchitis

ICD-9-CM Code: _____

15 Group B streptococcal pneumonia

ICD-9-CM Code: _____

16 Alzheimer's disease

ICD-9-CM Code: _____

17 Hypertension with end-stage renal disease

ICD-9-CM Codes: _____,

_____

18 Enteritis due to Norwalk virus

ICD-9-CM Code: _____

19 *Pneumocystis* pneumonia in patient with HIV

ICD-9-CM Codes: _____,

_____

20 Diabetic foot ulcer in patient with diabetes mellitus, type I, out of control

ICD-9-CM Codes: _____,

_____

21 Inanition

ICD-9-CM Code: _____

22 Neutropenic fever

ICD-9-CM Codes: _____,

_____

23 Anemia due to gastric cancer

ICD-9-CM Code(s): _____

24 Withdrawal from heroin, daily use

ICD-9-CM Code(s): _____

25 Seizure disorder

ICD-9-CM Code(s): _____

26 Acute renal failure in patient with hypertension

ICD-9-CM Code(s): _____

27 COPD with emphysema

ICD-9-CM Code(s): _____

28 Aspiration pneumonia

ICD-9-CM Code(s): _____

29 Mr. Jensen is status post colon resection 3 months ago for sigmoid colon cancer and is now admitted for adjunct chemotherapy.

ICD-9-CM Code(s): _____

CASE STUDY 1

History of Present Illness

This 50-year-old disabled male is a resident of a nursing home who has been admitted because of marked congestion and respiratory distress. He is known to have mental retardation and frequent urinary tract and pulmonary infections. He has a recurrent epileptic disorder that is well controlled on Dilantin.

Physical Examination

On admission, vital signs include a temperature of 101° F, respiratory rate of 32 breaths per minute, heart rate of 82 beats per minute, and blood pressure of 120/70 mm Hg. Examination of the chest reveals bilateral crepitations. There is moderate redness and edema of the scrotal skin.

Laboratory Data and Course in Hospital

His white blood cell count is 8.5; hemoglobin, 12.9 g/dl; polymorphonuclear leukocytes, 64; bands, 19; lymphocytes, 10; monocytes, 6; and eosinophils, 1. Urinalysis shows moderate bacterial and 1+ white blood cell count. Urine culture shows mixed flora. The repeat urine culture shows *Providencia stuartii* sensitive to Fortaz. Sputum culture reveals the presence of methicillin-resistant *Staphylococcus aureus,* sensitive to vancomycin. Chest x-ray film shows bilateral pulmonary infiltrates. Arterial blood gases on room air show a Po_2 of 48, Pco_2 of 30, and pH of 7.50. When repeated with the patient on oxygen, Po_2 is 66, Pco_2 is 36, and pH is 7.45. The patient is treated with intravenous vancomycin and intravenous Fortaz. His pulmonary infiltrate decreases. His oral intake has been somewhat poor, and he has been given intravenous fluids off and on. The nursing staff at the nursing home note that his intake, in terms of eating and taking fluids, is much better. His medications at the nursing home include Dilantin, 200 mg twice a day; Tegretol, 400 mg at 8 AM and 4 PM, and 200 mg at 8 PM; and Cipro, 500 mg twice a day; and his maintenance medications are continued. This patient is being discharged today.

Final Diagnosis

Acute respiratory insufficiency (2)

Bilateral pneumonia (1) due to staph auerus (MRSA) (5)

Mental retardation (3)

Epilepsy (6); UTI (4) due to *Providencia stuartii* (gram-negative bacilli)

30 ICD-9-CM Codes: (1)_____,

    (2)_____, (3)_____,

    (4)_____, (5)_____,

    (6)_____

CASE STUDY 2

History of Present Illness

The patient is an 80-year-old female with a known history of advanced metastatic carcinoma of the breast, which was the primary site. (The breast cancer is no longer present but has metastasized to other unspecified areas, which represents a secondary generalized neoplasm.) The patient has been admitted because of increased shortness of breath and severe pain. The pain is worse in her left chest, and this is associated with increased shortness of breath. At the time of admission, the patient is in so much pain that she is unable to remember her history. The patient initially presented for congestive heart failure more than a year earlier. This was subsequently found to be secondary to metastatic breast cancer, after left mastectomy, 3 years ago. The patient had previously been on chemotherapy.

Course in Hospital

The patient is treated initially with intravenous pain medication to control her pain, and subsequently her condition becomes stable on oral medication. By the time of discharge, the patient is stable on oral Vicodin. She is able to eat. Admission blood urea nitrogen (BUN) was

38 mg/dl with creatinine of 1.3 mg/dl secondary to dehydration. By the time of discharge, these levels have improved. Admission glucose of 225 mg/dl is down to 110 mg/dl at discharge.

Discharge Diagnoses

Uncontrolled pain, secondary to widely metastatic breast carcinoma

Dehydration

Type II diabetes mellitus, uncontrolled

31 What is the first-listed diagnosis and the code for the first-listed diagnosis for this patient?

First-listed Diagnosis Terms and Code:

_____

32 What are the other diagnoses for this patient and what are the codes for these other diagnoses?

Additional Diagnosis Codes:

_____

_____

_____

_____

QUICK CHECK ANSWERS

QUICK CHECK 5-1
1. 229.9 (Neoplasm, unknown site or unspecified, Benign)

"Qualities that best describe a successful coder would include meticulous attention to detail, a strong sense of honesty and integrity, and perseverance."

Patricia Cordy Henricksen, MS, CPC-I, CPC, CCP

Vice President; Senior Auditor; PMCC Instructor

Soterion Medical Services

Lexington, Kentucky

Chapter-Specific Guidelines (ICD-9-CM Chapters 9-17)

Chapter Topics

Diseases of the Digestive System

Diseases of the Genitourinary System

Complications of Pregnancy, Childbirth, and the Puerperium

Diseases of the Skin and Subcutaneous Tissue

Diseases of the Musculoskeletal System and Connective Tissue

Congenital Anomalies and Certain Conditions Originating in the Perinatal Period

Signs, Symptoms, and Ill-Defined Conditions

Injury and Poisoning

Chapter Review

Quick Check Answers

Learning Objectives

After completing this chapter you should be able to

1 Examine the digestive system coding.

2 Analyze the genitourinary system coding.

3 Review the pregnancy, childbirth, and puerperium coding.

4 Review the skin and subcutaneous tissue coding.

5 Examine the congenital anomalies and certain conditions originating in the perinatal period coding.

6 Define the rules of symptoms, signs, and ill-defined conditions coding.

7 Identify the elements of coding injuries and poisonings.

Make sure to check

evolve
learning system

for the latest content updates

DISEASES OF THE DIGESTIVE SYSTEM

Chapter 9, Diseases of the Digestive System, in the Tabular of the ICD-9-CM describes diseases or conditions affecting the digestive system. Digestion starts when food is taken into the mouth and follows the gastrointestinal tract until it leaves the body through the anus. The categories are sequenced in a manner that follows that path, starting with disorders of the teeth.

Throughout the chapter, as in other chapters, you must pay close attention to fifth-digit assignment, the use of combination codes, and carefully read the *Excludes* notes and any other instructions. Also important in the chapter is the presence of **hemorrhage** (bleeding) associated with the diseases. Codes from category 578, Gastrointestinal hemorrhage, are not assigned when codes for bleeding of any sites mentioned are available. Use this category only when the physician states clearly that the bleeding is due to another condition. The physician may not always indicate the presence of hemorrhage, and the coder must review the record and then clarify the documentation with the physician, then assign the appropriate code(s).

Example

Diagnosis: Diverticulitis of the colon with hemorrhage

Index: **Diverticulitis** (acute), colon (perforated) without hemorrhage 562.11, with hemorrhage 562.13

Note that the presence of hemorrhage makes a difference in the code assignment: without hemorrhage, 562.11; with hemorrhage, 562.13.

Tabular: **562 Diverticula of intestine**

562.13 Diverticulitis of colon with hemorrhage
(a combination code)

Code: 562.13 Diverticulitis of the colon with hemorrhage

If you begin your search for the above diagnosis of "Diverticulitis of the colon with hemorrhage" using the main term "Hemorrhage, gastrointestinal," you will find 578.9. When you reference 578.9 in the Tabular, you will find a long list of *Excludes* under the category code 578. Note that in the list of *Excludes* is "diverticulitis, intestine: large (562.13)" (see arrow below). This means that you cannot assign 578.9, gastrointestinal hemorrhage, when there is a mention of diverticulitis of the large intestine (562.13).

578 Gastrointestinal hemorrhage

 that with mention of:
    angiodysplasia of stomach and duodenum (537.83)
    angiodysplasia of intestine (569.85)
    diverticulitis, intestine:
→   *large (562.13)*
       small (562.03)
    diverticulosis, intestine:
       large (562.12)
       small (562.02)
    gastritis and duodenitis (535.0-535.6)
    ulcer:
       duodenum, gastric, gastrojejunal, or peptic (531.00-534.91)

If you are coding a diagnosis of gastrointestinal (GI) hemorrhage with any of the diagnoses listed in the *Excludes* and if the hemorrhage is due to that GI condition, only the combination code would be assigned.

From the Trenches

"Education is an ongoing process in the field of coding . . . . Success as a coder involves a thorough understanding of the code set guidelines, as well as knowledge of medical terminology and anatomy."

PATRICIA

Example

Diagnosis: Gastrointestinal hemorrhage due to acute antral ulcer

Index: **Ulcer,** antral—*see* Ulcer, stomach

Ulcer, stomach (eroded) (peptic) (round) 531.9

acute, with, hemorrhage 531.0

Tabular: **531 Gastric ulcer**

531.0 Acute with hemorrhage

Code 531.0 is not a complete code. You must assign a fifth digit based on if there was or was not a mention of obstruction. There is no mention of obstruction in the diagnosis, so the fifth digit assigned would be 0, without mention of obstruction, 531.00.

You must now determine if there is any further directive to report the hemorrhage with yet another code. Referencing hemorrhage in the Index, you are directed to 578 again and you note that the *Excludes* notes indicate not to code gastrointestinal hemorrhage with mention of gastric ulcer. So no further code is needed, as the hemorrhage is included in the code for the ulcer (531.00).

Index: **Hemorrhage, hemorrhagic** (nontraumatic) 459.0

gastrointestinal (tract) 578.9

Tabular: **578 Gastrointestinal hemorrhage**

> **EXCLUDES** *that with mention of:*
> *ulcer:*
> *duodenal, gastric, gastrojejunal, or peptic (531.00-534.91)*

Code: 531.00 Gastrointestinal hemorrhage due to acute antral ulcer

---

CODING SHOT

For a hemorrhage to be reported, there does not have to be **active** bleeding; however, there must be documentation in the medical record that supports the fact that active bleeding has occurred and the physician must identify the source of bleeding for the combination code to be assigned.

It is so important to verify code assignment in the Tabular. It is only when you check the Tabular that you can know for certain about the Includes and *Excludes,* which are not listed anywhere else. This is also where you will find if a fourth or fifth digit to the code is needed. Be certain to always, always check the Tabular before assigning a code.

EXERCISE 6-1   *Diseases of the Digestive System*

Assign ICD-9-CM codes for the following:

1 Appendicitis with generalized peritonitis

   ICD-9-CM Code: _____

2 Gastrointestinal bleeding due to acute duodenal ulcer

   ICD-9-CM Code: _____

3 Acute and chronic cholecystitis with cholelithiasis

   ICD-9-CM Codes: _____, _____

4 Gastroenteritis

   ICD-9-CM Code: _____

5 Gastroesophageal reflux

   ICD-9-CM Code: _____

DISEASES OF THE GENITOURINARY SYSTEM

Chapter 10, Diseases of the Genitourinary System, in the Tabular of the ICD-9-CM includes conditions and diseases of the male and female genital organs and urinary tract. There are several types of diseases of the kidney (580-589) that are also included in this chapter. For example, nephritis (inflammation of the kidney), nephritic syndrome (proteinuria and water retention), and the stages of kidney disease and failure. Also in this chapter are codes for diseases of the male genital organs (600-608), including codes for disorders and diseases of the prostate. Disorders of the breast (610-612) are also included in this chapter.

When you are reporting infections of the urinary tract or the genital organs, you are instructed to use an additional code to identify the organism.

REPORTING THE INFECTIOUS ORGANISM

Example

Diagnosis: Acute prostatitis due to *Streptococcus*

Index: **Prostatitis** (congestive) (suppurative) 601.9

       acute 601.0

Tabular: **601 Inflammatory diseases of prostate**

       601.0 Acute prostatitis

Index: **Infection, infected, infective** (opportunistic)

       streptococcal NEC 041.00

Tabular: **041 Bacterial infection in conditions classified elsewhere and of unspecified site**

       041.0 Streptococcus

          041.00 Streptococcus, unspecified

Codes: 601.0, 041.00 Acute prostatitis due to *Streptococcus*

EXERCISE 6-2 *Diseases of the Genitourinary System*

Assign ICD-9-CM codes for the following diagnostic statements:

1 Pelvic inflammatory disease (PID)

   ● ICD-9-CM Code(s): _____

2 Hematuria

   ● ICD-9-CM Code(s): _____

3 Acute and chronic pyelonephritis

   ● ICD-9-CM Code(s): _____

4 Benign prostatic hypertrophy (BPH)

   ● ICD-9-CM Code(s): _____

5 Fibrocystic breast disease

   ● ICD-9-CM Code(s): _____

COMPLICATIONS OF PREGNANCY, CHILDBIRTH, AND THE PUERPERIUM

Chapter 11, Complications of Pregnancy, Childbirth, and the Puerperium, of the Tabular of the ICD-9-CM is probably the most difficult chapter from which to code. One reason is that pregnancy and childbirth are natural functions, and physicians often overlook documentation of diagnoses that should be reported. Another reason the coding is complex is that there is extensive use of multiple coding in the chapter. Also, fifth-digit assignment for pregnancy is often difficult to determine. There are instructions throughout this chapter that must be read thoroughly. Obstetric coding can also be difficult because you may not use this chapter as frequently as some of the other chapters, so you won't be as familiar with the special notes and coding instructions. Any condition that occurs during pregnancy, childbirth, or the puerperium is considered to be a complication unless the attending physician specifically documents that it neither affects the pregnancy nor is affected by the pregnancy.

CODING SHOT An ectopic pregnancy is one in which the fertilized ovum implants outside the uterus, usually in the fallopian tube. Ectopic and Molar Pregnancy (630-633) contains instructions to use an additional code from category 639 to identify any complication(s).

Category 639, Complications following abortion and ectopic and molar pregnancies, reports genital tract and pelvic infection (639.0), delayed or excessive hemorrhage (639.1), damage to pelvic organs and tissues (639.2), kidney failure (639.3), metabolic disorders (639.4), shock (639.5), embolism (639.6), and other specified complications (639.8), or unspecified complications (639.9). You cannot assign 639, Complications, with any code from categories 634-638 (abortion) because the complications for the abortion are classified according to the fourth-digit subcategory codes. Examples are 635, Legally induced abortion and 635.1, Complicated by delayed or excessive hemorrhage. As stated previously, you assign 639, Complications, to identify any complications related to codes 630-633. You also assign 639, Complications, when the complication is the reason for the medical care, and the abortion, ectopic, or molar pregnancy was treated during a previous episode.

Complications mainly related to pregnancy (640-649) require fifth-digit subclassifications that are of special note:

0 unspecified as to episode of care or not applicable

1 delivered, with or without mention of antepartum condition

2 delivered, with mention of postpartum complication

3 antepartum condition or complication

4 postpartum condition or complication

The fifth digit 0 reports an abortion due to or associated with a complication. To assign the fifth digits 1 and 2, a delivery must have occurred during that inpatient stay. The 1 is assigned to cases in which an antepartum condition has or has not been noted. The fifth digits 3 and 4 are reported when no delivery has occurred during that encounter. The 3 is reported for antepartum conditions, and the 4 is reported for postpartum conditions. When you review the categories and subcategories throughout the chapter, you will note that many subcategories may indicate that you can use only certain fifth digits with a particular code. For example, with code 641.1, Hemorrhage from placenta previa, the only fifth digits that can be used are 0, 1, or 3. Neither 2 nor 4 can be used because placenta previa occurs **before** a baby is delivered and 2 and 4 are assigned **after** delivery.

When reporting multiple diagnoses from one inpatient stay, certain combinations of fifth digits are used to classify that stay or visit. These fifth-digit combinations are:

1 only, or with 2; NOT with 0, 3, or 4

2 only, or with 1; NOT with 0, 3, or 4

3 only, NOT with 0, 1, 2, or 4

4 only, NOT with 0, 1, 2, or 3

Category 650, Normal delivery, cannot be assigned with any other code within the range 630-676 because these codes refer to other than normal delivery. Code 650 is assigned only when all of the following are documented:

- A full-term, single liveborn infant is delivered.

- There are no antepartum or postpartum conditions classifiable to 630-676 (other than normal delivery).

- The presentation is cephalic, requiring minimal assistance and without fetal manipulation or the use of instrumentation.

- An episiotomy may or may not have been performed.

Most deliveries do not meet the requirements for a 650 Normal Delivery code assignment.

Category V27, Outcome of delivery, can be assigned as an additional code to the **mother's record.** Code V27 is indexed under the term "Outcome."

ICD-9-CM OFFICIAL GUIDELINES FOR CODING AND REPORTING

SECTION I.C.11.

b. Selection of OB Principal or First-listed Diagnosis

> **3) Episodes when no delivery occurs**
> In episodes when no delivery occurs, the principal diagnosis should correspond to the principal complication of the pregnancy, which necessitated the encounter. Should more than one complication exist, all of which are treated or monitored, any of the complication codes may be sequenced first.

COMPLICATING PREGNANCY

Example

Diagnosis: Iron deficiency anemia complicating pregnancy, antepartum

Index: **Pregnancy** (single) (uterine) (without sickness) V22.2

> complicated (by) 646.9
>> anemia (conditions classifiable to 280-285) 648.2

Tabular: **648.2 Anemia**

This code is not complete because it does not have a fifth-digit assignment and in the Tabular there are instructions to "Use additional code(s) to identify the **condition**," which means to identify the type of anemia. The Tabular directs you to assign fifth digits 0-4. No delivery has occurred and the condition is stated as being antepartum; therefore, the fifth digit 3 is assigned, 648.23. Next report an additional code to identify the type of anemia.

Index: **Anemia** 285.9, deficiency 281.9, iron (Fe) 280.9

Tabular: **280.9 Iron deficiency anemia, unspecified**

Codes: 648.23, 280.9 Iron deficiency anemia complicating pregnancy, antepartum

The first code, 648.23, indicates that the anemia is a complication of the pregnancy, and the second code, 280.9, identifies the type of anemia (iron deficiency anemia).

Read the following Guidelines that provide direction to the coder regarding sequencing and first-listed diagnosis.

ICD-9-CM OFFICIAL GUIDELINES FOR CODING AND REPORTING

SECTION I.C.

11. Chapter 11: Complications of Pregnancy, Childbirth, and the Puerperium (630-679)

> **a. General Rules for Obstetric Cases**
>
> > **1) Codes from chapter 11 and sequencing priority**
> > Obstetric cases require codes from Chapter 11, codes in the range 630-679, Complications of Pregnancy, Childbirth, and the Puerperium. Chapter 11 codes have sequencing priority over codes from other chapters. Additional codes from other chapters may be used in conjunction with chapter 11 codes to further specify conditions. Should the provider document that the pregnancy is incidental to the encounter, then code V22.2 should be used in place of any chapter 11 codes. It is the provider's responsibility to state that the condition being treated is not affecting the pregnancy.
> >
> > **2) Chapter 11 codes used only on the maternal record**
> > Chapter 11 codes are to be used only on the maternal record, never on the record of the newborn.

3) Chapter 11 fifth-digits

Categories 640-648, 651-676 have required fifth-digits, which indicate whether the encounter is antepartum, postpartum and whether a delivery has also occurred.

4) Fifth-digits, appropriate for each code

The fifth-digits, which are appropriate for each code number, are listed in brackets under each code. The fifth-digits on each code should all be consistent with each other. That is, should a delivery occur all of the fifth-digits should indicate the delivery.

b. Selection of OB Principal or First-Listed Diagnosis

1) Routine outpatient prenatal visits

For routine outpatient prenatal visits when no complications are present codes V22.0, Supervision of normal first pregnancy, and V22.1, Supervision of other normal pregnancy, should be used as the first-listed diagnoses. These codes should not be used in conjunction with chapter 11 codes.

2) Prenatal outpatient visits for high-risk patients

For routine prenatal outpatient visits for patients with high-risk pregnancies, a code from category V23, Supervision of high-risk pregnancy, should be used as the first-listed diagnosis. Secondary chapter 11 codes may be used in conjunction with these codes if appropriate.

3) Episodes when no delivery occurs

In episodes when no delivery occurs, the principal diagnosis should correspond to the principal complication of the pregnancy, which necessitated the encounter. Should more than one complication exist, all of which are treated or monitored, any of the complications codes may be sequenced first.

4) When a delivery occurs

When a delivery occurs, the principal diagnosis should correspond to the main circumstances or complication of the delivery. In cases of cesarean delivery, the selection of the principal diagnosis should be the condition established after study that was responsible for the patient's admission. If the patient was admitted with a condition that resulted in the performance of a cesarean procedure, that condition should be selected as the principal diagnosis. If the reason for the admission/encounter was unrelated to the condition resulting in the cesarean delivery, the condition related to the reason for the admission/encounter should be selected as the principal diagnosis, even if a cesarean was performed.

5) Outcome of delivery

An outcome of delivery code, V27.0-V27.9, should be included on every maternal record when a delivery has occurred. These codes are not to be used on subsequent records or on the newborn record.

c. Fetal Conditions Affecting the Management of the Mother

1) Codes from category 655

Known or suspected fetal abnormality affecting management of the mother, and category 656, Other fetal and placental problems affecting the management of the mother, are assigned only when the fetal condition is actually responsible for modifying the management of the mother, i.e., by requiring diagnostic studies, additional observation, special care, or termination of pregnancy. The fact that the fetal condition exists does not justify assigning a code from this series to the mother's record.

See I.C.18.d. for suspected maternal and fetal conditions not found

2) In utero surgery

In cases when surgery is performed on the fetus, a diagnosis code from category 655, Known or suspected fetal abnormalities affecting management of the mother, should be assigned identifying the fetal condition. Procedure code 75.36, Correction of fetal defect, should be assigned on the hospital inpatient record.

No code from Chapter 15, the perinatal codes, should be used on the mother's record to identify fetal conditions. Surgery performed in utero on a fetus is still to be coded as an obstetric encounter.

d. HIV Infection in Pregnancy, Childbirth and the Puerperium

During pregnancy, childbirth or the puerperium, a patient admitted because of an HIV-related illness should receive a principal diagnosis of 647.6X, Other specified infectious and parasitic diseases in the mother classifiable elsewhere, but complicating the pregnancy, childbirth or the puerperium, followed by 042 and the code(s) for the HIV-related illness(es).

Patients with asymptomatic HIV infection status admitted during pregnancy, childbirth, or the puerperium should receive codes of 647.6X and V08.

e. Current Conditions Complicating Pregnancy

Assign a code from subcategory 648.x for patients that have current conditions when the condition affects the management of the pregnancy, childbirth, or the puerperium. Use additional secondary codes from other chapters to identify the conditions, as appropriate.

f. Diabetes mellitus in pregnancy

Diabetes mellitus is a significant complicating factor in pregnancy. Pregnant women who are diabetic should be assigned code 648.0x, Diabetes mellitus complicating pregnancy, and a secondary code from category 250, Diabetes mellitus, or category 249, Secondary diabetes to identify the type of diabetes.

Code V58.67, Long-term (current) use of insulin, should also be assigned if the diabetes mellitus is being treated with insulin.

g. Gestational diabetes

Gestational diabetes can occur during the second and third trimester of pregnancy in women who were not diabetic prior to pregnancy. Gestational diabetes can cause complications in the pregnancy similar to those of pre-existing diabetes mellitus. It also puts the woman at greater risk of developing diabetes after the pregnancy. Gestational diabetes is coded to 648.8x, Abnormal glucose tolerance. Codes 648.0x and 648.8x should never be used together on the same record.

Code V58.67, Long-term (current) use of insulin, should also be assigned if the gestational diabetes is being treated with insulin.

h. Normal Delivery, Code 650

1) Normal delivery

Code 650 is for use in cases when a woman is admitted for a full-term normal delivery and delivers a single, healthy infant without any complications antepartum, during the delivery, or postpartum during the delivery episode. Code 650 is always a principal diagnosis. It is not to be used if any other code from chapter 11 is needed to describe a current complication of the antenatal, delivery, or perinatal period. Additional codes from other chapters may be used with code 650 if they are not related to or are in any way complicating the pregnancy.

2) Normal delivery with resolved antepartum complication

Code 650 may be used if the patient had a complication at some point during her pregnancy, but the complication is not present at the time of the admission for delivery.

3) V27.0, Single liveborn, outcome of delivery

V27.0, Single liveborn, is the only outcome of delivery code appropriate for use with 650.

i. The Postpartum and Peripartum Periods

1) Postpartum and peripartum periods

The postpartum period begins immediately after delivery and continues for six weeks following delivery. The peripartum period is defined as the last month of pregnancy to five months postpartum.

2) Postpartum complication

A postpartum complication is any complication occurring within the six-week period.

3) Pregnancy-related complications after 6-week period

Chapter 11 codes may also be used to describe pregnancy-related complications after the six-week period should the provider document that a condition is pregnancy related.

4) Postpartum complications occurring during the same admission as delivery

Postpartum complications that occur during the same admission as the delivery are identified with a fifth digit of "2." Subsequent admissions/encounters for postpartum complications should be identified with a fifth digit of "4."

5) Admission for routine postpartum care following delivery outside hospital

When the mother delivers outside the hospital prior to admission and is admitted for routine postpartum care and no complications are noted, code V24.0, Postpartum care and examination immediately after delivery, should be assigned as the principal diagnosis.

6) Admission following delivery outside hospital with postpartum conditions

A delivery diagnosis code should not be used for a woman who has delivered prior to admission to the hospital. Any postpartum conditions and/or postpartum procedures should be coded.

7) Puerperal sepsis

Code 670.2x, Puerperal sepsis, should be assigned with a secondary code to identify the causal organism (e.g., for a bacterial infection, assign a code from category 041, Bacterial infections in conditions classified elsewhere and of unspecified site.) A code from category 038, Septicemia, should not be used for puerperal sepsis. Do not assign code 995.91, Sepsis, as code 670.2x describes the sepsis. If applicable, use additional codes to identify severe sepsis (995.92) and any associated acute organ dysfunction.

j. Code 677, Late effect of complication of pregnancy

1) Code 677

Code 677, Late effect of complication of pregnancy, childbirth, and the puerperium is for use in those cases when an initial complication of a pregnancy develops a sequelae requiring care or treatment at a future date.

2) After the initial postpartum period

This code may be used at any time after the initial postpartum period.

3) Sequencing of Code 677

This code, like all late effect codes, is to be sequenced following the code describing the sequelae of the complication.

k. Abortions

1) Fifth-digits required for abortion categories

Fifth-digits are required for abortion categories 634-637. Fifth digit assignment is based on the status of the patient at the beginning (or start) of the encounter. Fifth-digit 1, incomplete, indicates that all of the products of conception have not been expelled from the uterus. Fifth-digit 2, complete, indicates that all products of conception have been expelled from the uterus.

2) Code from categories 640-648 and 651-659

A code from categories 640-648 and 651-659 may be used as additional codes with an abortion code to indicate the complication leading to the abortion.

Fifth digit 3 is assigned with codes from these categories when used with an abortion code because the other fifth digits will not apply. Codes from the 660-669 series are not to be used for complications of abortion.

3) Code 639 for complications

Code 639 is to be used for all complications following abortion. Code 639 cannot be assigned with codes from categories 634-638.

4) Abortion with Liveborn Fetus

When an attempted termination of pregnancy results in a liveborn fetus assign code 644.21, Early onset of delivery, with an appropriate code from category V27, Outcome of Delivery. The procedure code for the attempted termination of pregnancy should also be assigned.

5) Retained Products of Conception following an abortion

Subsequent admissions for retained products of conception following a spontaneous or legally induced abortion are assigned the appropriate code from category 634, Spontaneous abortion, or 635 Legally induced abortion, with a fifth digit of "1" (incomplete). This advice is appropriate even when the patient was discharged previously with a discharge diagnosis of complete abortion.

EXERCISE 6-3 *Complications of Pregnancy, Childbirth, and the Puerperium*

Assign ICD-9-CM codes for the following:

1 Blighted ovum

ICD-9-CM Code: _____

2 Incomplete spontaneous abortion; dilation and curettage (D&C) performed

ICD-9-CM Code: _____

3 False labor of 38-week pregnancy, undelivered

ICD-9-CM Code: _____

4 Vaginal delivery of liveborn single infant with fourth-degree perineal laceration; obstetric laceration repaired (include appropriate V code for outcome of delivery)

ICD-9-CM Codes: _____ (laceration), _____ (outcome)

5 Obstructed labor due to cephalopelvic disproportion; liveborn single infant delivered by lower segment cesarean section

ICD-9-CM Codes: _____, _____, _____

DISEASES OF THE SKIN AND SUBCUTANEOUS TISSUE

Chapter 12, Diseases of the Skin and Subcutaneous Tissue, in the Tabular of the ICD-9-CM describes diseases or conditions of the integumentary system. This chapter is one of the shorter chapters in the ICD-9-CM manual. Conditions affecting the nails, sweat glands, hair, and hair follicles are included in this chapter. Congenital conditions of skin, hair, and nails are classified in category 757, Congenital anomalies of the integument. Neoplasms of skin are classified in Chapter 2 of ICD-9-CM. When reviewing the first categories, such as 681, 682, and 683, you will note that multiple coding may be necessary for some conditions.

Example

MULTIPLE CODING

Diagnosis: Cellulitis right small finger due to Staphylococcus aureus

Index: **Cellulitis** (diffuse) (with lymphangitis) (*see also* Abscess) 682.9
finger (intrathecal) (periosteal) (subcutaneous) (subcuticular) 681.00

Tabular: **681 Cellulitis and abscess of finger and toe**

681.0 Finger

681.00 Cellulitis and abscess, unspecified

There is an instructional note that directs you to identify the **organism** when assigning code 681.00. To locate the code for the causative organism reference the main term "Infection" in the Index.

Index: **Infection, infected, infective** (opportunistic) 136.9
staphylococcal, NEC 041.10
aureus 041.11

Tabular: **041 Bacterial infection in conditions classified elsewhere and of unspecified site**

041.1 Staphylococcus

041.11 Methicillin susceptible Staphylococcus aureus

The Tabular states, "Use additional code to identify organism, such as Staphylococcus (041.1)." Code 041.1 must have a fifth-digit assignment before it can be reported, and you would know this only if you verified the code in the Tabular and found that the five-digit code 041.11 specifies Staphylococcus aureus.

Code(s): 681.00, 041.11 Cellulitis right small finger due to Staphylococcus aureus

The code for the organism is assigned as an additional code and is sequenced after the disease or condition.

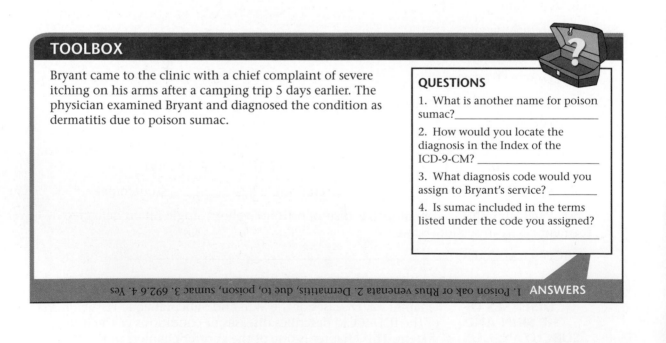

TOOLBOX

Bryant came to the clinic with a chief complaint of severe itching on his arms after a camping trip 5 days earlier. The physician examined Bryant and diagnosed the condition as dermatitis due to poison sumac.

QUESTIONS

1. What is another name for poison sumac?_____

2. How would you locate the diagnosis in the Index of the ICD-9-CM? _____

3. What diagnosis code would you assign to Bryant's service? _____

4. Is sumac included in the terms listed under the code you assigned?
_____

ANSWERS 1. Poison oak or Rhus venenata 2. Dermatitis, due to, poison, sumac 3. 692.6 4. Yes

EXERCISE 6-4 *Diseases of the Skin and Subcutaneous Tissue*

Assign ICD-9-CM codes for the following:

1 Pruritus

     ICD-9-CM Code: _____

2 Heat rash

     ICD-9-CM Code: _____

3 Psoriasis

     ICD-9-CM Code: _____

4 Decubitus ulcer buttock

     ICD-9-CM Codes: _____, _____

5 Dermatitis due to poison ivy

     ICD-9-CM Code: _____

DISEASES OF THE MUSCULOSKELETAL SYSTEM AND CONNECTIVE TISSUE

Chapter 13, Diseases of the Musculoskeletal System and Connective Tissue, in the ICD-9-CM Tabular describes diseases or conditions of the bone, joints, and muscles. It is important to refer to the note at the beginning of the chapter because that is where you will locate the information on the fifth-digit subclassifications used for categories 711-712, 715-716, 718-719, and 730. If you turn to category 711, you will see the fifth-digit subclassifications again, but not in the same detail as is found at the beginning of the chapter. Most arthropathies (disorders of the joint) are classified in categories 710 through 719 and most dorsopathies (disorders of the back) in categories 720 through 724 in ICD-9-CM.

Example
FIFTH DIGIT

Diagnosis: Pyogenic arthritis of the wrist

Index: **Arthritis**, arthritic (acute) (chronic) (subacute), 716.9
                pyogenic organism 711.0

Tabular: **711 Arthropathy associated with infections**

           711.0 Pyogenic arthritis

Code 711.0 is not valid until you assign a fifth digit to indicate the site of the arthritis. When reviewing the subclassifications, you must know whether the wrist is part of the forearm or part of the hand. Refer to that note at the beginning of the chapter, where you will note that fifth digit "3" reports the forearm includes the radius, ulna, and wrist joint.

Code: 711.03 Pyogenic arthritis of the wrist

Pathologic or spontaneous fracture codes are also located in Chapter 13. A pathologic or spontaneous fracture is a break in a bone that occurs because of bone disease or a change surrounding the bone tissue that makes the bone weak. For a pathologic fracture, you report the fracture and the disease process responsible for the fracture, such as osteoporosis or metastatic cancer of the bone. It is also possible to have a small trauma associated with a pathologic fracture. Suppose, for example, an elderly woman with severe osteoporosis bumps her hip against the doorway and sustains a fractured hip. This may be classifiable as a pathologic fracture because a person with healthy bones would not have fractured a hip as the result of a small trauma such as bumping the hip on a doorway. If there is any question about whether a fracture is pathologic or due to trauma, ask the physician what caused the fracture.

A pathologic fracture is serious because healing may be delayed by the underlying bone disease. Also, if a pathologic fracture is documented and no other disease process is indicated, review the record or clarify with the physician the underlying cause of the fracture. You should never assign a code for a traumatic fracture and a pathologic fracture of the same bone; only code one or the other.

Example

PATHOLOGIC FRACTURE

Diagnosis:	Pathologic fracture of the hip due to severe osteoporosis
Index:	**Fracture** (abduction) (adduction) (avulsion) (compression) (crush) (dislocation) (oblique) (separation) (closed) 829.0
	pathologic (cause unknown) 733.10
	hip 733.14
Tabular:	**733.1 Pathologic fracture**
	733.14 Pathologic fracture of neck of femur

A second code will be assigned to identify the underlying disease.

Index:	**Osteoporosis** (generalized) 733.00
Tabular:	**733.0 Osteoporosis**
	733.00 Osteoporosis, unspecified
Codes:	733.14, 733.00 Pathologic fracture of the hip due to severe osteoporosis

---

The instructions for category 730, Osteomyelitis, periostitis, and other infections involving bone, direct you to identify any organism with an additional code. It is easy to miss the instructions between an *Excludes* note and the list of fifth-digit subclassifications. Highlight these instructions in your ICD-9-CM until you become familiar with their use when coding in this area. If any additional information you add to your code book makes you a better coder—add it.

EXERCISE 6-5 *Diseases of the Musculoskeletal System and Connective Tissue*

Assign ICD-9-CM codes for the following:

1 Rheumatoid arthritis

    ICD-9-CM Code: _____

2 Pain in the neck

    ICD-9-CM Code: _____

3 Recurrent dislocation, right shoulder

    ICD-9-CM Code: _____

4 Spontaneous fracture left humerus due to metastatic bone cancer; history of cancer of the breast previously excised

    ICD-9-CM Code(s): _____ (fracture), _____ (neoplasm),

    _____ (history of)

CONGENITAL ANOMALIES AND CERTAIN CONDITIONS ORIGINATING IN THE PERINATAL PERIOD

Chapters 14 and 15, Congenital Anomalies and Certain Conditions Originating in the Perinatal Period, in the ICD-9-CM Tabular describe congenital anomalies and conditions that originate in the perinatal period. An **anomaly** is an abnormality of a structure or organ. **Congenital** means that it is an abnormality that one was born with. Some anomalies are noticeable and discovered at birth. In cases of other anomalies, it may be a number of months or even years before they are discovered. If there is any question about whether a condition is acquired or congenital, you can review the record or clarify the case with the physician.

The perinatal period extends through the 28 days following birth. The term **perinatal** applies only to the baby and **postpartum** applies to the mother. Codes from this chapter can still be assigned beyond that time frame, but as the chapter title indicates, the condition must have originated during the perinatal period.

ICD-9-CM OFFICIAL GUIDELINES FOR CODING AND REPORTING

SECTION I.C.

15. Chapter 15: Newborn (Perinatal) Guidelines (760-779)

For coding and reporting purposes the perinatal period is defined as before birth through the 28th day following birth. The following guidelines are provided for reporting purposes. Hospitals may record other diagnoses as needed for internal data use.

a. General Perinatal Rules

1) Chapter 15 Codes

They are <u>never</u> for use on the maternal record. Codes from Chapter 11, the obstetric chapter, are never permitted on the newborn record. Chapter 15 code may be used throughout the life of the patient if the condition is still present.

2) **Sequencing of perinatal codes**

Generally, codes from Chapter 15 should be sequenced as the principal/first-listed diagnosis on the newborn record, with the exception of the appropriate V30 code for the birth episode, followed by codes from any other chapter that provide additional detail. The "use additional code" note at the beginning of the chapter supports this guideline. If the index does not provide a specific code for a perinatal condition, assign code 779.89, Other specified conditions originating in the perinatal period, followed by the code from another chapter that specifies the condition. Codes for signs and symptoms may be assigned when a definitive diagnosis has not been established.

3) **Birth process or community acquired conditions**

If a newborn has a condition that may be either due to the birth process or community acquired and the documentation does not indicate which it is, the default is due to the birth process and the code from Chapter 15 should be used. If the condition is community-acquired, a code from Chapter 15 should not be assigned.

4) **Code all clinically significant conditions**

All clinically significant conditions noted on routine newborn examination should be coded. A condition is clinically significant if it requires:

- clinical evaluation; or
- therapeutic treatment; or
- diagnostic procedures; or
- extended length of hospital stay; or
- increased nursing care and/or monitoring; or
- has implications for future health care needs

Note: The perinatal guidelines listed above are the same as the general coding guidelines for "additional diagnoses", except for the final point regarding implications for future health care needs. Codes should be assigned for conditions that have been specified by the provider as having implications for future health care needs. Codes from the perinatal chapter should not be assigned unless the provider has established a definitive diagnosis.

b. **Use of Codes V30-V39**

When coding the birth of an infant, assign a code from categories V30-V39, according to the type of birth. A code from this series is assigned as a principal diagnosis, and assigned only once to a newborn at the time of birth.

c. **Newborn Transfers**

If the newborn is transferred to another institution, the V30 series is not used at the receiving hospital.

d. **Use of Category V29**

1) **Assigning a code from category V29**

Assign a code from category V29, Observation and evaluation of newborns and infants for suspected conditions not found, to identify those instances when a healthy newborn is evaluated for a suspected condition that is determined after study not to be present. Do not use a code from category V29 when the patient has identified signs and symptoms of a suspected problem; in such cases, code the sign or symptom.

A code from category V29 may also be assigned as a principal code for readmissions or encounters when the V30 code no longer applies. Codes from category V29 are for use only for healthy newborns and infants for which no condition after study is found to be present.

2) **V29 code on a birth record**

A V29 code is to be used as a secondary code after the V30, Outcome of delivery, code.

e. Use of other V codes on perinatal records

V codes other than V30 and V29 may be assigned on a perinatal or newborn record code. The codes may be used as a principal or first-listed diagnosis for specific types of encounters or for readmissions or encounters when the V30 code no longer applies.

See Section I.C.18 for information regarding the assignment of V codes.

f. Maternal Causes of Perinatal Morbidity

Codes from categories 760-763, Maternal causes of perinatal morbidity and mortality, are assigned only when the maternal condition has actually affected the fetus or newborn. The fact that the mother has an associated medical condition or experiences some complication of pregnancy, labor or delivery does not justify the routine assignment of codes from these categories to the newborn record.

g. Congenital Anomalies in Newborns

For the birth admission, the appropriate code from category V30, Liveborn infants according to type of birth, should be used, followed by any congenital anomaly codes, categories 740-759. Use additional secondary codes from other chapters to specify conditions associated with the anomaly, if applicable.

Also, see Section I.C.14 for information on the coding of congenital anomalies.

h. Coding Additional Perinatal Diagnoses

1) **Assigning codes for conditions that require treatment**

Assign codes for conditions that require treatment or further investigation, prolong the length of stay, or require resource utilization.

2) **Codes for conditions specified as having implications for future health care needs**

Assign codes for conditions that have been specified by the provider as having implications for future health care needs.

Note: This guideline should not be used for adult patients.

3) **Codes for newborn conditions originating in the perinatal period**

Assign a code for newborn conditions originating in the perinatal period (categories 760-779), as well as complications arising during the current episode of care classified in other chapters, only if the diagnoses have been documented by the responsible provider at the time of transfer or discharge as having affected the fetus or newborn.

i. Prematurity and Fetal Growth Retardation

Providers utilize different criteria in determining prematurity. A code for prematurity should not be assigned unless it is documented. The 5th digit assignment for codes from category 764 and subcategories 765.0 and 765.1 should be based on the recorded birth weight and estimated gestational age.

A code from subcategory 765.2, Weeks of gestation, should be assigned as an additional code with category 764 and codes from 765.0 and 765.1 to specify weeks of gestation as documented by the provider in the record.

j. Newborn sepsis

Code 771.81, Septicemia [sepsis] of newborn, should be assigned with a secondary code from category 041, Bacterial infections in conditions classified elsewhere and of unspecified site, to identify the organism. A code from category 038, Septicemia, should not be used on a newborn record. Do not assign 995.91, Sepsis, as code 771.81 describes the sepsis. If applicable, use additional codes to identify severe sepsis (995.92) and any associated acute organ dysfunction.

As Guideline Section I.C.15.b. states, code the birth from categories V30-V39, Liveborn infant according to type of birth. The birth code is assigned only once and that is on the birth record of the baby because it indicates the type of birth.

On the baby's birth record the appropriate V code is sequenced first as the first-listed diagnosis. If any other conditions or congenital anomalies are documented, they are reported as secondary diagnoses.

NEWBORN CONGENITAL ANOMALIES

Example

Diagnosis:	Newborn male delivered in the hospital by cesarean section and with Down's syndrome
Index:	**Newborn** (infant) (liveborn), single, born in hospital (without mention of cesarean delivery or section) V30.00 with cesarean delivery or section V30.01
Tabular:	**V30 Single liveborn**

The code is not complete until you add a fourth and fifth digit. The fourth digit is "0" for born in the hospital and the fifth digit is "1" for delivered by cesarean delivery. The code would be V30.01. Next, code the Down's syndrome.

Index:	**Syndrome**—*see also* Disease, Down's (mongolism) 758.0
Tabular:	**758 Chromosomal anomalies**
	758.0 Down's syndrome
Codes:	V30.01, 758.0 Newborn male delivered by cesarean section in the hospital; Down's syndrome

---

In the preceding example, if the baby was transferred to a second facility for treatment of the Down's syndrome, no V code would be assigned by the second facility to identify delivery. The V code can be assigned only once, as the first-listed diagnosis at the birthing facility on the baby's record. The first-listed diagnosis code at the second facility would be Down's syndrome (758.0).

You have to be careful about assigning codes from the 760-763 categories, Maternal Causes of Perinatal Morbidity and Mortality. Many times the mother has a condition, but that condition has no untoward (negative) effect on the baby or fetus. Codes from these categories are to be assigned only when the maternal condition has **affected** the health of the newborn.

EXERCISE 6-6 *Congenital Anomalies and Certain Conditions Originating in the Perinatal Period*

Assign ICD-9-CM codes for the following:

1 Congenital absence of the earlobe

   ICD-9-CM Code: _____

2 Newborn male delivered in the hospital via vaginal delivery; undescended left testicle (will reevaluate in 6 weeks)

   ICD-9-CM Codes: _____, _____

3 Three-year-old diagnosed with fragile X syndrome

   ICD-9-CM Code: _____

4 Newborn transferred to a facility because of congenital dislocation of right hip (code as the facility transferred to)

   ICD-9-CM Code: _____

SIGNS, SYMPTOMS, AND ILL-DEFINED CONDITIONS

Chapter 16, Signs, Symptoms, and Ill-Defined Conditions, in the Tabular of the ICD-9-CM includes symptoms, signs, abnormal results of investigations and other ill-defined conditions. Signs and symptoms codes are assigned for encounters until there is a definitive diagnosis. A sign is defined as objective evidence of disease that can be observed by the physician. A symptom is a subjective observation reported by the patient but not confirmed objectively by the physician.

You assign the codes from Chapter 16 when:

- No more specific diagnosis can be made after investigation.
- Signs and symptoms existing at the time of the initial encounter prove to be transient or a cause cannot be determined.
- A patient fails to return and you have only a provisional diagnosis.
- A case is referred elsewhere before a definitive diagnosis is made.
- A more precise diagnosis is not available for any other reason.
- Certain symptoms that represent important problems in the medical care exist and it may be desirable to classify them in addition to the known cause.

You do not code from Chapter 16 when a definitive diagnosis is available. Consider, for example, this diagnostic statement: "Right lower quadrant abdominal pain due to acute appendicitis." The code for right lower quadrant abdominal pain is 789.03, located in Chapter 16. But because the reason for the pain is the acute appendicitis, you would not include the code for the symptom of abdominal pain, rather you would assign 540.9 for the acute appendicitis—the definitive diagnosis.

You do not code from Chapter 16 when the symptom is considered to be routinely associated with a disease process. Consider, for example, this diagnostic statement: "Cough and fever with pneumonia." Both cough and fever are symptoms of the pneumonia; therefore, you would not assign codes for either symptom. The only code you would assign would be 486 for the pneumonia.

A disease reference book comes in handy until you become more familiar with disease symptoms. If you do not know the symptoms associated with a disease, consult reference material or ask a colleague.

Finding the codes for **abnormal investigations** in the Index is tricky. The codes are located under the main term "Findings, abnormal, without diagnosis (examination) (laboratory test)." Some entries may also be located under the main term "Elevation," such as blood pressure and body temperature.

ABNORMAL FINDINGS

Example

Diagnosis:	Abnormal liver scan

Index:	**Findings, abnormal, without diagnosis** (examination) (laboratory test) 796.4
	    scan NEC 794.9
	        liver 794.8

Tabular:	**794 Nonspecific abnormal results of function studies** **794.8 Liver**
Code:	794.8 Abnormal liver scan

When reporting complications of surgical or medical care, you must be certain the complications are present. A surgical complication is one that takes place as a result of the procedure. Just because a complication occurs following a procedure does not mean the complication is a surgical complication. Do not assume a cause-and-effect relationship. Clarify any doubt or questions with the physician. The term complication as used in ICD-9-CM does not imply that improper or inadequate care is responsible for the problem. There is no time limit defined for the development of a complication. At what time it presents will dictate the way in which it is coded. Be sure to use the Index carefully and follow all instructional notes. Exclusion notes are extensive in this section and often direct the coder elsewhere.

EXERCISE 6-7 *Symptoms, Signs, and Ill-Defined Conditions*

Assign ICD-9-CM codes for the following:

1 Fussy infant

     ICD-9-CM Code: _____

2 Pleuritic-type chest pain

     ICD-9-CM Code: _____

3 Abnormal mammogram

     ICD-9-CM Code: _____

4 Seizure

     ICD-9-CM Code: _____

5 Elevated blood pressure reading

     ICD-9-CM Code: _____

INJURY AND POISONING

ICD-9-CM OFFICIAL GUIDELINES FOR CODING AND REPORTING

SECTION I.C.

19. Supplemental Classification of External Causes of Injury and Poisoning (E codes, E800-E999)

Introduction: These guidelines are provided for those who are currently collecting E codes in order that there will be standardization in the process. If your institution plans to begin collecting E codes, these guidelines are to be applied. The use of E codes is supplemental to the application of ICD-9-CM diagnosis codes.

External causes of injury and poisoning codes (categories E000 and E800-E999) are intended to provide data for injury research and evaluation of injury prevention strategies. Activity codes (categories E001-E030) are intended to be used to describe the activity of a person seeking care for injuries as well as other health conditions, when the injury or other health condition resulted from an activity or the activity contributed to a condition. E codes capture how the injury, poisoning, or adverse effect happened (cause), the intent (unintentional or accidental; or intentional, such as suicide or assault), the person's status (e.g. civilian, military), the associated activity and the place where the event occurred.

Some major categories of E codes include:

> transport accidents
> poisoning and adverse effects of drugs, medicinal substances and biologicals
> accidental falls
> accidents caused by fire and flames
> accidents due to natural and environmental factors
> late effects of accidents, assaults or self-injury
> assaults or purposely inflicted injury
> suicide or self inflicted injury

These guidelines apply for the coding and collection of E codes from records in hospitals, outpatient clinics, emergency departments, other ambulatory care settings and provider offices, and nonacute care settings, except when other specific guidelines apply.

a. **General E Code Coding Guidelines**

1) **Used with any code in the range of 001-V89**
   An E code from categories E800-E999 may be used with any code in the range of 001-V89, which indicates an injury, poisoning, or adverse effect due to an external cause.

   An activity E code (categories E001-E030) may be used with any code in the range of 001-V89 that indicates an injury, or other health condition that resulted from an activity, or the activity contributed to a condition.

2) **Assign the appropriate E code for all initial treatments**
   Assign the appropriate E code for the initial encounter of an injury, poisoning, or adverse effect of drugs, not for subsequent treatment.

   External cause of injury codes (E-codes) may be assigned while the acute fracture codes are still applicable.
   See Section I.C.17.b.1 for coding of acute fractures.

3) **Use the full range of E codes**
   Use the full range of E codes (E800-E999) to completely describe the cause, the intent and the place of the occurrence, if applicable, for all injuries, poisonings, and adverse effects of drugs.
   See a.1.), j.), and k.) in this section for information on the use of status and activity E codes.

4) **Assign as many E codes as necessary**
   Assign as many E codes as necessary to fully explain each cause.

5) **The selection of the appropriate E code**
   The selection of the appropriate E code is guided by the Index to External Causes, which is located after the alphabetical index to diseases and by Inclusion and Exclusion notes in the Tabular List.

6) **E code can never be a principal diagnosis**
   An E code can never be a principal (first listed) diagnosis.

7) **External cause code(s) with systemic inflammatory response syndrome (SIRS)**
   An external cause code is not appropriate with a code from subcategory 995.9, unless the patient also has another condition for which an E code would be appropriate (such as an injury, poisoning, or adverse effect of drugs.

8) **Multiple Cause E Code Coding Guidelines**
   More than one E-code is required to fully describe the external cause of an illness, injury or poisoning. The assignment of E-codes should be sequenced in the following priority:

   If two or more events cause separate injuries, an E code should be assigned for each cause. The first listed E code will be selected in the following order:

E codes for child and adult abuse take priority over all other E codes. *See Section I.C.19.d. Child and adult abuse guidelines.*

E codes for terrorism events take priority over all other E codes except child and adult abuse.

E codes for cataclysmic events take priority over all other E codes except child and adult abuse and terrorism.

E codes for transport accidents take priority over all other E codes except cataclysmic events and child and adult abuse and terrorism.

Activity and external cause status codes are assigned following all causal (intent) E codes.

The first-listed E code should correspond to the cause of the most serious diagnosis due to an assault, accident, or self-harm, following the order of hierarchy listed above.

9) If the reporting format limits the number of E codes
If the reporting format limits the number of E codes that can be used in reporting clinical data, report the code for the cause/intent most related to the principal diagnosis. If the format permits capture of additional E codes, the cause/intent, including medical misadventures, of the additional events should be reported rather than the codes for place activity or external status.

b. Place of Occurrence Guideline
Use an additional code from category E849 to indicate the Place of Occurrence. The Place of Occurrence describes the place where the event occurred and not the patient's activity at the time of the event.

Do not use E849.9 if the place of occurrence is not stated.

c. Adverse Effects of Drugs, Medicinal, and Biological Substances Guidelines

1) Do not code directly from the Table of Drugs
Do not code directly from the Table of Drugs and Chemicals. Always refer back to the Tabular List.

2) Use as many codes as necessary to describe
Use as many codes as necessary to describe completely all drugs, medicinal or biological substances.

3) If the same E code would describe the causative agent
If the same E code would describe the causative agent for more than one adverse reaction, assign the code only once.

4) If two or more drugs, medicinal or biological substances
If two or more drugs, medicinal or biological substances are reported, code each individually unless the combination code is listed in the Table of Drugs and Chemicals. In that case, assign the E code for the combination.

5) When a reaction results from the interaction of a drug(s)
When a reaction results from the interaction of a drug(s) and alcohol, use poisoning codes and E codes for both.

If there are different fourth digit codes in the same three digit category, use the code for "Other specified" of that category. If there is no "Other specified" code in that category, use the appropriate "Unspecified" code in that category.

If the codes are in different three digit categories, assign the appropriate E code for other multiple drugs and medicinal substances.

6) Codes from the E930-E949 series
Codes from the E930-E949 series must be used to identify the causative substance for an adverse effect of drug, medicinal and biological substances, correctly prescribed and properly administered. The effect, such as tachycardia, delirium, gastrointestinal

hemorrhaging, vomiting, hypokalemia, hepatitis, renal failure, or respiratory failure, is coded and followed by the appropriate code from the E930-E949 series.

d. Child and Adult Abuse Guideline

1) Intentional injury

When the cause of an injury or neglect is intentional child or adult abuse, the first listed E code should be assigned from categories E960-E968, Homicide and injury purposely inflicted by other persons (except category E967). An E code from category E967, Child and adult battering and other maltreatment, should be added as an additional code to identify the perpetrator, if known.

2) Accidental intent

In cases of neglect when the intent is determined to be accidental E code E904.0, Abandonment or neglect of infant and helpless person, should be the first listed E code.

e. Unknown or Suspected Intent Guideline

1) If the intent (accident, self-harm, assault) of the cause of an injury or poisoning is unknown

If the intent (accident, self-harm, assault) of the cause of an injury or poisoning is unknown or unspecified, code the intent as undetermined E980-E989.

2) If the intent (accident, self-harm, assault) of the cause of an injury or poisoning is questionable

If the intent (accident, self-harm, assault) of the cause of an injury or poisoning is questionable, probable or suspected, code the intent as undetermined E980-E989.

f. Undetermined Cause

When the intent of an injury or poisoning is known, but the cause is unknown, use codes E928.9, Unspecified accident, E958.9, Suicide and self-inflicted injury by unspecified means, and E968.9, Assault by unspecified means.

These E codes should rarely be used, as the documentation in the medical record, in both the inpatient outpatient and other settings, should normally provide sufficient detail to determine the cause of the injury.

g. Late Effects of External Cause Guidelines

1) Late effect E codes

Late effect E codes exist for injuries and poisonings but not for adverse effects of drugs, misadventures, and surgical complications.

2) Late effect E codes (E929, E959, E969, E977, E989, or E999.1)

A late effect E code (E929, E959, E969, E977, E989, or E999.1) should be used with any report of a late effect or sequela resulting from a previous injury or poisoning (905-909).

3) Late effect E code with a related current injury

A late effect E code should never be used with a related current nature of injury code.

4) Use of late effect E codes for subsequent visits

Use a late effect E code for subsequent visits when a late effect of the initial injury or poisoning is being treated. There is no late effect E code for adverse effects of drugs. Do not use a late effect E code for subsequent visits for follow-up care (e.g., to assess healing, to receive rehabilitative therapy) of the injury or poisoning when no late effect of the injury has been documented.

h. Misadventures and Complications of Care Guidelines

1) Code range E870-E876

Assign a code in the range of E870-E876 if misadventures are stated by the provider. When applying the E code guidelines pertaining to sequencing, these E codes are considered causal codes.

2) Code range E878-E879

Assign a code in the range of E878-E879 if the provider attributes an abnormal reaction or later complication to a surgical or medical procedure, but does not mention misadventure at the time of the procedure as the cause of the reaction.

i. Terrorism Guidelines

1) Cause of injury identified by the Federal Government (FBI) as terrorism

When the cause of an injury is identified by the Federal Government (FBI) as terrorism, the first-listed E-code should be a code from category E979, Terrorism. The definition of terrorism employed by the FBI is found at the inclusion note at E979. The terrorism E-code is the only E-code that should be assigned. Additional E codes from the assault categories should not be assigned.

2) Cause of an injury is suspected to be the result of terrorism

When the cause of an injury is suspected to be the result of terrorism a code from category E979 should not be assigned. Assign a code in the range of E codes based circumstances on the documentation of intent and mechanism.

3) Code E979.9, Terrorism, secondary effects

Assign code E979.9, Terrorism, secondary effects, for conditions occurring subsequent to the terrorist event. This code should not be assigned for conditions that are due to the initial terrorist act.

4) Statistical tabulation of terrorism codes

For statistical purposes these codes will be tabulated within the category for assault, expanding the current category from E960-E969 to include E979 and E999.1.

Alphabetic Index to External Causes (E Code)

Alphabetic Index to External Causes of Injuries is the **index** for the E codes. The index classifies environmental events (tornadoes, floods), circumstances, and other conditions as the cause of injury and other adverse effects alphabetically. **E codes are never used as a first-listed diagnosis.** Rather, E codes are used to clarify injury or adverse effects.

E code terms describe the external circumstances under which an accident, injury, or act of violence occurred. The main terms in the E code index usually represent the type of accident or violence (e.g., assault, collision), with the specific agent or other circumstance listed below the main term. "Collision" in Fig. 6–1 is the type of accident, and listed below Collision are the circumstances of the accident.

✋ **CAUTION** *E codes have their own index. You can locate the E code index only in Volume 2, Section III, Index to External Causes of Injury, and then turn to the codes you're directed to in the E code Supplementary Classification of Volume 1 (they follow the V codes).*

You must be sure to read all the information under a term in the E code index before locating the code in the Tabular. Be sure to check for fourth-digit specificity for railway accidents, motor vehicle traffic and nontraffic accidents, other road vehicle accidents, water transport accidents, and air and space transport accidents shown in the Index of the External Causes.

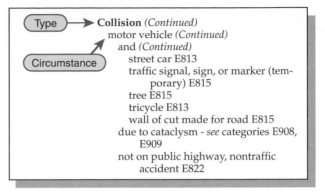

FIGURE 6–1 Section 3, Index to External Causes. (Modified from Buck CJ: *2010 ICD-9-CM, Volumes 1, 2, & 3, Professional Edition*, St. Louis, 2010, Saunders.)

When a code from the E code section is reported, it is **in addition** to an injury code from the Tabular List of the ICD-9-CM. The E code classification is an additional code for greater detail. Most groups of E codes have Includes or *Excludes* notes that provide further detail about assigning the codes. For example, for E845, Accident involving spacecraft, the Includes note states that launching-pad accidents are included and the *Excludes* note states that the effects of weightlessness in a spacecraft are not included. Be sure to read these notes as you become familiar with what is included or excluded.

The use of the additional digit adds specificity as to who was injured in the accident. For example, if the injured person was the driver of a car involved in a motor vehicle accident, the fifth digit would be 0. If the injured person was a passenger in the vehicle, the fifth digit would be 1.

E codes also permit the classification of environmental events, circumstances, and conditions as the cause of injury, poisoning, and other adverse effects. With E codes, anything that can injure or have an adverse effect on a human body can be coded. The E codes can supply a code if a person is injured while pearl diving (E910.3), injured when a window of a railroad car falls on someone's head (E806.9), or hurt when pecked by a bird (E906.8). They are all in the E codes! These are rather far-fetched examples, granted, but they show how extensive and specific the codes are.

CODING SHOT Place of occurrence E codes are reported to provide further specificity as to where the accident/external cause occurred. If the place of occurrence is unknown, no code is assigned in accordance with coding guidelines.

Some states have made the assignment of E codes mandatory, and the general use of E codes has increased significantly. At the beginning of Chapter 17, Injury and Poisoning (800-999), the note directs you to "Use E code(s) to identify the cause and intent of the injury or poisoning (E800-E999)." The Occupational Safety and Health Administration (OSHA) and Workers' Compensation are two entities that track the data from E codes to identify the causes of accidents. In states where E code assignment is not mandatory, each facility decides if it will or will not require assignment of E codes.

EXERCISE 6-8 E Codes

Using the ICD-9-CM manual, locate the correct E code for each of the following in Volume 2, Alphabetic Index, and then in Volume 1, Tabular List.

1 Railway (E800-E807)

Railway accident involving derailment without antecedent collision, injuring a porter

E code index term(s): _____

ICD-9-CM Code: _____

2 Motor Vehicle Traffic (E810-E819)

Motor vehicle traffic accident due to tire blowout; driver of the car was injured

E code index term(s): _____

ICD-9-CM Code: _____

3 Motor Vehicle Nontraffic (E820-E825)

Driver of an ATV (off-road vehicle) is injured when he collides with a fence

E code index term(s): _____

ICD-9-CM Code: _____

4 Other Road Vehicle (E826-E829)

Horse being ridden, rider injured, and non-motor vehicle collision

E code index term(s): _____

ICD-9-CM Code: _____

5 Water Transport (E830-E838)

Accident to watercraft causing other injury; occupant of small powered boat injured due to collision

E code index term(s): _____

ICD-9-CM Code: _____

Table of Drugs and Chemicals

Section II follows the Index in the ICD-9-CM and contains the Table of Drugs and Chemicals, which is an alphabetical listing of poisoning and external causes of adverse effects of drugs and other chemicals. The table headings pertaining to external cause are illustrated in Fig. 6–2.

Accident (E850-E869): Instances of accidental overdose of a drug, wrong substance given or taken, drug taken inadvertently, accidents in the use of drugs and biological agents during medical and surgical procedures, and external causes of poisonings classifiable to 980-989.

ACCIDENT

Example

A 35-year-old male is brought to the emergency department with memory disturbance after an accidental exposure to lead paint.

Lead paint	984.0
Memory disturbance	780.93
Accident, intention	E861.5

Substance	External Cause (E-Code)					
	Poisoning	Accident	Therapeutic Use	Suicide Attempt	Assault	Undetermined
Acrolein (gas)	987.8	E869.8	—	E952.8	E962.2	E982.8
liquid	989.89	E866.8	—	E950.9	E962.1	E980.9
Actaea spicata	988.2	E865.4	—	E950.9	E962.1	E980.9

FIGURE 6–2   Table headings pertaining to external cause. (Modified from Buck CJ: *2010 ICD-9-CM, Volumes 1, 2, & 3, Professional Edition,* St. Louis, 2010, Saunders.)

Therapeutic Use (E930-E949): Instances in which a correct substance properly administered in a therapeutic (treatment) or prophylactic (preventive) dosage has been the external cause of adverse effects.

THERAPEUTIC USE

Example

A 2-year-old male is taken by his mother to the pediatrician for a routine vaccination. That evening the child's temperature is 104°F, and he is taken by the mother to the emergency department.

Fever	780.60
Unspecified vaccine	E949.9

Suicide Attempt (E950-E959): Instances in which self-inflicted injuries or poisonings have been involved.

SUICIDE

Example

Rachael broke up with her boyfriend of 6 years. She became so despondent in the days that followed that she wrote a note indicating she was ending her life and took the entire bottle of her mother's prescription of Valium. She was found unconscious later by her mother.

Poisoning, Valium (diazepam)	969.4
Unconscious	780.09
Suicide, intention	E950.3

Assault (E960-E969): Instances in which injury or poisoning has been inflicted by another person with the intent to injure or kill.

ASSAULT

Example

A 42-year-old male presents to his physician with complaints of severe abdominal cramping and pain. After extensive laboratory tests, the physician identifies the source of the problem as high levels of arsenic in the patient's system. The patient's wife was charged with the attempted murder of her husband.

Poisoning, arsenic	985.1
Abdominal pain and cramps	789.00
Assault, intention	E962.1

Undetermined (E980-E989): Instances in which it cannot be determined whether the poisoning or injury was intentional or accidental.

UNDETERMINED

Example

A transient is found comatose under a freeway overpass. Later at the emergency department the patient is found to have high levels of heroin in his system. It is unknown at this time if the overdose was intentional or accidental.

Adult abuse	995.85
Poisoning, heroin	965.01
Coma	780.01
Undetermined, intention	E980.0

A thorough review of the documentation would be done to identify any indication of drug addiction and report if documented in the medical record.

Although certain substances are indexed in the Table of Drugs and Chemicals with one or more subentries, the majority are listed according to one use or state (i.e., solid, liquid, or gas). It is recognized that many substances may be used in various ways, in medicine and in industry, and may cause adverse effects or poisoning. In cases in which the reported data indicate a use or state not in the table, or one that is clearly different from those listed, an attempt should be made to classify the substances in the category that most nearly expresses the reported facts.

Adverse Effects

The coding of adverse effects and poisonings is probably the most difficult part of this chapter. It takes some practice to distinguish between an adverse effect and a poisoning. Because the physician is probably not going to use those specific terms in the diagnostic statement, you must question the physician if you are uncertain whether the diagnosis is an adverse effect or a poisoning.

ICD-9-CM OFFICIAL GUIDELINES FOR CODING AND REPORTING

SECTION I.C.17.
e. Adverse Effects, Poisoning, and Toxic Effects

The properties of certain drugs, medicinal and biological substances, or combinations of such substances, may cause toxic reactions. The occurrence of drug toxicity is classified in ICD-9-CM as follows:

1) Adverse Effect

When the drug was correctly prescribed and properly administered, code the reaction plus the appropriate code from the E930-E949 series. Codes from E930-E949 series must be used to identify the causative substance for adverse effect of drug, medicinal and biological substances, correctly prescribed and properly administered. The effect, such as tachycardia, delirium, gastrointestinal hemorrhaging, vomiting, hypokalemia, hepatitis, renal failure, or respiratory failure, is coded and followed by the appropriate code from E930-E949 series.

Adverse effects of therapeutic substances correctly prescribed and properly administered (toxicity, synergistic reaction, side effect, and idiosyncratic reaction) may be due to (1) differences among patients, such as age, sex, disease, and genetic factors, and (2) drug-related factors, such as type of drug, route of administration, duration of therapy, dosage, and bioavailability.

An **adverse effect** occurs when a drug has been correctly prescribed and properly administered and the patient develops a reaction. Everything has been done correctly by the physician and the patient, but a reaction or adverse effect has occurred because of the drug.

When reporting adverse effects, you code the **effect** first, followed by the E code from the **therapeutic** column in the Table of Drugs and Chemicals. (You use the therapeutic column because the medication was prescribed by the physician as a therapy for a condition.)

ADVERSE EFFECT

Example

Diagnosis: Urticaria due to penicillin (properly taken and prescribed)

Index: **Urticaria 708.9, due to, drugs 708.0**

Tabular: **708 Urticaria**

              708.0 Allergic urticaria

You also report the drug using the Table of Drugs and Chemicals.

Table of Drugs: Penicillin (any type) E930.0

Tabular: **E930 Antibiotics**

              E930.0 Penicillins

Codes: 708.0, E930.0 Urticaria due to penicillin

The code for the effect (urticaria, 708.0) is listed first and the cause (penicillin, E930.0) next.

The E codes from this section (E930-E949) are considered required E codes. Thus, therapeutic E codes for adverse effects must be assigned. E codes are never assigned as a first-listed diagnosis but are always considered an additional code.

In Fig. 6–3, the Table of Drugs and Chemicals shows that column 1 (Substance) contains the name of the drug or chemical. Column 2 (Poisoning)

TABLE OF DRUGS AND CHEMICALS

Substance	Poisoning	External Cause (E-Code)				
		Accident	Therapeutic Use	Suicide Attempt	Assault	Undetermined
Acrolein (gas)	987.8	E869.8	—	E952.8	E962.2	E982.8
liquid	989.89	E866.8	—	E950.9	E962.1	E980.9
Actaea spicata	988.2	E865.4	—	E950.9	E962.1	E980.9
Acterol	961.5	E857	E931.5	E950.4	E962.0	E980.4
ACTH	962.4	E858.0	E932.4	E950.4	E962.0	E980.4
Acthar	962.4	E858.0	E932.4	E950.4	E962.0	E980.4
Actinomycin (C) (D)	960.7	E856	E930.7	E950.4	E962.0	E980.4
Adalin (acetyl)	967.3	E852.2	E937.3	E950.2	E962.0	E980.2
Adenosine (phosphate)	977.8	E858.8	E947.8	E950.4	E962.0	E980.4
Adhesives	989.89	E866.6	—	E950.9	E962.1	E980.9
ADH	962.5	E858.0	E932.5	E950.4	E962.0	E980.4
Adicillin	960.0	E856	E930.0	E950.4	E962.0	E980.4
Adiphenine	975.1	E855.6	E945.1	E950.4	E962.0	E980.4
Adjunct, pharmaceutical	977.4	E858.8	E947.4	E950.4	E962.0	E980.4
Adrenal (extract, cortex or medulla) (glucocorticoids) (hormones) (mineralocorticoids)	962.0	E858.0	E932.0	E950.4	E962.0	E980.4
ENT agent	976.6	E858.7	E946.6	E950.4	E962.0	E980.4
ophthalmic preparation	976.5	E858.7	E946.5	E950.4	E962.0	E980.4
topical NEC	976.0	E858.7	E946.0	E950.4	E962.0	E980.4
Adrenalin	971.2	E855.5	E941.2	E950.4	E962.0	E980.4
Adrenergic blocking agents	971.3	E855.6	E941.3	E950.4	E962.0	E980.4
Adrenergics	971.2	E855.5	E941.2	E950.4	E962.0	E980.4
Adrenochrome (derivatives)	972.8	E858.3	E942.8	E950.4	E962.0	E980.4
Adrenocorticotropic hormone	962.4	E858.0	E932.4	E950.4	E962.0	E980.4
Adrenocorticotropin	962.4	E858.0	E932.4	E950.4	E962.0	E980.4
Adriamycin	960.7	E856	E930.7	E950.4	E962.0	E980.4
Aerosol spray - see Sprays	—	—	—	—	—	—
Aerosporin	960.8	E856	E930.8	E950.4	E962.0	E980.4
ENT agent	976.6	E858.7	E946.6	E950.4	E962.0	E980.4
ophthalmic preparation	976.5	E858.7	E946.5	E950.4	E962.0	E980.4
topical NEC	976.0	E858.7	E946.0	E950.4	E962.0	E980.4
Aethusa cynapium	988.2	E865.4	—	E950.9	E962.1	E980.9
Afghanistan black	969.6	E854.1	E939.6	E950.3	E962.0	E980.3
Aflatoxin	989.7	E865.9	—	E950.9	E962.1	E980.9
African boxwood	988.2	E865.4	—	E950.9	E962.1	E980.9
Agar (-agar)	973.3	E858.4	E943.3	E950.4	E962.0	E980.4
Agricultural agent NEC	989.89	E863.9	—	E950.6	E962.1	E980.7
Agrypnal	967.0	E851	E937.0	E950.1	E962.0	E980.1
Air contaminant(s), source or type not specified	—	—	—	—	—	—
specified type - see specific substance	987.9	E869.9	—	E952.9	E962.2	E982.9
Akee	988.2	E865.4	—	E950.9	E962.1	E980.9
Akrinol	976.0	E858.7	E946.0	E950.4	E962.0	E980.4
Alantolactone	961.6	E857	E931.6	E950.4	E962.0	E980.4
Albamycin	960.8	E856	E930.8	E950.4	E962.0	E980.4
Albumin (normal human serum)	964.7	E858.2	E934.7	E950.4	E962.0	E980.4
Albuterol	975.7	E858.6	E945.7	E950.4	E962.0	E980.4
Alcohol	980.9	E860.9	—	E950.9	E962.1	E980.9
absolute	980.0	E860.1	—	E950.9	E962.1	E980.9
beverage	980.0	E860.0	E947.8	E950.9	E962.1	E980.9
amyl	980.3	E860.4	—	E950.9	E962.1	E980.9
antifreeze	980.1	E860.2	—	E950.9	E962.1	E980.9
butyl	980.3	E860.4	—	E950.9	E962.1	E980.9
dehydrated	980.0	E860.1	—	E950.9	E862.1	E980.9
beverage	980.0	E860.0	E947.8	E950.9	E962.1	E980.9
denatured	980.0	E860.1	—	E950.9	E962.1	E980.9
deterrents	977.3	E858.8	E947.3	E950.4	E962.0	E980.4
diagnostic (gastric function)	977.8	E858.8	E947.8	E950.4	E962.0	E980.4
ethyl	980.0	E860.1	—	E950.9	E962.1	E980.9
beverage	980.0	E860.0	E947.8	E950.9	E962.1	E980.9
grain	980.0	E860.1	—	E950.9	E962.1	E980.9
beverage	980.0	E860.0	E947.8	E950.9	E962.1	E980.9

How adverse effect occurred

Drug/chemical name

Poisoning code **+** How the poisoning occurred

FIGURE 6–3 Section 2, Table of Drugs and Chemicals. (Modified from Buck CJ: *2009 ICD-9-CM, Volumes 1, 2, & 3, Professional Edition*, St. Louis, 2009, Saunders.)

contains the list of poisoning codes. The remaining five columns are the E codes that are assigned to indicate how the poisoning or adverse effect occurred.

There is a code available for an **unknown adverse effect.** For example, if the physician has documented a reaction due to penicillin and you cannot determine from the record what the exact adverse effect has been, you would report an unknown adverse effect. Adverse effects can be located in the Index under the main term "Effect, adverse," and the subterm "drugs and medicinals correct substance properly administered 995." The correct codes for an unknown adverse effect due to penicillin are 995.20 and E930.0.

A **poisoning** occurs when drugs or other chemical substances are taken not according to a physician's instruction. Poisonings occur in a variety of ways:

- The wrong dosage is given in error, either during medical treatment or by nonmedical personnel such as the mother or the patient herself or himself.

- The medication is given to the wrong person.

- The medication is taken by the wrong person.

- A medication overdose has occurred.

- Medications (prescription or over-the-counter) have been taken in combination with alcohol or recreational drugs.

- Over-the-counter medications have been taken in combination with prescription medications without physician approval.

ICD-9-CM OFFICIAL GUIDELINES FOR CODING AND REPORTING

SECTION I.C.17.e.

2. Poisoning

(a) Error was made in drug prescription

Error made in drug prescription or in the administration of the drug by provider, nurse, patient, or other person, use the appropriate poisoning code from the 960-979 series.

(b) Overdose of a drug intentionally taken

If an overdose of a drug was intentionally taken or administered and resulted in drug toxicity, it would be coded as a poisoning (960-979 series).

(c) Nonprescribed drug taken with correctly prescribed and properly administered drug

If a nonprescribed drug or medicinal agent was taken in combination with a correctly prescribed and properly administered drug, any drug toxicity or other reaction resulting from the interaction of the two drugs would be classified as a poisoning.

(d) Interaction of drug(s) and alcohol

When a reaction results from the interaction of a drug(s) and alcohol, this would be classified as poisoning.

(e) Sequencing of poisoning

When coding a poisoning or reaction to the improper use of a medication (e.g., wrong dose, wrong substance, wrong route of administration) the poisoning code is sequenced first, followed by a code for the manifestation. If there is also a diagnosis of drug abuse or dependence to the substance, the abuse or dependence is coded as an additional code.
See Section I.C..3.a.6.b. if poisoning is the result of insulin pump malfunctions and Section I.C.19 for general use of E-codes.

Poisoning codes are found in the Table of Drugs and Chemicals. You must always sequence the poisoning code first, then code any manifestation of the poisoning, such as coma, second. You also assign the corresponding E code from the Table of Drugs and Chemicals. If there is no documentation to indicate the intent so the intent is unknown or if the intent is questionable, code the intent as undetermined E980-E989.

> **CAUTION** *You CANNOT use an E code from the therapeutic column (E930-E949) with a poisoning code because they are mutually exclusive (can't be reported together). Something that is therapeutic (intended for treatment) could not be a poisoning (harmful).*

POISONING

Example

Diagnosis: Coma due to accidental overdose of Valium (Valium is the brand name for benzodiazepine)

When you reference the main term "Overdose" in the Index, you are directed to the Table of Drugs and Chemicals.

Table of Drugs: Valium 969.4 (poisoning)

                    E853.2 (accidental)

Tabular: **969 Poisoning by psychotropic agents**

                        969.4 Benzodiazepine-based tranquilizers

Tabular: **E853 Accidental poisoning by tranquilizers**

                        E853.2 Benzodiazepine-based tranquilizers

Index: **Coma 780.01**

Tabular: **780 General symptoms**

                        780.01 Coma

Codes: 969.4, 780.01, E853.2 Coma due to accidental overdose of Valium. Note that the poisoning code (969.4) is sequenced first, followed by the manifestation (780.01) and then the E code (E853.2).

If there has been no manifestation (coma, in the above case) of the poisoning, you would assign only the poisoning code (969.4) with the appropriate E code. When a patient undergoes a poisoning that involves more than one drug or chemical, there could be a different poisoning code and E code for each drug or chemical.

EXERCISE 6-9 *Poisoning/Table of Drugs and Chemicals*

Using the ICD-9-CM manual, assign poisoning codes and E codes to the following:

1 Poisoning by the ingestion of the beverage grain alcohol

     ICD-9-CM Codes: _____ (poisoning), _____ (E code)

2 Undetermined poisoning by antifreeze

     ICD-9-CM Codes: _____ (poisoning), _____ (E code)

3 Accidental overdose due to therapeutically prescribed valium

      ICD-9-CM Code(s): _____

Manifestations (symptoms or signs) of poisonings and adverse effects of drugs and chemicals are found in Section 1, under the specific symptom or disease. For example, Fig. 6–4 illustrates the location of the symptom Rash in Volume 2, the Alphabetic Index. If the symptom of the drug poisoning or adverse effect is a rash, the subterm "drug (internal use)" directs you to 693.0.
    Turn to code 693.0 in Volume 1, Tabular List.

4 What does the description of the ICD-9-CM code state? _____

Note the statement below the code: "Use additional E code to identify drug." In this case the condition is a rash. So when you see this statement, you know you have to identify the drug that caused the rash.

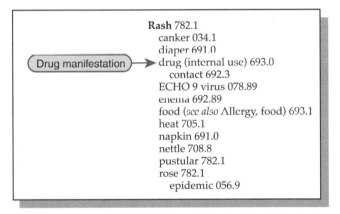

FIGURE 6–4   Index to Diseases, Rash. (Modified from Buck CJ: *2010 ICD-9-CM, Volumes 1, 2, & 3, Professional Edition,* St. Louis, 2010, Saunders.)

Burns   There are numerous guidelines that pertain to injuries and poisonings. It is within this chapter that the codes to report burns are located. First, read the Guidelines on burns:

ICD-9-CM OFFICIAL GUIDELINES FOR CODING AND REPORTING

SECTION I.C.17.

c. Coding of Burns

Current burns (940-948) are classified by depth, extent and by agent (E code). Burns are classified by depth as first degree (erythema), second degree (blistering), and third-degree (full-thickness involvement).

1) **Sequencing of burn and related condition codes**
   Sequence first the code that reflects the highest degree of burn when more than one burn is present.

   a. When the reason for the admission or encounter is for treatment of external multiple burns, sequence first the code that reflects the burn of the highest degree.

   b. When a patient has both internal and external burns, the circumstances of admission govern the selection of the principal diagnosis or first-listed diagnosis.

   c. When a patient is admitted for burn injuries and other related conditions such as smoke inhalation and/or respiratory failure, the circumstances of admission govern the selection of the principal or first-listed diagnosis.

2) **Burns of the same local site**
   Classify burns of the same local site (three-digit category level, 940-947) but of different degrees to the subcategory identifying the highest degree recorded in the diagnosis *[as is illustrated in Fig. 6–5].*

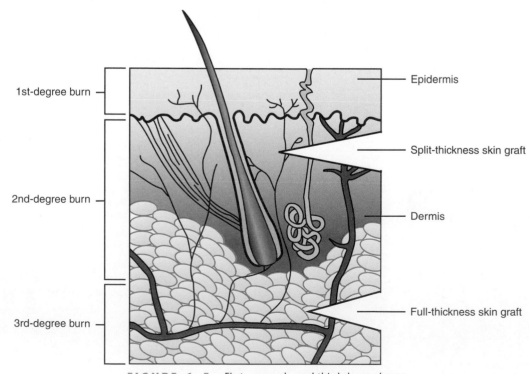

FIGURE 6–5   First-, second-, and third-degree burns.

ICD-9-CM OFFICIAL GUIDELINES FOR CODING AND REPORTING

SECTION I.C.17.

c. Coding of Burns

3) Non-healing burns

Non-healing burns are coded as acute burns. Necrosis of burned skin should be coded as a non-healed burn.

4) Code 958.3, Posttraumatic wound infection

Assign code 958.3, Posttraumatic wound infection, not elsewhere classified, as an additional code for any documented infected burn site.

5) Assign separate codes for each burn site

When coding burns, assign separate codes for each burn site. Category 946 Burns of Multiple specified sites, should only be used if the locations of the burns are not documented.

Category 949, Burn, unspecified, is extremely vague and should rarely be used.

6) Assign codes from category 948, Burns

Burns classified according to extent of body surface involved, when the site of the burn is not specified or when there is a need for additional data. It is advisable to use category 948 as additional coding when needed to provide data for evaluating burn mortality, such as that needed by burn units. It is also advisable to use category 948 as an additional code for reporting purposes when there is mention of third-degree burn involving 20 percent or more of the body surface.

In assigning a code from category 948:

Fourth-digit codes are used to identify the percentage of total body surface involved in a burn (all degree).

Fifth-digits are assigned to identify the percentage of body surface involved in third-degree burn.

Fifth-digit zero (0) is assigned when less than 10 percent or when no body surface is involved in a third-degree burn.

Category 948 is based on the classic "rule of nines" *[refer to Figs. 6–6 and 6–7]* in estimating body surface involved: head and neck are assigned nine percent, each arm nine percent, each leg 18 percent, the anterior trunk 18 percent, posterior trunk 18 percent, and genitalia one percent. Providers may change these percentage assignments when necessary to accommodate infants and children who have proportionately larger heads than adults and patients who have large buttocks, thighs, or abdomen that involve burns.

7) Encounters for treatment of late effects of burns

Encounters for the treatment of the late effects of burns (i.e., scars or joint contractures) should be coded to the residual condition (sequelae) followed by the appropriate late effect code (906.5-906.9). A late effect E code may also be used, if desired.

8) Sequelae with a late effect code and current burn

When appropriate, both a sequelae with a late effect code, and a current burn code may be assigned on the same record (when both a current burn and sequelae of an old burn exist).

d. Coding of Debridement of Wounds, Infection, or Burn

Excisional debridement involves surgical removal or cutting away, as opposed to a mechanical (brushing, scrubbing, washing) debridement.

For coding purposes, excisional debridement is assigned to code 86.22.

Nonexcisional debridement is assigned to code 86.28.

The guidelines for **burns** direct you to sequence the highest degree of burn first. If you are coding a third-degree burn of the hand and a second-degree burn of the chest wall, you would sequence the code for the third-degree burn of the hand first, followed by the second-degree burn of the chest.

If different degrees of burns are documented at the same site, assign a code to the highest degree only. For example, if the patient has first- and second-degree burns to the hand, you would code only the second-degree burn to the hand because that is the highest level of specificity and the most severe.

Facilities may choose to capture data regarding the extent of body area burned. In this case, the rule of nines is applied (Figs. 6–6 and 6–7). The Index entry is "Burn...948.0" with a note indicating that the fifth digit is added to indicate the extent of body surface involved (in percentage).

Burns are located in the Index by referring to the main term "Burn," subterms according to the site (abdomen or thigh), and finally to the degree of burn (second or third).

Codes from the 948 category can be assigned alone or in combination with other specific burn codes. The inclusion of codes from 948 are important for statistical purposes and may affect reimbursement. The use of the three-digit code 948 indicates a burn condition. The **fourth** digit indicates the **total percentage** of the body that has been burnt—including all first-, second-, and third-degree burns. The **fifth** digit (0-9) indicates the percentage of the body that received **third-degree** burns. It is not the coder's job to calculate the percentages, but you should seek clarification from the physician if documentation is missing or unclear regarding the percentages. Codes 940 through 949 are used for current unhealed burns excluding friction burns and sunburn; these are classified as dermatitis and superficial injury. Necrosis and non-healing burns are coded to acute current burns. Remember it is possible for a patient to have both healed and unhealed burns coded from the same episode of care because burns can heal at a different rate.

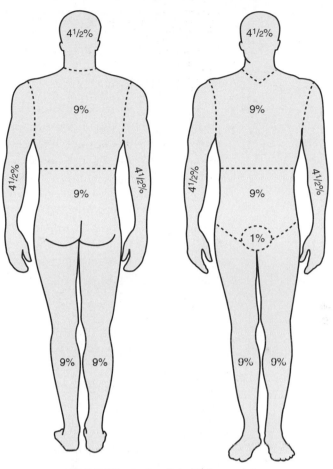

FIGURE 6–6   Rule of nines, adult.

Relative percentage of body surface areas (% BSA) affected by growth

	0 yr	1 yr	5 yr	10 yr	15 yr
a – 1/2 of head	9 1/2	8 1/2	6 1/2	5 1/2	4 1/2
b – 1/2 of 1 thigh	2 3/4	3 1/4	4	4 1/4	4 1/2
c – 1/2 of lower leg	2 1/2	2 1/2	2 3/4	3	3 1/4

FIGURE 6–7   Lund-Browder chart for estimating the extent of burns on children.

Examples:

Diagnosis: First- and second-degree burn to the back

Index: **Burn**, back, second degree 942.24

Tabular: **942 Burn of trunk**

   942.2 Blisters, epidermal loss [second degree]

A fifth digit is used to indicate the specific location of the burn to the trunk. In this case, the fifth digit 4 is used to indicate the location, back, 942.24.

Code(s):   942.24 First- and second-degree burn to the back

Note that the diagnosis includes first- and second-degree burns and the code assigned indicates second-degree burns. You code only the highest degree when the burns are at the same site.

Diagnosis: Second-degree burn, 1%, chin, and third-degree burn, 3%, scapular region, for a total of 4% of the body surface

Index: **Burn**, chin, second 941.24

Tabular: **941 Burn of face, head, and neck**

   941.2 Blisters, epidermal loss [second degree]

A fifth digit is used to indicate the specific location of the burn to the face, head, or neck. In this case, the fifth digit 4 is used to indicate the location, chin, 941.24. Now, to code the burn to the scapular region:

Index: **Burn**, scapular region, third degree 943.36

Tabular: **943 Burn of upper limb, except wrist and hand**

   943.3 Full-thickness skin loss [third degree NOS]

A fifth digit is used to indicate the specific location of the burn. In this case, the fifth digit 6 is used to indicate the location, scapular region, 943.36.

   But wait! You need one more code to finish coding this example—one to indicate the total body surface involved.

Index: **Burn**, extent, less than 10%, 948.0

Tabular: **948.0 Burn [any degree] involving less than 10% of body surface**

The fifth digit "0" is required to indicate less than 10% total body surface was involved in a third-degree burn, 948.00.

Code(s):   943.36, 941.24, 948.00 Third-degree burn, scapular region, and second-degree burn, chin; with the 948.00 indicating that there is less than 10% third-degree burn on less than 10% of the body surface.

E codes for burns are assigned, as per facility policy, for all initial treatments.

EXERCISE 6-10 *Burns*

Code the burn, extent of the body surface involved, and percentage of body surface burned using the rule of nines.

1 A 3-year-old receives third-degree burns of the abdomen, 10%, and second-degree burns of the thigh, 5% after pulling a pot of hot water on herself

Third-degree Code: ___942.33___ Second-degree Code: ___945.26___

E Code: ___E924.0___ Degree and Percentage (extent) Code: ___948.11___

2 Infected third-degree burn, left thigh, 4½%, subsequent treatment

ICD-9-CM Codes: ___945.36___ (third degree), ___958.3___ (infected burn), ___948.00___ (extent)

3 First- and second-degree burn, right foot, 2¼%, due to bonfire

ICD-9-CM Codes: ___945.22___ (second degree), ___948.00___ (extent), ___E897___ (E code)

4 Non-healing third-degree burn, right hand, 2¼%; excisional debridement performed by physician; patient seen 10 days ago for initial treatment

ICD-9-CM Codes: ___944.30___ (third degree), ___948.00___ (extent)

5 Second-degree burn, right forearm, 2%; first-degree burn, right hand, 1%, and third-degree burn, chest wall, 8%, subsequent treatment

ICD-9-CM Codes: ___942.32___, ___943.21___, ___944.10___, ___948.10___

Fractures Now it is time to learn how to report fractures, so begin by reading the Guidelines on fracture reporting:

ICD-9-CM OFFICIAL GUIDELINES FOR CODING AND REPORTING

SECTION I.C.

17. **Chapter 17: Injury and Poisoning (800-999)**

a. **Coding of Injuries**

When coding injuries, assign separate codes for each injury unless a combination code is provided, in which case the combination code is assigned. Multiple injury codes are provided in ICD-9-CM, but should not be assigned unless information for a more specific code is not available. These traumatic injury codes are not to be used for normal, healing surgical wounds or to identify complications of surgical wounds.

The code for the most serious injury, as determined by the provider and the focus of treatment, is sequenced first.

1) **Superficial injuries**

Superficial injuries such as abrasions or contusions are not coded when associated with more severe injuries of the same site.

2) **Primary injury with damage to nerves/blood vessels**

When a primary injury results in minor damage to peripheral nerves or blood vessels, the primary injury is sequenced first with additional code(s) from categories 950-957, Injury to nerves and spinal cord, and/or 900-904, Injury to blood vessels. When the primary injury is to the blood vessels or nerves, that injury should be sequenced first.

b. Coding of Traumatic Fractures

The principles of multiple coding of injuries should be followed in coding fractures. Fractures of specified sites are coded individually by site in accordance with both the provisions within categories 800-829 and the level of detail furnished by medical record content. Combination categories for multiple fractures are provided for use when there is insufficient detail in the medical record (such as trauma cases transferred to another hospital), when the reporting form limits the number of codes that can be used in reporting pertinent clinical data, or when there is insufficient specificity at the fourth-digit or fifth-digit level. More specific guidelines are as follows:

1) Acute Fractures vs. Aftercare

Traumatic fractures are coded using the acute fracture codes (800-829) while the patient is receiving active treatment for the fracture. Examples of active treatment are: surgical treatment, emergency department encounter, and evaluation and treatment by a new physician.

Fractures are coded using the aftercare codes (subcategories V54.0, V54.1, V54.8, or V54.9) for encounters after the patient has completed active treatment of the fracture and is receiving routine care for the fracture during the healing or recovery phase. Examples of fracture aftercare are: cast change or removal, removal of external or internal fixation device, medication adjustment, and follow up visits following fracture treatment.

Care for complications of surgical treatment for fracture repairs during the healing or recovery phase should be coded with the appropriate complication codes.

Care of complications of fractures, such as malunion and nonunion, should be reported with the appropriate codes.

Pathologic fractures are not coded in the 800-829 range, but instead are assigned to subcategory 733.1. *See Section I.C.13.a for additional information.*

2) Multiple fractures of same limb

Multiple fractures of same limb classifiable to the same three-digit or four-digit category are coded to that category.

3) Multiple unilateral or bilateral fractures of same bone

Multiple unilateral or bilateral fractures of same bone(s) but classified to different fourth-digit subdivisions (bone part) within the same three-digit category are coded individually by site.

4) Multiple fracture categories 819 and 828

Multiple fracture categories 819 and 828 classify bilateral fractures of both upper limbs (819) and both lower limbs (828), but without any detail at the fourth-digit level other than open and closed type of fracture.

5) Multiple fractures sequencing

Multiple fractures are sequenced in accordance with the severity of the fracture. The provider should be asked to list the fracture diagnoses in the order of severity.

Fracture is the first section in the chapter and it contains the codes assigned for fractures caused by trauma. A fracture not indicated as closed or open should be classified as **closed**. If you have any doubt, check with the physician as to the nature of the fracture. A dislocation and fracture of the same bone would be coded to the fracture site because that is the highest level of specificity and fracture is more severe than dislocation. You are also instructed in the Index, under the main term dislocation to *see* Fracture, by site. The cross-reference *"see"* is a mandatory instruction that tells you to go to "Fracture" and not to code the dislocation separately. You locate fractures in the Index under "Fracture" and then on the basis of the anatomic location of the fracture.

Examples

Diagnosis: Fracture, right patella with abrasions of the site

Index: **Fracture**, patella (closed) 822.0

Tabular: **822 Fracture of patella**

822.0 Closed

Code(s):   822.0 Fracture, right patella with abrasions of the site

When a fracture is not specified as open or closed, assign a code that indicates a **closed** fracture. You would not assign a code for the dislocation when there is a more severe injury (the fracture) at the same site, as in the following example.

Diagnosis: Fractured hip with dislocation

Index: **Dislocation**, with fracture—*see* Fracture by site.

The *"see* Fracture by site" means the dislocation is included with the fracture code.

Index: **Fracture**, hip (closed) 820.8

Tabular: **820 Fracture of neck of femur**

820.8 Unspecified part of neck of femur, closed

Code(s):   820.8 Fractured hip with dislocation

Wounds

Wounds (lacerations) are found under the main term "Wound." There are three subcategories in some of the wound codes. These injuries can be classified as:

1. Without mention of complication
2. Complicated
3. With tendon involvement

A **complicated wound** is one that includes documentation of delayed healing, delayed treatment, foreign body, or primary infection.

These codes are for traumatic injuries and should not be reported to identify surgical wounds or ulceration including decubitus and stasis ulcers.

Example

Diagnosis: Infected wound of the right knee

Index: **Wound**, knee 891.0
   complicated 891.1

Tabular: **891 Open wound of knee, leg [except thigh], and ankle**

891.1 Complicated

Codes: 891.1 Infected wound of the right knee

QUICK CHECK 6-1

In the Index under Wound, there is information included for coding:

a. Penetrating wounds of internal organs
b. Insect bites
c. Crush injuries
d. All of the above

Complications　　When a patient is admitted for a complication that resulted from medical care or a surgical procedure, the complication is the first-listed. Read the Guideline on complications:

ICD-9-CM OFFICIAL GUIDELINES FOR CODING AND REPORTING

SECTION II.
G. Complications of surgery and other medical care

When the admission is for treatment of a complication resulting from surgery or other medical care, the complication code is sequenced as the principal diagnosis. If the complication is classified to the 996-999 series and the code lacks the necessary specificity in describing the complication, an additional code for the specific complication should be assigned.

EXERCISE 6-11　*Complications*

In the Index, you will find complications of medical and surgical procedures under the main term "Complications."

Code the following complications:

1 Breast implants, infection

ICD-9-CM Code: _____

2 Bone marrow graft, rejection

ICD-9-CM Code: _____

3 Surgical procedures, stitch abscess

ICD-9-CM Codes: _____, _____

4 Cardiac pacemaker, (device) mechanical complication

ICD-9-CM Code: _____

CHAPTER REVIEW

CHAPTER 6, PART I, THEORY

Circle the correct answer in each of the following:

1 In order to code a gastrointestinal condition with hemorrhage, active bleeding must be present.

   True   False

2 It is common to use a fifth digit of 0 when coding complications related to pregnancy.

   True   False

3 A pathologic fracture occurs in a bone that is weakened by disease.

   True   False

4 The perinatal period extends for 6 weeks following birth.

   True   False

5 Generally you do not assign a code from Chapter 16 if a definitive diagnosis is documented.

   True   False

6 When an accident occurs, an E code should be the first-listed diagnosis.

   True   False

7 If a fracture and dislocation are present at the same site, assign only the fracture code.

   True   False

8 An infected laceration should be coded as a complicated wound.

   True   False

9 A poisoning occurs when a drug has been correctly prescribed and properly administered and the patient develops a reaction.

   True   False

10 When coding a poisoning, the poisoning code is sequenced before any manifestation code.

   True   False

CHAPTER 6, PART II, PRACTICAL

Using an ICD-9-CM manual, answer the following questions:

11 Nephrogenic diabetes insipidus

ICD-9-CM Code: _____588.1_____

12 Ovarian cyst

ICD-9-CM Code: _____620.2_____

13 Uterine fibroids complicating pregnancy, 23 weeks' gestation

ICD-9-CM Codes: _____654.13_____, _____621.8_____

14 Dehiscence cesarean wound. Patient delivered one week ago at another facility.

ICD-9-CM Code: _____674.14_____

15 Term birth, 2268 grams, delivered by cesarean section, with intrauterine growth retardation

ICD-9-CM Codes: _____764.98_____, _____V30.01_____

16 Anal fistula

ICD-9-CM Code: _____565.1_____

17 Lower gastrointestinal bleeding due to angiodysplasia of colon

ICD-9-CM Code: _____569.85_____

18 Kidney stone

ICD-9-CM Code: _____592.0_____

19 Paronychia toe

ICD-9-CM Code: _____681.11_____

20 Pilonidal cyst with abscess

ICD-9-CM Code: _____685.0_____

21 Osteoarthritis, right knee

ICD-9-CM Code: _____715.96_____

22 Postlaminectomy syndrome, lumbar

ICD-9-CM Code: _____722.83_____

23 Bicuspid aortic valve

ICD-9-CM Code: _____746.4_____

24 Patent ductus arteriosus

ICD-9-CM Code: _____747.0_____

25 Palpitations

ICD-9-CM Code: _____785.1_____

26 Lack of appetite

ICD-9-CM Code: _____783.0_____

27 Infected mosquito bites, both legs

ICD-9-CM Codes: _____916.5_____, _____E906.4_____

28 Sunburn

ICD-9-CM Codes: _____692.71_____, _____E926.2_____

29 Hives due to prescription penicillin, which was properly taken

ICD-9-CM Codes: _____708.9_____, _____E930.0_____

30 Chest pain due to cocaine

ICD-9-CM Codes: _____970.8_____, _____786.50_____, _____E854.3_____, _____305.60_____

Assign the ICD-9-CM codes for the following cases:

31 Mr. Jones presents to the emergency department with acute abdominal pain. After a thorough examination and diagnostic x-ray film, Mr. Jones is diagnosed with acute small bowel obstruction and taken immediately to surgery.

ICD-9-CM Code: _____560.9_____

32 Mrs. Smith is at 32 weeks' gestation and is admitted with severe bleeding with abdominal cramping. An emergency ultrasound is done and fetal monitors are applied. She is diagnosed with total placenta previa with indications of fetal distress. An emergency cesarean section is done, with delivery of a viable male infant.

ICD-9-CM Codes: _____641.11_____, _____656.81_____, _____644.21_____, _____V27.0_____

33 Miss Halliday is an 80-year-old woman who presents to the emergency department with a history of abdominal pain, fever, and burning with urination. Urine culture is obtained, and Miss Halliday is admitted for workup to rule out urosepsis. Urosepsis was ruled out.

❀ ICD-9-CM Code(s): _____789.00_____, _____780.60_____, _____788.1_____

34 Mr. Johnson is admitted to the hospital with chest and epigastric pain. He is evaluated by the emergency department physician with a diagnosis of rule out myocardial infarction. Mr. Johnson is then transferred to a larger facility for further workup.

🌐 ICD-9-CM Code(s): _786.50, 789.06_

CASE STUDY 1

History of Present Illness

The patient is a 68-year-old female, status post motor vehicle accident 3 months ago. The patient had an open fracture that was treated initially with traction for 6 to 8 weeks. After initial treatment with traction, the patient was placed in a cast brace. She presents with a complaint of pain in the left femur and inability to bear weight on her leg. The patient was referred from an orthopedic surgeon. The past medical history was significant for no history of myocardial infarction or renal disease and no asthma. The patient had undergone no previous procedures with the exception of debridement of the open fracture. Otherwise the patient's history was unremarkable. The patient was taking no medications and had no known allergies. She underwent a preoperative workup that included a gallium scan.

Physical Examination

The heart, lungs, and abdomen were benign. The left knee had a 30-degree extension lag. There was motion with the knee approximately 30 degrees from horizontal axis to 90 degrees of flexion. The patella was difficult to palpate, and it was very difficult to tell at the time of examination whether motion was occurring at the fracture or whether it was occurring at the knee joint. The vascular examination was unremarkable.

Laboratory Data and Course in Hospital

The x-ray film showed nonunion of the left femur. The gallium scan obtained preoperatively was negative, and there was no evidence of infection.

Treatment

On May 14, the patient underwent open reduction and internal fixation of the left femur fracture with a 90-degree dynamic condylar screw and side plate. The patient tolerated the procedure well. She received two units of her own autologous blood at the time of surgery. Postoperatively she was quite anemic due to acute blood loss, with hemoglobin of 6 to 7 mg/dl. The patient was asymptomatic clinically, and her vascular examination was intact. On postoperative day 2, she had motion in the left knee from 0 to 30 degrees of flexion. She was placed in continuous passive motion and was up with physical therapy but non-weight-bearing on the left leg. Physical therapy was tolerated well. The hospital course was benign. The wound was clean and dry, and the neurovascular examination was unchanged. The x-ray films obtained before discharge showed maintenance of alignment of the left femur. The patient's staples were removed on postoperative day 7. She was placed in a cast brace and was discharged home after being independent in physical therapy.

Final Diagnosis

Nonunion of the left femur

Procedure

Open reduction and internal fixation of the left femur with 90-degree screw and site plate

35 ICD-9-CM Codes: _733.82, 285.1, 905.4, E929.0_

"ICD-10-CM will most likely be 'messy' at first, but be prepared and start educating yourself now. It will take longer than a few short training sessions to comprehend a whole new system and 100,000 more codes!"

Lynne Padilla, CPC
Medical Course Developer
Allied Business Schools
Laguna Hills, California

ICD-10-CM

Chapter Topics

Development of the
ICD-10-CM

Development of the
ICD-10-PCS

Chapter Review

Learning Objectives

After completing this chapter you should be able to

1 Explain the format of ICD-10-CM.

2 Examine the ICD-10-PCS system.

Make sure to check
evolve
learning system
**for the latest
content updates**

DEVELOPMENT OF THE ICD-10-CM

The tenth revision of the *International Classification of Diseases* (ICD-10) was issued in 1993 by the World Health Organization (WHO), and WHO is responsible for maintaining it. The ICD-10 does not include a procedure classification (Volume 3). Each world government is responsible for adapting the ICD-10 to suit its own country's needs. For example, Australia uses the ICD-10-AM, that is, the ICD-10-Australian Modification. Each government is responsible for ensuring that its modification conforms with the WHO's conventions in the ICD-10. In the United States, the Centers for Medicare and Medicaid Services is responsible for developing the procedure classification entitled the ICD-10-PCS (PCS stands for Procedure Coding System). The ICD-10-PCS will replace the volume 3 of the current ICD-9-CM manual. The National Center for Health Statistics (NCHS) is responsible for the disease classification system (Volumes 1 and 2) entitled ICD-10-CM (CM stands for Clinical Modification) (refer to the figures on pages 196-199 for examples of the ICD-10-CM and the ICD-10-PCS).

The ICD-10 is already widely used in Europe. The ICD-10 is available in the six official languages of Arabic, Chinese, English, French, Russian, and Spanish as well as in 36 other languages and used in over 190 countries. Conversion to the new edition in the United States has taken a great deal of time to implement. The date proposed for the International Classification of Diseases, Tenth Revision, Clinical Modification (ICD-10-CM) implementation will be effective October 1, 2013. Conversion to ICD-10 is critical to development of a nationwide electronic health information environment.

The ICD-9 was developed more than 30 years ago, and currently contains over 17,000 codes. With the publication of the ICD-10-CM over 155,000 will be available. In addition, Medicare Severity Diagnosis Related Groups (MS-DRGs) is the prospective payment system in place for reimbursement of Medicare hospital inpatient stays, and the MS-DRG system is based on the ICD-9-CM.

Development of the ICD-10-CM to Replace the ICD-9-CM, Volumes 1 and 2

The ICD-10-CM will replace ICD-9-CM, Volumes 1 and 2, currently the coding system utilized to report diagnoses. Prior to the implementation of the new edition, extensive consultation and review must take place with physician groups, clinical coders, third-party payers, clearinghouses, and others who transmit any electronic health information. The NCHS established a 20-member Technical Advisory Panel of representatives of the health care and coding communities to provide input during the development of the 10th revision.

From the Trenches

"Make sure you are comfortable with ICD-9 before moving on to ICD-10. Start looking at the information now available on ICD-10 so that you aren't bombarded later. A slow, thoughtful process will make the conversion easier."

LYNNE

In July 2007, the International Classification of Disease, 10th revision, Clinical Modification (ICD-10-CM) was released. This replaced the "pre-release draft of June 2003." This release of ICD-10-CM is intended for public viewing, but the codes are not currently valid for any purpose or use and no comments are being solicited at this time. Guidance for the use of ICD-10-CM is available at www.cms.hhs.gov/ICD10/01_Overview.asp#TopOfPage. The preface of the July 2009 ICD-10-CM is illustrated in Fig. 7–1.

In addition to using a new coding system, physician offices and facilities will need to update their billing software. Under the Health Insurance Portability and Accountability Act (HIPAA), the Department of Health and Human Services (HHS) establishes standards for electronic healthcare transactions. The current standard cannot accommodate the additional characters of the ICD-10-CM and ICD-10-PCS coding sets. HHS is confident that the new upgrade will reduce the need for manual intervention and will also increase the use of electronic claims submission.

Improvements in the ICD-10-CM. Notable improvements in the content and format of the ICD-10-CM include the:

- Addition of information relevant to ambulatory and managed care encounters
- Extensive expansion of the injury codes allows for greater specificity For example, S50.351 is the code for superficial foreign body of right elbow.

ICD-10-CM PREFACE
2009

Introduction This 2009 update of the International Classification of Diseases, 10th revision, Clinical Modification (ICD-10-CM) is being published by the United States Government in recognition of its responsibility to promulgate this classification throughout the United States for morbidity coding. The International Statistical Classification of Diseases and Related Health Problems, 10th Revision (ICD-10), published by the World Health Organization (WHO), is the foundation of ICD-10-CM. ICD-10 continues to be the classification used in cause-of-death coding in the United States. The ICD-10-CM is comparable with the ICD-10. The WHO Collaborating Center for the Family of International Classifications in North America, housed at the National Center for Health Statistics (NCHS), has responsibility for the implementation of ICD and other WHO-FIC classifications and serves as a liaison with the WHO, fulfilling international obligations for comparable classifications and the national health data needs of the United States. The historical background of ICD and ICD-10 can be found in the Introduction to the International Classification of Diseases and Related Health Problems (ICD-10), Second Edition, World Health Organization, Geneva, Switzerland, 2005.

ICD-10-CM is the United States' clinical modification of the World Health Organizations's ICD-10. The term clinical is used to emphasize the modification's intent: to serve as a useful tool in the area of classification of morbidity data for indexing of medical records, medical care review, and ambulatory and other medical care programs, as well as for basic health statistics. To describe the clinical picture of the patient the codes must be more precise than those needed only for statistical groupings and trend analysis.

Characteristics of ICD-10-CM
ICD-10-CM far exceeds its predecessors in the number of concepts and codes provided. The disease classification has been expanded to include health-related conditions and to provide greater specificity at the sixth digit level and with a seventh digit extension. The sixth and seventh characters are not optional; they are intended for use in recording the information documented in the clinical record.

FIGURE 7–1 ICD-10-CM Preface, 2009 Release. (Courtesy U.S. Department of Health and Human Services, Centers for Disease Control and Prevention.)

■ Creation of combination diagnosis/symptom codes to reduce the number of codes needed to fully describe a condition
  For example, I25.110 is the code for atherosclerotic heart disease with unstable angina. Under the ICD-9-CM, two codes are required to classify both diagnoses.

■ Greater specification on the depth of a decubitus ulcer
  For example, through the skin, to the muscle, or to the bone.

■ Addition of a sixth character
  For example, S06.336 is the code for contusion and laceration of brainstem with prolonged [>24 hrs.] loss of consciousness...

■ Incorporation of common fourth- and fifth-digit subclassifications
  For example, F10.150 is the code for alcohol abuse with alcohol-induced psychotic disorder with delusions.

■ Updating and greater specificity of diabetes mellitus codes
  For example, E11.21 is the code for Type 2 diabetes mellitus with diabetic nephropathy.

These notable improvements will provide facilitation of providing greater specificity when assigning codes.

Structure of the System. ICD-10-CM contains 21 chapters and excludes the Supplementary Classifications found in ICD-9-CM. The E and V codes of ICD-9-CM have been incorporated throughout the ICD-10-CM. Chapter titles in the ICD-10-CM remain the same except for the presence of two new chapters: Chapter VII, Diseases of the Eye and Adnexa, and Chapter VIII, Diseases of the Ear and Mastoid Process.

Mapping. As a part of the conversion, a Diagnosis Code Set General Equivalence Mappings has been developed. This mapping is a crosswalk that converts ICD-9-CM codes to ICD-10-CM codes. Fig. 7–2 illustrates a section of

ICD-9-CM to ICD-10-CM Conversion
Diseases of the Blood and Blood-forming Organs
(pound sign (#) following ICD-10-CM code indicates the best match of one to many matches)

ICD-9-CM Code	ICD-9-CM Abbreviated Title	ICD-10-CM Code	Best Match	ICD-10-CM Abbreviated Title
280	IRON DEFICIENCY ANEMIAS			
280.0	IRON DEF ANEM DT BL LOSS	D50.0		CHRONIC BLOOD LOSS ANEMIA
280.1	IRON DEF ANEM DT DIET	D50.8		FE DEFICIENCY ANEMIA NEC
280.8	IRON DEFICIT ANEMIAS NEC	D50.1		SIDEROPENIC DYSPHAGIA
280.8	IRON DEFICIT ANEMIAS NEC	D50.8	#b	FE DEFICIENCY ANEMIA NEC
280.9	IRON DEFICIT ANEMIA NOS	D50.9		FE DEFICIENCY ANEMIA NOS
281	OTHER DEFICIENCY ANEMIAS			
281.0	PERNICIOUS ANEMIA	D51.0		PERNICIOUS ANEMIA
281.1	VIT B12 DEFIC ANEMIA NEC	D51.3		DIETARY B12 DEF ANEM NEC
281.1	VIT B12 DEFIC ANEMIA NEC	D51.8		B12 DEFICIENC ANEM NEC
281.1	VIT B12 DEFIC ANEMIA NEC	D51.1	#a	B12 DEFICIENC ANEM NOS

ICD-10-CM Best Match for 281.1

Best Match Designation

FIGURE 7–2 ICD-9-CM to ICD-10-CM Conversion (crosswalk). (Courtesy U.S. Department of Health and Human Services, Centers for Medicare and Medicaid Services.)

the crosswalk. Sometimes, more than one ICD-10-CM code crosswalks from the ICD-9-CM code. In these instances, the possible matches are noted in a Best Match column. For example, in Fig. 7–2 the ICD-9-CM code 281.1, Vitamin B$_{12}$ deficiency anemia NEC, has three possible matches with ICD-10-CM codes. In the Best Match column, the symbol "#a" indicates that the best match for 281.1 is ICD-10-CM code D51.1. Every ICD-9-CM code is crosswalked to ICD-10-CM code(s) in this way.

CHECK THIS OUT ☞ The crosswalk (General Equivalence Mapping Files) is available on the CMS website at www.cdc.gov/nchs/about/otheract/icd9/icd10cm.htm

Index. The Index for the ICD-10-CM is alphabetic, as illustrated in Fig. 7–3. As in the ICD-9-CM, the ICD-10-CM index presents the main terms in bold type, and subterms indented under the main term. After the index entry, a code is provided. Sometimes, only the first four digits of the code are given. To ensure that you have chosen the correct code and/or to obtain the remaining digits, you must refer to the Tabular. As always you do not code from the index.

Tabular. The 21 chapters of the Tabular are arranged in numeric order after the first letter assigned to the chapter. For example, the letter R is assigned to the chapter regarding symptoms. Fig. 7–4 illustrates a portion of the chapter concerning symptoms. Note that in the index (see Fig. 7–3) the main entry is Abdomen, abdominal, and the first subterm is "acute," directing the coder to the Tabular location, R10.0. Now, note in the Tabular (see Fig. 7–4) the location of R10.0 as Acute abdomen.

FIGURE 7–3 ICD-10-CM Index. (Modified from Buck CJ: *ICD-10-CM, Volumes 1 and 2, Professional Editon*, St. Louis, 2010, Saunders.)

R10 **Abdominal and pelvic pain**

    Excludes1: *renal colic (N23)*

    Excludes2: *dorsalgia (M54.-)*
                 flatulence and related conditions (R14.-)

R10.0 **Acute abdomen**

    Severe abdominal pain (generalized) (with abdominal rigidity)

    Excludes1: *abdominal rigidity NOS (R19.3)*
                 generalized abdominal pain NOS (R10.84)
                 localized abdominal pain (R10.1-R10.3-)

R10.1 **Pain localized to upper abdomen**

    R10.10 **Upper abdominal pain, unspecified**

    R10.11 **Right upper quadrant pain**

    R10.12 **Left upper quadrant pain**

    R10.13 **Epigastric pain**

R10.2 **Pelvic and perineal pain**

    Excludes1: *vulvodynia (N94.81)*

Tabular location R10.0 →

FIGURE 7–4 ICD-10-CM Tabular. (Modified from Buck CJ: *ICD-10-CM, Volumes 1 and 2, Professional Editon,* St. Louis, 2010, Saunders.)

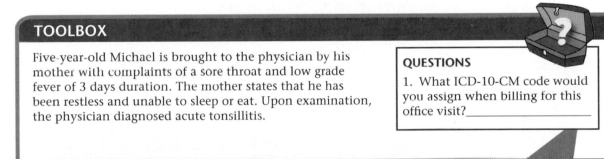

TOOLBOX

Five-year-old Michael is brought to the physician by his mother with complaints of a sore throat and low grade fever of 3 days duration. The mother states that he has been restless and unable to sleep or eat. Upon examination, the physician diagnosed acute tonsillitis.

QUESTIONS

1. What ICD-10-CM code would you assign when billing for this office visit?_____

ANSWERS 1. J35.01

DEVELOPMENT OF THE ICD-10-PCS

The new structure will allow more expansion than was possible with Volume 3 of the ICD-9-CM because it lacks specificity (exactness) and does not provide for sufficient expansion to support government payment systems and data needs. CMS contracted with 3M Health Information Systems to develop the ICD-10-PCS to replace the ICD-9-CM procedure codes (Volume 3) for reporting **inpatient** procedures.

Four major objectives guided the development of ICD-10-PCS:

1. **Completeness.** There is a unique code for all substantially different procedures. Currently, procedures performed on different body parts, using different approaches or of different types, are sometimes assigned the same code.

2. **Expandability.** As new procedures are developed, the structure of the ICD-10-PCS should allow for incorporation of these new procedures as unique codes.

3. **Multiaxial** (more than one part). ICD-10-PCS should have a structure such that each code character has, as much as possible, the

same meaning, both within the specific procedure section and across procedure sections.

4. **Standardized terminology.** Although the meaning of a specific word may vary in common usage, ICD-10-PCS should not include multiple meanings for the same term; each term should be assigned a specific meaning, and ICD-10-PCS should include definitions of the terminology.

A complete, expandable, multiaxial ICD-10-PCS with standardized terminology allows coding specialists to determine the accurate code with minimal effort.

The Seven Characters of the ICD-10-PCS

The ICD-10-PCS has a seven-character alphanumeric code structure. Each character has as many as 34 different values: 10 digits (0-9) and 24 letters (A-H, J-N, and P-Z) may be assigned to each character. The letters O and I are not used in order to avoid confusion with the digits 0 and 1. In the ICD-10-PCS, the term "procedure" refers to the complete designation of the seven characters. Procedures are divided into sections according to the type of procedure.

Character 1 Identifies the Section. The first character of the procedure code identifies the section. To assign an ICD-10-PCS code, the section where the procedure is coded must be identified. For example, a chest x-ray is in the Imaging section, a breast biopsy is in the Medical and Surgical section, and crisis intervention is in the Mental Health section. Each section is identified by a specific character—number or letter. Section titles and numbers/letters are shown in Fig. 7–5.

SECTIONS

0	Medical and Surgical
1	Obstetrics
2	Placement
3	Administration
4	Measurement and Monitoring
5	Extracorporeal Assistance and Performance
6	Extracorporeal Therapies
7	Osteopathic
8	Other Procedures
9	Chiropractic
B	Imaging
C	Nuclear Medicine
D	Radiation Oncology
F	Physical Rehabilitation and Diagnostic Audiology
G	Mental Health
H	Substance Abuse Treatment

FIGURE 7–5   Sections of ICD-10-PCS. (From Buck CJ: *ICD-10-PCS, Professional Edition,* St. Louis, 2010, Saunders.)

EXERCISE 7-1 *ICD-10-PCS First Character*

Using Fig. 7–5, identify the first section character that would be assigned to the following procedures. For example, chiropractic would be "9."

1 _____ Gait training (Physical Rehabilitation)

2 _____ Cesarean section (Obstetrics)

3 _____ Computerized tomography, spine (Imaging)

4 _____ Cholecystectomy (Medical and Surgical)

5 _____ Insertion of radium into cervix (brachytherapy) (Radiation Oncology)

6 _____ Cranioplasty (Medical and Surgical)

Changing Characters. Characters 2 through 7 have a standard meaning within each section but may have different meanings across sections. The meanings for each character are described in each section. For example, Fig. 7–6 shows the meanings of the seven characters for the Medical and Surgical sections, and Fig. 7–7 shows the meanings for the Imaging section. Notice that several characters have different meanings across these sections. For instance, the third character in medical and surgical procedures (see Fig. 7–6) is used to define the root *operation* (extraction, insertion, removal, etc.), whereas the third character in imaging procedures (see Fig. 7–7) is used to define the root *type* (fluoroscopy, MRI, CT, ultrasonography, etc.).

⬤ **STOP** *Each code must include seven characters. If a character is not applicable to a specific procedure, the letter Z is assigned.*

Character 2 Is the Body System. The second character identifies the body system in all sections except Rehabilitation and Mental Health. In these two sections, the second character identifies the type of procedure performed.

Character 3 Is the Root Operation. The third character identifies the root operation in all sections except Radiation Oncology, Rehabilitation,

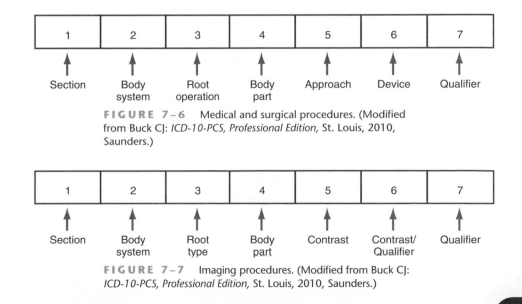

FIGURE 7–6 Medical and surgical procedures. (Modified from Buck CJ: *ICD-10-PCS, Professional Edition,* St. Louis, 2010, Saunders.)

FIGURE 7–7 Imaging procedures. (Modified from Buck CJ: *ICD-10-PCS, Professional Edition,* St. Louis, 2010, Saunders.)

and Mental Health. In many sections, only a few root operations are performed, and these operations are defined in that section. The Medical and Surgical section uses an extensive list of root operations. The Obstetrics and Placement sections use some of these same root operations as well as section-specific root operations. See Table 7–1 (p. 201) for a list of the Medical and Surgical root operations definitions, explanations, and examples.

EXERCISE 7-2   *Root Operation*

Using Table 7–1, place the character for the root operation term before its definition:

1 _____ Taking or letting out fluids and/or gases from a body part

2 _____ Freeing a body part

3 _____ Taking out or off a device from a body part

4 _____ Visually and/or manually exploring a body part

5 _____ Restoring, to the extent possible, a body part to its natural anatomic structure and function

6 _____ Altering the route of passage of the contents of a tubular body part

7 _____ Cutting out or off, without replacement, all of a body part

8 _____ Physical eradication of all or a portion of a body part by direct use of energy, force, or a destructive agent

9 _____ Correcting, to the extent possible, a malfunctioning or displaced device

10 _____ Cutting out or off, without replacement, a portion of a body part

1 Bypass

5 Destruction

7 Drainage

8 Excision

L Release

M Removal

N Repair

R Resection

G Inspection

T Revision

A Closer Look at Root Operations.   The root operation is described by one of the main terms, as outlined on page 201 in Table 7–1 (e.g., Alteration, Change, Bypass). These root operations can be grouped into types of operations, such as operations that always involve devices: insertion, replacement, removal, change. Table 7–2 (p. 204) shows the root operations grouped by types.

EXERCISE 7-3   *Root Operation Terms*

Using Table 7–2, identify the root operation term for each example:

1 _____ Tendon transfer

2 _____ Sigmoid polypectomy

3 _____ Diagnostic arthroscopy

4 _____ Heart transplant

5 _____ Pacemaker insertion

6 _____ Cardiac pacemaker removal

7 _____ Lithotripsy, gallstones

8 _____ Fallopian tube ligation

9 _____ Hip prosthesis adjustment

10 _____ Peritoneal adhesiolysis

TABLE 7–1

MEDICAL AND SURGICAL ROOT OPERATION DEFINITIONS (SELECT)

Alteration	**Definition:**	Modifying the anatomic structure of a body part without affecting the function of the body part
	Explanation:	Principal purpose is to improve appearance
	Examples:	Face lift, breast augmentation
Bypass	**Definition:**	Altering the route of passage of the contents of a tubular body part
	Explanation:	Rerouting contents around an area of a body part to another distal (downstream) area in the normal route; rerouting the contents to another different but similar route and body part; or to an abnormal route and another dissimilar body part. It includes one or more concurrent anastomoses with or without the use of a device such as autografts, tissue substitutes and synthetic substitutes.
	Examples:	Coronary artery bypass, colostomy formation
Change	**Definition:**	Taking out or off a device from a body part and putting back an identical or similar device in or on the same body part without cutting or puncturing the skin or a mucous membrane
	Explanation:	All Change procedures are coded using the approach External
	Example:	Urinary catheter change, gastrostomy tube change
Control	**Definition:**	Stopping, or attempting to stop, postprocedural bleeding
	Explanation:	The site of the bleeding is coded as an anatomical region and not to a specific body part.
	Examples:	Control of post-prostatectomy hemorrhage, control of post-tonsillectomy hemorrhage
Creation	**Definition:**	Making a new genital structure that does not physically take the place of a body part
	Explanation:	Used only for sex change operations
	Examples:	Creation of vagina in a male, creation of penis in a female
Destruction	**Definition:**	Physical eradication of all or a portion of a body part by the direct use of energy, force or a destructive agent
	Explanation:	None of the body part is physically taken out
	Examples:	Fulguration of rectal polyp, cautery of skin lesion
Detachment	**Definition:**	Cutting off all or a portion of the upper or lower extremities
	Explanation:	The body part value is the site of the detachment, with a qualifier if applicable to further specify the level where the extremity was detached
	Examples:	Below knee amputation, disarticulation of shoulder
Dilation	**Definition:**	Expanding an orifice or the lumen of a tubular body part
	Explanation:	The orifice can be a natural orifice or an artificially created orifice. Accomplished by stretching a tubular body part using intraluminal pressure or by cutting part of the orifice or wall of the tubular body part
	Examples:	Percutaneous transluminal angioplasty, pyloromyotomy
Division	**Definition:**	Cutting into a body part without draining fluids and/or gases from the body part in order to separate or transect a body part
	Explanation:	All or a portion of the body part is separated into two or more portions.
	Examples:	Spinal cordotomy, osteotomy
Drainage	**Definition:**	Taking or letting out fluids and/or gases from a body part
	Explanation:	The qualifier Diagnostic is used to identify drainage procedures that are biopsies.
	Examples:	Thoracentesis, incision and drainage
Excision	**Definition:**	Cutting out or off, without replacement, a portion of a body part
	Explanation:	The qualifier Diagnostic is used to identify excision procedures that are biopsies
	Examples:	Partial nephrectomy, liver biopsy
Extirpation	**Definition:**	Taking or cutting out solid matter from a body part
	Explanation:	The solid matter may be an abnormal byproduct of a biological function or a foreign body. The solid matter is imbedded in a body part, or is in the lumen of a tubular body part. The solid matter may or may not have been previously broken into pieces. No appreciable amount of the body part is taken out
	Examples:	Thrombectomy, choledocholithotomy

Continued

TABLE 7–1

MEDICAL AND SURGICAL ROOT OPERATION DEFINITIONS (SELECT) (Continued)

Extraction	**Definition:**	Pulling or stripping out or off all or a portion of a body part by the use of force
	Explanation:	The qualifier Diagnostic is used to identify extractions that are biopsies
	Examples:	Dilation and curettage, vein stripping
Fragmentation	**Definition:**	Breaking solid matter in a body part into pieces
	Explanation:	The solid matter may be an abnormal byproduct of a biological function or a foreign body. Physical force (e.g., manual, ultrasonic) applied directly or indirectly through intervening body parts is used to break the solid matter into pieces. The pieces of solid matter are not taken out, but are eliminated or absorbed through normal biological functions
	Examples:	Extracorporeal shockwave lithotripsy, transurethral lithotripsy
Fusion	**Definition:**	Joining together portions of an articular body part rendering the articular body part immobile
	Explanation:	The body part is joined together by fixation device, bone graft, or other means
	Examples:	Spinal fusion, ankle arthrodesis
Insertion	**Definition:**	Putting in a nonbiological appliance that monitors, assists, performs or prevents a physiological function, but does not physically take the place of a body part
	Explanation:	N/A
	Examples:	Insertion of radioactive implant, insertion of central venous catheter
Inspection	**Definition:**	Visually and/or manually exploring a body part
	Explanation:	Visual exploration may be performed with or without optical instrumentation. Manual exploration may be performed directly or through intervening body layers
	Examples:	Diagnostic arthroscopy, exploratory laparotomy
Map	**Definition:**	Locating the route of passage of electrical impulses and/or locating functional areas in a body part
	Explanation:	Applicable only to the cardiac conduction mechanism and the central nervous system
	Examples:	Cardiac mapping, cortical mapping
Occlusion	**Definition:**	Completely closing an orifice or lumen of a tubular body part
	Explanation:	The orifice can be a natural orifice or an artificially created orifice
	Examples:	Fallopian tube ligation, ligation of inferior vena cava
Reattachment	**Definition:**	Putting back in or on all or a portion of a separated body part to its normal location or other suitable location
	Explanation:	Vascular circulation and nervous pathways may or may not be reestablished
	Examples:	Reattachment of hand, reattachment of avulsed kidney
Release	**Definition:**	Freeing a body part from an abnormal physical constraint by cutting or by use of force
	Explanation:	Some of the restraining tissue may be taken out but none of the body part is taken out
	Examples:	Adhesiolysis, carpal tunnel release
Removal	**Definition:**	Taking out or off a device from a body part
	Explanation:	If the device is taken out and a similar device is put in without cutting or puncturing the skin or mucous membrane, the procedure is coded to the root operation CHANGE. Otherwise, the procedure for taking out the device is coded to the root operation REMOVAL and the procedure for putting in the new device is coded to the root operation performed
	Examples:	Drainage tube removal, cardiac pacemaker removal
Repair	**Definition:**	Restoring, to the extent possible, a body part to its normal anatomic structure and function
	Explanation:	Used only when the method to accomplish the repair is not one of the other root operations
	Examples:	Herniorrhaphy, suture of laceration
Replacement	**Definition:**	Putting in or on biological or synthetic material that physically takes the place and/or function of all or a portion of a body part
	Explanation:	The biological material is non-living, or the biological material is living and from the same individual. The body part may have been previously taken out, previously replaced, or may be taken out concomitantly with the Replacement procedure. If the body part has been previously replaced, a separate Removal procedure is coded for taking out the device used in the previous replacement
	Examples:	Total hip replacement, bone graft, free skin graft

TABLE 7-1

MEDICAL AND SURGICAL ROOT OPERATION DEFINITIONS (SELECT) (Continued)

Reposition	**Definition:**	Moving to its normal location or other suitable location all or a portion of a body part
	Explanation:	The body part is moved to a new location from an abnormal location, or from a normal location where it is not functioning correctly. The body part may or may not be cut out or off to be moved to the new location
	Examples:	Reposition of undescended testicle, fracture reduction
Resection	**Definition:**	Cutting out or off, without replacement, all of a body part
	Explanation:	N/A
	Examples:	Total nephrectomy, total lobectomy of lung
Restriction	**Definition:**	Partially closing the orifice or lumen of a tubular body part
	Explanation:	The orifice can be a natural orifice or an artificially created orifice
	Examples:	Esophagogastric fundoplication, cervical cerclage
Revision	**Definition:**	Correcting, to the extent possible, a malfunctioning or displaced device
	Explanation:	Revision can include correcting a malfunctioning or displaced device by taking out or putting in components of the device such as a screw or pin
	Examples:	Adjustment of pacemaker lead, adjustment of hip prosthesis
Supplement	**Definition:**	Putting in or on biologic or synthetic material that physically reinforces and/ or augments the function of a portion of a body part
	Explanation:	The biological material is non-living, or the biological material is living and from the same individual. The body part may have been previously replaced. If the body part has been previously replaced, the Supplement procedure is performed to physically reinforce and/or augment the function of the replaced body part
	Examples:	Herniorrhaphy using mesh, free nerve graft, mitral valve ring annuloplasty, put a new acetabular liner in a previous hip replacement
Transfer	**Definition:**	Moving, without taking out, all or a portion of a body part to another location to take over the function of all or a portion of a body part
	Explanation:	The body part transferred remains connected to its vascular and nervous supply
	Examples:	Tendon transfer, skin pedicle flap transfer
Transplantation	**Definition:**	Putting in or on all or a portion of a living body part taken from another individual or animal to physically take the place and/or function of all or a portion of a similar body part
	Explanation:	The native body part may or may not be taken out, and the transplanted body part may take over all or a portion of its function
	Examples:	Kidney transplant, heart transplant

TABLE 7–2

COMPARISON OF MEDICAL AND SURGICAL ROOT OPERATIONS (SELECT)

Operation	Action	Target	Clarification	Example
Procedures that take out or eliminate all or a portion of a body part:				
Excision	Cutting out or off	Portion of a body part	Without replacing body part	Sigmoid polypectomy
Resection	Cutting out or off	All of a body part	Without replacing body part	Total nephrectomy
Extraction	Pulling out or off by physical force	All or a portion of a body part	Without replacing body part	Toenail extraction
Destruction	Eradicating	All or a portion of a body part	Without taking out or replacing body part	Rectal polyp fulguration
Detachment	Cutting off	All or a portion of an extremity	Without replacing extremity	Below knee amputation
Procedures that involve putting in or on, putting back, or moving living body parts:				
Transplantation	Putting in or on	All or a portion of a living body part from other individual or animal	Physically takes the place and/or function of all or a portion of a body part	Heart transplant
Reattachment	Putting back in or on	All or a portion of a separated body part	Put in its normal or other suitable location.	Finger reattachment
Reposition	Moving	All or a portion of a body part	Put in its normal or other suitable location. Body part may or may not be cut out or off	Reposition undescended testicle
Transfer	Moving	All or a portion of a body part	Without taking out body part; assumes function of similar body part and remains connected to its vascular and nervous supply	Tendon transfer
Procedures that take out or eliminate solid matter, fluids, or gases from a body part:				
Drainage	Taking or letting out	Fluids and/or gases from a body part	Without taking out any of the body part	Incision and drainage
Extirpation	Taking or cutting out	Solid matter in a body part	Without taking out any of the body part	Thrombectomy
Fragmentation	Breaking down	Solid matter in a body part	Without taking out any of the body part or any solid matter	Lithotripsy of gallstones
Procedures that only involve examination of body parts and regions:				
Inspection	Visual and/or manual exploration	A body part	Performed with or without optical instrumentation, directly or through body layers	Diagnostic arthroscopy
Map	Locating	Route of passage of electrical impulses or functional areas in a body part	Applicable only to cardiac conduction mechanism and central nervous system	Cardiac mapping
Procedures that can be performed only on tubular body parts:				
Bypass	Altering the route of passage	Contents of tubular body part	May include use of living tissue, non-living biological material or synthetic material which does not take the place of the body part	Gastrojejunal bypass
Dilation	Expanding	Orifice or lumen of tubular body part	By application of intraluminal pressure or by cutting the wall or orifice	Anal sphincter dilation
Occlusion	Completely closing	Orifice or lumen of tubular body part	N/A	Fallopian tube ligation
Restriction	Partially closing	Orifice or lumen of tubular body part	N/A	Cervical cerclage

TABLE 7–2

COMPARISON OF MEDICAL AND SURGICAL ROOT OPERATIONS (SELECT) (Continued)

Operation	Action	Target	Clarification	Example
Procedures that always involve devices:				
Insertion	Putting in	Device in or on a body part	Does not physically take the place of a body part	Pacemaker insertion
Replacement	Putting in or on	Biological or synthetic material; living tissue taken from same individual	Physically takes the place of all or a portion of a body part	Total hip replacement
Supplement	Putting in or on	Biological or synthetic material; living tissue taken from same individual	Physically reinforces or augments a portion of a body part	Herniorrhaphy using mesh
Removal	Taking out or off	Device from a body part	N/A	Cardiac pacemaker removal
Change	Taking out or off and putting back	Identical or similar device in or on a body part	Without cutting or puncturing skin or mucous membrane	Drainage tube change
Revision	Correcting	Malfunctioning or displaced device in or on a body part	To the extent possible	Hip prosthesis adjustment
Procedures involving cutting or separation only:				
Division	Separating	A body part	Without taking out any of the body part	Osteotomy
Release	Freeing	A body part	Eliminating abnormal constraint without taking out any of the body part	Peritoneal adhesiolysis
Procedures involving other repairs:				
Control	Stopping or attempting to stop	Postprocedural bleeding	Limited to anatomic regions and extremities	Control of postprostatectomy bleeding
Repair	Restoring	A body part to its normal structure	To the extent possible	Hernia repair
Procedures with other objectives:				
Alteration	Modifying	Anatomic structure of a body part	Without affecting function of body part, performed for cosmetic purposes	Face lift
Creation	Making	New genital structure	Does not physically take the place of a body part, used for sex change operations	Artificial vagina creation
Fusion	Joining together	An articular body part	Rendering body part immobile	Spinal fusion

The Index   ICD-10-PCS codes are described in both the Index and the Tabular List. The Index is used to locate codes by means of an alphabetic lookup. The Index is arranged according to root operation terms and has subentries based on:

- Body System
- Body Part
- Operation (for Revision)
- Device (for Change)

The Index may also be consulted for a specific operation term such as "Hysterectomy," where a cross-reference directs you to "*see* Resection, Female Reproductive System, OUT." Although you need to become very familiar with the root operations, you may be able to locate a code for a specific operation such as an appendectomy more rapidly by looking under the term "Appendectomy" than by consulting the root operation term "Resection," subterms "by Body Part," and "Appendix." See Fig. 7–8 for an example of the Index of the ICD-10-PCS.

Codes may also be located in the Index by specific procedures such as X-ray—*see* Imaging. The Index refers you to a specific entry in the Tabular List by providing the first three or four digits of the procedure code. It is always necessary to refer to the Tabular List to obtain the complete code because the Index contains only the first few numbers and letters.

The Tabular List Completes the Code

The Tabular List provides the remaining characters needed to complete the code listed in the Index. The Tabular List is arranged by sections, and most sections are subdivided by body systems. For each body system, the Tabular List begins with a list of the operations performed, that is, the root operations. When a procedure involves distinct parts, multiple codes are provided. For example, a section of the listing of operations performed in respect to the central nervous system is as follows:

- Bypass
- Change
- Destruction
- Division
- Drainage
- Excision

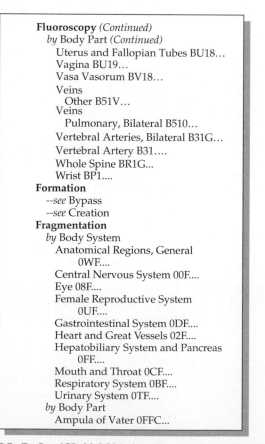

FIGURE 7–8 ICD-10-PCS Index. (From Buck CJ: *ICD-10-PCS, Professional Edition*, St. Louis, 2010, Saunders.)

The Tabular List for each body system also includes a list of the body parts, approaches, devices, and qualifiers for that system. These lists are followed by tables for each root operation in that body system. At the top of each of the tables is the name of the section, body system, and root operation as well as the definition of the root operation. The list is formatted as a grid, with rows and columns. The four columns in the grid represent the last four characters of the code (which are labeled Body Part, Approach, Device, and Qualifier in the Obstetrics and Medical and Surgical sections). Each row in the grid specifies the allowable combinations of the last four characters. For example, referring to the grid in Fig. 7–9, you see that the code for delivery of retained products of conception is 10E0XZZ:

1 Obstetrics (Section)

0 Pregnancy (Body System)

E Delivery (Root Operation)

0 Products of Conception, Retained (Body Part, Character 4)

X External (Approach, Character 5)

Z None (Device, Character 6)

Z None (Qualifier, Character 7)

Code 10E0XZZ would be the only allowable code for Products of Conception, using an external approach with no devices, because you may not complete a code by choosing entries from different rows (a row may consist of multiple entries in a box). Thus the code 10E0XZ6 is not permitted because the qualifier 6 is not an option. If you begin the code with 0, Products of Conception, you must continue to choose from the available numbers or letters in that same line.

FIGURE 7–9 ICD-10-PCS Tabular. (Modified from Buck CJ: *ICD-10-PCS, Professional Edition,* St. Louis, 2010, Saunders.)

From the Trenches

"Books are out and several training courses have started to give a heads up on ICD-10. Also the CMS website has information for download to help coders learn ICD-10."

MELONY

EXERCISE 7-4   ICD-10-PCS Format

Complete the following:

Achievement of the four major objectives guiding the development of the ICD-10-PCS will result in a classification system that is

1 _____

2 _____

3 _____

4 _____

Provide the requested information about the ICD-10-PCS code structure:

5 The ICD-10-PCS has a _____ character code structure.

6 The characters in ICD-10-PCS are _____.

7 Each character has up to _____ different values.

8 The letters _____ are not used as character values.

9 The complete specification of seven characters describes a _____ in the ICD-10-PCS.

CHAPTER REVIEW

CHAPTER 7, PART I, THEORY

Answer the following:

1 ICD-10-CM codes are alphanumeric.

   True   False

2 ICD-10-CM is indexed in a similar manner to ICD-9-CM.

   True   False

3 Like ICD-9-CM, ICD-10-CM contains 17 chapters.

   True   False

4 The American Medical Association is responsible for the development of ICD-10-PCS.

   True   False

5 In ICD-10-PCS, if a character is not applicable, the letter X is used.

   True   False

6 When implemented, the United States will be the first nation to use ICD-10.

   True   False

7 The term "fusion" means the freeing of a body part.

   True   False

8 An example of a procedure that involves inspection is:

   a. gastrojejunal bypass
   b. control of postprocedural bleeding
   c. diagnostic arthroscopy
   d. incision and drainage of abscess

9 Altering the route of passage of the contents of a tubular body part is a:

   a. resection
   b. bypass
   c. revision
   d. drainage

10 ICD-10 was issued in 1993 by:

   a. CMS
   b. AHIMA
   c. AHA
   d. WHO

CHAPTER 7, PART II, PRACTICAL

Using the ICD-10-CM Index and Tabular, assign ICD-10-CM codes to the following:

11 Long-term use of anticoagulant

ICD-10-CM Code: _____

12 Bacteremia

ICD-10-CM Code: _____

13 Idiopathic scoliosis, thoracic, adolescent

ICD-10-CM Code: _____

14 Asthma in a patient with chronic obstructive bronchitis with an acute exacerbation

ICD-10-CM Code: _____

15 Myasthenia gravis with acute exacerbation

ICD-10-CM Code: _____

16 Second-degree burns of multiple sites (5%) on the right hand and wrist

Burn: _____

Extent of the burn: _____

17 Congenital macrocephaly (enlarged head)

ICD-10-CM Code: _____

18 Osteoporosis in a 92-year-old female

ICD-10-CM Code: _____

19 Gastroesophageal reflex in a 23-year-old male, without esophagitis

ICD-10-CM Code: _____

20 Secondary and primary syphilis of the anus in 30-year-old male

ICD-10-CM Code: _____

"Teamwork is an essential requirement in our profession. We learn from each other . . . then pass the knowledge on. It is an unbroken cycle."

Nancy Maguire, ACS, PCS, FCS, CPC, CPC-H, HCS-D, CRT
Physician Coding
Consultant/Auditor
San Antonio, Texas

Introduction to the CPT and Level II National Codes (HCPCS)

Chapter Topics

The Purpose of the CPT Manual

Updating the CPT Manual

CPT Manual Format

Starting with the Index

History of National Level Codes

Chapter Review

Quick Check Answers

Learning Objectives

After completing this chapter you should be able to

1 Identify the uses of the CPT manual.

2 Name the developers of the CPT manual.

3 Know the importance of using the current-year CPT manual.

4 Identify placement of CPT codes on the CMS-1500 insurance form.

5 Recognize the symbols used in the CPT manual.

6 Identify the content of the CPT appendices.

7 List the major sections found in the CPT manual.

8 Interpret the information contained in the section Guidelines and notes.

9 Describe the CPT code format.

10 Append modifiers.

11 Describe what is meant by unlisted procedures/services.

12 State the purposes of a special report.

13 Review Category II and III CPT codes.

14 Locate the terms in the CPT index.

15 List the major features of Level II National Codes, HCPCS.

16 Demonstrate the ability to assign HCPCS codes.

Make sure to check
evolve
learning system
for the latest content updates

THE PURPOSE OF THE CPT MANUAL

Current Procedural Terminology (CPT), also known as CPT-4, is a coding system developed by the American Medical Association (AMA) to convert widely accepted, uniform descriptions of medical, surgical, and diagnostic services rendered by health care providers into five-digit numeric codes. The use of the CPT codes enables health care providers to communicate both effectively and efficiently with third-party payers (i.e., commercial insurance companies, Medicare, Medicaid) about the procedures and services provided to the patient. For example, on an insurance form you can report a service by entering 21182 rather than "Reconstruction of orbital walls, rims, forehead, nasoethmoid complex following intra- and extracranial excision of benign tumor of the cranial bone (e.g., fibrous dysplasia) with multiple autografts (includes obtaining grafts); total area of bone grafting less than 40 sq cm." By using 21182, you are able to communicate not only quickly but also exactly about a very detailed service.

The majority of CPT codes are referred to as Category I codes and have been approved by the Editorial Panel of the AMA. Category II codes are optional performance measures (e.g., 3014F, screening mammography). Category III codes are temporary codes that identify emerging technologies, services, and procedures (e.g., 0092T, arthroplasty).

Health care providers are reimbursed for the procedures and services rendered based on the codes submitted on a claim form. For an example of placement of the CPT codes on a claim form, refer to arrow on Fig. 8–1 (24D).

Reporting the correct code is essential because incorrect coding can result in a provider being reimbursed incorrectly or in some cases being penalized by the government for submitting inappropriate claims. The CPT coding system is used by clinics, outpatient hospital departments, ambulatory surgery centers, and third-party payers to describe health care services. Although there are differences in the rules governing coding in various health care settings, CPT codes offer increased compatibility and comparability of data among users and providers, allowing for comparative analysis, research, and reimbursement.

The CPT coding system was first developed and published by the AMA in 1966 as a method of reporting medical and surgical procedures and services using standard terminology. Three editions of *Current Procedural Terminology* were published in the 1970s, and updates and revisions reflected changes in the technology and practices of health care. Use of the CPT manual was increased in 1983 when the Centers for Medicare and Medicaid Services (CMS), formerly the Health Care Financing Administration (HCFA), incorporated CPT codes into the Healthcare Common Procedural Coding System (HCPCS) to provide a uniform system of reporting services, procedures, and supplies. CPT codes are Level I codes and, for the most part, define professional services. Level II National Codes (HCPCS) are alphanumeric codes that are used by providers to report services, supplies, and equipment provided to Medicare and Medicaid patients for which no CPT codes exist.

HCPCS codes may be required even if a CPT Level I is available. Some third-party payers follow Medicare and Medicaid guidelines and may also require HCPCS Level II codes be assigned (e.g., J codes), so HCPCS may be required on non-Medicare and Medicaid patients. Certain HCPCS Level II codes are required by all payers, such as the drug codes, J codes.

UPDATING THE CPT MANUAL

Because the practice of medicine is ever changing, the CPT manual is ever changing. It is updated annually to reflect technologic advances and editorial revisions. It is very important to use the most current CPT manual available so as to provide quality data and ensure appropriate reimbursement. Many revisions to the CPT were necessary to address requirements of the Health Insurance Portability and Accountability Act of 1996 (HIPAA). HIPAA requires the Secretary of Health and Human Services to adopt national uniform standards for the electronic transmission of financial and

CARRIER

1500

HEALTH INSURANCE CLAIM FORM

APPROVED BY NATIONAL UNIFORM CLAIM COMMITTEE 08/05

| | PICA | | | | | | | | PICA | |

1. MEDICARE ☐ (Medicare #)   MEDICAID ☐ (Medicaid #)   TRICARE CHAMPUS ☐ (Sponsor's SSN)   CHAMPVA ☐ (Member ID#)   GROUP HEALTH PLAN ☐ (SSN or ID)   FECA BLK LUNG ☐ (SSN)   OTHER ☐ (ID)

1a. INSURED'S I.D. NUMBER   (For Program in Item 1)

2. PATIENT'S NAME (Last Name, First Name, Middle Initial)

3. PATIENT'S BIRTH DATE   MM | DD | YY   SEX   M ☐   F ☐

4. INSURED'S NAME (Last Name, First Name, Middle Initial)

5. PATIENT'S ADDRESS (No., Street)

6. PATIENT RELATIONSHIP TO INSURED   Self ☐   Spouse ☐   Child ☐   Other ☐

7. INSURED'S ADDRESS (No., Street)

CITY   STATE

8. PATIENT STATUS   Single ☐   Married ☐   Other ☐   Employed ☐   Full-Time Student ☐   Part-Time Student ☐

CITY   STATE

ZIP CODE   TELEPHONE (Include Area Code) (   )

ZIP CODE   TELEPHONE (Include Area Code) (   )

9. OTHER INSURED'S NAME (Last Name, First Name, Middle Initial)

10. IS PATIENT'S CONDITION RELATED TO:

11. INSURED'S POLICY GROUP OR FECA NUMBER

a. OTHER INSURED'S POLICY OR GROUP NUMBER

a. EMPLOYMENT? (Current or Previous)   YES ☐   NO ☐

a. INSURED'S DATE OF BIRTH   MM | DD | YY   SEX   M ☐   F ☐

b. OTHER INSURED'S DATE OF BIRTH   MM | DD | YY   SEX   M ☐   F ☐

b. AUTO ACCIDENT?   PLACE (State)   YES ☐   NO ☐

b. EMPLOYER'S NAME OR SCHOOL NAME

c. EMPLOYER'S NAME OR SCHOOL NAME

c. OTHER ACCIDENT?   YES ☐   NO ☐

c. INSURANCE PLAN NAME OR PROGRAM NAME

d. INSURANCE PLAN NAME OR PROGRAM NAME

10d. RESERVED FOR LOCAL USE

d. IS THERE ANOTHER HEALTH BENEFIT PLAN?   YES ☐   NO ☐   If yes, return to and complete item 9 a-d.

READ BACK OF FORM BEFORE COMPLETING & SIGNING THIS FORM.
12. PATIENT'S OR AUTHORIZED PERSON'S SIGNATURE I authorize the release of any medical or other information necessary to process this claim. I also request payment of government benefits either to myself or to the party who accepts assignment below.

SIGNED_____   DATE_____

13. INSURED'S OR AUTHORIZED PERSON'S SIGNATURE I authorize payment of medical benefits to the undersigned physician or supplier for services described below.

SIGNED_____

PATIENT AND INSURED INFORMATION

14. DATE OF CURRENT: MM | DD | YY   ◄ ILLNESS (First symptom) OR INJURY (Accident) OR PREGNANCY(LMP)

15. IF PATIENT HAS HAD SAME OR SIMILAR ILLNESS. GIVE FIRST DATE   MM | DD | YY

16. DATES PATIENT UNABLE TO WORK IN CURRENT OCCUPATION   FROM MM | DD | YY   TO MM | DD | YY

17. NAME OF REFERRING PROVIDER OR OTHER SOURCE

17a.
17b.

18. HOSPITALIZATION DATES RELATED TO CURRENT SERVICES   FROM MM | DD | YY   TO MM | DD | YY

19. RESERVED FOR LOCAL USE

20. OUTSIDE LAB?   YES ☐   NO ☐ $ CHARGES

21. DIAGNOSIS OR NATURE OF ILLNESS OR INJURY (Relate Items 1, 2, 3 or 4 to Item 24E by Line)

1. |___ . ___   3. |___ . ___
2. |___ . ___   4. |___ . ___

22. MEDICAID RESUBMISSION CODE   ORIGINAL REF. NO.

23. PRIOR AUTHORIZATION NUMBER

24. A. DATE(S) OF SERVICE		B. PLACE OF SERVICE	C. EMG	D. PROCEDURES, SERVICES, OR SUPPLIES (Explain Unusual Circumstances)		E. DIAGNOSIS POINTER	F. $ CHARGES	G. DAYS OR UNITS	H. EPSDT Family Plan	I. ID. QUAL.	J. RENDERING PROVIDER ID. #
From MM DD YY	To MM DD YY			CPT/HCPCS	MODIFIER						
1											
2											
3											
4											
5											
6											

25. FEDERAL TAX I.D. NUMBER   SSN ☐ EIN ☐

26. PATIENT'S ACCOUNT NO.

27. ACCEPT ASSIGNMENT? (For govt. claims, see back)   YES ☐   NO ☐

28. TOTAL CHARGE $

29. AMOUNT PAID $

30. BALANCE DUE $

31. SIGNATURE OF PHYSICIAN OR SUPPLIER INCLUDING DEGREES OR CREDENTIALS (I certify that the statements on the reverse apply to this bill and are made a part thereof.)

SIGNED   DATE

32. SERVICE FACILITY LOCATION INFORMATION

a.   b.

33. BILLING PROVIDER INFO & PH # (   )

a.   b.

PHYSICIAN OR SUPPLIER INFORMATION

NUCC Instruction Manual available at: www.nucc.org   **PLEASE PRINT OR TYPE**   APPROVED OMB-0938-0999 FORM CMS-1500 (08-05)

FIGURE 8-1   The CMS-1500 Health Insurance Claim Form was revised to accommodate reporting of the National Provider Identifier (NPI) number mandated for April 2007. (Courtesy U.S. Department of Health and Human Services, Centers for Medicare and Medicaid Services.)

administrative health information. These standards include a wide variety of health care information. One item that HIPAA requires is a common, concise coding system with clear, expandable definitions. The AMA is meeting this requirement by continuing to make the code definitions more precise.

From the Trenches

"Beginners think that if you have the coding books (CPT, ICD-9-CM) you're good to go. I tell them there is a story and history behind each code . . . . They must investigate codes, modifiers, HCPCS codes, and more before a final decision can be made. It is never boring!"

NANCY

Updated editions of the CPT manual are available for purchase in November for use beginning the following January 1.

CHECK THIS OUT ☞ The American Medical Association (AMA) has a website located at www.ama-assn.org

EXERCISE 8-1 *The Purpose of the CPT Manual*

Complete the following:

1 The CPT manual was developed by the _____, _____, _____.

2 CPT stands for _____, _____, _____.

3 Providers of health care are paid based on the codes submitted for _____ or procedures provided to the patient.

4 The first CPT was published in this year: _____.

5 In which year were CPT codes incorporated as Level I codes into the Healthcare Procedure Coding System (HCPCS)? _____.

CPT MANUAL FORMAT
The symbols used in the CPT manual are noted on the bottom of each page along with a short description of the symbol.
In the CPT manual, **new** codes are identified by the bullet (●) symbol that is placed in front of the code. Note the location of this symbol in Fig. 8–2.

Important Symbols and Appendices
A triangle (▲) placed in front of a code indicates that the description for the code has been **changed** or modified since the previous edition. Changes may be additions, deletions, or revisions in code descriptions (Fig. 8–3).
When the text has changed, a right and a left triangle (► ◄) indicate the beginning and end of the text changes, as illustrated in Fig. 8–4.

New code for service/procedure symbol

●3XXXX Exchange of a previously placed arterial catheter during thrombolytic therapy

FIGURE 8–2 New CPT code symbol.

Changed code description

▲3XXXX Arteriovenous anastomosis, direct, any site (e.g., Cimino type)

FIGURE 8–3   Changed CPT code symbol.

Pacemaker or ►Pacing Cardioverter-◄ Defibrillator

A pacemaker system includes a pulse generator containing electronics and a battery, and one or more electrodes (leads). Pulse generators ►are◄ placed in a subcutaneous "pocket" created in either a subclavicular site ►or underneath the abdominal muscles just below the ribcage.◄ Electrodes may be inserted through a vein (transvenous) or ►they may be placed◄ on the surface of the heart (epicardial).► The epicardial . . .

FIGURE 8–4   Changed CPT text symbols.

The plus symbol (+) placed in front of a code indicates an **add-on code** (Fig. 8–5), while a circle symbol (○) is placed in front of any reinstated or recycled code (Fig. 8–6).

Add-on codes are never used alone; rather, they are reported with another primary procedure or service code. For example, code 11000 describes a debridement (removal of contaminated tissue) of up to 10% of the body surface. Add-on code 11001 is reported for each additional 10% of the body surface debrided or part thereof. Code 11001 cannot be reported unless code 11000 is used first. Also notice in Fig. 8–5 that there is a note in parentheses that indicates that code 11001 can be used only in conjunction with code 11000. **Appendix D** in the CPT manual lists all add-on codes.

The circle with a line through it (⊘) identifies a **modifier -51 exempt** code (Fig. 8–7).

Modifier -51 indicates that more than one (multiple) procedure was performed. **Appendix E** in the CPT manual contains the complete list of modifier -51 exempt codes.

11000 Debridement of extensive eczematous or infected skin; up to 10% of body surface

+ ▲**11001**   each additional 10% of the body surface or part thereof (List separately in addition to code for primary procedure)

►(Use 11001 in conjunction with code 11000)◄

Add-on code symbol   Note

FIGURE 8–5   Add-on CPT code symbol.

✚ ○ **0054T**   Code Reinstated/Recycled

✚ ○ **0055T**   Code Reinstated/Recycled

FIGURE 8–6   Reinstated or recycled CPT code symbol.

48510   External drainage, pseudocyst of pancreas; open

⊘ 48511   percutaneous

Modifier -51 exempt code symbol

FIGURE 8–7   Modifier -51 exempt CPT code symbol.

Modifier -51 is discussed later in greater detail in Chapter 9.

QUICK CHECK 8-1

1. Symbols with definitions are located at the bottom of the page in the CPT.
   True or False?

Appendix A lists all modifiers that are used to alter or modify codes. Modifiers will be discussed in detail later in the chapter and in greater detail in Chapter 9.

Appendix B of the CPT manual contains a complete list of the additions to, deletions from, and revisions of the CPT manual. When a code is listed in Appendix B, the type of change is also listed (Fig. 8–8).

Appendix C of the CPT manual contains clinical examples of many of the Evaluation and Management (E/M) codes (Fig. 8–9).

The examples in Appendix C are meant to offer a broad idea of the type of presenting problem that each code could represent. But a word of caution: Only the patient's record and the services rendered by the physician to a patient determine the level of service provided. Appendix C is not meant to be an exhaustive list of E/M services.

Appendix F of the CPT manual contains the summary of CPT codes that are Modifier -63 exempt. Modifier -63 identifies procedures that are performed on infants who weigh less than 4 kg or 8.8 pounds and represents a significant increase in the physician's work and complexity of service/procedure. Services/Procedures submitted with modifier -63 may be reviewed for an increase in reimbursement.

	Appendix B
2XXXX Code deleted. To report, use 2XXXX	2XXXX Code deleted. To report, use 2XXXX

Deletion

	Appendix B
3XXXX Terminology revised	3XXXX Nasal/sinus endoscopy code added

Revisions   Additions

FIGURE 8–8   CPT manual Appendix B, showing types of changes.

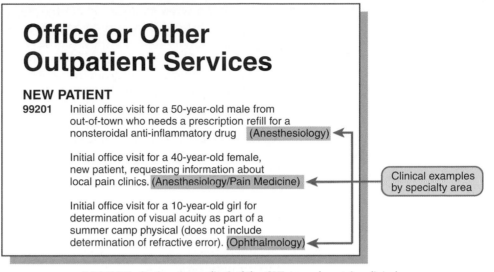

Office or Other Outpatient Services

NEW PATIENT

99201 Initial office visit for a 50-year-old male from out-of-town who needs a prescription refill for a nonsteroidal anti-inflammatory drug (Anesthesiology)

Initial office visit for a 40-year-old female, new patient, requesting information about local pain clinics. (Anesthesiology/Pain Medicine)

Initial office visit for a 10-year-old girl for determination of visual acuity as part of a summer camp physical (does not include determination of refractive error). (Ophthalmology)

Clinical examples by specialty area

FIGURE 8–9 Appendix C of the CPT manual contains clinical examples in the use of E/M codes.

Appendix G is a summary of Moderate (Conscious) Sedation codes identified with a bullseye (⊙) that denotes a procedure that includes moderate (conscious) sedation. For example, 32201, Pneumonostomy with percutaneous drainage of abscess or cyst, has a bullseye before the code indicating that bundled into the code is both the insertion of the catheter and any conscious sedation provided. Moderate or conscious sedation is the type that leaves the patient alert enough to follow directions but still sedated enough to alleviate pain.

Appendix H is the Alphabetic Index of Performance Measures by Clinical Condition or Topic and lists the Category II codes. Category II codes are optional tracking codes that are used to identify performance measures of clinical components that may be typically included in evaluation and management services. The codes make it easier to collect data about certain services or test results that contribute to the health and quality of care of the patient. You learn more about Category II codes later in this chapter.

Appendix I lists the Genetic Testing Code Modifiers. The modifiers in this appendix are reported with molecular laboratory procedures that are related to genetic testing. The first digit is a number that indicates the disease category and the second digit is a letter that denotes the gene type. For example, 0M is the modifier that indicates retinoblastoma (Rb).

Appendix J is the Electrodiagnostic Medicine Listing of Sensory, Motor and Mixed Nerves that identifies the sensory, motor, and mixed nerves with the corresponding conduction study code (95900, 95903, and 95904). Codes 95900 and 95903 are used to report motor nerve conduction studies, and 95904 is used to report sensory nerve conduction studies. Appendix J identifies the nerves in each of the nerve groups. Sensory and motor nerves are part of the peripheral nervous system (PNS) and run from the stimulus receptors to the central nervous system (CNS). A table in Appendix J lists the "reasonable maximum number of studies performed per diagnostic category necessary for a physician to arrive at a diagnosis in 90% of the patients with that final diagnosis." The recommended number of studies for each indication (condition) is identified. For example, if the indication was myopathy, it is recommended that the physician perform two needle electromyographies (EMGs), two motor nerve conduction studies (NCS), two sensory NCS, and two neuromuscular junction testings.

Appendix K, Products Pending FDA Approval, contains the lightning bolt symbol (⚡) that identifies codes that are being tracked by the AMA to monitor Food and Drug Administration (FDA) status for approval of a drug.

The internet site www.ama-assn.org/ama/pub/category/10902.html provides updates to the list of FDA pending approval codes.

Appendix L, Vascular Families, is a helpful listing of the orders of the vascular families. Listed are the first order, second order, third order branches, and beyond third order branches. The assumption is made that the starting point is the aorta. If the vessel is accessed at some other location, the branches, of course, would not be correct. You will find this appendix very helpful when you are coding catheterizations in the later chapters.

Appendix M, Summary of Crosswalk Deleted CPT Codes, lists the current-year code to replace a deleted code.

In 2010, the American Medical Association introduced a new initiative for the CPT that was termed **resequencing**. Historically, the codes within a CPT section have been in numeric order, but with the publication of the 2010 CPT, that was no longer the case for 27 codes. The pound symbol (#) appears before the resequenced codes. An example of this resequencing is in the 51725-51798 range where the code and code description for 51797 follow 51729, which is not in numeric order. Code 51797 also appears in correct numeric order in the CPT, but next to the code a note states "Code is out of numerical sequence. See 51725-51798." The following are the codes that are affected in the 2010 CPT:

> 21552, 21554, 23071, 23073, 24071, 24073, 25071, 25073, 26111, 26113, 27043, 27045, 27059, 27329, 27337, 27339, 27632, 27634, 28039, 28041, 49645, 49646, 46220, 46320, 46947, 51797, 82652

EXERCISE 8-2 *Symbols*

Match the following code symbols with the correct definition:

1 ▲ _____   a. beginning and end of text changes

2 ►◄ _____   b. modifier -51 exempt

3 ● _____   c. revised description

4 ⊘ _____   d. add-on

5 + _____   e. moderate (conscious) sedation included

6 ⊙ _____   f. pending FDA approval status

7 ✗ _____   g. new

8 Where is a complete list of additions, deletions, and revisions located in the CPT manual? _____

9 Which CPT manual appendix contains a complete list of all modifier -51 exempt codes? _____

10 Which CPT manual appendix contains a complete list of add-on codes? _____

CPT Sections

The CPT manual is composed of six chapters into which all codes and descriptions are categorized. These chapters are called **sections.**

THE SECTIONS OF THE CPT MANUAL

- Evaluation and Management   99201-99499
- Anesthesia   00100-01999, 99100-99140
- Surgery   10021-69990
- Radiology   70010-79999
- Pathology and Laboratory   80047-89398
- Medicine   90281-99199, 99500-99607

The sections are further divided into subsections, subheadings, categories, and subcategories. A **section** is a chapter that covers one of the six topics included in the CPT manual: Evaluation/Management (E/M), Anesthesia, Surgery,

Radiology, Pathology/Laboratory, and Medicine codes. The CPT codes are arranged in numerical order in each section. Let's review these six sections.

Sections are divided into **subsections.** For example, the Surgery section includes subsections of Integumentary, Musculoskeletal, Respiratory, Cardiovascular, and so forth.

Subsections, **subheadings, categories,** and **subcategories** are divisions of sections that are based on anatomy, procedure, condition, description, or approach.

Example

Section:	Surgery
Subsection:	Cardiovascular System
Subheading:	Arteries and Veins
Category:	Embolectomy/Thrombectomy
Subcategory:	Arterial, With or Without Catheter

Example

Section:	Surgery
Subsection:	Nervous System
Subheading:	Skull, Meninges, and Brain
Category:	Approach Procedures
Subcategory:	Anterior Cranial Fossa

EXERCISE 8-3   *Section, Subsection, Subheading, and Category*

To see an example of section, subsection, subheading, and category, locate the code 19000 Puncture aspiration of cyst of breast in the CPT in the Surgery section.

With a CPT beside you, open to the page where CPT code 19000 is located, or referring to Fig. 8–10 find the information on the top of the CPT manual page:

Section. At the top of the page, the word "Surgery" indicates the section. Note that this word is followed by a range of numbers, which is a list of all the code numbers located on that page.

Subsection. Also at the top of the page, the phrase "Integumentary System" indicates the subsection.

Subheading. The word "Breast" indicates the subheading.

Category. The word "Incision" indicates the category.

In summary, the divisions for the previous example are

Section:	Surgery
Subsection:	Integumentary System
Subheading:	Breast
Category:	Incision

Now you try one.

With a CPT manual open to the page that contains code 30100, locate the following information for the 30100 code:

1 Section: _____

2 Subsection: _____

3 Subheading: _____

4 Category: _____

FIGURE 8–10   Section, subsection, subheading, and category.

Using the section, subsection, subheading, and category information makes it much faster and easier to get around in the CPT manual.

CPT Guidelines   Each section in the CPT manual includes Guidelines. The Guidelines provide specific information about coding in that section and contain valuable information for the coder. Guidelines that are applicable to all codes in the section are found at the beginning of each section (Fig. 8–11).

Notes pertaining to specific codes or groups of codes are listed before or after the codes (Fig. 8–12).

The Guidelines and notes may contain definitions of terms, applicable modifiers, subsection information, unlisted services, special reports information, or clinical examples. Always read the Guidelines and notes before coding to help ensure accurate assignment of the CPT codes.

FIGURE 8–11   Section Guidelines.

FIGURE 8–12   Specific notes.

EXERCISE 8-4 *Guidelines*

Using the Guidelines for each of the sections, answer the following questions:

1 Write the definition of a chief complaint using the E/M Guidelines.

_____

_____

_____

2 According to the Surgery Guidelines, surgical destruction is a part of a surgical procedure and

_____ methods of destruction are not ordinarily listed separately.

3 According to the Radiology Guidelines, who must sign a written report to have the report

considered part of the radiologic procedure? _____

4 Under whose supervision are Pathology and Laboratory services provided? _____

5 What is the code listed in the Medicine Guidelines that is to be used to identify materials supplied

by the physician that are beyond those ordinarily included in the service provided? _____

Code Format Procedure and service descriptions are located after the code (Fig. 8-13). These are commonly accepted descriptions of procedures or services that are provided to patients.

There are two types of codes: **stand-alone codes** and **indented codes** (Fig. 8-14).

Only the stand-alone codes have the full description; indented codes are listed under associated stand-alone codes. It is understood that descriptions for indented codes include that portion of the stand-alone code description that precedes the semicolon. The purpose of the semicolon is to save space.

✋ **CAUTION** *You may not have realized it, but you've just been given a critical clue to coding—the semicolon. The following information will help you understand why the semicolon is so important.*

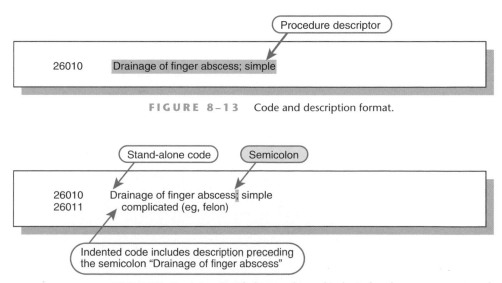

Procedure descriptor

26010   Drainage of finger abscess; simple

FIGURE 8-13   Code and description format.

Stand-alone code   Semicolon

26010   Drainage of finger abscess; simple
26011   complicated (eg, felon)

Indented code includes description preceding the semicolon "Drainage of finger abscess"

FIGURE 8-14   Stand-alone codes and indented codes.

In Fig. 8–14, the code 26011 is an indented code—the indentation serves to represent the words "Drainage of finger abscess," which appear before the semicolon in CPT code 26010. The semicolon is a powerful tool in the CPT manual; when you see it, be sure to read the words before it carefully.

The words following the semicolon can indicate alternative anatomic sites, alternative procedures, or a description of the extent of the service.

Example

ALTERNATIVE ANATOMIC SITE:

27705	Osteotomy; tibia
27707	fibula
27709	tibia and fibula

ALTERNATIVE PROCEDURE:

31505	Laryngoscopy, indirect; diagnostic (separate procedure)
31510	with biopsy
31511	with removal of foreign body
31512	with removal of lesion
31513	with vocal cord injection

DESCRIPTION OF EXTENT OF THE SERVICE:

20520	Removal of foreign body in muscle or tendon sheath; simple
20525	deep or complicated

CAUTION *Before assigning an indented code, make sure you refer to the preceding stand-alone code and read the words that precede the semicolon. That is the only way to ensure a full description and select a correct code.*

EXERCISE 8-5 *Code Format*

Complete the following:

1 Describe a stand-alone code.

_____

_____

2 Describe an indented code.

_____

_____

3 Words following the semicolon in stand-alone codes can indicate the following three things:

a _____

b _____

c _____

Modifiers

Modifiers provide additional information to the third-party payer about services provided to a patient. At times, the five-digit CPT code may not reflect completely the service or procedure provided. Because numeric codes, not written procedure descriptions, are required by third-party payers, additional numbers or letters may be added to the basic five-digit code to modify the CPT code and provide further specificity. These additional modifiers may be two numbers, two letters, or a letter and a number and are appended, or "tacked on," to the basic five-digit CPT code. In the HCPCS manual, two-place modifiers such as -RC and -F1 are used. Notice the HCPCS modifiers are alpha characters or alphanumeric.

In the CPT system, a modifier is an appended two-digit number, such as:

Example

-62, two surgeons
or
-51, multiple procedures

The two-digit modifier is added to the five-digit CPT code.

Example

Code 43820 is the CPT procedure code for a gastrojejunostomy, without vagotomy (removal of part of the vagus nerve). If two surgeons with different surgical skills participated as primary surgeons, each performing a specific part of the procedure, the procedure code 43820 could be altered by the addition of the modifier -62 to indicate co-surgeons (Fig. 8–15).

The code would be 43820-62 for a gastrojejunostomy, without vagotomy, in which two surgeons participated as primary surgeons. Each physician would submit his or her own bill, indicating code 43820-62.

For a complete listing of all modifiers, see Appendix A in the CPT manual. Refer to Fig. 8–16 for an example of the information found in Appendix A. Further information regarding modifiers is presented throughout the following chapters of this text.

CPT modifiers are listed first in descending numeric order (e.g., -62-50), and CPT modifiers are listed before HCPCS modifiers (e.g., -62-RT).

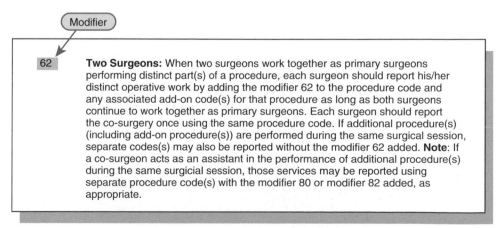

Modifier

62　**Two Surgeons:** When two surgeons work together as primary surgeons performing distinct part(s) of a procedure, each surgeon should report his/her distinct operative work by adding the modifier 62 to the procedure code and any associated add-on code(s) for that procedure as long as both surgeons continue to work together as primary surgeons. Each surgeon should report the co-surgery once using the same procedure code. If additional procedure(s) (including add-on procedure(s)) are performed during the same surgical session, separate codes(s) may also be reported without the modifier 62 added. **Note**: If a co-surgeon acts as an assistant in the performance of additional procedure(s) during the same surgical session, those services may be reported using separate procedure code(s) with the modifier 80 or modifier 82 added, as appropriate.

FIGURE 8–15 Two-digit modifier.

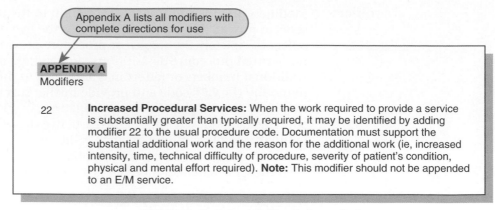

FIGURE 8-16   Modifiers in Appendix A.

EXERCISE 8-6   *Modifiers*

Using Appendix A of the CPT manual and the information you just learned, answer the following:

1 What is the two-digit modifier that indicates two primary surgeons? _____

2 If the CPT code is 43820 (gastrojejunostomy without vagotomy) and two primary surgeons

performed the service, the service could be stated this way: _____, by each surgeon.

Use Appendix A of the CPT manual to list the correct two-digit modifier in the following examples:

3 Bilateral inguinal herniorrhaphy: _____

4 A postoperative ureterotomy patient has to be returned to the operating room (unplanned) for a

complication related to the initial procedure during the postoperative period: _____

5 A decision to perform surgery is made during an evaluation and management service on the day

before or the day of surgery: _____

6 Multiple procedures performed during the same surgical session: _____

7 A surgical team is required: _____

8 Physician A actively assists physician B during a surgical procedure: _____

Unlisted Procedures   When developing the CPT manual, the AMA realized that not every surgical and diagnostic procedure could be listed. There may not be a code for many procedures that are considered experimental, newly approved, or seldom used. In addition, medical advancements often create a variation of procedures currently performed. A procedure or service not found in the CPT manual can be coded as an unlisted procedure if no Category I or III exists to describe the procedure/service provided. For example, when the first heart transplant was performed, there was no code to report the new surgical procedure. Until a code was available, the unlisted code for cardiac surgery was used to report this procedure (Fig. 8–17).

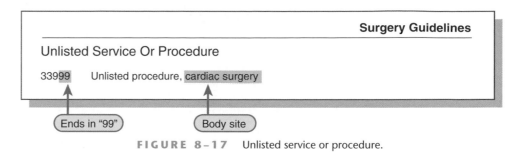

FIGURE 8-17   Unlisted service or procedure.

The Surgery Guidelines have unlisted procedure codes listed by body site or type of procedure. Individually unlisted procedure codes are also at the end of the subsection or subheading to which they refer. For example, at the end of the Cardiovascular System subsection, Heart and Pericardium subheading, is the unlisted cardiac procedure code 33999, and at the end of the Respiratory System subsection, Lungs and Pleura subheading is the unlisted lungs/pleura code 32999.

EXERCISE 8-7   *Unlisted Procedures*

Assuming there is no Category III code available for the procedure you are reporting, using the Guidelines in the front of the sections indicated below, locate the five-digit unlisted procedure code for each of the following:

1 Surgery

Unlisted procedure; middle ear: Code: _____

    arthroscopy: Code: _____

    esophagus: Code: _____

2 Pathology and Laboratory

Unlisted procedure; cytogenetic study: Code: _____

    urinalysis procedure: Code: _____

    chemistry procedure: Code: _____

3 Medicine

Unlisted special service, procedure, or report: Code: _____

4 Radiology

Unlisted procedure; clinical brachytherapy: Code: _____

Unlisted miscellaneous procedures;
diagnostic nuclear medicine: Code: _____

Category II Codes

Earlier in the chapter you were introduced to Category II codes located in Appendix H of the CPT manual. Now it is time to take a closer look at the purpose of these codes and how they are reported.

In December of 2006, Congress enacted a law that established a voluntary program within Medicare that paid physicians a bonus for reporting these quality measures. The pay-for-reporting program is the Physicians

Quality Reporting Initiative (PQRI). The measures have been established to determine if the physician is performing certain elements that are considered to be necessary elements of care. For example, patients with diabetes mellitus are at a high risk for heart attack and stroke and it is very important that these patients control not only their diabetes but also their blood pressure and cholesterol levels. The instruction in the PQRI measure for blood pressure management indicates that at a minimum the diabetic patient's blood pressure is to be reported once in a 12-month period for each patient with diabetes 18-75 years of age. According to the measure, a controlled pressure is less than 140/80 mm Hg.

The **systolic** pressure would be reported with one of the following codes:

3074F	<130 mm Hg
3075F	130-139 mm Hg
3077F	≥140 mm Hg (≥ means equal to or greater than)

The **diastolic** pressure would be reported with one of the following codes:

3078F	<80 mm Hg
3079F	80-89 mm Hg
3080F	≥90 mm Hg

If the documentation indicated the patient's blood pressure reading was 138/100, you would report 3075F for the systolic pressure and 3080F for the diastolic pressure.

In addition to the code, a modifier may be assigned. There are only 4 modifiers approved for use with Category II codes, and they all report the reason the performance measure was not performed.

1P	medical reasons, such as contraindicated due to adverse drug interaction
2P	patient reason, such as the patient declined for religious reasons
3P	system reasons, such as the equipment to perform the service was not available
8P	not otherwise specified

The measures also state that an E/M code from the CPT or a G code from the HCPCS coding system are the two types of codes permissible with these Category II codes. For example, if 99201 (new patient, office or other patient visit) was reported for a patient with a diagnosis of diabetes and whose blood pressure reading was 128/87 mm Hg. The Category II codes 3074F (<130 mm Hg) and 3078F (<80 mm Hg) would be reported with 99201 because Category II codes are supplemental codes. HCPCS codes G0270/G0271 (Medical nutrition therapy) may also be reported with the codes in the range 3074F-3080F.

The ICD-9-CM diagnosis codes that may be submitted with 3074F-3080F are also listed in the standards for the PQRI measure. For example, 250.00-250.09, Diabetes mellitus, and 648.00-648.04, Complications of pregnancy, are ranges of diagnoses codes that are acceptable for submitting with 3074F-3080F.

The Category II codes are reported in field 24D on the CMS1500 paper claim and on the electronic claim (ASC X12N 837) in segment SV1, the professional services segment.

You might wonder why physicians would agree to do all this additional tracking and coding! CMS pays a bonus to physicians who report at least 80% of encounters for each of the quality measures. The physician's submissions are tracked by the NPI (national provider identification number) because that is the unique physician identification that never changes. Even if a physician moves from one clinic to another, the NPI for that physician moves right with him or her. The bonus is paid not only on those patients that the physician submits quality measures for but on all Medicare services provided during that 12-month period. For example, if a physician receives $200,000 of Medicare revenue for the year and has reported on at least 80% of his or her encounters for the year with a maximum of three measures per patient (or less if applicable), that physician would receive a $3,000 bonus from CMS. This is a significant amount of money, especially when you consider that this is for reporting measures that the physician would usually perform anyway. The numbers get even more impressive, when applied to a group practice. For example, a clinic has 40 physicians and each generated about $200,000 annually in Medicare revenue. The PQRI bonus could mean an additional $120,000 for the practice. That is a big financial incentive to record, code, and submit the measures. Further, there is nothing a coder likes more than additional codes—it is, after all, great job security!

You can anticipate that these measures will move from voluntary to mandatory and tracking these measures will be just another element of the ever-changing world of coding.

CHECK THIS OUT ☞ For more information on PQRI, check out www.cms. hhs.gov/pqri/

Category III Codes

Category III codes report emerging technology and are temporary codes used for up to 5 years. If there is a Category III code for the service or procedure you are reporting, you must use the Category III code, not the Category I unlisted code.

Category I codes (Level 1) are those that are widely used to describe services and procedures that have been approved by the Food and Drug Administration (FDA), if appropriate. Category I codes also relate to services and procedures that have been proven to have clinical effectiveness. Category III codes describe services and procedures that may not have been approved by the FDA, may not be widely offered, and may not have been proven to be clinically effective. The use of the Category III codes allows physicians, other health care professionals, third-party payers, researchers, and health policy experts to identify emerging trends in health care.

Format of Category III Codes. The codes have five digits—four numbers and a letter: for example, 0030T (antiprothrombin). Prior to the existence of Category III codes, you would have reported this procedure using an unlisted code, because there was no specific code that described the antiprothrombin. But because there now is a Category III code available that describes it, you must report the antiprothrombin using the Category III code, not an unlisted code from Category I.

Category III codes may or may not eventually receive Category I code status and be placed in the main part of the CPT.

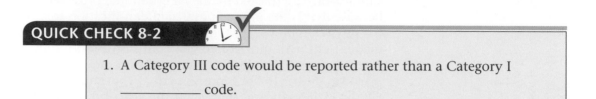

QUICK CHECK 8-2

1. A Category III code would be reported rather than a Category I _____ code.

Publication of Category III Codes. New Category III codes are released twice a year (January and July) via the AMA website. The full set of temporary codes is published in the next edition of the CPT in a section following the Medicine section.

Special Reports   Special reports must accompany claims when an unusual, new, seldom used, or Category I unlisted code, or Category III code is submitted. The special report should include an adequate definition or description of the **nature, extent,** and **need** for the procedure or service and the **time, effort,** and **equipment** necessary to provide the service. The special report helps the third-party payer determine the appropriateness of the care and the medical necessity of the service provided.

From the Trenches

What advice do you give to a coder looking to advance or move up?
"Enlarge your circle of influence, investigate other specialties, look to areas of coding compliance, attend workshops, become certified, and continue to learn."
NANCY

QUICK CHECK 8-3

1. Special reports must be submitted with claims for procedures that are unusual, new, seldom used, or use Category I _____ codes or Category _____ codes.

STARTING WITH THE INDEX

Locating the Terms

The CPT index is located at the back of the CPT manual and is arranged alphabetically. Index headings located at the top right and left corners of the index pages direct the coder to the entries that are included on that page, much like a dictionary. Use of index headings speeds location of the term (Fig. 8–18).

Code numbers are displayed in the CPT index in one of the ways shown in the following example.

Example

single code:	38115
multiple codes:	26645, 26650
range:	22305-22325

See Fig. 8–19 for an example of the display in the index using the single, multiple, and range formats.

Single Code

When only one code is stated, you should verify the code in the main (tabular) portion of the CPT manual to ensure its accuracy.

Multiple Codes

The use of a **comma** between code numbers indicates the presence of only those numbers displayed. If more than one code is listed, then all codes must be reviewed in the tabular to make an accurate choice.

Range of Codes

A range is indicated by a **hyphen.** When a range is given in the index, you must look up each code within the range in the tabular of the CPT manual to select the appropriate code from the range. There may even be multiple ranges listed.

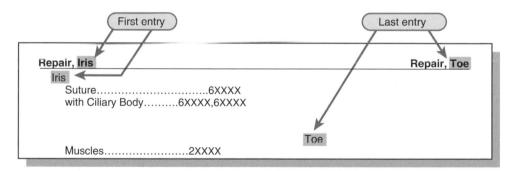

FIGURE 8–18 CPT manual index headings.

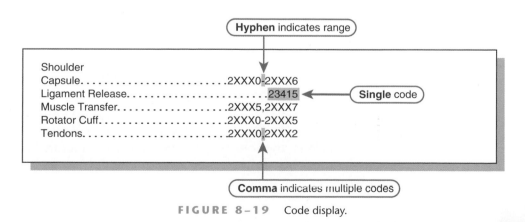

FIGURE 8–19 Code display.

CAUTION *Never code directly from the index. You can't be sure you have the right code until you have located the code in the main portion of the CPT manual and read the information presented there regarding the specifics of the code.*

The index is in alphabetic order by main terms and is further divided by subterms. Fig. 8–20 illustrates the main term and subterm as used in the index. Having identified the main term of the service or procedure, you can locate the term in the index. When you are just beginning to use the CPT manual, it may be difficult to locate the main term. Not being able to locate a term in the index can be very frustrating, but don't be discouraged if you don't identify the main term on the first try. This is a skill that is learned by practice, and part of the practice is making mistakes. Soon you'll be locating those main terms quickly. Just keep thinking about the service or procedure and looking up the words in the index.

Some basic location methods will help you to locate these main terms.

LOCATION METHODS

- Service or Procedure
- Anatomic Site
- Condition or Disease
- Synonym
- Eponym
- Abbreviation

Let's take these location methods and apply each one to locating "repair of a fracture of a femur" in the following exercise.

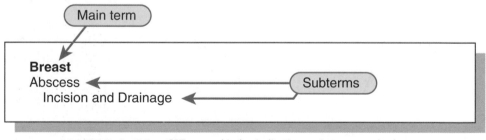

FIGURE 8–20   CPT manual index indicating main terms and subterms.

EXERCISE 8-8   *Term Practice*

SERVICE OR PROCEDURE

1 When using the service or procedure location method, "repair" would be the main term in "**repair** of a fracture of a femur."

  a Locate "Repair" in the index of the CPT manual. Using this location method, "Repair" is the main term and the subterms are "Fracture" and "Femur."

  b Under the main term "Repair," locate the subterm "Femur." If you were to look under "Repair" and then look for the term "Fracture," you wouldn't find "Fracture," because listed under "Repair" are the anatomic divisions that can be repaired. "Fracture" isn't an anatomic division, so it isn't located under "Repair." It can be just as difficult to locate the correct subterm as it is to find the main term.

Right now, don't be concerned with looking up the codes in the main part of the CPT manual. Concentrate on learning how to locate the main term and subterms in the index of the CPT manual.

ANATOMIC SITE

2 The second method of locating an anatomic site uses the word **"femur"** as the main term, and the subterms are "fracture" and "repair."

    a Locate "Femur" in the index of the CPT manual.

    b Under the main term "Femur," locate the subterm "Fracture."

    c Notice that the entry "Fracture" is further divided based on repair type (e.g., closed treatment) or anatomic location (e.g., distal).

CONDITION OR DISEASE

3 The third location method focuses on the condition or disease. In this instance you would use the main term **"fracture"** as a condition.

    a Locate the main term "Fracture" in the index.

    b Locate the subterm "Femur."

The use of the first three location methods will usually get you to the applicable codes in the index. If you try each of the first three methods and still can't locate the codes in the index, don't despair; try one of the other location methods: synonym, eponym, or abbreviation.

SYNONYM

4 The fourth location method involves synonyms. Synonyms are words with similar meanings.

    a Toe joint is a **synonym** for interphalangeal joint or metatarsophalangeal joint. Suppose, then, you couldn't think of the correct medical term, but you could think of the word "toe." In that case, you could look up "Toe" in the CPT manual index, and that entry would direct you to:

    See Interphalangeal Joint, Toe; Metatarsophalangeal Joint; Phalanx

EPONYM

5 The fifth location method uses **eponyms.** Eponyms are things that are named after people. For example, the Barr Procedure—a tendon-transfer procedure—was named after the person who developed it.

    a Locate "Barr Procedure" in the CPT manual index. You are directed to:

    See Tendon, Transfer, Leg, Lower

ABBREVIATION

6 The sixth location method uses **abbreviations.** Abbreviations are common in medicine for names of drugs, diseases, and procedures.

    a Locate the abbreviation "INH" in the index of the CPT manual. You are directed to:

    See Drug Assay

Medicine uses many synonyms, eponyms, and abbreviations. A good medical dictionary that contains the most common synonyms, eponyms, and abbreviations will be a necessity for you.

Locate each of the following main terms in the CPT manual index, and then locate the subterms and secondary subterms and fill in the code(s) you find there:

MAIN TERM	SUBTERM	SECONDARY SUBTERM	
1 Repair	Abdomen	Suture	Code: _____
2 Femur	Abscess	Incision	Code: _____
3 Fracture	Ankle	Lateral	Codes: _____

You are now ready to put your term location skills to work by doing the next exercise.

EXERCISE 8-9 *Main Term Location*

Identify the main terms in the following examples and write the main term on the line provided. Then locate the main terms and any subterms in the CPT manual index. Write the code listed in the index for that service or procedure on the line provided.

1 Description: Emergency Department Services, Physician Direction of Advanced Life Support

    a Main term: _____.

    b Locate the code available in the index of the CPT manual for Emergency Department Services, Physician Direction of Advanced Life Support.

       Code: _____

2 Condition/Disease: Intertrochanteric femoral fracture (closed treatment)

    a Main term: _____

    b Locate the code available in the index of the CPT manual for intertrochanteric femoral fracture (closed treatment).

       Code: _____

3 Procedure: Removal of gallbladder calculi

    a Main term: _____

    b Locate the code available in the index of the CPT manual for removal of gallbladder calculi.

       Code: _____

4 Anatomic site: Lung, bullae excision

    a Main term: _____

    b Locate the code available in the index of the CPT manual for excision of bullae of lung.

       Code: _____

As you can probably see from this exercise, there are often many ways to locate an item in the index. The same word can serve as a main term or a subterm, depending on the location method you are using. In addition, the annual updating of the CPT results in numerous changes within the index.

You will be locating terms in the CPT manual index throughout your study of this text. For your ready reference, there is also a guideline at the beginning of the index in the CPT manual that contains directions for the use of the CPT manual index. **Appendix B of this text will list not only the correct code answer, but also one index location for that code.** For example, if the correct answer is 99203, the following appears after the code: (Office and/or Other Outpatient Services, New Patient). It is difficult to locate items in the CPT index when you begin coding, so if you get stuck and just cannot locate the index entry, you will be able to find one location following each code in Appendix B of this text.

QUICK CHECK 8-4

1. In the CPT manual there are instructions for using the index. These instructions appear just before the index. The heading on this page is Index, Instruction for the _____ of the _____ Index.

See   "See" is a **cross-reference** term found in the index of the CPT manual. The term directs you to another term or other terms.

    "*See*" indicates that the correct code will be found elsewhere.

Example

Anticoagulant   *See* Clotting Inhibitors

EXERCISE 8-10   *See*

Complete the following:

1 Locate the term "Renal Disease Services" in the CPT index. You are directed to

_____.

2 Locate the abbreviation "ANA" in the CPT index. The entry you find is _____.

3 Locate the term "Arm" in the CPT index. You are directed to _____.

HISTORY OF NATIONAL LEVEL CODES

CPT coding is only one of a two-part coding system called HCPCS (pronounced hick-picks). The Centers for Medicare and Medicaid Services (CMS), formerly the Health Care Financing Administration, developed the Healthcare Common Procedure Coding System in 1983. The HCPCS is a collection of codes that represent procedures, supplies, products, and services that may be provided to Medicare and Medicaid beneficiaries and to individuals enrolled in private health insurance programs.

Two Levels of Codes

HCPCS is divided into two levels or groups.

    Level I codes are CPT codes in the CPT manual, which was developed and is maintained and copyrighted by the AMA. The CPT is the primary coding system used in the outpatient setting to code professional services provided to patients.

Level II codes (National Codes) are approved and maintained jointly by the Alpha-Numeric Workgroup, consisting of the CMS, the Health Insurance Association of America, and the Blue Cross and Blue Shield Association. Level II codes are five-position alphanumeric codes representing physician and nonphysician services that are not represented in the Level I codes.

There used to be **Level III** codes (Local Codes) that were developed by Medicare carriers or state payers for use at the local (carrier) level. These were five-position alphanumeric codes representing physician and nonphysician services that were not represented in the Level I or Level II codes. Local codes are no longer available since the implementation of HIPAA (Health Insurance Portability Accountability Act). Some local codes were integrated into the National Codes (HCPCS).

CPT codes do not cover all services that are provided to patients. Allied health care professionals—such as dentists, orthodontists, and various technical support services, such as ambulance services—are not specifically reportable with the CPT coding system. There are also no codes in the CPT system for many of the supplies that are used in patient care (e.g., drugs, durable medical equipment, and orthoses). Reporting of National Codes is mandatory on all Medicare and Medicaid claims submitted for payment for services of the previously listed professionals. Although many of the National Codes were developed for use when reporting for services rendered to Medicare patients, many third-party payers now require that providers use the National Codes when submitting bills for non-Medicare patients too, because the system allows for continuity and specificity. This uniformity also helps the effort to collect uniform health service data.

QUICK CHECK 8-5

1. What is the code range for Drugs? _____
2. In what publication are these codes (from Question 1) published?
   a. HCPCS
   b. CPT
   c. CMT
   d. ICD

The first digit in a national code is a letter such as, A, B, C, D, E, G, H, J, K, L, M, P, Q, R, S, T, or V—that is followed by four numbers. Codes beginning with the letters K, G, Q, and S are for temporary assignment until a definitive decision can be made about appropriate code assignment. The K codes are temporary codes for durable medical equipment, the G codes are temporary codes for procedures and professional services, and the Q codes are temporary codes for procedures, services, and supplies. S codes are temporary Blue Cross/Blue Shield codes that are not valid for Medicare or Medicaid patients. All codes and descriptions are updated annually by the CMS in November for use the following January 1. The alphanumeric listing contains headings of groups of codes, as illustrated in Fig. 8–21.

> Note: In Figs. 8–21 through 8–27, and 8–30, the HCPCS codes are samples for the purpose of illustration only. They may not be displayed as such in the current HCPCS manual.

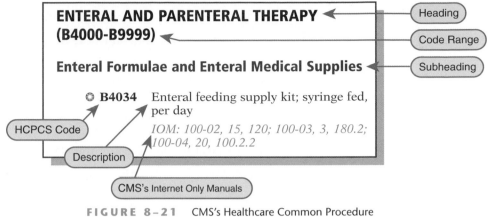

FIGURE 8–21 CMS's Healthcare Common Procedure Coding System (HCPCS), National Codes. (Modified from Buck CJ: *2010 HCPCS Level II, Professional Edition,* St. Louis, 2010, Saunders.)

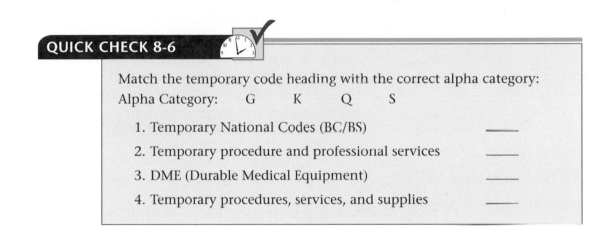

QUICK CHECK 8-6

Match the temporary code heading with the correct alpha category:

Alpha Category: G   K   Q   S

1. Temporary National Codes (BC/BS) _____

2. Temporary procedure and professional services _____

3. DME (Durable Medical Equipment) _____

4. Temporary procedures, services, and supplies _____

Note that following the heading (in Fig. 8–21) is the range of codes available for assignment in the category. There are also subheadings preceding the codes to identify the type of codes that follow.

National Codes are not used by health care facilities to report services provided to inpatients. Inpatient health care facilities use the diagnosis (from ICD-9-CM) as the basis of payment for their services and assign codes from ICD-9-CM, Volume 3, for inpatient procedures. The two levels of National Codes are used in outpatient settings (including physicians' offices) where the basis of payment is the service rendered, not the diagnosis.

General Guidelines. The HCPCS manual includes the general guidelines for use of the National Codes, a list of modifiers, the codes, a Table of Drugs, and an index. We begin our study of the HCPCS manual at the index. Publishers of HCPCS manuals have a variety of entries in their individual manuals, so expect to see variations in the number and type of index entries. You have to be able to locate items in the index in order to be able to identify the correct code. The main index terms include tests, services, supplies, orthoses, prostheses, medical equipment, drugs, therapies, and some medical and surgical procedures. The subterms of the index are listed under the main term to which they apply, along with the code.

Example

Blood glucose monitor is found under the entry:
Monitor
   blood glucose, E0607

You then locate the code in the main part of the manual and read any notes that are listed with the code.

General rules for coding using the National Codes are as follows:

1. Never code directly from the index. Always use both the alphanumeric listing and the index.

2. Analyze the statement or description provided that designates the item that requires a code.

3. Identify the main term in the index.

4. Check for relevant subterms under the main term. Verify the meaning of any unfamiliar abbreviations.

5. Note the code(s) found after the selected main term or subterm.

6. After locating the term and the code in the index, verify the code in the tabular to ensure the specificity of the code.

7. In most cases, for each entry a specific code is provided. In some cases, you are referred to a range of codes among which you can locate the required code. You must review the entire range of codes in the tabular to locate the correct entry.

   If you are referred to a single code, locate that code in the tabular. Verify the code and description to be sure that you have selected the correct code to describe the item you are reporting.

8. In all cases, when locating an entry in the index, it is necessary to look at all descriptors under the main term and subterms in order to identify the correct entry and to locate the code in the tabular.

QUICK CHECK 8-7

In the HCPCS index, locate the main term Aerosol. Identify the subterms that represent:
a. compressor E0571, E0572
b. compressor filter K0178-K0179
c. mask K0180

1. A single code   _____

2. A range of codes   _____

3. Multiple codes   _____

CODE GROUPINGS

■ A Codes	Transportation Services, including Ambulance
	Medical and Surgical Supplies
	Administrative, Miscellaneous, and Investigational
■ B Codes	Enteral and Parenteral Therapy
■ C Codes	Hospital Outpatient Prospective Payment System (OPPS)

- ▪ D Codes   Dental Procedures (published in Current Dental Terminology, CDT)
- ▪ E Codes   Durable Medical Equipment
- ▪ G Codes   Temporary (Procedures/Professional Services)
- ▪ H Codes   Alcohol and/or Drug Services
- ▪ J Codes   Drugs Administered Other Than Oral Method
- ▪ K Codes   Temporary (Durable Medical Equipment)
- ▪ L Codes   Orthotics and Prosthetics
- ▪ M Codes   Medical Services
- ▪ P Codes   Pathology and Laboratory Services
- ▪ Q Codes   Temporary (Procedures, Services, and Supplies)
- ▪ R Codes   Diagnostic Radiology Services
- ▪ S Codes   Temporary National Codes (developed by BC/BS)
- ▪ T Codes   State Medicaid Agencies
- ▪ V Codes   Vision/Hearing Services

Index.   The index is in alphabetical order and includes main terms and subterms (Fig. 8–22). The entries in the index of the National Codes may be listed under more than one main term. For example, surgical kit can be found under the two entries "Kits" and "Surgical," as illustrated in Fig. 8–23.

From the index, you turn to the code in the alphanumeric listing. The entries in the alphanumeric listing further explain what is included in the code.

The venous pressure clamps codes are shown as they appear in the alphanumeric listing in Fig. 8–24. Note that A4918 specifies "each."

There are more than 50 alphabetical modifiers available for assignment to add further specificity to the five-digit national code. For example, modifiers can be used to specify the service provider, specify the anatomic site, or add specificity (Fig. 8–25). Appendix A of the CPT contains some of the Level II, HCPCS/National modifiers.

FIGURE 8–22   HCPCS index, National Codes. (Modified from Buck CJ: *2010 HCPCS Level II Professional Edition,* St. Louis, 2010, Saunders.)

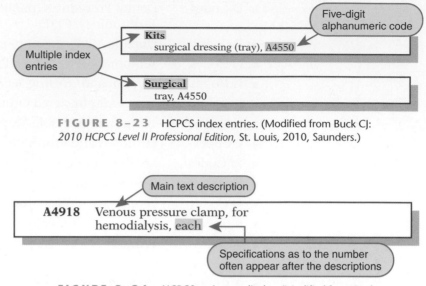

FIGURE 8–23 HCPCS index entries. (Modified from Buck CJ: *2010 HCPCS Level II Professional Edition,* St. Louis, 2010, Saunders.)

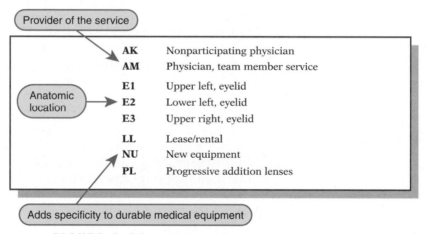

FIGURE 8–24 HCPCS main text display. (Modified from Buck CJ: *2010 HCPCS Level II Professional Edition,* St. Louis, 2010, Saunders.)

Provider of the service		
	AK	Nonparticipating physician
	AM	Physician, team member service
	E1	Upper left, eyelid
Anatomic location	**E2**	Lower left, eyelid
	E3	Upper right, eyelid
	LL	Lease/rental
	NU	New equipment
	PL	Progressive addition lenses
Adds specificity to durable medical equipment		

FIGURE 8–25 HCPCS modifiers. (Modified from Buck CJ: *2010 HCPCS Level II Professional Edition,* St. Louis, 2010, Saunders.)

> ✋ **CAUTION** *HCPCS manuals vary considerably depending on publisher.*

Table of Drugs. J codes identify the drugs administered and the amounts or dosages given. The National Codes contain a Table of Drugs (Fig. 8–26) to direct the user to the appropriate drug titles and the corresponding codes. J codes refer to drugs only by generic name. However, if a drug is known only by a brand or trade name, you will be directed to the generic name of the drug and then to the associated J code by a cross-reference system within the table. A *Physicians' Desk Reference* (PDR) is a publication that contains prescribing information on prescription drugs and lists the drugs by generic and brand names. The PDR is a valuable resource for the coder when using the Table of Drugs.

Diazepam	up to 5 mg	IM, IV	J3360
Diazoxide	up to 300 mg	IV	J1730
Dibent	up to 20 mg	IM	J0500
Dicyclocot	up to 20 mg		J0500
Dicyclomine HCl	up to 20 mg	IM	J0500
Didronel	per 300 mg	IV	J1436
Diethylstilbestrol diphosphate	250 mg	IV	J9165
Diflucan	200 mg	IV	J1450
Digibind	per vial		J1162
DigiFab	per vial		J1162
Digoxin	up to 0.5 mg	IM, IV	J1160
Digoxin immune fab (ovine)	per vial		J1162
Dihydrex	up to 50 mg	IV, IM	J1200
	50 mg	ORAL	Q0163
Dihydroergotamine mesylate	per 1 mg	IM, IV	J1110
Dilantin	per 50 mg	IM, IV	J1165

(Annotations: "Generic drug name" points to Digoxin; "Route" points to IM, IV column; "HCPCS Code" points to J1162 column)

FIGURE 8–26 Example from Table of Drugs. (Modified from Buck CJ: *2010 HCPCS Level II Professional Edition,* St. Louis, 2010, Saunders.)

The Route of Administration column (see Fig. 8–26) lists the most common methods of delivering the referenced generic drug. The official definitions for Level II J codes generally describe administration other than by the oral method. Orally given drugs are not usually provided in a physician's office but are bought at a pharmacy after the visit. Therefore, with a few exceptions, orally delivered drugs are omitted from the Route of Administration column. The following abbreviations and listings are used in the Route of Administration column:

INJ	Injection
IT	Intrathecal
IV	Intravenous
IM	Intramuscular
SC	Subcutaneous
INH	Inhalant solution
VAR	Various routes
OTH	Other routes

QUICK CHECK 8-8

1. Medication Administration Route information is provided with the Table of Drugs and Chemicals.
   True or False?

EXERCISE 8-11 *Table of Drugs*

Define the following routes of administration for drugs:

1 Intrathecal _____

_____

2 Intravenous _____

_____

3 Intramuscular _____

_____

4 Subcutaneous _____

_____

5 Inhalant solution _____

_____

Routes of Administration of Drugs. Intravenous administration includes all methods, such as gravity infusion, injections, and timed pushes. When several routes of administration are listed, the first listing is the most common method. A "VAR" posting denotes various routes of administration and is used for drugs that are commonly administered into joints, cavities, or tissues, and as topical applications. Listings posted with "OTH" alert the coder to other administration methods, for example, suppositories or catheter injections. Fig. 8–27 illustrates J code information as listed in the tabular.

J1120	Injection, acetazolamide sodium, **up to 500 mg**
	Other: Diamox, Acetazolamid Sodium
	IOM: 100-02, 15, 50
J1160	Injection, digoxin, **up to 0.5 mg**
	NDC: Digoxin, Lanoxin
	IOM: 100-02, 15, 50
J1162	Injection, digoxin immune Fab (ovine), **per vial**
	NDC: Digibind; DigiFab
	Other: Digoxin immune Fab (ovine)
	IOM: 100-02, 15, 50
J1165	Injection, phenytoin sodium, **per 50 mg**
	Other: Dilantin; Phenytoin sodium
	IOM: 100-02, 15, 50
J1170	Injection, hydromorphone, **up to 4 mg**
	NDC: Dilaudid, Hydromorphone HCl
	Other: Dilaudid-5; Dilaudid-HP, Hydromorphone Hcl/Sodium Chloride
	IOM: 100-02, 15, 50

FIGURE 8–27 HCPCS J codes. (Modified from Buck CJ: *2010 HCPCS Level II Professional Edition*, St. Louis, 2010, Saunders.)

Durable Medical Equipment. Durable medical equipment (DME) is equipment used by a patient with a chronic disabling condition, and the term also includes some equipment that is used only temporarily until the patient has healed. Claims for DME and related supplies can be paid only if the items meet the Medicare definition of covered DME and are medically necessary. The determination of medical necessity is made using documentation written by the physician. The documentation can include medical records, a plan of care, discharge plans, and prescriptions or forms explicitly designed to document medical necessity. These forms are referred to as Certificates of Medical Necessity (CMN). An example of a CMN is CMS-848 for a transcutaneous electrical nerve stimulator (Fig. 8–28) on page 243.

Claims for other items require the use of the CMN, for example, power-operated vehicles, air-fluidized beds, decubitus care pads, seat-lift mechanisms, and paraffin baths.

Physician completion of the required medical documentation ensures that the DME items furnished to a Medicare beneficiary are those specifically needed for the unique medical condition of the patient. The CMS also requires the use of form CMS-484 on page 244 for the Certification of Medical Necessity—Oxygen (Fig. 8–29).

CHECK THIS OUT ☞ The forms download website of CMS is www.cms.hhs. gov/cmsforms/

National Physician Fee Schedule. Each fall, the Centers for Medicare and Medicaid Services produces the National Physician Fee Schedule, which lists all HCPCS and CPT codes along with the amount allocated for each services and the covered/noncovered status of each service. A list of fees for drugs is produced on a quarterly basis based on the current Average Sales Price (ASP) of each drug. Fig. 8–30 illustrates a portion of the National Physician Fee Schedule.

CHECK THIS OUT ☞ The Physician Fee Schedule is on the CMS website at www.cms.hhs.gov/PhysicianFeeSched/PFSRVF/list.asp#TopOfPage

EXERCISE 8-12 *National Codes*

With information provided in this chapter, complete the following:

1 HCPCS is divided into two levels. List the names of the levels, in order, and the level numbers:

a _____

Level _____

b _____

Level _____

2 There are four groups of codes that are used by CMS for temporary assignment until a definitive decision can be made about the correct code assignment. What are the alphabetic letters of these four groups of codes? _____, _____, _____, and _____

3 Are all HCPCS modifiers numeric? _____

4 What alphabetic group of codes is used to reference drugs in the HCPCS? _____

5 The term "route of administration" generally describes the administration of drugs by methods other than _____.

6 What group of codes is used to reference durable medical equipment in the National Codes?

_____

Use Fig. 8–24 through Fig. 8–26 to answer the following questions:

7 What is the modifier for each of the following (Fig. 8–25)?

a New equipment _____

b Lower left eyelid _____

c The services of a physician who was a member of a team that provided service _____

8 What is the route of administration of dicyclomine (HCI) (Fig. 8–26)? _____

9 What is the amount of diazepam for code J3360 (Fig. 8–26)? _____

10 What is the J code for an injection of diazoxide (Fig. 8–26)? _____

11 What is the code available for a venous pressure clamp (Fig. 8–24)?_____

DEPARTMENT OF HEALTH AND HUMAN SERVICES
CENTERS FOR MEDICARE & MEDICAID SERVICES

Form Approved
OMB No. 0938-0679

CERTIFICATE OF MEDICAL NECESSITY
CMS-848 — TRANSCUTANEOUS ELECTRICAL NERVE STIMULATOR (TENS)

DME 06.03B

SECTION A   Certification Type/Date: INITIAL ___/___/___   REVISED ___/___/___   RECERTIFICATION___/___/___

PATIENT NAME, ADDRESS, TELEPHONE and HIC NUMBER

SUPPLIER NAME, ADDRESS, TELEPHONE and NSC or applicable NPI NUMBER/LEGACY NUMBER

(___ ___ ___) ___ ___ ___ - ___ ___ ___ ___ HICN _____

(___ ___ ___) ___ ___ ___ - ___ ___ ___ ___ NSC or NPI #_____

PLACE OF SERVICE_____ | HCPCS CODE | PT DOB ___/___/___ Sex ____ (M/F) Ht. ____(in) Wt ____(lbs.)

NAME and ADDRESS of FACILITY
if applicable (see reverse)

PHYSICIAN NAME, ADDRESS, TELEPHONE and applicable NPI NUMBER or UPIN

(___ ___ ___) ___ ___ ___ - ___ ___ ___ ___ UPIN or NPI #_____

SECTION B   **Information in this Section May Not Be Completed by the Supplier of the Items/Supplies.**

EST. LENGTH OF NEED (# OF MONTHS): _____ 1-99 *(99=LIFETIME)* | DIAGNOSIS CODES (ICD-9): _____ _____ _____ _____

ANSWERS	ANSWER QUESTIONS 1-6 for purchase of TENS (Circle Y for Yes, N for No,)
Y N	1. Does the patient have chronic, intractable pain?
_____ Months	2. How long has the patient had intractable pain? (Enter number of months, 1 - 99.)
1 2 3 4 5	3. Is the TENS unit being prescribed for any of the following conditions? (Circle appropriate number) 1 - Headache 2 - Visceral abdominal pain 3 - Pelvic pain 4 - Temporomandibular joint (TMJ) pain 5 - None of the above
Y N	4. Is there documentation in the medical record of multiple medications and/or other therapies that have been tried and failed?
Y N	5. Has the patient received a TENS trial of at least 30 days?
____/____/____	6. What is the date that you reevaluated the patient at the end of the trial period?

NAME OF PERSON ANSWERING SECTION B QUESTIONS, IF OTHER THAN PHYSICIAN (Please Print):
NAME: _____ TITLE: _____ EMPLOYER:_____

SECTION C   **Narrative Description of Equipment and Cost**

(1) Narrative description of all items, accessories and options ordered; (2) Supplier's charge; and (3) Medicare Fee Schedule Allowance for each item, accessory, and option. (see instructions on back)

SECTION D   **PHYSICIAN Attestation and Signature/Date**

I certify that I am the treating physician identified in Section A of this form. I have received Sections A, B and C of the Certificate of Medical Necessity (including charges for items ordered). Any statement on my letterhead attached hereto, has been reviewed and signed by me. I certify that the medical necessity information in Section B is true, accurate and complete, to the best of my knowledge, and I understand that any falsification, omission, or concealment of material fact in that section may subject me to civil or criminal liability.

PHYSICIAN'S SIGNATURE_____ DATE ____/____/____

Form CMS-848 (09/05)

FIGURE 8-28   CMS Certificate of Medical Necessity—TENS. (Courtesy U.S. Department of Health and Human Services, Public Health Service, Centers for Medicare and Medicaid Services.)

DEPARTMENT OF HEALTH AND HUMAN SERVICES
CENTERS FOR MEDICARE & MEDICAID SERVICES

Form Approved
OMB No. 0938-0534

CERTIFICATE OF MEDICAL NECESSITY
CMS-484 — OXYGEN

DME 484.03

SECTION A   Certification Type/Date: **INITIAL** ___/___/___   **REVISED** ___/___/___   **RECERTIFICATION** ___/___/___

PATIENT NAME, ADDRESS, TELEPHONE and HIC NUMBER	SUPPLIER NAME, ADDRESS, TELEPHONE and NSC or applicable NPI NUMBER/LEGACY NUMBER
(_ _ _) _ _ _ - _ _ _ _ HICN _____	(_ _ _) _ _ _ - _ _ _ _ NSC or NPI #_____

PLACE OF SERVICE_____	HCPCS CODE	PT DOB ___/___/___ Sex ____ (M/F)
NAME and ADDRESS of FACILITY *if applicable (see reverse)*	_____ _____ _____ _____	PHYSICIAN NAME, ADDRESS, TELEPHONE and applicable NPI NUMBER or UPIN (_ _ _) _ _ _ - _ _ _ _ UPIN or NPI #_____

SECTION B   **Information in This Section May Not Be Completed by the Supplier of the Items/Supplies.**

EST. LENGTH OF NEED (# OF MONTHS): _____ 1-99 *(99=LIFETIME)*   DIAGNOSIS CODES (ICD-9): _____ _____ _____ _____

ANSWERS	ANSWER QUESTIONS 1-9. (Circle Y for Yes, N for No, or D for Does Not Apply, unless otherwise noted.)
a)_____mm Hg b)_____% c)___/___/___	1. Enter the result of most recent test taken on or before the certification date listed in Section A. Enter (a) arterial blood gas PO2 and/or (b) oxygen saturation test; (c) date of test.
1 2 3	2. Was the test in Question 1 performed (1) with the patient in a chronic stable state as an outpatient, (2) within two days prior to discharge from an inpatient facility to home, or (3) under other circumstances?
1 2 3	3. Circle the one number for the condition of the test in Question 1: (1) At Rest; (2) During Exercise; (3) During Sleep
Y N D	4. If you are ordering portable oxygen, is the patient mobile within the home? If you are not ordering portable oxygen, circle D.
_____LPM	5. Enter the highest oxygen flow rate ordered for this patient in liters per minute. If less than 1 LPM, enter a "X".
a)_____mm Hg b)_____% c)___/___/___	6. If greater than 4 LPM is prescribed, enter results of most recent test taken on 4 LPM. This may be an (a) arterial blood gas PO2 and/or (b) oxygen saturation test with patient in a chronic stable state. Enter date of test (c).
	ANSWER QUESTIONS 7-9 **ONLY** IF PO2 = 56–59 OR OXYGEN SATURATION = 89 IN QUESTION 1
Y N	7. Does the patient have dependent edema due to congestive heart failure?
Y N	8. Does the patient have cor pulmonale or pulmonary hypertension documented by P pulmonale on an EKG or by an echocardiogram, gated blood pool scan or direct pulmonary artery pressure measurement?
Y N	9. Does the patient have a hematocrit greater than 56%?

NAME OF PERSON ANSWERING SECTION B QUESTIONS, IF OTHER THAN PHYSICIAN (Please Print):
NAME: _____ TITLE: _____ EMPLOYER:_____

SECTION C   **Narrative Description of Equipment and Cost**

(1) Narrative description of all items, accessories and options ordered; (2) Supplier's charge and (3) Medicare Fee Schedule Allowance for each item, accessory and option. (See instructions on back.)

SECTION D   **Physician Attestation and Signature/Date**

I certify that I am the treating physician identified in Section A of this form. I have received Sections A, B and C of the Certificate of Medical Necessity (including charges for items ordered). Any statement on my letterhead attached hereto, has been reviewed and signed by me. I certify that the medical necessity information in Section B is true, accurate and complete, to the best of my knowledge, and I understand that any falsification, omission, or concealment of material fact in that section may subject me to civil or criminal liability.

PHYSICIAN'S SIGNATURE _____ DATE ___/___/___

Form CMS-484 (09/05)

FIGURE 8–29   CMS Certificate of Medical Necessity—Oxygen. (Courtesy U.S. Department of Health and Human Services, Public Health Service, Centers for Medicare and Medicaid Services.)

HCPCS	Description	Status Code	Conversion Factor
A0021	Outside state ambulance serv	I	$36.0666
A0080	Noninterest escort in non er	I	$36.0666
A0090	Interest escort in non er	I	$36.0666
A0100	Nonemergency transport taxi	I	$36.0666
A0110	Nonemergency transport bus	I	$36.0666
A0120	Noner transport mini-bus	I	$36.0666
A0130	Noner transport wheelch van	I	$36.0666
A0140	Nonemergency transport air	I	$36.0666
A0160	Noner transport case worker	I	$36.0666
A0170	Noner transport parking fees	I	$36.0666
A0180	Noner transport lodgng recip	I	$36.0666
A0190	Noner transport meals recip	I	$36.0666
A0200	Noner transport lodgng escrt	I	$36.0666
A0210	Noner transport meals escort	I	$36.0666
A0380	Basic life support mileage	X	$36.0666
A0382	Basic support routine suppls	X	$36.0666
A0384	Bls defibrillation supplies	X	$36.0666
A0390	Advanced life support mileag	X	$36.0666
A0392	Als defibrillation supplies	X	$36.0666

FIGURE 8-30   Example of CMS's National Physician Fee Schedule Relative Value File indicates HCPCS code and description along with the conversion factor for that code for the following year. (Courtesy U.S. Department of Health and Human Services, Centers for Medicare and Medicaid Services.)

CHAPTER REVIEW

CHAPTER 8, PART I, THEORY

Do not use your CPT manual for this part of the review.

1 CPT stands for

_____ .

2 The CPT manual often reflects the technologic advances made in medicine with these codes:

_____

3 The CPT manual is ever changing and is updated annually to reflect technologic advances and

editorial _____ .

4 What type of code ends with 99?

_____

5 Coding information that pertains to an entire

section is located in the _____ .

6 These codes provide supplemental information and do not substitute for a Category I code.

_____

7 What is the name of the two-digit number or a digit and a number that is located after the CPT code number and provides more detail about the code?

_____

8 Where is a list of all the modifiers located?

_____

9 When using an unlisted or Category III code, third-party payers usually require the submission of what?

_____ , _____

10 Additions, deletions, and revisions are listed in which Appendix? _____

11 A listing of all add-on codes is located in which Appendix? _____

12 The symbol used between two code numbers to indicate that a range is available is a

_____ .

Using Fig. 8–31, identify the category, section, subheading, and subsection.

13 _____

14 _____

15 _____

16 _____

17 The symbol that indicates a product is pending FDA approval is the _____ .

18 A complete list of the codes designated with the symbol that indicates a product is pending FDA approval is listed in this appendix of the CPT manual.

_____

19 The Genetic Testing Code Modifiers are listed in this appendix of the CPT manual.

_____

FIGURE 8–31 Identify the section, subsection, subheading, and category.

CHAPTER 8, PART II, PRACTICAL

Use your CPT manual for this part of the review. Using Appendix A of the CPT manual, list the correct two-digit modifiers for the following services:

20 Repeat procedure by the same physician:

_____

21 Surgical care only: _____

22 Anesthesia by the surgeon: _____

23 Bilateral procedure: _____

Assuming there is no Category III code for the unlisted procedure you are reporting, locate the following unlisted procedure codes using the Surgery Guidelines:

24 Orbit: Code: _____

25 Rectum: Code: _____

26 Lips: Code: _____

27 General musculoskeletal:

Code: _____

Using the index of the CPT manual, locate and write on the line an example of each of the following types of code display:

28 Single code _____

29 Multiple code _____

30 Range _____

Using the index of the CPT manual, locate the following terms and write what the index note directs you to do:

31 T4 Total _____

32 SHBG _____

33 Radius _____

34 Physical Therapy _____

Using the index of the CPT manual, locate the code(s) for the following (you do not need to check the codes in the tabular for this exercise):

35 Repair, Abdomen _____

36 Bypass Graft, Excision, Abdomen

_____

37 Catheterization, Arteriovenous Shunt, Initial

_____

38 Cystotomy, with Drainage _____

39 Fracture, Femur, Intertrochanteric, Closed

Treatment _____

40 Alveoloplasty _____

41 Duodenotomy _____

Using the index of the HCPCS manual, locate the code(s) following these terms:

42 Enoxaparin sodium _____

43 Cast, hand restoration _____

44 Ice, collar _____

45 Positioning seat _____

46 Speech assessment _____

47 Whirlpool equipment _____

48 Transportation, corneal tissue _____

49 Orthotic devices, Legg-Perthes _____

50 Contraceptive, cervical cap _____

QUICK CHECK ANSWERS

QUICK CHECK 8-1
1. True

QUICK CHECK 8-2
1. unlisted

QUICK CHECK 8-3
1. unlisted, III

QUICK CHECK 8-4
1. Use, CPT

QUICK CHECK 8-5
1. J0120-J9999
2. a. HCPCS

QUICK CHECK 8-6
1. S
2. G
3. K
4. Q

QUICK CHECK 8-7
1. c
2. b
3. a

QUICK CHECK 8-8
1. True

"As you develop your skills, you can move into dozens of different areas of specialization. Pay close attention to the areas of your work where you feel most inclined to excel and explore. You're likely to be very happy there!"

Jane A. Tuttle, CPC-I, CCS-P
Coding Education Endeavors
Westford, Massachusetts

Modifiers

Chapter Topics

CPT Modifiers

Modifier -22

Modifier -23

Modifier -24

Modifier -25

Modifier -26

Modifier -32

Modifier -47

Modifier -50

Modifier -51

Modifier -52

Modifier -53

Modifier -54

Modifier -55

Modifier -56

Modifier -57

Modifier -58

Modifier -59

Modifier -62

Learning Objectives

After completing this chapter you should be able to

1 Recognize modifiers.

2 Understand the purpose of modifiers.

3 Assign Increased Procedural Services modifier -22.

4 Assign Unusual Anesthesia modifier 23.

5 Assign Unrelated E/M Services by the Same Physician During a Postoperative Period modifier -24.

6 Assign Significant Separately Identifiable E/M Service by the Same Physician on the Same Day of the Procedure or Other Service modifier -25.

7 Assign the Professional Component modifier -26.

8 Assign Mandated Services modifier -32.

9 Assign Anesthesia by Surgeon modifier -47.

10 Assign Bilateral Procedure modifier -50.

11 Assign Multiple Procedures modifier -51.

12 Assign Reduced Services modifier -52.

13 Assign Discontinued Procedure modifier -53.

14 Assign Surgical Care Only modifier -54.

15 Assign Postoperative Management Only modifier -55.

16 Assign Preoperative Management Only modifier -56.

17 Assign Decision for Surgery modifier -57.

18 Assign Staged or Related Procedure or Service by the Same Physician During the Postoperative Period modifier -58.

19 Assign Distinct Procedural Service modifier -59.

20 Assign Two Surgeons modifier -62.

Make sure to check
evolve
learning system
for the latest
content updates

Modifier -63

Modifier -66

Modifier -76

Modifier -77

Modifier -78

Modifier -79

Modifier -80

Modifier -81

Modifier -82

Modifier -90

Modifier -91

Modifier -92

Modifier -99

Chapter Review

Quick Check Answers

21 Assign Procedure Performed on Infants Less than 4 kg modifier -63.

22 Assign Surgical Team modifier -66.

23 Assign Repeat Procedure or Service by Same Physician modifier -76.

24 Assign Repeat Procedure by Another Physician modifier -77.

25 Assign Unplanned Return to the Operating/Procedure Room by the Same Physician Following Initial Procedure for a Related Procedure During the Postoperative Period modifier -78.

26 Assign Unrelated Procedure or Service by the Same Physician During the Postoperative Period modifier -79.

27 Assign Assistant Surgeon modifier -80.

28 Assign Minimum Assistant Surgeon modifier -81.

29 Assign Assistant Surgeon (When Qualified Resident Surgeon Not Available) modifier -82.

30 Assign Reference (Outside) Laboratory modifier -90.

31 Assign Repeat Clinical Diagnostic Laboratory Test modifier -91.

32 Assign Alternative Laboratory Platform Testing modifier -92.

33 Assign Multiple Modifiers modifier -99.

CPT MODIFIERS   Modifiers inform third-party payers of circumstances that may affect the way payment is made. Appendix A of the CPT manual lists the full description for all modifiers and the circumstances for their use.

Modifiers indicate the following types of information:

- Altered service

    service greater than usually required

    unusual circumstances

    part of a service

- Bilateral procedure

- Multiple procedures

- Professional part of the service/procedure only

- More than one physician/surgeon

Modifiers complete the story for insurance carriers to determine reimbursement. Consider using a modifier when the CPT code does not complete the story.

CODING SHOT   When there are multiple CPT modifiers assigned to one code, list the modifiers from highest to lowest. For example, -78-50.

The CPT modifiers are shown in Fig. 9–1.

CPT Modifiers

-22	-50	-58	-79
-23	-51	-59	-80
-24	-52	-62	-81
-25	-53	-63	-82
-26	-54	-66	-90
-32	-55	-76	-91
-47	-56	-77	-92
	-57	-78	-99

FIGURE 9–1   CPT modifiers.

-22, Increased Procedural Services

Modifier -22 indicates that the service was greater than usual and required increased physician work above and beyond normal. A special report must accompany the use of modifier -22 to explain how the service was greater. Documentation should indicate the time it usually takes to perform the service and the significant increase in that time due to documented factors. For example, if it normally takes 15 minutes to provide the service, but because of the extent and complications 90 minutes was required. Modifier -22 is reported with surgical codes. Turn to Appendix A in the CPT manual and read the description of this modifier.

The use of modifier -22 indicates that the service provided was significantly greater than the service described in the CPT code. A few additional minutes spent on a procedure does not warrant the use of this modifier. The medical record must contain documentation that substantiates that the service was unusual in some way, such as statements about the increased risk to the patient, the difficulty of the procedure, excessive blood loss, or other statements to indicate the occurrence of an unusually difficult situation. Examples include:

- Excessive blood loss.
- Extensive well-documented adhesions in abdominal surgery.
- Trauma extensive enough to complicate the procedure and the complication is not reported separately.
- Other pathologies, tumors, malformations that directly interfere with the procedure but are not reported separately.
- The service rendered was significantly more complex than described for the code description.

Modifier -22 is overused, so it comes under particularly close scrutiny by third-party payers, especially as there is usually a payment increase of 20% to 30% for services that qualify for the use of modifier -22. When reporting modifier -22, be sure that you have the documentation to support the claim. When the third-party payer receives a claim that includes a service to which modifier -22 has been added, the claim is sent to an individual who reviews the claim. Appropriate documentation must, therefore, accompany the claim—an operative report, a pathology report, office notes, hospital chart notes, and so forth.

When assigning modifier -22, additional charges are added based on the increase in physician work, and the documentation that supports the higher charge is contained in the medical record.

Avoid routine use of modifier -22, as the modifier should be reported only when a surgeon provides a service that is greater than usually required and a secondary code that would claim the additional work cannot be reported. The use of specialized technology (e.g., laparoscope or laser) does not automatically qualify for use of modifier -22. Abuse of the modifier will attract unwanted scrutiny. Repeated misuse could trigger an audit.

CMS developed the National Correct Coding Initiative (NCCI) to promote national correct coding methods and to control improper coding leading to inappropriate payment in Part B claims. CMS developed the coding policies based on the CPT manual, national and local policies, coding guidelines developed by national societies, analysis of standard medical and surgical practices, and a review of current coding practices. NCCI guidelines are only for beneficiaries of government programs, such as Medicare, but many third-party payers have adopted many of the guidelines. Within this text, reference will be made to the NCCI guidelines as follows:

NCCI

The Medicare Claims Processing Manual 100-04, Chapter 12, 20.4.6 (www.cms.hhs.gov/manuals/downloads/clm104c12.pdf) states that the fees for services represent the average work effort and practice expenses required to provide a service. For any given procedure code, there would be a typical range of work effort and practice expense required to provide a service. There is an increase or decrease in the payment for a service only under very unusual circumstances based upon review of medical records and other supporting documentation.

Modifier -22 is valid for codes with global periods of 0, 10, or 90 days. Modifier -22 is not valid for "XXX" global period indicators, which includes E/M, radiology, laboratory, pathology, and most medicine codes.

QUICK CHECK 9-1

1. According to The Medicare Claims Processing Manual 100-04, Chapter 12, 20.6, Updating Factor for Fee Schedule Services (www.cms.hhs.gov/manuals/downloads/clm104c12.pdf), "Physicians and suppliers are subject to a _____ percent reduction if their claims are processed more than _____ months after the services are rendered."

-23, Unusual Anesthesia

Modifier -23 is used by an anesthesiologist to indicate a service for which general anesthesia was used when normally the anesthesia would have been local or regional. Turn to Appendix A in the CPT manual and read the description of this modifier.

This modifier can only be assigned with codes in the Anesthesia section (00100-01999) and only by the physician providing the general anesthesia that would usually be provided by an anesthesiologist. This modifier is added to the primary procedure that would not usually require general anesthesia. For example, 62270-23 (diagnostic lumbar spinal puncture) would not usually require general anesthesia. When modifier -23 is reported, the claim must be accompanied by a written report explaining the circumstance that required general anesthesia instead of the normally used local or regional anesthesia.

QUICK CHECK 9-2

1. Which of the following may be an example of "unusual anesthesia" circumstances?
   a. Simple open wound repair on the face of a 2-year-old who is unable to sit still for the repair
   b. Pelvic exam on a developmentally challenged woman who is unable to cooperate
   c. Cast application for fracture care of a combative Alzheimer's patient
   d. All of the above

-24, Unrelated Evaluation and Management Service by the Same Physician During a Postoperative Period

Modifier -24 is used only with E/M codes. Turn to Appendix A in the CPT manual and read the description of this modifier.

Modifier -24 reports services that were performed during a postoperative period but were unrelated to recovery from the surgical procedure. Surgical procedures have a package of services, such as preoperative, procedure (intraoperative), and normal follow-up care. If an E/M service unrelated to the surgical procedure is provided to a patient during the postoperative period, the third-party payer would think that the service was part of the surgical package. Modifier -24 is added to indicate that the E/M service was not part of the surgical package (global period) but was an unrelated service. The postoperative period of a major surgical procedure is usually 90 days; a minor surgery, 10 days. Payment for the surgical procedure includes postoperative care of the patient during these periods.

You can also use modifier -24 with the General Ophthalmological Service codes 92002-92014 for eye evaluations, even though these codes are located in the Medicine section. Ophthalmologists report new and established medical examinations using 92002-92014.

CODING SHOT Modifier -24 requests payment for an unassociated E/M within a global period. The diagnosis code would indicate that the reason for the service was unrelated to the surgical procedure.

For example, a male patient is within the 10-day global period for an incision and drainage of a skin abscess. The patient presents to the physician's office for a wound check and also to ask the physician to evaluate a mole on his chest that has changed color. The postoperative visit is reported with 99024 (no charge code), and the evaluation of the mole is reported with 9921X-24 to indicate a medically necessary E/M service unrelated to the incision and drainage of the skin abscess. The diagnosis code reported with the E/M service for the mole would indicate the medical necessity of the service, such as 236.1 for a malignant hydatiform mole.

-25, Significant Separately Identifiable E/M Service by the Same Physician on the Same Day of the Procedure or Other Service

Modifier -25 is used to report an E/M service on a day when another service was provided to the patient by the same physician. Turn to Appendix A in the CPT manual and read the description of this modifier.

NCCI

> If reporting services for a Medicare patient, modifier -25 could be added to an E/M code when a decision for surgery was made on the same day as a procedure with a global surgical package of 0-10 days. Modifier -57 would be added to an E/M code when the service resulted in a decision for surgery on the day before or the day of a procedure with a global surgical package of 90 days.

To assign modifier -25 correctly, there must be a medical necessity to provide a separate, additional E/M service on the same day a procedure was performed or another service was provided. The medical necessity for this additional E/M service must be documented in the patient's medical record. If you do not add modifier -25 to the additional E/M code for service on the day of a procedure, the third-party payer would disallow the charge because it would be thought to be the evaluation/management portion of the procedure. By adding modifier -25, you are stating that the service was separate from the procedure or original service. Use of modifier -25 increases the potential of receiving payment for the service. For example, a physician provided a dialysis service to a hospital inpatient. In addition, the physician provided a separate discharge service (not related to the dialysis). You would report the dialysis service (procedure) and also report the inpatient service (discharge), adding the modifier -25 to the discharge service.

The modifier can also be assigned when additional E/M services are provided on the same day to the same patient. For example, if a patient came into the office for a visit early in the day and then later in the day returned for a separate unrelated E/M service. You report both services using E/M codes and add modifier -25 to the second E/M code. If the services were for the same related condition as seen in the earlier service, documentation for both services would be considered to assign only one E/M code for that day.

Let's review a couple other examples of the use of modifier -25. A patient presents for repair of a laceration (12042, intermediate laceration repair) and the questions asked by the physician were related only to the laceration repair. In this case, the E/M service is included in the laceration repair service and not reported separately. However, if the physician documented the patient had elevated blood pressure and a history of hypertension and the physician evaluated and treated the hypertensive condition, modifier -25 would be added to the E/M code. Diagnosis code 401.X (hypertension) would be reported as the diagnosis for the E/M service. The laceration repair would have a trauma diagnosis for open wound, and as such, the diagnosis code would support the medical necessity for the laceration repair. In this example, both the E/M service (with -25) and the laceration repair are reported with diagnoses codes that indicate the medical necessity of both services.

-26, Professional Component

Modifier -26 is used to designate a physician (professional) component of diagnostic services. Turn to Appendix A in the CPT manual and read the description of this modifier.

Modifier -26 is usually used with radiology service because radiology services often have two components—professional component and technical component. An example of the technical component is an independent radiology facility that takes the x-rays (technical component) and sends them to a private radiologist who reads the x-rays and writes a report of the findings (professional component). The physician's services would be reported with modifier -26 added to the code for the x-ray, indicating that only the professional component of the x-ray service was provided, as in the following:

A 35-year-old white female was seen in the emergency department following a fall from a horse. She complained of pain in her right clavicle and shoulder. The emergency physician ordered a complete x-ray of the clavicle and did an independent interpretation for a diagnosis of a fracture clavicle. The physician component of the x-ray would be reported with 73000-26.

EXERCISE 9-1   *Modifiers -22 through -26*

Using the CPT manual, code the following:

1 The surgeon performed a repair of an enterocele using an abdominal approach (57270) on a morbidly obese patient, and because of the patient's obesity the procedure took a significant amount of additional time to perform (50 minutes added to the normal time usually required).

   CPT Code and Modifier: _____

2 During a radical orchiectomy for an extensive primary, malignant neoplasm (54535) of the testes, the patient began to hemorrhage (a complication). After considerable time and effort, which extended the surgery by 60 minutes, the hemorrhage was controlled.

   CPT Code and Modifier: _____

   ICD-9-CM Codes: _____, _____

3 An extremely anxious and combative elderly man presented to the outpatient same-day surgery unit for a gastroscopy due to hematemesis and suspected peptic ulcer. The patient was unable to cooperate. The physician determined that, because of the patient's advanced Alzheimer's, general anesthesia during this procedure, which usually does not require anesthesia, was the best approach to use with the patient. What modifier would you report when reporting this service?

   Modifier: _____

   ICD-9-CM Codes: _____, _____, _____

4 Dr. Foster admitted a patient to a skilled nursing facility because of the patient's advanced dementia (during the global period for a herniorrhaphy that Dr. Foster performed). What modifier would be added to the admission service?

   Modifier: _____

   ICD-9-CM Code: _____

5 A patient came to the office twice in one day to see the same physician for unrelated problems. What modifier would be added to the code for the second office visit?

   Modifier: _____

6 A 60-year-old female patient is referred to a radiology laboratory by her general physician. The laboratory takes the x-rays requested and sends them on to a radiologist to interpret and to develop the written report that is sent to the general physician. If you were coding for the radiologist, what modifier would you add to indicate the service provided by the radiologist?

   Modifier: _____

-32, Mandated Services

Modifier -32 indicates a service that is required by some third-party entity. Turn to Appendix A in the CPT manual and read the description of this modifier.

This modifier is **not** used to report a second opinion requested by a patient, a family member, or another physician. Modifier -32 is reported only when a service is mandated. For example, the police require a suspected rape or abuse victim to have certain tests. These are mandated services to which modifier -32 would be added. Another common use of modifier -32 is to indicate that a third-party payer or Workers' Compensation mandated a physical examination of a covered patient. The third-party payer usually waives the deductible and copayment for the patient and usually pays 100% of these mandated services.

-47, Anesthesia by Surgeon

Modifier -47 is used to report a surgical procedure in which the surgeon administered regional or general anesthesia to the patient. Turn to Appendix A in the CPT manual and read the description of this modifier.

There are times, although they occur infrequently, when a physician acts as both the anesthesiologist and the surgeon. For example, a closed reduction of a mandibular fracture performed in the office under intravenous sedation/general anesthesia would be reported with 21451 for the procedure and 21451-47 as a separate line item for the anesthesia/sedation.

NCCI

Medicare does not reimburse the surgeon for anesthesia service when he/she is the performing surgeon.

If the third-party payer allowed payment for modifier -47, payment would be made based on the **time** spent administering the anesthetic. The surgeon acting as an anesthesiologist would report modifier -47 with the surgery code. Modifier -47 is added only to surgery codes and is never added to anesthesia codes.

-50, Bilateral Procedures

If the same procedure is performed on a mirror-image part of the body (such as two knees or two arms), modifier -50, indicating a bilateral procedure, would be reported. Turn to Appendix A in the CPT manual and read the description of this modifier.

For example, an arthroplasty (total knee replacement, 27447 and 27447-50) for both left and right knees at the same operative session would be reported using the modifier -50.

Another example in which the same services may be performed on two sides would be a bilateral breast procedure (e.g., bilateral, simple complete mastectomy, 19303 and 19303-50).

It is very important to determine how the third-party payer wants bilateral procedures submitted on the claim form, on a single line or multiple lines. One payer may require two codes to be displayed for the bilateral procedure (such as 27447 and 27447-50) for which they would reimburse 100% for the first code and 50% for the second code. Another payer may require that bilateral procedures be reported with only one code (27447-50) and would reimburse 150% based on that one code with modifier -50 representing two services. Still other payers want the service reported as 27447-RT and 27447-LT.

Medicare does not accept two line items to describe a bilateral procedure. Medicare rules direct the coder to use one line with modifier -50 and 1 unit of service. For example, submit 27447-50 rather than 27447, 27447-50.

Be sure to find out whether your third-party payer wants the surgical code to be used once with the modifier (code plus modifier -50) or used twice (code alone and code plus modifier -50) or whether the procedure should be listed twice.

CAUTION *Some CPT codes are for bilateral procedures and do not require a bilateral modifier. For example, 27395 is for bilateral lengthening of the hamstring tendon. It would be incorrect to place a bilateral modifier on 27395. Code 92020 (gonioscopy) is also a bilateral procedure and use of modifier -50 would be inappropriate.*

-51, Multiple Procedures

During any given operative session, more than one procedure may be performed. This is referred to as "multiple procedures" and is indicated by modifier -51. Turn to Appendix A in the CPT manual and read the description of this modifier.

Assign modifier -51 when multiple procedures, other than the E/M services, are performed on the same day or at the same session by the same provider. When reporting multiple surgeries, the primary procedure (the procedure with the highest relative value unit) should be listed first on the claim.

For example, a benign skin lesion is excised from a patient's chest (diameter over 4.0 cm) and closure of the defect using layered closure. The service is reported with **11406** (Excision, benign lesion including margins, except skin tag [unless listed elsewhere], trunk, arms or legs; excised diameter over 4.0 cm) and **12032-51** (Layer closure of wounds of scalp, axillae, trunk and/or extremities [excluding hands and feet]; 2.6 cm to 7.5 cm).

NCCI

After the first eligible procedure is reimbursed at 100% of Medicare's allowance, the remaining procedures are reimbursed at 50% up to five procedures. No documentation is required. After the fifth procedure, the procedures will be considered 'by report' and documentation is then required.

(Source: Bulletin of the American College of Surgeons, Volume 92, Number 5.)

You have to be careful when coding multiple procedures because CPT codes include many different procedures bundled together in one code. For example, code 58200 is a total abdominal hysterectomy, but it also includes a partial vaginectomy (removal of the vagina) with para-aortic and pelvic lymph node sampling, with or without removal of tube(s), and with or without removal of ovary(ies). It would be incorrect to report each service separately because they are included (bundled) in the description for code 58200. Listing the subsequent procedures separately (unbundling) is considered fraud by a third-party payer. Unbundling is assigning multiple codes when one code would fully describe the service or procedure. The assigning of multiple codes results in increased reimbursement.

1. What is the symbol in the CPT manual that indicates modifier -51 should not be used? _____

However, if one code does not describe all of the procedures performed, and the secondary procedure is not considered a minor procedure that is incidental to the major procedure (and therefore bundled into the major procedure), each additional procedure may be reported by using the multiple procedure modifier (-51). For example, if a patient has a laminectomy with lumbar disc removal (for a herniated disc) reported with 63030. The patient also has an arthrodesis (stabilization of the area where the disc was removed) reported with 22612. Both services would be reported, and modifier -51 would be added to the lesser of the two services.

There are three significant times when multiple procedures are reported:

1. Same Operation, Different Site
2. Multiple Operation(s), Same Operative Session
3. Procedure Performed Multiple Times

Same Operation, Different Site. Multiple procedures are reported using modifier -51 when the same procedure is performed on different sites. For example, a patient has an excision of a 1.5-cm benign lesion from the forearm and at the same time has an excision of a 3-cm benign lesion from the neck. In this case, the reporting would be 11423 for the 3-cm lesion and 11402-51 for the 1.5-cm lesion. List the most resource-intensive (expensive) procedure first, without a modifier.

Example

The payer reimburses $175.96 for 11423 and $140.54 for 11402. The difference in reimbursement is significant based on the order of the codes.

   11423, 11402-51 = $175.96 + $70.27 (50% of $140.54) payment is **$246.23**

   11402, 11423-50 = $140.54 + $87.98 (50% of $175.96) payment is **$228.52**

   The difference in reimbursement is $17.71 for submission of just these two services in an incorrect order.

Multiple Operation(s), Same Operative Session. Multiple procedures (-51) are also reported when more than one procedure is performed during the same operative session.

The primary procedure during the surgical session would be paid at the full fee, the second procedure during the same session would usually be paid at 50% of the fee, and the third procedure would usually be paid at 25% of the fee. Again, when you are coding procedures for payment, it is important that you put the most resource-intensive procedure first, without a modifier, and then list the subsequent procedures in order of complexity, remembering to use the -51 modifier for all subsequent procedures. This process of assigning the -51 modifier helps to ensure that optimal reimbursement occurs.

Procedure Performed Multiple Times.   Multiple procedures are also reported when the same procedure code identifies a service performed more than once during a single operative session. There are two ways to report procedures performed multiple times, depending on the requirements of the third-party payer. One way is to use the code number only once but to list the number of times it is performed (number of units). For example, if a patient had a repair of two flexor tendons of the leg, you would report 27658 × 2 units. Units are used because the code description states "each" tendon, and two tendons were repaired. The other way to code this would be to list 27658 once without a modifier and again with modifier -51 (i.e., 27658-51).

Third-party payers require submission of codes in various formats with various modifiers. HCPCS (Healthcare Common Procedure Coding System) modifiers indicate the right side (-RT) and left side (-LT) and the system also has modifiers that indicate the digits of the foot and hand:

-FA	Left hand, thumb	-TA	Left foot, great toe
-F1	Left hand, second digit	-T1	Left foot, second digit
-F2	Left hand, third digit	-T2	Left foot, third digit
-F3	Left hand, fourth digit	-T3	Left foot, fourth digit
-F4	Left hand, fifth digit	-T4	Left foot, fifth digit
-F5	Right hand, thumb	-T5	Right foot, great toe
-F6	Right hand, second digit	-T6	Right foot, second digit
-F7	Right hand, third digit	-T7	Right foot, third digit
-F8	Right hand, fourth digit	-T8	Right foot, fourth digit
-F9	Right hand, fifth digit	-T9	Right foot, fifth digit

NCCI

For all Medicare claims, the digit-specific modifiers must be reported.

You will find some of the more common HCPCS modifiers on the front inside cover of the Professional Edition of the CPT manual and in Appendix A of the CPT manual. HCPCS modifiers add specificity and, for that reason, are required by many payers.

CODING SHOT

HCPCS modifiers are listed in ascending alphabetic order when added to a code. For example, -AK-GT. If there are also CPT modifiers added to the code, list the CPT modifiers first (highest to lowest) followed by the HCPCS modifiers (ascending alphabetic order).

All of the variations in format can be a bit confusing when you begin coding, so let's stop here for a moment and review a few of the more common configurations that affect -50, -51, and reporting of units (times symbol).

Examples

MODIFIER -50 (BILATERAL)

The physician performs a surgical sinus endoscopy with total ethmoidectomy, 31255, on the left and right ethmoid sinuses (bilateral).

1. Using modifier -50, the service would be usually reported:
   31255 and 31255-50
2. Using the HCPCS modifiers for sides (-LT, left side, and -RT, right side), the service would be reported:
   31255-LT and 31255-RT
3. Using the one-line format, the service would be reported:
   31255-50

The most specific method of reporting is the second format, as it indicates not only the number of procedures, but also the side of the body.

MODIFIER -51 (MULTIPLE)

The physician percutaneously repairs a distal phalangeal fracture of the second and third fingers of the left hand, with skeletal fixation (26756).

1. Using modifier -51, the service would be reported:
   26756 and 26756-51
2. Using the HCPCS modifiers for fingers (-F1, left hand, second digit, and F2, left hand, third digit), the service would be reported:
   26756-F1 and 26756-F2
3. Using the times symbol, the service would be reported:
   26756 × 2

You can see that the most specific method of reporting is again the second format, as it indicates the procedure, hand, and digit.

The use of the times symbol is another area of confusion when you first begin coding.

TIMES SYMBOL (×)

The physician performs a skin biopsy on five skin lesions.

11100 (first lesion) and 11101 × 4 (second through fifth lesions)

Look for the word **"each"** in the code description as a hint to use the times symbol. The code description for 11101 states **"each** separate/additional lesion . . . ,"** with the "each" being the hint to use the times symbol.

Another example of the use of the times symbol is in pathology codes because some payers want multiple specimens reported in units. For example, the pathologist examines three tissue specimens.

88302 (first specimen) and 88302 × 2 (second and third specimens)

The number of units is placed in Block 24G (Units) on the CMS-1500 form.

CAUTION *Modifier -51 is not used with add-on codes that specify "each additional. . . . " For example, 19290 is for the placement of one wire into a breast lesion. If two wires were placed, the first wire would be reported 19290 and the second wire would be reported 19291 for the additional wire.*

CODING SHOT

As always, be aware that the payers dictate how providers are to submit for payment of services. For example, some payers may not want providers to submit modifier -51 for the same operation performed on different sites but instead, modifier -59 (Distinct Procedural Service). Usually, however, the standard is to require -51 for the three significant times when multiple procedures are provided.

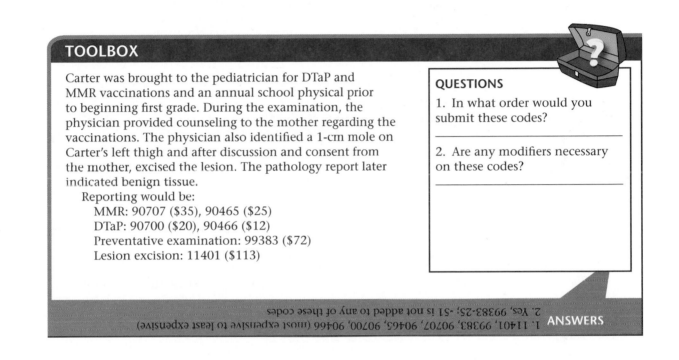

TOOLBOX

Carter was brought to the pediatrician for DTaP and MMR vaccinations and an annual school physical prior to beginning first grade. During the examination, the physician provided counseling to the mother regarding the vaccinations. The physician also identified a 1-cm mole on Carter's left thigh and after discussion and consent from the mother, excised the lesion. The pathology report later indicated benign tissue.

Reporting would be:
MMR: 90707 ($35), 90465 ($25)
DTaP: 90700 ($20), 90466 ($12)
Preventative examination: 99383 ($72)
Lesion excision: 11401 ($113)

QUESTIONS

1. In what order would you submit these codes?

2. Are any modifiers necessary on these codes?

ANSWERS 1. 11401, 99383, 90707, 90465, 90700, 90466 (most expensive to least expensive) 2. Yes, 99383-25; -51 is not added to any of these codes

-52, Reduced Services

Modifier -52 is used to indicate that a service was provided but was reduced in comparison to the full description of the service. Turn to Appendix A in the CPT manual and read the description of this modifier.

An example of a circumstance in which modifier -52 would be reported is a surgical procedure for the removal of an abdominal carcinoma in which the patient was anesthetized and the excision begun but then was terminated by the physician because the metastasis was too far advanced. When modifier -52 is reported, additional documentation, such as operative reports and/or physician explanation of the reason for the reduced service, will speed the reimbursement process, as the third-party payer usually wants to know the reason for the reduction before making payment.

CODING SHOT

Modifier -52 may or may not affect reimbursement. Some payers decrease the payment if the procedure was not completed, and others pay in full once anesthesia has been administered to the patient.

Example

A physician performed a hammer toe correction (28285) but the tendon was already split (the surgeon usually has to perform this), thereby decreasing the work necessary by the surgeon. In this case, only a portion of the usual procedure was completed. The service would be reported with 28285 with modifier -52.

Example

The operative report indicates: "Excision of ischial pressure ulcer, without ostectomy." Assign 15946 (Excision, ischial pressure ulcer, with ostectomy) with modifier -52. Modifier -52 indicates that all the procedure components were not entirely completed because the code indicated "with ostectomy" and the operative reported stated "without ostectomy."

NCCI

Do not assign modifier -52 with E/M services. Medicare does not recognize the modifier for this purpose, according to the Medicare Carriers Manual Section 15501. Instead, use unspecified E/M code 94999 and submit documentation that explains why less than the normal service was completed.

EXERCISE 9-2   *Modifiers -32 through -52*

Using the CPT manual, code the following using the two code format for codes to which you add -50 or -51:

1 Workers' Compensation referred a patient to a physician for a mandatory examination to determine the legitimacy of a claim (insurance certification). What modifier would be added to the code for the examination service?

   Modifier: _____

   ICD-9-CM Code: _____

2 Dr. Ramus administers regional anesthesia by intravenous injection (also known as Bier's local anesthesia) for a surgical procedure on the patient's lower arm. Dr. Ramus then performs the surgical procedure. What modifier would be added to the surgical code?

   Modifier: _____

3 A patient underwent bilateral carpal tunnel surgery. When you assign a code, what modifier would you be certain to use?

   Modifier: _____

   ICD-9-CM Code: _____

4 Destruction of primary, malignant lesion of neck, 4 cm in diameter (17274, $142.43), with destruction of primary, malignant lesion of arm, 4 cm in diameter (17264, $78.40).

   CPT Codes and Modifier: _____, _____

   ICD-9-CM Codes: _____, _____

5 Two bilateral supratentorial burr holes (each, 61250) for chronic, subdural hematomas.

   CPT Codes and Modifier: _____, _____

   ICD-9-CM Code: _____

6 Treatment of two tarsal bone fractures, without manipulation (each 28450).

   CPT Codes and Modifier: _____, _____

7 What is the code for a bilateral total knee replacement (arthroplasty)?

   CPT Codes and Modifier: _____, _____

8 Which modifier describes a procedure that was reduced at the direction of the physician?

   Modifier: _____

For questions 9 and 10, list the three formats that may be required by third-party payers.

9 What are the codes for bilateral arthrotomy of the elbows (24006)?

   One code listed twice with CPT modifier: _____, _____

   One code listed once with CPT modifier: _____

   One code listed twice with HCPCS modifiers: _____, _____

10 The code for a radical mastectomy is 19305. List two ways the bilateral modifier could be used to indicate that a bilateral procedure was performed, depending on the third-party payer's preferences.

   One code listed twice with CPT modifier: _____, _____

   One code listed once with CPT modifier: _____

   One code listed twice with HCPCS modifiers: _____, _____

-53, Discontinued Procedure

Modifier -52 describes circumstances in which services were reduced at the direction of the physician, whereas modifier -53 describes circumstances in which a procedure was stopped because of the patient's status. Turn to Appendix A in the CPT manual and read the description of this modifier.

An example of the correct assignment of modifier -53 would be when a patient had received anesthesia and the procedure was underway. The patient then developed arrhythmia that could not be controlled. The physician discontinued the procedure because of the risk continuation presented to the patient. The code for the surgical procedure would be reported along with modifier -53 to indicate that although the procedure was begun, it was discontinued due to the patient's status. The key to proper reporting of modifier -53 is that the patient has been prepared for surgery, anesthetized, and the surgeon discontinued the procedure.

Modifier -53 is **not** used to report services:

■ When the patient cancels the procedure

■ With E/M codes

■ With any code that is based on time (e.g., critical care codes)

Attach a cover note and state the percentage of the procedure that was completed and why the procedure had to be stopped. For example, "Only 50% of procedure was completed. The procedure was stopped because patient developed arrhythmia that could not be controlled."

NCCI

Modifier -53 should be used to report a failed or terminated colonoscopy. When a colonoscopy is attempted, but not completed, it should not be reported as a sigmoidoscopy but as discontinued colonoscopy procedure 45378-53.

Modifiers -54, -55, and -56

There may be times when a surgeon performs only the surgery (modifier -54) and requests another physician to perform the preoperative evaluation (modifier -56) and/or the postoperative care (modifier -55). When reporting his or her own individual services, each physician would use the same procedure code for the surgery, letting the modifier indicate to the third-party payer the part of the surgical package that each personally performed.

Example

19303	Mastectomy, simple, complete
19303-54	Mastectomy, simple, complete, **surgery** (intraoperative) only
19303-56	Mastectomy, simple, complete, **preoperative** evaluation only
19303-55	Mastectomy, simple, complete, **postoperative** care only

---

-54, Surgical Care Only

Modifier -54 indicates the surgical care portion of a surgical procedure (intraoperative). Use modifier -54 only with codes from the Surgery section (10021-69990). Turn to Appendix A in the CPT manual and read the description of this modifier.

Modifier -54 is used correctly only when there has been a **transfer** of responsibility for care from one physician to another. This transfer takes place by means of a transfer order that is signed by both physicians and kept in the patient's medical record. Modifier -54 is not used for minor surgical procedures but for major procedures that involve follow-up care as a part of the service of the surgery (surgery package). Although third-party payers vary, the payment for only the surgical procedure is usually about 70% of the total payment for the procedure, with 10% for the physician who provides the preoperative service, and 20% for the physician who provides the postoperative care.

CODING SHOT Modifier -54 usually results in reimbursement to the surgeon for the intraoperative percentage of the global package payment. However, some payers also include the preoperative service as a part of the intraoperative care portion. In these cases, you will submit a statement to indicate the preoperative service was provided by another physician.

-55, Postoperative Management Only

Another part of a surgical package is the postoperative care. The amount of postoperative care that is considered part of a surgery varies according to the complexity of the surgery, with 0, 10, or 90 days being the most commonly used number of postoperative days. Turn to Appendix A in the CPT manual and read the description of this modifier.

Modifier -55 is used only for services provided to the patient after discharge from the hospital. To report services by another physician provided while the patient is still in the hospital, you would use E/M codes (99231-99233, subsequent hospital care) because the payment to the operating physician (70%) assumes that the operating physician provides the care until the patient is discharged from the hospital.

You report the postoperative services by adding modifier -55 to the surgical code. For example, a patient had a nephrolithotomy (calculus removed from kidney), reported with 50060, and then the operating physician transferred to a second physician the postoperative care after the patient's discharge from the hospital. The operating physician would report services using 50060-54, and the physician providing the postoperative care would report 50060-55, with the date of the surgery. The claim is not submitted until after the first postoperative office visit. The physicians use the same surgery code (50060). In this way, the third-party payer knows that the two physicians are splitting the care of the patient into surgical care and postoperative care after discharge.

Modifier -55 should result in reimbursement of the postoperative percentage for the global package. This percentage is based on how many days had passed after the operation before the care was transferred from the first physician to the second physician. Care must be officially transferred from the physician providing the surgical care to the physician providing the postoperative care by way of a transfer order that is kept in the medical record.

When different physicians in a group practice participate in the care of a patient, the group reports the entire global package (no modifier). The physician who performs the surgery is indicated on the claim as the performing physician.

-56, Preoperative Management Only

The third part of a surgical service is the preoperative care. If a physician provides only the preoperative management to a patient in preparation for surgery, the service is reported with modifier -56 added to the surgical code. Turn to Appendix A in the CPT manual and read the description of this modifier.

Before a patient undergoes surgery, a physical examination is performed to determine whether the patient is physically able to withstand the procedure. This examination is the preoperative workup or preop. When one physician performs the preoperative workup and another physician performs the surgery, both physicians report the services using the surgical procedure code with the correct modifier. For example, in preparation for a nephrolithotomy, the patient's local physician performs the preoperative care (50060-56), an itinerate (visiting) surgeon performs the surgery (50060-54), and the local physician performs the postoperative care (50060-55).

NCCI
Modifier -56 is never used for services reported to Medicare, as Medicare considers the preoperative service to be part of the surgery and bundles the payment into the surgical payment.

-57, Decision for Surgery

Modifier -57 is reported with an E/M code to indicate the day the decision to perform a major surgery was made. Turn to Appendix A in the CPT manual and read the description of this modifier.

Modifier -57 can be reported not only with E/M codes (99201-99499) to indicate the initial decision to perform a procedure or service but also with the ophthalmologic codes (92002-92014) located in the Medicine section. Modifier -57 requests payment for an E/M service outside of the global package for a major procedure when the decision to perform the surgery was made during the E/M service.

At the present time, not all modifiers are recognized by all third-party payers. Some third-party payers have agreed to pay a physician separately from the surgical package for the initial evaluation of a condition during which the decision to perform surgery was made. Modifier -57 is used to let the payer know that payment for this initial evaluation should be made in addition to payment for surgery.

E/M services provided the **day before** or the **day of** a major surgery are included in the global package. There are some exceptions, such as when the service is the patient's initial visit to the physician. To receive payment for these initial visits, modifier -57 is reported to indicate the day before or the day of the **major** procedure and modifier -25 is used to indicate the day of the **minor** procedure.

CAUTION *Don't make the all too common mistake of adding -57 to codes from the Surgery section. Modifier -57 is never added to surgical codes; rather, it is added only to E/M codes.*

CODING SHOT
Note that the description of modifier -57 does not indicate whether the decided-upon procedure is diagnostic or therapeutic, minor or major. These guidelines are established by the third-party payers.

NCCI
Medicare Carriers Manual Section 15501C states that the carrier is only to pay for an E/M service on the day of or on the day before a procedure with a 90-day global surgical period.

-58, Staged or Related Procedure or Service by the Same Physician During the Postoperative Period

Modifier -58 notifies the payer that a subsequent surgery was planned or staged at the time of the first surgery. Turn to Appendix A in the CPT manual and read the description of this modifier.

The procedure must have been intended to include the original procedure plus one or more subsequent procedures. For example, multiple skin grafts are often done in stages to allow adequate healing time between procedures. The modifier is added to the subsequent submissions of the code when the second or related service is performed during the global period to inform the third-party payer that the service was staged. Modifier -58 can also be used if a therapeutic procedure is performed because of the findings of a diagnostic procedure. For example, a patient may have a surgical breast biopsy, and if the pathology report indicates that the specimen is malignant, the patient may elect to have an immediate radical mastectomy. The mastectomy may be performed during the postoperative period of the biopsy. Modifier -58 indicates to the third-party payer that the second surgery was therapeutic treatment that followed the original diagnostic procedure, and full payment would usually be made for the mastectomy. A new postoperative period would start after the mastectomy, and any postoperative care provided to the patient would be part of the surgical package for the mastectomy.

CAUTION *There are some codes that include multiple sessions in the code description. For example, 67141 and 67145 include the "1 or more sessions" in the code description. Modifier -58 is not appropriate with these multiple session codes.*

CODING SHOT Modifier -58 requests full payment for a subsequent procedure that may have been planned in follow-up, at the time of the first surgery, or performed as a more extensive procedure subsequent to the first surgery. A new global period begins with each subsequent procedure modified with -58.

Example

A lesion was excised and determined to be malignant. The patient was returned to the operating room a few days later for a re-excision of the malignancy. Report the re-excision with modifier -58 because the second procedure was performed within the global period of the first procedure and related to the first procedure.

Example

A patient required a toe amputation due to gangrene. On follow-up, the surgeon determined the patient requires further amputation, this time of his entire foot because the original procedure did not completely remove the gangrenous tissue. If the second amputation occurs within the postoperative period of the first amputation, the second amputation would be reported with modifier -58 as it is related to the first procedure.

-59, Distinct Procedural Service

Modifier -59 is reported to indicate that services that are usually bundled into one payment were provided as separate services. Turn to Appendix A in the CPT manual and read the description of this modifier.

As the code description notes, modifier -59 is used to identify the following:

- Different session
- Different procedure or surgery
- Different site or organ system
- Separate incision/excision
- Separate lesion
- Separate injury or area of injury in extensive injuries

Modifier -59 is reported with codes from all sections of the CPT manual except E/M codes.

NCCI

Medicare has lists of codes that cannot be reported together and they are termed **edits**. These edits have been established to ensure that providers do not report services that are included in a pre-established bundle. For example, the same physician would not report a standard preoperative visit related to a major surgical procedure and then report separately the surgery and follow-up care. All three services—preoperative, intraoperative, postoperative—are bundled together in one major surgical CPT code. The use of modifier -59 indicates that the service was not a part of another service but, indeed, was a distinct service. For example, a colonoscopy utilizing a snare (45385) and a colonoscopy with hot biopsy forceps (45384) would usually not be reported together because both codes would be in the edits, but if -59 was appended to 45384, the surgeon would be indicating that distinct services were provided.

CODING SHOT

Modifier -59 requests payment for a procedure performed on the same day as another procedure that normally would not be reimbursed separately, e.g., a biopsy of one site and an excision of another site.

A note of caution is that modifier -59 has been abused by providers and excessively submitted. The Office of the Inspector General has targeted the submission of this modifier for the years 2004 and 2005. That means random audits of physician claim submission will be conducted.

EXERCISE 9-3 *Modifiers -53 through -59*

Using the CPT manual, code the following:

1 Mrs. Knight has a diagnostic surgical biopsy of deep cervical lymph nodes on May 8, and the pathology report comes back showing primary malignancy. Mrs. Knight elects to have a lymphadenectomy on May 11. What modifier would be used with the lymphadenectomy code?

    Modifier: _____

    ICD-9-CM Code: _____

2 The intraoperative service for a total esophagectomy without reconstruction (43124)

    CPT Code and Modifier: _____

3 The postoperative care only for a radical mastectomy including pectoral muscles, axillary, and internal mammary lymph nodes (19306)

    CPT Code and Modifier: _____

4 The procedure in question 3 when only the preoperative service is provided

    CPT Code and Modifier: _____

-62, Two Surgeons Modifier -62 indicates two surgeons acted as co-surgeons. Turn to Appendix A in the CPT manual and read the description of this modifier.

From the Trenches

"Learning to use the CPT manual effectively as a tool is one of the best skills I can teach my students to develop . . . . I always advise them to start with a strong foundation by taking classes in medical terminology, anatomy, and physiology."

JANE

To assign modifier -62 correctly, two physicians of different specialties must have worked together as co-surgeons and each surgeon must have dictated his/her own operative report. If one physician assists another physician, the service cannot be reported using modifier -62. Co-surgeons use different skills during the surgery. Many third-party payers require documentation showing the medical necessity of co-surgeons. The operative reports document each surgeon's participation and clearly show the distinct services each performed. Modifier -62 is correctly reported when two physicians are necessary to complete one surgical procedure, each completing a distinct portion of the procedure. For example, a cardiologist and a general surgeon may install a pacemaker, with the general surgeon preparing the implantation site, the cardiologist inserting and activating the pacemaker, and the general surgeon closing the site. Each physician would report his/her service using the pacemaker insertion code with modifier -62.

CODING SHOT — Modifier -62 will usually cue the payer to reimburse at 125% of the fee schedule, which is then divided, half for each surgeon.

Example

A patient diagnosed with bladder cancer undergoes a radical cystectomy and ilia conduit (passage from the kidney to the exterior). A general surgeon opens the surgical area to view, then a urologist removes the bladder. The general surgeon creates an ilia conduit and both surgeons close the incisions. Each physician reports 51575 (removal of bladder and nodes) with modifier -62. The surgeons would be paid a combined 125% of the fee schedule amount for the code (62.5% each).

-63, Procedure Performed on Infants Less than 4 kg

Modifier -63 is used to identify procedures provided to a neonate or infant up to 4 kg (8.8 lbs). Turn to Appendix A in the CPT manual and read the description of this modifier.

Do not use modifier -63 with the Integumentary System codes (10040-19499). Parenthetical notes also follow some codes in the 20000-69990 range and direct the coder not to report -63 with certain codes.

Procedures on neonates or infants with a body weight of less than 4 kg (8.8 lbs) are more complex than procedures that are performed on neonates or infants with a body weight of more than 4 kg.

QUICK CHECK 9-4

1. Would modifier -63 be reported with codes 49491-49496? Why or why not? _____

-66, Surgical Team

Modifier -66 is used with very complex surgical procedures that require several physicians, usually of different specialty, to complete the procedure. Turn to Appendix A in the CPT manual and read the description of this modifier.

A surgical team consists of physicians (more than two), technicians, and other trained personnel who function together to complete a complex procedure. For example, teams are usually used in organ transplant surgeries, with each member of the team completing the same function at each surgery. Each physician on the team reports the procedure code with modifier -66. Third-party payers will often increase the total reimbursement for a team. The reimbursement is divided among the physicians on the basis of a prearranged agreement.

CODING SHOT — Modifier -66 will cue the payer that payment for a procedure should be increased by whatever the contract allows to be divided by all surgeons involved.

Example

A patient is admitted for an artificial heart transplant (33935, heart-lung transplant with recipient cardiectomy-pneumonectomy). A team of cardiologists, general surgeons, and thoracic surgeons performs the surgery and each dictates a description of the procedure. Each surgeon would report 33935 with modifier -66. Each surgeon not only dictates his or her portion of the surgery but also submits his or her own claim.

-76, Repeat Procedure or Service by Same Physician

Modifier -76 is assigned to report services or procedures that are being repeated by the same physician. Turn to Appendix A in the CPT manual and read the description of this modifier.

The modifier is reported to indicate to third-party payers that the services are not duplicate services and the bill is not a duplicate bill. Sometimes these repeat services are provided on the same day as the previous service, and without the use of modifier -76, the third-party payer would assume a duplicate bill had been submitted. When modifier -76 has been submitted, documentation to establish medical necessity must accompany the claim.

CODING SHOT Modifier -76 requests payment for a service that was repeated. If the modifier was not used, the subsequent service would be denied as a duplicate service.

-77, Repeat Procedure by Another Physician

Modifier -77 reports services or procedures that are repeated and are provided by a physician other than the physician who originally provided the service or procedure. Turn to Appendix A in the CPT manual and read the description of this modifier.

Modifier -77 reports to the third-party payer that the services are not duplicate services and, therefore, the bill is not a duplicate bill. Sometimes these repeat services are provided on the same day as the original service or during the postoperative period. Without the use of modifier -77, the third-party payer would assume a duplicate bill had been submitted. When modifier -77 has been assigned, documentation must accompany the claim in order to establish the medical necessity for the procedure.

CODING SHOT Modifier -77 requests payment for a service that was repeated. If the modifier was not used, the subsequent service would be denied as a duplicate service.

If only a portion of the original service or procedure is repeated, you would also assign modifier -52 to indicate a reduced service.

CAUTION *CMS stated that the increased use of both -76 and -77 indicates possible inappropriate assignment with E/M services and closer monitoring will be given to the submission of these two modifiers.*

-78, Unplanned Return to the Operating/ Procedure Room by the Same Physician Following Initial Procedure for a Related Procedure During the Postoperative Period

Modifier -78 is assigned to indicate a circumstance in which a patient is returned to the operating room for surgical treatment of a complication that resulted from the first procedure. Turn to Appendix A in the CPT manual and read the description of this modifier.

Modifier -78 is appended to the subsequent procedure code to indicate to the third-party payer that the second surgery was necessary because of complications resulting from the first operation. For many third-party payers, only the surgery portion (intraoperative) of the surgical package is paid when the -78 modifier is reported. The patient remains within the postoperative period of the first operation for any further preoperative or postoperative care. For example, if the patient were to develop a second set of complications stemming from the original surgery, you would again report the procedure performed to treat the second complication and add modifier -78 to the code. In this way, the third-party payer continues to know that the complication requiring surgery originated from the original surgery.

✋ **CAUTION** *If there were a complication, you would report -78 (Unplanned Return to the Operating/Procedure Room) and -76 (Repeat Procedure or Service by Same Physician). For example, a patient who has an open heart coronary artery bypass graft procedure (Service 1) returns to the operating room for tamponade (fluid accumulation in the pericardium) twice on the same day (Services 2 and 3).*

Service 1	
33510	Coronary artery bypass graft
Service 2	
35820-78	Exploration for postoperative hemorrhage, chest
Service 3	
35820-78-76	Repeat exploration for postoperative hemorrhage, chest

Services 2 and 3 procedures should be reimbursed at the intraoperative rate but the global period would continue from the first session and would not start over again.

CODING SHOT 🖊 Modifier -78 will cue the payer to reimburse the procedure at the intraoperative percent of the service. The patient remains in the global period for the initial surgery.

An "operating/procedure" room is defined as a place of service specifically equipped and staffed for the sole purpose of performing procedures. For example a cardiac catheterization suite, a laser suite, and an endoscopy suite. It does not include a patient's room, a minor treatment room, a recovery room, or intensive care unit (unless the patient's condition was so critical there was insufficient time for transport to an operating room).

-79, Unrelated Procedure or Service by the Same Physician During the Postoperative Period

Modifier -79 explains that a patient requires surgery for a condition totally unrelated to the condition for which the first operation was performed. Turn to Appendix A in the CPT manual and read the description of this modifier.

For example, the patient had an appendectomy and 2 weeks later had a gallbladder episode that necessitates removal of the gallbladder. Modifier -79 would be placed on the cholecystectomy code, indicating that the subsequent procedure was unrelated to the first procedure. The diagnosis codes for the two procedures would also be different, further indicating the two procedures were unrelated.

🖐 **CAUTION** *Do not use modifier -79 with staged procedures (use modifier -58) or with procedures that are related to the original procedure. If the service is provided during the postoperative period of a major surgical procedure, billing separately for services included in the surgical package is fraudulent.*

 CODING SHOT Modifier -79 requests payment for the full fee of the subsequent service because it was unassociated with the first procedure. A new global period should start when -79 is submitted.

-80, Assistant Surgeon

A surgical assistant is one who provides service (an extra pair of hands) to the primary surgeon during a surgical procedure. Turn to Appendix A in the CPT manual and read the description of this modifier.

The assistant surgeon's services are reported using the same code as the primary surgeon's, but modifier -80 is added to alert the third-party payer to the assistant surgeon's status. Usually, the assistant receives only 15% to 30% of the usual charge for a surgery when acting in the assistant capacity. Not all payers allow for a surgical assistant on all procedures. A preauthorization for surgery should be completed before surgery to determine if the payer will reimbursement for a surgical assistant.

 CODING SHOT Preauthorization does not guarantee payment, as the payer can always deny the approval upon review.

🖐 **CAUTION** *A physician assistant providing assist at surgery would use the HCPCS modifier -AS, not modifier -80.*

-81, Minimum Assistant Surgeon

Modifier -81 indicates an assistant surgeon who provides services that are less extensive than those described by modifier -80. Turn to Appendix A in the CPT manual and read the description of this modifier.

Modifier -81 is not commonly used, although there are times when an assistant surgeon is present and assists for only a portion of the procedure. This minimal assistant surgeon service is then reported by adding -81 to the surgical code. Some third-party payers define a minimal assistant surgeon as a nurse practitioner, physician's assistant, or other specialized clinical nursing personnel, but according to the CPT definition, the service is provided by a physician acting in a minimal capacity. You should receive written directives from the third-party payer before reporting -81 for individuals other than a physician.

Many third-party payers do not pay for a minimum assistant surgeon. For example, Medicare will pay for a minimum assistant only on rare occasions in which medical necessity can be proven. Usually, the minimum assistant surgeon receives 10% of the usual charge for a surgery.

-82, Assistant Surgeon (When Qualified Resident Surgeon Not Available)

Modifier -82 is assigned when the hospital in which the procedure was performed has an affiliation with a medical school and has a residency program, but no resident was available to serve as an assistant surgeon. Residents are medical students who are completing a required surgical training period in the hospital during which the residents serve as employees of the hospital who are there to receive training and provide assistance to physicians as part of the hospital's agreement with the medical school. Hospitals that have affiliations with medical schools are considered teaching facilities. Turn to Appendix A in the CPT manual and read the description of this modifier.

Do not confuse modifier -80 (assistant surgeon) with -82 when reporting services.

CODING SHOT Medicare does not pay for an assistant surgeon if the hospital has a residency program.

Modifier -82 has very limited use and requires supporting documentation that the patient's condition was such that the service required an assistant and that a qualified resident was not available.

EXERCISE 9-4 *Modifiers -62 through -82*

Using the CPT manual, indicate the correct modifier:

1 Dr. Edwards, a cardiologist, and Dr. Mathews, a general surgeon, worked together as primary surgeons on a complex surgical case. What modifier would be added to the CPT surgery codes for

   the services of both Dr. Edwards and Dr. Mathews? _____

2 A team of physicians with different specialties, along with a highly skilled team of technical personnel, performed a liver transplant for a patient with chronic viral hepatitis C that has resulted in cirrhosis of the liver. Using which modifier would indicate the surgical team concept?

   Modifier: _____

   ICD-9-CM Codes: _____, _____

3 Dr. Stenopolis served as a surgical assistant to Dr. Edwards in a quadruple bypass procedure. Dr. Stenopolis' services were reported by using this modifier:

   Modifier: _____

4 In the middle of the bypass procedure in Question 3, the patient experienced severe complications. Dr. Edwards asked Dr. Loren to come into the operating room to temporarily assist in stabilizing the patient. What modifier would be used when reporting the service Dr. Loren provided?

   Modifier: _____

5 A patient has a hernia repair and two days later must be returned to the operating room for a related repair. When coding the secondary hernia repair, which modifier would you add onto the surgical code?

   Modifier: _____

6 If Mr. Smith undergoes an appendectomy on June 8, and then a cholecystectomy is performed on August 16 by the same surgeon, what modifier would be placed on the cholecystectomy code?

   Modifier: _____

7 What modifier would you add to a code to indicate that a basic procedure performed by another physician was repeated?

   Modifier: _____

-90, Reference (Outside) Laboratory

Modifier -90 is used to indicate that services of an outside laboratory were used. Turn to Appendix A in the CPT manual and read the description of this modifier.

This modifier is reported with Pathology and Laboratory codes to report that the procedures were performed by someone other than the treating or reporting physician.

NCCI

Medicare does not allow physicians to bill for outside laboratory services and then reimburse the outside laboratory for those services. If the outside laboratory provides the services, the outside laboratory must report the services.

-91, Repeat Clinical Diagnostic Laboratory Test

Modifier -91 reports a laboratory test that was performed on the same day as the original laboratory test. Turn to Appendix A in the CPT manual and read the description of this modifier.

This modifier is correctly assigned when a laboratory test has been repeated so as to produce multiple test results. It cannot be assigned if the lab equipment malfunctioned or if there was a problem with the specimen, because this would result in third-party payers' paying for laboratory errors. Also, do not assign the modifier for services performed because a subsequent test was done to confirm the results of the initial test. The modifier also cannot be assigned when there is a series of test results, such as those performed in allergy testing.

-92 Alternative Laboratory Platform Testing

Modifier -92 reports those incidents when a kit or transportable instrument is used in a laboratory test. For example, a single-use, disposable HIV kit (86701-86703). Turn to Appendix A in the CPT manual and read the description of this modifier.

-99 Multiple Modifiers

Modifier -99 is needed only if the third-party payer does not accept multiple modifiers. This is the case with some computerized insurance submissions. Turn to Appendix A in the CPT manual and read the description of this modifier.

On the CMS-1500 (08/05) there is space for multiple modifiers (Fig. 9–2). Third-party payers vary in terms of how they require multiple modifiers to be reported, so be certain to check with the payer before submitting multiple modifiers.

EXERCISE 9-5 *Modifiers -90 through -99*

Using the CPT manual, code the following:

1 What is the modifier that indicates that multiple modifiers apply? _____

2 What modifier would be added to the laboratory procedure code to indicate testing by an outside laboratory? _____

3 The medical record indicated that the physician had an established patient go to the lab for a blood panel in the morning, and in the afternoon had the patient return to the lab for another blood panel so as to produce multiple test results. What modifier would you add to the code for the panel? _____

---

24. A.	DATE(S) OF SERVICE						B.	C.	D. PROCEDURES, SERVICES, OR SUPPLIES		E.
	From			To			PLACE OF		(Explain Unusual Circumstances)		DIAGNOSIS
	MM	DD	YY	MM	DD	YY	SERVICE	EMG	CPT/HCPCS	MODIFIER	POINTER
1									19306		

FIGURE 9–2   Multiple modifiers on CMS-1500 (08/05).

CHAPTER REVIEW

CHAPTER 9, PART I, THEORY

Complete the following:

1 When more than two physicians, with technicians and specialized equipment, work together to complete a complicated procedure and each physician has a specific portion of the surgery to complete, they are termed what?

_____

2 Can modifier -22 be assigned to 99291, 99292 codes?

Yes   No

3 This modifier indicates an increased service and is overused and results in an increase in payment of 20% to 30%. As such, the assignment of this modifier comes under particularly close scrutiny by third-party payers. What is this modifier?

_____

4 When modifier -54 is assigned, payment for

the _____ portion of the surgical procedure is being requested.

5 Joan is a new coder at the local clinic. You have been assigned to review her coding before it is submitted to the third-party payer. You note that she assigned modifier -32 to E/M consultation code 99244. The medical record indicates that the request for the second opinion was made by the patient's spouse. Is Joan correct in modifier -32 assignment? Why or why not?

_____

_____

_____

6 Which of these statements is true about modifier -59?

   a. it is only appended to E/M codes
   b. it is only appended to other than E/M codes

7 What is the weight in pounds of a 4-kilogram infant?

   a. 7.9
   b. 8.8
   c. 8.9
   d. 9.1

8 Which of the following statements is NOT true about modifier -53?

   a. describes circumstances based on the patient's condition
   b. may be used to describe those times when the physician elects to terminate a procedure due to the well-being of the patient
   c. describes circumstances in which the patient cancelled the procedure
   d. may be used to describe ASC reporting of previously scheduled procedure that is partially reduced as a result of extenuating circumstances

9 Modifier -57 can be added to Surgery section codes?

True   False

10 When adding multiple CPT modifiers to a code, you would list the modifiers from:

   a. highest to lowest
   b. lowest to highest
   c. makes no difference which is listed first

CHAPTER 9, PART II, PRACTICAL

Using your CPT manual, identify the modifier for the following descriptions:

11 Repeat procedure or service by same physician _____

12 Two surgeons _____

13 Professional component _____

14 Multiple modifiers _____

15 Distinct procedural service _____

16 Mandated service _____

17 Significant identifiable E/M service provided by the same physician on the same day as another service or procedure _____

18 Minimum assistant surgeon _____

19 Repeat procedure by another physician _____

20 Unrelated procedure or service by the same physician during the postoperative period _____

21 Unusual anesthesia _____

22 Unplanned return to the operating room for a related procedure during the postoperative period _____

23 Surgical care only _____

24 Reduced service _____

25 Surgical team _____

QUICK CHECK ANSWERS

QUICK CHECK 9-1
1. 10, 12

QUICK CHECK 9-2
1. d. All of the above

QUICK CHECK 9-3
1. ⊘ Symbol preceding a code indicates it is modifier -51 exempt.

QUICK CHECK 9-4
1. No. Parenthetical notes following codes indicate modifier -63 is not reported with these codes.

"I think having a goal of being a lifelong learner is important. One also has to have a great degree of integrity. It takes knowledge and character to adhere to the correct way to do things, and not be swayed by other factors, such as how to 'get it paid.'"

Joan E. Wolfgang, BA, CPC, CPC-H, CPC-I
Coding QI & Provider Education Director
Lakeshore Medical Clinics
South Milwaukee, Wisconsin

Evaluation and Management (E/M) Services

Chapter Topics

Contents of the E/M Section

Three Factors of E/M Codes

Various Levels of E/M Service

An E/M Code Example

Using the E/M Codes

Documentation Guidelines

Chapter Review

Quick Check Answers

Learning Objectives

After completing this chapter you should be able to

1 Identify and explain the three factors of E/M code assignment.

2 Differentiate between a new and an established patient.

3 Differentiate between an inpatient and an outpatient.

4 Explain the levels of E/M service.

5 Review the key components.

6 Analyze the key component history.

7 Analyze the key component examination.

8 Analyze the key component medical decision making.

9 List contributory factors.

10 Analyze code information.

11 Analyze the types of E/M codes.

12 Identify CMS Documentation Guidelines.

13 Demonstrate the ability to code E/M services.

Make sure to check
evolve
learning system
**for the latest
content updates**

CONTENTS OF THE E/M SECTION

The information in Chapter 8 described the basic format of the CPT manual. The information and exercises in this chapter will familiarize you with the first section of the CPT manual, Evaluation and Management (E/M). Locate Table 1, Categories and Subcategories of Service, in the E/M Guidelines of the CPT manual, which indicates all the E/M categories/subcategories.

Office or Other Outpatient Services		**Prolonged Services**	
New Patient	99201-99205	With Direct (Face-To-Face) Patient Contact	99354-99357
Established Patient	99211-99215	Without Direct (Face-To-Face) Patient Contact	99358-99359
Hospital Observation Services		Physician Standby Services	99360
Observation Care Discharge Services	99217	**Case Management Services**	
Initial Observation Care	99218-99220	Anticoagulation Management	99363, 99364
Hospital Inpatient Services		Medical Team Conferences	99366-99368
Initial Hospital Care	99221-99223	**Care Plan Oversight Services**	99374-99380
Subsequent Hospital Care	99231-99236	**Preventive Medicine Services**	
Hospital Discharge Services	99238-99239	New Patient	99381-99387
Consultations		Established Patient	99391-99397
Office Consultations or Other Outpatients	99241-99245	Individual Counseling	99401-99404
Inpatient Consultations	99251-99255	Group Counseling	99411-99412
Emergency Department Services	99281-99288	Other	99420-99429
Critical Care Services		**Non-Face-to-Face Physician Services**	
Adult (over 24 months of age)	99291-99292	Telephone Services	99441-99443
Nursing Facility Services		Online Medical Evaluation	99444
Initial Nursing Facility Care	99304-99306	**Special E/M Services**	99450-99456
Subsequent Nursing Facility Care	99307-99310	**Newborn Care Services**	99460-99463
Nursing Facility Discharge Services	99315-99316	Delivery/Birthing Room Attendance	99464-99465
Other Nursing Facility Services	99318	**Inpatient Neonatal Intensive Care Services and Pediatric**	
Domiciliary, Rest Home (e.g., Boarding Home), or		**and Neonatal Critical Care Services**	
Custodial Care Services		Pediatric Critical Care Patient Transport	99466, 99467
New Patient	99324-99328	Inpatient Neonatal and Pediatric Critical Care	99468-99476
Established Patient	99334-99337	Initial and Continuing Intensive Care	99477-99480
Domiciliary, Rest Home (e.g., Assisted	99339-99340	Services	
Living Facility), or Home Care Plan		**Other E/M Services**	99499
Oversight Services			
Home Services			
New Patient	99341-99345		
Established Patient	99347-99350		

THREE FACTORS OF E/M CODES

Code assignment in the E/M section varies according to three factors:

1. Place of service
2. Type of service
3. Patient status

Place of Service

The first factor you must consider in code assignment is the place of service (Fig. 10–1).

Place of service explains the setting in which the services were provided to the patient. Codes vary depending on the place of the service. Places of

FACTORS

Place of Service ← Office, hospital, emergency department, nursing home
Type of Service
Patient Status

FIGURE 10–1 Place of service.

service can be a physician's office, hospital, emergency department, nursing home, and so on.

Type of Service

The second factor in code assignment is the type of service (Fig. 10–2).

Type of service is the reason the service is requested or performed. Examples of types of service are consultation, admission, newborn care, and office visit.

- **Consultation** is written or verbal request from one provider/physician to another to obtain an opinion and/or advice about a diagnosis or management options.
- **Admission** is attention to an acute illness or injury that results in admission to a hospital.
- **Newborn care** is the evaluation and determination of care management of a newly born infant.
- **Office visit** is a face-to-face encounter between a physician and a patient to allow for primary management of the patient's health care status.

Patient Status

The third factor in code assignment is patient status (Fig. 10–3).

The four types of patient **status** are new patient, established patient, outpatient, and inpatient. Codes are often grouped in the CPT manual according to the type of patient involved.

- **New** patient is one who has not received professional face-to-face services from the physician or another physician of the same specialty in the same group within the past 3 years.
- **Established** patient is one who has received professional face-to-face services from the physician or another physician of the same specialty in the same group within the past 3 years.
- **Outpatient** is one who has not been formally admitted to a health care facility or a patient admitted for observation.
- **Inpatient** is one who has been formally admitted to a health care facility.

FIGURE 10–2   Type of service.

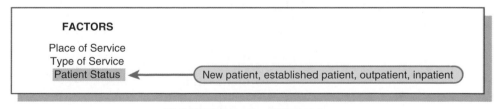

FIGURE 10–3   Patient status.

EXERCISE 10-1   *Three Factors of E/M Codes*

Using a CPT manual, locate the subsection Office and Other Outpatient Services and then the category New Patient in the E/M section to answer the following questions:

1 Where is the place of service? _____

2 What is the type of service? _____

3 What is the patient status? _____

4 What is the first code number listed under the subheading New Patient?

   CPT Code: _____

5 Each code represents a different level of service. How many codes are listed under Office or Other Outpatient Services for a new patient? _____

6 How many codes are listed for the established patient in the Office or Other Outpatient Services category? _____

Medical Records Documentation

Patient information is located in the medical record. This information is referred to as **documentation**. The documentation in the medical record has many uses, such as evaluation of the patient's treatment, communications regarding the patient's health care, reimbursement claims, review of the use of the health care facility, research/education, and legal documentation. Seven organizations (American Health Information Management Association, American Hospital Association, Managed Care and Review Association, American Medical Association, American Medical Peer Review Association, Blue Cross and Blue Shield Association, and the Health Insurance Association of America) developed minimum documentation guidelines, as follows:

1. The medical record should be complete and legible.
2. Documentation of each encounter should include the date, reason for encounter, appropriate history and physical examination, review of ancillary services, assessment, and plan of care with provider signature and date.
3. Past and present diagnoses should be accessible to the treating and/or consulting physician.
4. The reasons for and results of x-rays, lab tests, and other ancillary services should be clear.
5. Relevant risk factors should be identified.
6. The patient's progress and response to treatment, any change in treatment or change in diagnosis, and any patient noncompliance should be documented.
7. A written plan of treatment should include, when appropriate, treatments and medications, specifying frequency and dosage, any referrals or consultations, patient or family education, and any specific instructions for follow-up care.
8. Documentation should report the intensity of the patient evaluation and/or the treatment, including thought processes and the complexity of the medical decision making.
9. All entries should be dated and authenticated by provider or provider extender.

10. The CPT/ICD-9-CM codes reported on the insurance claim or billing statement should reflect **(support)** the documentation in the medical record.

VARIOUS LEVELS OF E/M SERVICE

The levels of E/M service are based on documentation located in the patient's medical record supporting various amounts of skill, effort, time, responsibility, and medical knowledge used by the physician to provide the service to the patient. The levels of service are based on **key components** (history, examination, and medical decision making complexity) and **contributory factors** (counseling, coordination of care, nature of presenting problem, and time). The components contain a great deal of information that you need to know before you learn about factors. Let's look at each of these components and factors individually.

Key Components

- History
- Examination
- Medical decision making

The key components of history, examination, and medical decision making reflect the clinical information that is recorded by the physician in the patient's medical record. Key components are present in every patient case except counseling encounters, which are discussed later in the chapter. Key components enable you to choose the appropriate level of service. New patient encounters, consultations, emergency-department visits, and admissions require documentation of all three of the key components. Subsequent visits such as daily hospital visits or outpatient visits for an established patient require that only two of the three key components be present for assignment to a given code. For example, to assign code 99214—established patient, office visit—at least two of the three key components must be documented in the patient's medical record.

Example

99214   Office or other outpatient visit for the evaluation and management of an established patient, which requires **at least two of these three key components:**

- **a detailed history;**
- **a detailed examination;**
- **medical decision making of moderate complexity.**

Office, New Patient

According to the E/M Guidelines, the following categories/subcategories must meet or exceed the stated level of the key components:

- Hospital Observation Services
- Initial Hospital Care
- Office Consultation
- Inpatient Consultation
- Emergency Department Services
- Initial Nursing Facility Care
- Domiciliary Care, New Patient
- Home, New Patient

QUICK CHECK 10-1

1. The above categories/subcategories must meet or _____
_____ of three key components.

Of the following categories/subcategories, **two** of the **three** key components must be met or exceeded before the code may be assigned:

■ Office, Established Patient
■ Subsequent Hospital Care
■ Subsequent Nursing Facility Care
■ Domiciliary Care, Established Patient
■ Home, Established Patient

History.   The history is the subjective information the patient tells the physician based on the four elements of a history—chief complaint (CC); history of present illness (HPI); review of systems (ROS); and past, family, and/or social history (PFSH). The history contains the information the physician needs to appropriately assess the patient's condition. Not all histories have all elements. The inclusion of each of the elements and the extent to which each of the elements is contained in a history are determined by the physician, based on the need for more or less subjective information, and will determine the extent of the history level. The documentation of the history is found in the patient's medical record and is recorded by the physician.

Ancillary staff (nurses, physician assistants, and so forth) are allowed to document some of the history, such as chief complaint and past, family, and social histories, but the physician must authenticate the entries (physician must evaluate the form and indicate in the medical record that the form has been reviewed). Also, a physician can have the patient complete a form composed of questions concerning the review of systems; however, the physician must authenticate the information.

QUICK CHECK 10-2

1. Some history elements may be documented by ancillary staff or the patient.
True or False?

THE FOUR ELEMENTS OF A HISTORY

■ Chief Complaint (CC)
■ History of Present Illness (HPI)
■ Review of Systems (ROS)
■ Past, Family, and/or Social History (PFSH)

History Elements.   You need to be able to identify the various elements and levels of a history by reading the notes entered into the medical record by the physician.

1. **Chief Complaint (CC)** is a concise statement describing the symptom, problem, condition, diagnosis, physician-recommended return, or other factor that is the reason for the encounter, usually stated in the patient's words.

2. **History of Present Illness (HPI)** is a chronological description of the development of the patient's present illness from the first sign and/or symptom or from the previous encounter to the present. The HPI may include the elements identified in the following example:

Example

Location: thoracic spine (site on body)

Quality: burning, throbbing (characteristics)

Severity: on a scale of 1 to 10, an 8 (intensity)

Duration: 3 days (how long is an episode or how long has the problem existed)

Timing: throughout the day, continuously, at night, in the morning, etc., the frequency (when does it occur)

Context: when bending over (under what circumstances does it occur)

Modifying factors: better when lying down (what circumstances make it better or worse)

Associated signs and symptoms: weakness (what else is present that relates to chief complaint)

The HPI must be documented in the medical record by the physician.

TOOLBOX

Juanita presents to her family physician today with complaints of sharp stomach pain (5/10, 5 on a severity scale of 10) for 6 days, usually in the afternoon after her afternoon coffee.

HISTORY OF PRESENT ILLNESS (HPI)
1. Location (site on body)
2. Quality (characteristic: throbbing, sharp)
3. Severity (1/10 or how intense)
4. Duration (how long for problem or episode)
5. Timing (when it occurs)
6. Context (under what circumstances does it occur)
7. Modifying factors (what makes it better or worse)
8. Associated signs and symptoms (what else is happening when it occurs)

QUESTIONS

An E/M audit form would have the HPI elements listed as in the audit form on the left. The coder checks off each element of the HPI as documented in the medical record. Check off the HPI elements on the audit form based on Juanita's record.

ANSWERS 1. ✓ (stomach) 2. ✓ (sharp) 3. ✓ (5/10) 4. ✓ (6 days) 5. ✓ (afternoon) 6. ✓ (afternoon coffee)

3. **Review of Systems (ROS)** is an inventory of body systems obtained through a series of questions seeking to identify signs and/or symptoms that the patient may be experiencing or has experienced. According to Huffman's *Health Information Management,** the "ROS is an inventory of systems to reveal subjective symptoms that the patient either forgot to describe or which at the time seemed relatively unimportant. In general, an analysis of the subjective findings will indicate the nature and extent of examination required." The inventory of systems may be made by means of a questionnaire filled out by the patient or ancillary staff; but the physician *must* evaluate the questionnaire and document in the medical record that the questionnaire has been reviewed in order for it to qualify as an ROS. For the purposes of an ROS, the following systems are recognized**:

- Constitutional symptoms

  Usual weight, recent weight changes, fever, weakness, fatigue

- Eyes (Ophthalmologic)

  Glasses or contact lenses, last eye examination, visual glaucoma, cataracts, eyestrain, pain, diplopia, redness, lacrimation, inflammation, blurring

- Ears, Nose, Mouth, Throat (Otolaryngologic)

  Ears: hearing, discharge, tinnitus, dizziness, pain

  Nose: head colds, epistaxis, discharges, obstruction, postnasal drip, sinus pain

  Mouth and Throat: condition of teeth and gums, last dental examination, soreness, redness, hoarseness, difficulty in swallowing

- Cardiovascular

  Chest pain, rheumatic fever, tachycardia, palpitation, high blood pressure, edema, vertigo, faintness, varicose veins, thrombophlebitis

- Respiratory

  Chest pain, wheezing, cough, dyspnea, sputum (color and quantity), hemoptysis, asthma, bronchitis, emphysema, pneumonia, tuberculosis, pleurisy, last chest radiograph (note: also shortness of breath)

- Gastrointestinal

  Appetite, thirst, nausea, vomiting, hematemesis, rectal bleeding, change in bowel habits, diarrhea, constipation, indigestion, food intolerance, flatus, hemorrhoids, jaundice

- Genitourinary

  Urinary: frequent or painful urination, nocturia, pyuria, hematuria, incontinence, urinary infection

  Genito-reproductive: male—venereal disease, sores, discharge from penis, hernias, testicular pain or masses; female—age at menarche and menstruation (frequency, type, duration, dysmenorrhea, menorrhagia; symptoms of menopause), contraception, pregnancies, deliveries, abortions, last Papanicolaou smear

- Musculoskeletal

  Joint pain or stiffness, arthritis, gout, backache, muscle pain, cramps, swelling, redness, limitation in motor activity

---

*Definitions from Huffman E: *Health Information Management,* 10th ed. Revised by the American Medical Record Association. Berwyn, IL, Physician's Record Company, 1994, pp 57–62.

**Modified from Huffman E: *Health Information Management,* 10th ed. Revised by the American Medical Record Association. Berwyn, IL, Physician's Record Company, 1994, pp 57–62.

■ Integumentary (skin and/or breast)

Skin: rashes, eruptions, dryness, cyanosis, jaundice, changes in skin, hair, or nails*

Breast: lumps, dimpling, nipple discharge*

■ Neurologic *(neurological)*

Faintness, blackouts, seizures, paralysis, tingling, tremors, memory loss

■ Psychiatric

Personality type, nervousness, mood, insomnia, headache, nightmares, depression

■ Endocrine

Thyroid trouble, heat or cold intolerance, excessive sweating, thirst, hunger, or urination, blood sugar levels

■ Hematologic/Lymphatic

Anemia, easy bruising or bleeding, past transfusions

■ Allergic/Immunologic

Sneezing, itching eyes, rhinorrhea, nasal obstruction, or recurrent infections

4. Past, Family, and/or Social History (PFSH)*

■ Past history is the patient's past experience with illnesses, operations, injuries, and treatments; that includes significant information about:

Prior major illnesses and injuries

Prior operations

Prior hospitalizations

Current medications

Allergies (e.g., drug, food)

Age-appropriate immunization status

Age-appropriate feeding/dietary status

■ Social history is an age-appropriate review of past and current activities that includes significant information about:

Marital status and/or living arrangements

Current employment

Occupational history

Use of drugs, alcohol, and tobacco

Level of education

Sexual history

Other relevant social factors

■ Family history is a review of medical events in the patient's family that includes significant information about:

The health status or cause of death of parents, siblings, and children

Specific diseases related to problems identified in the Chief Complaint or History of the Present Illness, and/or System Review

Diseases of family members that may be hereditary or place the patient at risk

---

*Definitions from 2010 CPT, Evaluation and Management Guidelines, p 4. CPT codes, descriptions, and materials only are © 2009 American Medical Association.

Three of the elements of a history (HPI, ROS, and PFSH) are included to varying degrees in all patient encounters. The degree or level of HPI, ROS, and PFSH is determined by the chief complaint or presenting problem of the patient.

History Levels. Now that you have reviewed the elements of a history you are prepared to choose a history level. There are four history levels; the level is based on the extent of the history during the history-taking portion of the physician-patient encounter.

The history of present illness (HPI) must be documented by the physician or NPP billing for the service.

HISTORY LEVELS

- Problem focused
- Expanded problem focused
- Detailed
- Comprehensive

1. **Problem focused:** The physician focuses on the chief complaint and a brief history of the present problem of a patient.

    A brief history would include a review of the history regarding pertinent information about the present problem or chief complaint. Brief history information would center around the severity, duration, and/or symptoms of the problem or complaint. The brief history does not have to include the past, family, or social history or a review of systems. A brief HPI includes 1-3 of the eight elements.

2. **Expanded problem focused:** The physician focuses on a chief complaint, obtains a brief history of the present problem, and also performs a problem pertinent review of systems. The expanded problem focused history does not have to include the past, family, or social history.

    This history would center around specific questions regarding the system involved in the presenting problem or chief complaint. The review of systems for this history would cover the organ system most closely related to the chief complaint or presenting problem and any related or associated organ system. For example, if the presenting problem or chief complaint is a red, swollen knee, the system reviewed would be the musculoskeletal system.

3. **Detailed:** The physician focuses on a chief complaint, obtains an extended history of the present problem (4 or more of the 8 elements), an extended review of systems, and a pertinent PFSH.

    The system review in this history is extended, which means that positive responses and pertinent negative responses relating to multiple organ systems should be documented.

4. **Comprehensive:** This is the most complex of the history types: the physician documents the chief complaint, obtains an extended history of the present problem, does a complete review of systems, and obtains a complete PFSH.

For a summary of the elements required for each level of history (according to the 1995 Documentation Guidelines), see Fig. 10–4.

Some third-party payers have established standards for the number of elements that must be documented in the medical record to qualify for a given level of service. For example, a third-party payer may state that to qualify as a comprehensive history the medical record must document

History Elements

Chief Complaint (CC)
Reason for the encounter in the patient's words

History of Present Illness (HPI)
Location
Quality
Severity
Duration*
Timing
Context
Modifying factors
Associated signs and symptoms

Review of Systems (ROS)
Constitutional symptoms (fever, weight loss, etc.)
Ophthalmologic (eyes)
Otolaryngologic (ears, nose, mouth, throat)
Cardiovascular
Respiratory
Gastrointestinal
Genitourinary
Musculoskeletal
Integumentary (skin and/or breast)
Neurological
Psychiatric
Endocrine
Hematologic/Lymphatic
Allergic/Immunologic

Past, Family, and/or Social History (PFSH)
Past major illnesses, operations, injuries, and treatments
Family medical history for heredity and risk
Social activities, both past and current

Elements Required for Each Level of History

		Problem Focused	Expanded Problem Focused	Detailed	Comprehensive
History	HPI	Brief 1-3	Brief 1-3	Extended 4+	Extended 4+
	ROS	None	Problem-pertinent 1	Extended 2-9	Complete 10+
	PFSH	None	None	Pertinent 1	Complete 2-3

* Duration is not listed in the CPT E/M Guidelines, but listed in the 1995 Documentation Guidelines.

FIGURE 10-4 History elements required for each level of history.

that an extended HPI was conducted and that it included four of the eight elements (e.g., location, quality, severity, duration), a complete ROS, including a review of at least 10 of the 14 organ systems, and a complete review of all three areas of the PFSH.

CODING SHOT When selecting a history level, the choice goes to the lowest level. For example, if the HPI is a level 2, the ROS is a level 2, but the PFSH is a level 1, the history level is 1. Another example is if the HPI is a level 3, the ROS is a level 2, and the PFSH is a level 2, the history is a level 2.

QUICK CHECK 10-3

1. Which levels of history require the documentation of the Chief Complaint (CC)?
   a. Problem focused
   b. Expanded problem focused
   c. Detailed
   d. Comprehensive
   e. All of the above

EXERCISE 10-2 *History Levels*

Using the CPT manual, locate the Office or Other Outpatient Services subsection, New Patient category, to identify the history level on each of the following codes:

CODE	HISTORY LEVEL
1 99201	_____
2 99202	_____
3 99203	_____
4 99204	_____
5 99205	_____

Examination. The patient has presented the physician with the **subjective** information regarding the complaint or problem in the history portion of the encounter; now the physician will do an examination of the patient to provide **objective** information, "hands-on" (those findings observed by the physician) about the complaint or problem. The physician then documents the objective findings in the patient record.

Examination Levels. The examination levels have the same titles as the history levels—problem focused, expanded problem focused, detailed, and comprehensive. The four levels are used to indicate the extent and complexity of the patient examination.

EXAMINATION LEVELS
- Problem focused
- Expanded problem focused
- Detailed
- Comprehensive

1. **Problem focused:** Examination is limited to the affected body area or organ system identified by the chief complaint.
2. **Expanded problem focused:** A limited examination is made of the affected body area or organ system and other symptomatic or related body area(s)/organ system(s).
3. **Detailed:** An extended examination is made of the affected body area(s) and other symptomatic or related organ system(s).

4. **Comprehensive:** This is the most extensive examination; it encompasses a general multi-system examination and should include findings about 8 or more of the 12 organ systems.

Some third-party payers, such as Medicare, have guidelines for the comprehensive examination that state that only organ systems qualify when determining the level for the comprehensive examination and that body areas do not qualify.

Fig. 10–5 summarizes the elements required for each level of examination. These elements include various body areas (BAs) and organ systems (OSs). The elements also include an assessment of a patient's general condition, which is indicated by the patient's general appearance, vital signs, and the like.

Examination Elements

Constitutional* (OS)
Blood pressure, sitting
Blood pressure, lying
Pulse
Respirations
Temperature
Height
Weight
General appearance

Body Areas (BA)
Head (including the face)
Neck
Chest (including breasts and axillae)
Abdomen
Genitalia, groin, buttocks
Back
Each extremity

Organ System (OS)
Ophthalmologic (eyes)
Otolaryngologic (ears, nose, mouth, throat)
Cardiovascular
Respiratory
Gastrointestinal
Genitourinary
Musculoskeletal
Integumentary (skin)
Neurologic
Psychiatric
Hematologic/Lymphatic/Immunologic

Elements Required for Each Level of Examination

	Problem Focused	Expanded Problem Focused	Detailed	Comprehensive
Examination	Limited to affected BA or OS	Limited to affected BA or OS and other related OS(s)	Extended of affected BA(s) and other related OS(s)	General multi-system (OSs only)
# of OS/BA	1	2-7 limited	2-7 extended	8+

*Constitutional is NOT in the CPT manual but is in the 1995 Documentation Guidelines (DGs). In the DGs, constitutional is listed as the first organ system for a total of 12 organ systems. Most third-party payers allow for the counting of the constitutional elements to identify the level of the examination. The constitutional examination is placed at the top of the examination elements in this text to provide a list of the various constitutional elements.

FIGURE 10–5 Examination elements required for each level of examination.

EXERCISE 10-3 *Examination Levels*

Using the CPT manual, locate the Office or Other Outpatient Services subsection, New Patient category, to identify the examination levels for each of the following codes:

CODE	EXAMINATION LEVELS
1 99201	_____
2 99202	_____
3 99203	_____
4 99204	_____
5 99205	_____

The patient's medical record will reflect the number of systems examined in a brief statement of the findings. The examination would include the examination elements and the number and extent of elements required for the physician to arrive at the diagnosis. For example, if a patient came to a physician with the complaint of a small foreign object lodged in the eye, the physician would not usually need to do a cardiologic examination. The extent of the examination is based on what needs to be done to treat the patient.

Now you need to pull all the information on history and examination together so that it is usable information. What better way to do that than to use the information in the practical application of an exercise?

EXERCISE 10-4 *Examination Elements*

Label each of the following as body area (BA) or organ system (OS):

1 Skin _____

2 Head _____

3 Eyes _____

4 Ears _____

5 Nose _____

6 Mouth _____

7 Throat _____

8 Neck _____

9 Thorax, anterior and posterior _____

10 Breasts _____

11 Lungs _____

12 Heart _____

13 Abdomen _____

14 Genitourinary _____

15 Vaginal _____

16 Arm _____

17 Musculoskeletal _____

18 Lymphatics _____

19 Psychiatric _____

20 Neurologic _____

Read the following patient record:

21 A new patient, an 8-year-old female, is brought into the office by her mother, who states that the child has an earache in her right ear. Mother reports that the child has been complaining of pain in right ear with a severity of 8 of 10 for the past 2 days. Exam: Child appears to be in only minor distress. Vitals: Temperature, 101° F. Tympanic membrane red, fluid noted in right ear. Health history reviewed. Diagnosis: Acute serous otitis media.

From the patient record, we can identify the history elements as follows:

HISTORY ELEMENTS	PATIENT RECORD
CC:	Earache in the right ear
HPI:	Complaining of pain in the right ear with a severity of 8 of 10 for the past 2 days

	Location:	Right ear
	Quality:	Aching and ringing
	Severity:	8 of 10
	Duration:	Two days

PFSH:	Health history reviewed. (The patient information form completed by the mother contains the information that the physician reviewed, along with questions to the patient.)
ROS:	Ears (one organ system)

In this case, the physician focused on the chief complaint and did a brief history centered on gathering information about the present illness. Referring to the description of history levels summarized in Fig. 10–4 or discussed in the E/M Guidelines, answer the following question:

    a What is the history level for this case? _____

Now let's establish the level of examination:

EXAMINATION	PATIENT RECORD
General Survey:	Child appears to be in only minor distress
Vital Signs:	Temperature, 101° F
Body Areas/Organ Systems	Ears (one organ system)

In this case, the physician focused on constitutional (temperature and general appearance) and one organ system (ears). Referring to the description of examination levels summarized in Fig. 10–5 or discussed in the E/M Guidelines, answer the following question:

    b What is the examination level for this case? _____

That wasn't so difficult, was it? Okay, now you do one.

Read the following patient record:

22 A 68-year-old female established patient presents to the office today with a "cold" of 9 days' duration. Patient reports that she has had a dry, hacking cough and nasal congestion for the past 6 days and a fever for the past 3 days. She states that she is unable to sleep due to the cough, fever, and aching. She appears to be in minor distress. Personal and family history are negative for respiratory problems. Temperature is 100° F; blood pressure 150/90; pulse 93 and regular. Lungs clear to percussion and auscultation. Examination of head and ears, normal; nose, mucous membranes inflamed with postnasal phlegm. Diagnosis: Sinusitis. Plan: Patient was advised to drink fluids, take aspirin as needed for pain, obtain bed rest, and to return if symptoms have not improved in 5 days.

Continued

Locate the information in the patient record that matches the history element and place the information on the lines provided:

HISTORY ELEMENTS   **PATIENT RECORD**

CC:

_____

_____

_____

HPI:

_____

_____

_____

PFSH:

_____

_____

_____

ROS:

_____

_____

_____

With the information you placed on the preceding lines, choose the correct history level:

a What is the history level for this case? _____

Locate the information in the patient record that matches the examination, and place the information on the lines provided:

EXAMINATION   **PATIENT RECORD**

General Survey: _____

Vital Signs: _____

_____

_____

_____

Body Areas/Organ Systems: _____

With the information you placed on the preceding lines, choose the correct examination level:

b What is the examination level for this case? _____

Medical Decision Making. The key component of medical decision making (MDM) is based on the complexity of the decision the physician must make about the patient's diagnosis and care. Complexity of decision making is based on three elements:

1. Number of diagnoses or management options. The options can be minimal, limited, multiple, or extensive.

2. Amount or complexity of data to review. The data can be minimal or none, limited, moderate, or extensive.

3. Risk of complication or death if the condition goes untreated. Risk can be minimal, low, moderate, or high.

Levels. The extent to which each of these elements is considered determines the levels of MDM complexity.

MEDICAL DECISION MAKING COMPLEXITY LEVELS

- Straightforward
- Low
- Moderate
- High

1. **Straightforward decision making:** minimal diagnosis and management options, minimal or none for the amount and complexity of data to be reviewed, and minimal risk to the patient of complications or death if untreated.

2. **Low-complexity decision making:** limited number of diagnoses and management options, limited data to be reviewed, and low risk to the patient of complications or death if untreated.

3. **Moderate-complexity decision making:** multiple diagnoses and management options, moderate amount and complexity of data to be reviewed, and moderate risk to the patient of complications or death if untreated.

4. **High-complexity decision making:** extensive diagnoses and management options, extensive amount and complexity of data to be reviewed, and high risk to the patient for complications or death if the problem is untreated.

Management Options. According to the 1995 E/M Documentation Guidelines, documentation of management options in the medical record are as follows:

1. For each encounter, an assessment, clinical impression, or diagnosis should be documented. It may be explicitly stated or implied in documented decisions regarding management plans or further evaluation.

    - For a presenting problem with an established diagnosis, the record should reflect whether the problem is (a) improved, well controlled, resolving, or resolved; or (b) inadequately controlled, worsening, or failing to change as expected.

    - For a presenting problem without an established diagnosis, the assessment or clinical impression may be stated in the form of differential diagnoses or as a "possible," "probable," or "rule out" (R/O) diagnosis.

    - Note: Physician/Provider coders do not code "rule out," "possible," or "probable" diagnosis; rather they code the presenting symptoms and/or complaints unless there is a definitive diagnosis rendered.

2. The initiation of, or changes in, treatment should be documented. Treatment includes a wide range of management options, including patient instructions, nursing instructions, therapies, and medications.

3. If referrals are made, consultations requested, or advice sought, the record should indicate to whom or where the referral or consultation has been made or from whom the advice is requested.

Data to Be Reviewed. The following are some basic documentation guidelines for the amount and complexity of data to be reviewed:

1. If a diagnostic service (test or procedure) is ordered, planned, scheduled, or performed at the time of the E/M encounter, the type of service (e.g., laboratory or radiology) should be documented.

2. The review of laboratory, radiology, or other diagnostic tests should be documented. An entry in a progress note such as "WBC elevated" or "chest x-ray negative" is acceptable. Alternatively, the review may be documented by initialing and dating the report containing the test results.

3. A decision to obtain old records or to obtain additional history from the family, caregiver, or other source to supplement that obtained from the patient should be documented.

4. Relevant findings from the review of old records or the receipt of additional history from the family, caregiver, or other source should be documented. If there is no relevant information beyond that already obtained, that fact should be documented. A notation of "old records reviewed" or "additional history obtained from family" without elaboration is insufficient.

5. The results of discussion of laboratory, radiology, or other diagnostic tests with the physician who performed or interpreted the study should be documented.

6. The direct visualization and independent interpretation of an image, tracing, or specimen previously interpreted by another physician should be documented.

Risk. Some basic documentation guidelines for risk of significant complications, morbidity, or mortality include the following:

1. Comorbidities (secondary conditions), underlying diseases, or other factors that increase the complexity of medical decision making by increasing the risk of complications, morbidity, or mortality should be documented.

2. If a surgical or invasive diagnostic procedure is ordered, planned, or scheduled at the time of the E/M encounter, the type of procedure (e.g., laparoscopy) should be documented.

3. If a surgical or invasive diagnostic procedure is performed at the time of the E/M encounter, the specific procedure should be documented.

4. The referral for or decision to perform a surgical or invasive diagnostic procedure on an urgent basis should be documented or implied.

Examples of the levels of risk may be found in Table 10–1.

When you select one of the four types of complexity of medical decision making—straightforward, low, moderate, or high—the documentation in the medical record must support the selection in terms of the number of diagnoses or management options, amount and/or complexity of data to be reviewed, and risks. Two of the three elements in Fig. 10–6 must be met or exceeded to qualify for a level of medical decision making.

Refer to Fig. 10–6 for an overview of medical decision making. Given the information in the medical record, you would consider the information in the context of the complexity of the diagnosis and management options, data to be reviewed, and risks to the patient in order to choose the complexity of MDM. Let's look at an example of choosing the MDM level.

TABLE 10-1

LEVELS OF RISK

Level of Risk	Presenting Problem or Problems
Minimal (Level 1)	One self-limited or minor problem (e.g., insect bite, tinea corporis)
Low (Level 2)	Two or more self-limited or minor problems
	One stable chronic illness (e.g., well-controlled hypertension or non–insulin dependent diabetes, cataract, benign prostatic hypertrophy)
	Acute, uncomplicated illness or injury (e.g., cystitis, allergic rhinitis, simple sprain)
Moderate (Level 3)	One or more chronic illnesses with mild exacerbation, progression, or side effects of treatment
	Two or more stable chronic illnesses
	Undiagnosed new problem with uncertain prognosis (e.g., lump in breast)
	Acute illness with systemic symptoms (e.g., pyelonephritis, pneumonitis, colitis)
High (Level 4)	One or more chronic illnesses with severe exacerbation, progression, or side effects of treatment
	Acute or chronic illnesses or injuries that pose a threat to life or body function (e.g., multiple trauma, acute myocardial infarction, pulmonary embolus, severe respiratory distress, progressive severe rheumatoid arthritis, psychiatric illness with potential threat to self or others, peritonitis, acute renal failure)
	An abrupt change in neurologic status (e.g., seizure, transient ischemic attack, weakness, or sensory loss)

Medical Decision-Making Elements

Number of Diagnoses or Management Options
Minimal
Limited
Multiple
Extensive

Amount or Complexity of Data to Review
Minimal/None
Limited
Moderate
Extensive

Risk of Complications or Death if Condition Goes Untreated
Minimal
Low
Moderate
High

Elements Required for Each Level of Medical Decision-Making

	Straightforward	Low	Moderate	High
Number of DX or management options	Minimal	Limited	Multiple	Extensive
Amount or complexity of data	Minimal/None	Limited	Moderate	Extensive
Risks	Minimal	Low	Moderate	High

FIGURE 10-6 Decision making elements required for each level of medical decision making complexity. Two of the three elements must be met or exceeded to qualify for a level of medical decision making.

CODING SHOT

When selecting an MDM level, the choice is the majority. For example, if the number of diagnosis management options is a level 2, the amount of data is a level 2, but the risk is a level 1, the MDM level is 2. Another example is if the number of management options is a level 1, the amount of data is a level 3, and the risk is a level 2, the history is a level 2. This is different than the history in which the lowest level directed the level choice; in the MDM the level is the highest two.

Example 1

An established patient's outpatient medical record indicates the following: Female patient fell and scraped arm; problem focused history and examination were done. The patient states that she slipped on the ice on the walk outside her home approximately 3 hours earlier. The area of abrasion appears to be relatively clean, with no foreign materials imbedded. There appears to be only minimal cutaneous damage. The area was washed and a dressing applied.

1. **Diagnosis and management options** for an abrasion (clean and dress). (Options are minimal, limited, multiple, or extensive.)

    As a coder, you think about how many various options are open to the physician to diagnose the problem and decide how to manage this patient's care—minimal, limited, multiple, extensive? The management of an abrasion is fairly clear—clean and dress the wound; therefore, the diagnosis and management options are minimal.

2. **Data to review** to provide service. (Data can be minimal/none, limited, moderate, or extensive.)

    Think about how much and how complex would the information (data) be that the physician must obtain, review, and analyze to care for this patient—minimal/none, limited, moderate, or extensive? The amount of data to review would be minimal/none for an abrasion.

3. **Risk** if not treated. (Risk can be minimal, low, moderate, or high.)

    As a coder, you think about how great a risk there is that the patient would die or encounter severe complications (e.g., infection), morbidity (additional diseases such as gangrene), or mortality (death) if the abrasion was not treated—minimal, low, moderate, or high? The risk of death or of complications is minimal.

The diagnosis and management options are minimal, data are minimal/none, and risk is minimal. Consideration of these three elements has placed this patient's care into a straightforward MDM complexity level.

The history level is stated to be problem focused and the examination level is problem focused. The patient was an established patient seen as an outpatient. Carefully look at each of the items set in boldface type in code 99212 below. The place of service, type of service, type of history, type of examination, and complexity level of the MDM are identified in the description of the code.

99212   **Office or other outpatient** visit for the evaluation and management of an **established patient** that requires at least two of these three key components:

         ■ **a problem focused history**

         ■ **a problem focused examination**

         ■ **straightforward medical decision making**

CPT code 99212 is the correct code for this service.

Example 2

The patient's record states the following: Unknown (new) patient presenting to the office with chest pain **(786.50)** [ICD-10-CM: R07.9]. A comprehensive history was taken and a comprehensive examination performed. The physician ordered an electrocardiogram (ECG), laboratory reports, and x-rays.

The MDM complexity level must be chosen:

1. **Diagnosis and management options** for a cardiac origin could be myocardial infarction, angina, or heart block. Gastrointestinal origin could be reflux or an ulcer. Respiratory origin could be a pulmonary embolism or pleuritis. (Diagnosis and management options can be minimal, limited, multiple, or extensive.)

   What do you think it would take for the physician to decide on the diagnosis or management options for this patient? There are many possibilities of origin for the chest pain; therefore, the diagnosis and management options are extensive.

2. **Data to review** in order for the physician to provide service. (Data can be minimal/none, limited, moderate, or extensive.) How much data would the physician have to obtain through current tests and how much review and analysis of previous records would be necessary to provide services to the patient—minimal/none, limited, moderate, extensive? In this case, the patient's care requires moderate data review, including laboratory reports, radiology reports, and ECG. You very well may have chosen the data review level of extensive rather than moderate and that is acceptable. Once you are in the medical office and have the patient's full medical record available to review, the choice of the amount of data that was reviewed becomes easier to identify.

3. **Risk** if left untreated. (Risk can be minimal, low, moderate, or high.) If the patient's condition was not treated, what do you think the risk of death or serious complication would be—minimal, low, moderate, or high? This patient would have a high risk of death or severe complications if this condition was left untreated.

The extensive diagnosis and management options and high risk to the patient mean that two of the three elements have been met. So this patient's care is considered to have a high level of MDM complexity. A new patient with a comprehensive history and examination together with a high MDM complexity assigns this case to code 99205.

EXERCISE 10-5 *Medical Decision Making Complexity*

A new patient's record states that an initial office visit was made for the evaluation and management of a 48-year-old male with recurrent low back pain from a herniated disc, with pain radiating to the leg (myelopathy). A detailed history and a detailed examination were performed.

Using the information above, identify the following factors in the case:

1 Diagnosis and management options for recurrent low back pain radiating to the leg. (Options can be minimal, limited, multiple, or extensive.)

    _____

2 Data to review in order to provide service. (Data can be minimal/none, limited, moderate, or extensive.) Only the current record is available.

    _____

3 Risk if left untreated. (Risk can be minimal, low, moderate, or high.)

    _____

4 Two of the three elements have been met to qualify this patient for what level of MDM complexity? (Complexity can be straightforward, low, moderate, or high.)

    _____

5 The patient record indicates that a detailed history was taken and a detailed examination was performed. When this is combined with the level of MDM complexity you arrived at for this patient, what is the correct CPT code for the case?

    CPT Code: _____

    ICD-9-CM Code: _____ (ICD-10-CM Code: _____)

Now, let's look again at two cases for which you previously established the history and examination levels:

6 A new patient, an 8-year-old female, is brought into the office by her mother, who states that the child has an earache in the right ear. Mother reports that the child has been complaining of pain in right ear with a severity of 8 of 10 for the past 2 days. Child appears to be in only minor distress. Temperature, 101° F. Tympanic membranes red, fluid noted in right ear. Health history reviewed. Diagnosis: Acute serous otitis media.

    What is the MDM level for this patient? _____

    What ICD-9-CM code reports the diagnosis for this patient? _____

    (ICD-10-CM Code: _____)

7 A 68-year-old female established patient presents to the office today with a "cold" of 9 days' duration. Patient reports that she has had a dry, hacking cough and nasal congestion for the past 6 days and a fever for the past 3 days. She states that she is unable to sleep due to the cough, fever, and aching. She appears to be in minor distress. Personal and family history are negative for respiratory problems. Temperature is 100° F; blood pressure 150/90; pulse 93 and regular. Lungs clear to percussion and auscultation. Examination of head and ears, normal; nose, mucous membranes inflamed with postnasal phlegm. Diagnosis: Acute sinusitis. Plan: Patient was advised to drink fluids, take aspirin as needed for pain, obtain bed rest, and return if symptoms have not improved in 5 days.

    What is the MDM level for this patient? _____

    What ICD-9-CM code reports the diagnosis for this patient? _____

    (ICD-10-CM Code: _____)

There is certainly a great amount of information that must be considered in order to choose the correct E/M code! Only with practice can you expect to remember all of the various elements and levels within each component. Each medical facility has its own procedure for identifying the level of E/M service; some facilities require the physician to identify all the components of service, whereas other facilities require the component information to be abstracted from the medical record by support personnel. Either way, you need to be knowledgeable about all components of E/M codes and it really does get easier with practice!

From the Trenches

"I tell people that while the study and practice of medicine is considered a science, the coding is an art. There are often varying ways to do things, dependent on different circumstances. Attention to detail is important, but flexibility is also necessary."

JOAN

⬡ **STOP** *You have examined each of the three key components and seen how they apply to the assignment of an E/M code. You will be referring to the information as you are presented with additional cases. Make note of the important points and remember that the information about the key components is in the E/M Guidelines in the CPT manual.*

Now that you are familiar with the key components of history, examination, and medical decision making, let's review the contributory factors.

Contributory Factors

There are three contributory factors: counseling, coordination of care, and the nature of the presenting problem. Contributory factors are those conditions that help the physician determine the extent of the history, examination, and decision making (key components) necessary to treat the patient. Contributory factors may or may not be considered in every patient case.

CONTRIBUTORY FACTORS

- Counseling
- Coordination of care
- Nature of presenting problem

Counseling. Counseling is a service that physicians provide to patients and their families. It involves discussion of diagnostic results, impressions, and recommended diagnostic studies; prognosis; risks and benefits of treatment; instructions for treatment; importance of compliance with treatment; risk factor reduction; and patient and family education. Some form of counseling usually takes place in all physician-patient encounters, and this was factored into the codes when they were developed by the AMA. Only when counseling is the reason for the encounter or consumes most of the visit time (more than 50% of the total time) is counseling considered a component of code assignment. The following statement is made often within the codes in the E/M section:

Counseling and/or coordination of care with other providers or agencies are provided consistent with the nature of the problem(s) and the patient's and/or family's needs.

Coordination of Care. Coordination of care with other health care providers or agencies may be necessary for the care of a patient. In coordination of care, a physician might arrange for other services to be provided to the patient, such as arrangements for admittance to a long-term nursing facility.

Nature of the Presenting Problem. This is the foundation of the level assigned. The presenting problem is the patient's chief complaint or the situation that leads the physician to determining the level of care necessary to diagnose and treat the patient. The CPT describes the **presenting problem** as a disease, condition, illness, injury, symptom, sign, finding, complaint, or other reason for the encounter, with or without a diagnosis being established at the time of the encounter. There are five types of presenting problems:

- Minimal
- Self-limited
- Low severity
- Moderate severity
- High severity

1. **Minimal:** A problem may not require the presence of the physician, but a service is provided under the physician's supervision. A minimal problem is a blood pressure reading, a dressing change, or another service that can be performed without the physician's being immediately present.

2. **Self-limited:** Also called a minor presenting problem, a self-limited problem runs a definite and prescribed course, is transient (it comes and goes), and is not likely to permanently alter health status, or the presenting problem has a good prognosis with management and compliance.

3. **Low severity:** The risk of complete sickness (morbidity) without treatment is low, there is little or no risk of death without treatment, and full recovery without impairment is expected.

4. **Moderate severity:** The risk of complete sickness (morbidity) without treatment is moderate, there is moderate risk of death without treatment, and an uncertain prognosis or increased probability of impairment exists.

5. **High severity:** The risk of complete sickness (morbidity) without treatment is high to extreme, there is a moderate to high risk of death without treatment, or there is a strong probability of severe, prolonged functional impairment.

The patient's medical record should contain the physician's observation concerning the complexity of the presenting problem(s). Your responsibility is to identify the words that correctly indicate the type of presenting problem.

Direct face-to-face and **unit/floor time** are two measures of time. Outpatient visits are measured as direct face-to-face time. Direct face-to-face time is the time a physician spends directly with a patient during an office visit obtaining the history, performing an examination, and discussing the results. Inpatient time is measured as unit/floor time and is used to describe the time a physician spends in the hospital setting dealing with the patient's care. Unit/floor time includes care given to the patient at the bedside as well as at other settings on the unit or floor (e.g., the nursing station). It is an often-heard comment that physicians get paid a great deal of money just for stopping in to see a hospitalized patient. However, what is not realized is that the physician spends additional time reviewing the patient's records, test results, and writing orders for the patient's care.

Time in the E/M section is referred to in statements such as this one that is located with code 99203:

Usually, the presenting problem(s) are of moderate severity. Physicians typically spend 30 minutes face-to-face with the patient and/or family.

These statements concerning time are used when counseling or coordination of care represent more than **50% of the time spent with a patient.** The times referred to in these statements are the basis of the selection of the E/M code. For example: An established patient returns for an office visit to get the results of tests. The physician spends 25 minutes going over the unfavorable results of the tests. The physician discusses various treatment options, the prognosis, and the risks of treatment and of treatment refusal. The correct code would be 99214, in which the time statement is, "Physician typically spends 25 minutes face to face with the patient and/or family." The physician must either document the beginning and ending time in the patient's medical record or document the total time spent and how much was spent in counseling in order to be able to consider time in the code assignments.

CAUTION *Time was not included in the CPT manual before 1992 but was incorporated to assist with the selection of the most appropriate level of E/M services. The times indicated with the codes are only **averages** and represent a simple estimate of the possible duration of a service.*

EXERCISE 10-6 *Presenting Problem*

Match the presenting problem to the severity level in the patient:

a. minimal   b. self-limited   c. low   d. moderate   e. high

1 Four-year-old female established patient presents with slight pain in right ear, of 2 days' duration. Physician diagnosed a minor infection and prescribed antibiotic for acute exudative otitis media.

    Level of Presenting Problem: _____

    ICD-9-CM Code: _____ (ICD-10-CM Code: _____)

2 Eighty-six-year-old woman who has a history of chronic obstructive pulmonary disease (COPD) and is oxygen-dependent comes in because of dizziness and weakness. Diagnosis is acute exacerbation of COPD.

    Level of Presenting Problem: _____

    ICD-9-CM Code: _____ (ICD-10-CM Code: _____)

3 Established patient, 71 years old, with shortness of breath on exertion and a history of congestive cardiomyopathy.

    Level of Presenting Problem: _____

    ICD-9-CM Codes: _____ (shortness of breath), _____ (cardiomyopathy,

        congestive) (ICD-10-CM Codes: _____, _____)

4 Fourteen-year-old presents with moderate pain in left thumb after a fall from his skateboard. Diagnosis is sprain of left thumb.

    Level of Presenting Problem: _____

    ICD-9-CM Code: _____ (ICD-10-CM Code: _____)

5 Established patient, 34 years old, presents for a blood pressure check due to her malignant hypertension.

    Level of Presenting Problem: _____

    ICD-9-CM Code: _____ (ICD-10-CM Code: _____)

6 Physician recommends an over-the-counter medication for patient with seasonal grass allergic reaction.

    Level of Presenting Problem: _____

    ICD-9-CM Code: _____ (ICD-10-CM Code: _____)

AN E/M CODE EXAMPLE   With the CPT manual open to the first page of the E/M section, locate the notes above the 99201 code. These notes highlight the incidents in which codes in that particular category are appropriate for assignment. The notes above 99201 indicate that the codes that follow the notes are appropriate for use in coding services provided in a "physician's office or in an outpatient or other ambulatory facility."

The information also directs you to other code subsections if the patient classification is not correct. As an example of this directional feature, the notes above 99201 state, "For services provided by physicians in the emergency department, see 99281-99285."

Fig. 10–7 shows the first code for a new patient under the category New Patient under subsection Office or Other Outpatient Services. Review Fig. 10–7 carefully before continuing. Note the location of each important piece of information.

FIGURE 10-7 Code information.

Locate the following items in Fig. 10–7:

1. Three key components
2. Three contributory factors
3. Number of key components required
4. Place of service
5. Category of the code
6. Code

USING THE E/M CODES

Now you are going to use the information you have learned about codes in the E/M services section as you continue to identify the differences among the codes.

Office and Other Outpatient Services

New Patient.   The first subsection in the E/M section is Office and Other Outpatient Services, New Patient Category (99201-99205).

You will recall from information presented earlier that a new patient is defined as one who has not received any face-to-face professional services from the physician or another physician with the same specialty in the same group within the past 3 years. A physician must spend more time with a new patient—obtaining the history, conducting the examination, and considering the data—than with an established patient. Consider that the established patient is probably known to the physician, and the person's medical records are available, but with a new patient none of this is available to the physician. For these reasons, the cost of a new patient office visit is higher, so third-party payers reimburse the physician at a higher rate for new patient services than for the same type of service when it is provided to an established patient.

EXERCISE 10-7 *New Patient Services*

Using the CPT manual, fill in the blanks with the correct words:

1 For code 99203, the history level is _____, the examination is _____, and the MDM is of _____ complexity.

2 For code 99204, the history level is _____, the examination is _____, and the MDM complexity is _____.

3 For code 99205, the history level is _____, the examination is _____, and the MDM complexity is _____.

Code the following cases for new patients:

4 A 53-year-old new patient presents for an initial office visit to discuss a surgical vasectomy for sterilization. The history and examination are detailed and the MDM is of low complexity.

      CPT Code: _____

      ICD-9-CM Code: _____ (ICD-10-CM Code: _____)

5 A 4-year-old new patient presents for the removal of sutures made for an appendectomy 10 days earlier in another city. The physician conducts a brief history and examination prior to removing the stitches.

      CPT Code: _____

      ICD-9-CM Code: _____ (ICD-10-CM Code: _____)

6 A 23-year-old man who is a new patient has an initial office visit for severe depression *(report as first-listed diagnosis)* that has led to frequent thoughts of suicide in the past several weeks and is acute today. More than an hour is spent discussing the patient's problems and options. Past medical history is negative. The social history reveals that the patient suffers from sleeplessness *(report as an additional diagnosis)*; smokes between two and two and a half packs of unfiltered cigarettes a day and has for 5 years *(report as tobacco abuse)*; drinks 10 to 12 cups of coffee; and denies current use of drugs. (The actual patient record continues and indicates that a comprehensive history and examination was conducted; high MDM complexity.)

      CPT Code: _____

      ICD-9-CM Codes: _____, _____, _____

      (ICD-10-CM Codes: _____, _____, _____)

7 A new patient, a 10-year-old boy, is brought in by his father for a knee injury sustained in a hockey game. The knee is swollen and the patient is in apparent pain. A detailed history and examination are obtained. A diagnosis of medial collateral sprain of knee is made. Low MDM complexity.

      CPT Code: _____

      ICD-9-CM Code: _____ (ICD-10-CM Code: _____)

8 A 41-year-old woman, new to the office, complains of headache and rhinitis of 4 days' duration. The patient states that she has had a problem with her allergies during this season for years. An expanded problem focused history and examination are done. Straightforward MDM complexity. The diagnosis was grass pollen allergy.

      CPT Code: _____

      ICD-9-CM Code: _____ (ICD-10-CM Code: _____)

Established Patient. The second category of codes in subsection Office and Other Outpatient Services is for the established patient in an outpatient setting (99211-99215). You will recall that the definition of an established patient is one who has received face-to-face professional services from the physician or another physician of the same specialty in the same group within the past 3 years.

Code 99211 reports services provided in the office and for which the physician may not be present during the service but is in the office suite and is immediately available. Further, the employee providing the service must have the credentials necessary to provide the service, and the service must be part of a documented treatment plan. The physician should sign the documentation of the service.

QUICK CHECK 10-4

1. Could a physician assign 99211 to report a patient encounter? Yes or No?

EXERCISE 10-8 *Established Patient Services*

Fill in the blanks with information from codes in the Established Patient category:

1 99211: This minimal service level does not exist in the New Patient category because a new patient is seen by the physician. The established patient may or may not be seen by the physician. Read the description and information for code 99211 in the CPT manual. Would an established patient

returning for a simple blood pressure check be appropriately reported as 99211? _____

2 A 42-year-old established patient presents for an office visit with complaints of severe vaginal itching and moderate pain. During the expanded problem focused history, the patient states that several weeks earlier she had noted a slight itching, which has increased in severity. Yesterday, she noted a lesion on her genitalia. Burning and painful urination have increased over the past 5 days accompanied by rectal itching. She has tried a variety of over-the-counter ointments and creams, which induced no improvement. The patient states that she has had several yeast infections in the past that had been successfully treated by her previous physician. Personal history indicates several prior urinary infections. No discharge noted. A problem focused examination of the external genitalia reveals a lesion, which had previously ruptured, located on the vulva. Bacterial and viral smears are done. The MDM complexity is straightforward. The patient is advised that the smears would be back in 24 hours and that a treatment plan would be developed based on the reports. (The smear was positive for a bacterial infection, for which antibiotics were prescribed.)

   CPT Code: _____

3 A 17-year-old football player comes to the clinic for a 50 mg gold injection for an anterior cruciate knee sprain that occurred last week. The injection was given by the nurse. Only the nurse sees this established patient. (Code only the E/M service and diagnosis.)

   CPT Code: _____

   ICD-9-CM Code: _____ (ICD-10-CM Code: _____)

4 A 53-year-old established patient complains of frequent fainting. The history and examination are comprehensive, and the MDM is of high complexity.

   CPT Code: _____

   ICD-9-CM Code: _____ (ICD-10-CM Code: _____)

5 A 61-year-old established patient is seen for medication management of malaise and fatigue produced by hypertensive medication. An expanded problem focused history and examination are done, and the MDM is of moderate complexity.

   CPT Code: _____

   ICD-9-CM Codes: _____, _____, _____

   (ICD-10-CM Codes: _____, _____, _____)

6 An established 31-year-old patient presents with an irritated infected skin tag. A problem focused history and examination are done. MDM complexity is low.

   CPT Code: _____

   ICD-9-CM Code: _____ (ICD-10-CM Code: _____)

7 A 48-year-old woman has had diarrhea for the past 5 days. Her temperature is 101° F. An expanded problem focused history and examination are done. MDM complexity is low.

   CPT Code: _____

   ICD-9-CM Code: _____ (ICD-10-CM Code: _____)

Remember, it takes a lot of practice to learn to code. It is not a skill that is quickly acquired. You need to have patience and know that practice, practice, practice is the only thing that will make this skill yours.

Hospital Observation Services

The codes in the Hospital Observation subsection (99217-99220) identify initial observation care or observation discharge services. The services in the observation subsection are for patients who are in a hospital on observation status.

Observation is a status used for the classification of a patient who does not have an illness severe enough to meet acute inpatient criteria and does not require resources as intensive as an inpatient but does require hospitalization for a short period of time. Patients are also admitted to observation so further information can be obtained about the severity of the condition and to determine whether the patient can be treated on an outpatient basis. In some hospitals in some parts of the country, observation status is conducted in the temporary care unit (TCU).

The observation codes are for new or established patients. There are no time components with observation codes, as codes are based on the level of service. Each code from the range 99218-99220 requires all three of the key components to establish a level of service.

If a patient is admitted to the hospital as an inpatient after having been admitted earlier the same day as an observation patient, you do not report the observation status separately. The services provided during observation become part of (are bundled into) the initial inpatient hospital admission code.

QUICK CHECK 10-5

1. Are observation codes 99218-99220 reported for inpatient or outpatient services? _____

Observation Care Discharge Services. The Observation Care Discharge Services code (99217) includes the final examination of the patient upon discharge from observation status. Discussion of the hospital stay, instructions for continued care, and preparation of discharge records are also bundled into the Observation Care Discharge Services code. The code is used only with patients who are discharged on a day that follows the first day of observation.

Initial Observation Care. Initial Observation Care codes (99218-99220) designate the beginning of observation status in a hospital. Again, the hospital does not need to have a formal observation area, since the designation of observation status is dependent on the severity of illness of the patient. These codes also include development of a care plan for the patient and periodic reassessment while on observation status. Observation admission can be reported only for the first day of the service. If the patient is admitted and discharged on the same day, a code from the range 99234-99236, Observation or Inpatient Care Services, is assigned to report the service. If the patient is in the hospital overnight but remains there for a period that is **less than 48 hours,** the first day's service is reported with a code from the range 99218-99220, Initial Observation Care, and the second day's service is coded 99217, Observation Care Discharge Services. If the patient is on observation status for **longer than 48 hours**, the first day is reported with a code from the range 99218-99220, Initial Observation Care; the second day is reported with a code from the range 99212-99215, Established Office or Other Outpatient Services; and the third day is coded 99217, Observation Care Discharge Services.

Services performed in sites other than the observation area (e.g., clinic, nursing home, emergency department) and that precede admission to observation status are included in (bundled into) the Initial Observation Care codes and are not to be reported separately.

For example, an established patient was seen in the physician's office for frequent fainting of unknown origin. The history and examination were comprehensive and the MDM complexity was moderate. The code for the office visit would be 99215. But the physician decided to admit the patient immediately to observation status until a further determination could be made as to the origin of the fainting. You would assign a code from the Hospital Observation Services subsection, Initial Observation Care subheading, to report the physician's service of admission to observation status (99219) and would not separately report the office visit (99215).

If a patient is admitted to observation status and then becomes ill enough to be admitted to the hospital, an Initial Hospital Care code (99221-99223), not an observation code, is assigned to report services.

CAUTION *Observation or Inpatient Care Services (including admission and discharge service), codes 99234-99236, have a very specific purpose: to report services for a patient who is admitted to and discharged from observation or inpatient status on the **same day**. All the services provided to the patient—same-day office services, observation care, and discharge—are bundled into one code from the 99234-99236 range.*

NCCI

When reporting physician services (99234-99236), Medicare requires a patient to be admitted to observation status for **more than 8 hours** and discharged on the same date of service. A period of 8 hours or less is reimbursed as initial observation status (99218-99220), even if the patient is discharged on the same date.

EXERCISE 10-9 *Hospital Observation Services*

Using the CPT manual, code the following:

1 A patient was in an automobile accident and is complaining of a minor headache and no other apparent injuries. History gathered from bystanders states that patient was not wearing a seat belt and hit his head on the windshield. A 15-minute loss of consciousness was noted. The patient was diagnosed with a concussion. The patient was then admitted for 24-hour observation to rule out head injury. A comprehensive history and examination are done. The MDM is of moderate complexity.

  CPT Code: _____

  ICD-9-CM Code: _____ (ICD-10-CM Code: _____)

Hospital Inpatient Services

Hospital Inpatient Services codes (99221-99239) report a patient's status as an inpatient in a hospital or partial hospital setting and, therefore, to identify the hospital setting as the place where the physician renders service to the patient. An **inpatient** is one who has been formally admitted to an acute health care facility.

Note that within the subsection Hospital Inpatient Services, all the subheadings **except** Hospital Discharge Services are divided on the basis of the three key components of history, examination, and MDM complexity. Further, within this subsection only Subsequent Hospital Care codes do not require all three key components to be at the level described in the code. For example, the key components for code 99222 are a comprehensive history, a comprehensive examination, and a moderate level of MDM complexity. If the case you are coding has a comprehensive history and a comprehensive examination but a low complexity of MDM, you cannot assign code 99222 to the case; instead, you would have to assign the lower level code of 99221, which has a low complexity of MDM because the codes require three of the three key components to assign the code to a service.

The subsection of Hospital Inpatient Services is divided into two subheadings.

1. Initial Hospital Care
2. Subsequent Hospital Care

Initial Hospital Care.   Initial Hospital Care codes are used to report the initial service of admission to the hospital by the **admitting physician.** Only the admitting physician can report the Initial Hospital Care codes. These codes reflect services in any setting (office, emergency department, nursing home) that are provided in conjunction with the admission to the hospital. For example, if the patient is seen in the office and subsequently is admitted to the hospital the same day, the office visit is bundled into the initial hospital care service. All services provided in the office may be taken into account when selecting the appropriate level of hospital admission. This means that if the physician performed a comprehensive examination in the office, that level of examination is considered when determining the level of the hospital admission service.

EXERCISE 10-10 *Initial Hospital Care*

Fill in the missing words or codes for the following:

1 Which Initial Hospital Care code has a comprehensive history with a straightforward or low complexity of MDM?

CPT Code: _____

2 Which code has a time component of 70 minutes?

CPT Code: _____

3 Code 99222 has a _____ history and examination level and a _____ MDM complexity.

4 An 80-year-old woman has inflammation of the kidneys and renal pelvic area. She is complaining of hematuria, dysuria, and pyuria. She is in good general health other than this condition. She has had some previous workup for this condition as an outpatient but is now being admitted for a cystoscopy. In the patient's history, the physician noted the patient's chief complaints and described the bright red nature of the hematuria, the severe discomfort associated with the dysuria, including burning and itching, and her other symptoms of frequency and urgency. The patient had stated that her symptoms had begun gradually over the past 2 weeks but had become more intense in the past 48 hours. The physician documented the patient's positive responses and pertinent negative responses in his review of her cardiovascular, respiratory, genitourinary, musculoskeletal, neurologic, and endocrine systems. Her past history relating to urinary and renal problems was reviewed. The physical examination noted the complete findings relative to her reproductive system as well as to her urinary system. An examination of her back and related musculoskeletal structures was included because she complained of mild back pain as well. After completing the detailed history and examination, the physician concluded with a diagnosis of acute cystitis and acute pyelitis, possibly associated with endometritis. The MDM complexity was low. The patient was reassured and told to expect a short stay once the exact problem was pinpointed.

CPT Code: _____

ICD-9-CM Codes: _____, _____

(ICD-10-CM Codes: _____, _____)

Subsequent Hospital Care. Subsequent Hospital Care (99231-99239) is the second subheading of codes in the Hospital Inpatient Services subsection. The Subsequent Hospital Care codes are used by physicians to report daily hospital visits while the patient is hospitalized.

The first Subsequent Hospital Care code is 99231. Typically, the 99231 level implies that the patient is in stable condition and is responding well to treatment. Subsequent codes in the subsection indicate (in the "Usually, the patient…" area) the status of the patient, such as stable/unstable or recovering/unresponding. Be certain to read the contributory factors area for each code in this subheading.

A general rule of thumb for subsequent hospital services is as follows:

- Level 1 The patient is recovering and improving.
- Level 2 The patient has a minor complication or inadequate response to the current therapy.
- Level 3 The patient is unstable, has a significant complication, or has developed a new problem.

The patient's medical record should indicate the patient's progress from the status indicated in the previous note.

Several physicians, of different specialties, can report the subsequent care codes on the same day. This is called concurrent care. **Concurrent care** is being provided when more than one physician provides service to a patient on the same day for different conditions. An example of concurrent care is a circumstance in which physician A, a cardiologist, treats the patient for a heart condition and at the same time physician B, an oncologist, treats the patient for a cancer condition. The patient's attending (admitting) physician maintains the primary responsibility for the overall care of the patient, no matter how many other physicians are providing services to the patient, unless a formal transfer of care has occurred.

An **attending physician** is a doctor who, on the basis of education, training, and experience, is granted medical staff membership and clinical privileges by a health care organization to perform diagnostic and therapeutic procedures in the facility. An attending physician is legally responsible for the care and treatment provided to a patient. The attending physician may be a patient's personal physician or may be a physician assigned to a patient who has been admitted to a hospital through the emergency department. The attending physician is usually a provider of primary care, such as a family practitioner, internist, or pediatrician, but the attending physician may also be a surgeon or another type of specialist. In an academic medical center, the attending physician is a member of the academic or medical school staff who is responsible for the supervision of medical residents, interns, and medical school students and oversees the care the residents, interns, or students provide to the patients.

CODING SHOT

Note that there is no comprehensive history or comprehensive examination level in the codes in the Subsequent Hospital Care subheading because the comprehensive level of service would have been provided at the time of admission. Also note that only two of the three key components must be met or exceeded to assign a subsequent hospital code.

Observation or Inpatient Care Services (Including Admission and Discharge Services). Codes in the 99234-99236 range report services provided when the patient is admitted and discharged on the **same day**. For example, when the patient is admitted from observation status on the same day. Codes in this range require that all three of the key components must be at or exceed the level stated in the code description. These codes include both the admission service and the discharge service. Bundled into the admission are services that were provided in another location, such as the physician's office, nursing facility or emergency department. This means that the services provided in these other locations are considered when assigning a code from the 99234-99236 range.

Hospital Discharge Services. Inpatient Hospital Discharge Services (99238, 99239) are reported on the final day of services for a **multiple-day** stay in a hospital setting. The service reflects the final examination of the patient as appropriate, follow-up instructions to the patient, and arrangements for discharge, including completion of discharge records. The codes are based on the time spent by the physician in handling the final discharge of the patient and the time spent must be documented in the medical record.

The Hospital Discharge Services codes are not assigned if the physician is a consultant, unless the primary physician transfers complete care to the consultant. If a consulting physician is following the patient for a separate condition, those services would require a subsequent hospital care code. Only the attending physician, not the consultant, is responsible for completion of the final examination, follow-up instructions, and arrangements for discharge and discharge records. Because these additional services are included in the Hospital Discharge codes, only the attending physician's services can be reported using the codes.

Code 99239, discharge instructions greater than 30 minutes requires documentation of time spent performing the discharge instructions. If no indication of time is noted in the documentation, the lowest level of discharge service is reported.

QUICK CHECK 10-6

1. What is the one criterion for selecting a hospital discharge day management code? _____

EXERCISE 10-11 *Hospital Discharge Services*

Fill in the blanks:

1 What are the times indicated for each of the Hospital Discharge Services codes?

_____

2 According to the category notes in Hospital Discharge Services, does the time spent by the physician arranging for the final hospital discharge of the patient have to be continuous? _____

Consultation Services

We all need advice once in a while—maybe for a problem or situation that we cannot find a solution to. Perhaps we think we are doing the right thing but want another person's advice or view to make certain we are following the best course of action. Physicians need opinions and advice, too, and when they do, they ask another physician for an opinion or advice on the treatment, diagnosis, or management of a patient. The physician asking for the advice or opinion is making a **request for consultation** and is the **requesting** physician. The physician giving the advice is providing a consultation and is the **consultant.** Consultations can be provided to both outpatients and inpatients. The CPT manual has different codes for each of the two types of patient consultation—outpatient and inpatient.

"Request for consultation" used to be termed "referral"; making a referral means that the referring physician is asking for the advice or opinion of another physician (a consultation). However, some third-party payers have chosen to define **referral** to mean a total transfer of the care of a patient. In other words, if a patient is referred by physician A to physician B, physician A is expecting physician B to evaluate and treat (assume care for) the patient for the condition for which the patient is being referred. The services of physician B would then **not** be reported using consultation codes. On the other hand, if physician A makes a **request for a consultation** to physician B, it is expected that physician B will provide physician A with his or her advice or opinion and that the patient will return to physician A for any necessary treatment. Physician B would then report his or her services using consultation codes. Although these semantics (uses of words) may seem unimportant, they make a difference in the codes you assigned to report the services.

QUICK CHECK 10-7

1. The criteria required to report a consultation include:

_____ from the attending to the consultant to see the patient, evaluation of the patient by the consultant _____ back to the attending of the findings and recommendations of the consultant

In the Consultation subsection (99241-99255), there are two subheadings of consultations:

1. Office or Other Outpatient Consultations
2. Inpatient Consultations

These subheadings define the location in which the service is rendered; the patient is an outpatient or an inpatient.

Only one initial consultation is reported by a consultant for the patient on each admission, and any subsequent service is reported using codes from the Subsequent Hospital Care codes (99231-99233) or Office or Other Outpatient Services, established patient (99211-99215). If more than one consultation is ordered on an inpatient, each consultant may report the initial consultation using the Inpatient Consultation codes (99251-99255).

A **consultation** is a service provided by a physician whose opinion or advice regarding the management or diagnosis of a specific problem has been requested. The consultant provides a written report of the opinion or advice to the attending physician and documents the opinion and services provided in the medical record; the care of the patient is thus complete. Sometimes the attending physician will request the consultant to assume responsibility for a specific area of the patient's care. For example, a consultant may be asked by the attending physician to see an inpatient regarding the care of the patient's diabetes while the patient is hospitalized for gallbladder surgery. After the initial consultation, the attending physician may ask the consultant to continue to monitor the patient's diabetic condition. The consultant assumes responsibility for management of the patient in the specific area of diabetes. Subsequent visits made by the consultant would then be reported using the codes from the subheading Subsequent Hospital Care or Subsequent Nursing Facility Care.

Documentation in the medical record for a consultation must show a request from a physician for an opinion or the advice of a consultant for a specific condition. Findings and treatments rendered during the consultation must be documented in the medical record by the consulting physician and communicated to the requesting physician. The consulting physician can order tests and services for a patient, but the medical necessity of all tests and services must be indicated in the medical record.

Office or Other Outpatient Consultations. The Office or Other Outpatient Consultations codes (99241-99245) report consultative services provided to a patient in an office setting, including hospital observation services, home services, custodial care, and services that are provided in a domiciliary, rest home, or emergency department. Outpatient consultations include consultations provided in the emergency department because the patient is considered an outpatient in the emergency department setting. The codes are for both new and established patients. The codes in this subsection are of increasing complexity, based on the three key components and any contributory factors.

From the Trenches

"Keep the lines of communication open with fellow students, former instructors, co-workers, and the medical staff for whom you code. If you can establish yourself as someone who is dedicated to doing your work with integrity, interact with respect, and is always willing to help out, you will be successful."

JOAN

Inpatient Consultations.   The codes in the Inpatient Consultations subheading (99251-99255) report services by physicians in inpatient settings. This subheading is used for both new and established patients and can be reported only one time per patient admission, per consulting physician, per specialty.

After the initial consultation report, the subsequent hospital or nursing facility codes would be assigned to report services.

The office and inpatient consultation codes (99241-99255) require documentation in the medical record to support all three of the key components listed in the code description. For example, 99243, office consultation, requires a detailed history and examination as well as a low level of medical decision making complexity. Let's say the documentation indicated a detailed history and examination, but only a straightforward level of medical decision making. Code 99243 could not be reported because only two of the three key components were at the correct level. The lower level code, 99242, would be assigned.

Various people request consultations on a recommended treatment or diagnosis. Insurance companies or other third-party payers may request a consultation regarding a diagnosis, prognosis, or treatment plan for a patient. These types of consultations are also reported based on the location of the service—office or inpatient. If the consultation is mandated, such as those required by an insurance company or a required school physical, add modifier -32 (Mandated Service) to the code. This modifier is only added if the consultation is mandated by an official body.

For office consultations, a written or verbal request stating results is sent to the requesting physician. This is not necessary with an inpatient because the physicians share the patient's medical record and the inpatient consultant would dictate a consultation report to be included in the medical record.

QUICK CHECK 10-8

1. Can time be utilized to determine a consultation level of service rather than the key components?

   Yes or No?

EXERCISE 10-12 *Consultation Services*

Using the CPT manual, code the visit in the following scenarios:

1 A 56-year-old female was sent at the request of her primary care physician (PCP) to the oncologist for his opinion regarding the treatment options. The patient had had a right breast carcinoma 6 years earlier but over the past 4 months had developed progressively more painful back pain. In the physician's HPI it was noted that the pain was in the mid-back, with the patient rating it an 8 in intensity on a scale of 1 to 10. However, when the pain started, she thought it was about a 4 on the same scale. The pain has caused her to have neck and leg pains as well, as she has adjusted her walking stance in order to alleviate the pain. She responded to the physician's questions in the review of 10 of her organ systems. Her past medical and surgical history was noted, including the fact that her mother and one sister had also had breast cancer. A comprehensive history was taken. She had worked as a legal secretary up until 2 weeks earlier but is now on sick leave. The comprehensive physical examination performed by the physician was a complete multisystem review of 12 organ systems. The physician ordered a series of radiographic and laboratory tests and reviewed her recent spine x-ray series, which revealed multiple pathologic vertebral compression fractures. The MDM complexity was moderate.

    CPT Code: _____

    ICD-9-CM Codes: _____, _____

    (ICD-10-CM Codes: _____, _____)

2 A 45-year-old man was sent by his PCP to an orthopedic surgeon's office for acute pain and stiffness in his right elbow. In his problem focused history, the physician noted that the man was a farmer and used his right hand and arm repeatedly, lifting heavy objects. The patient had no other complaints and reported to be in otherwise excellent health. The patient described the pain as severe and unrelenting, and it prevented him from using his arm. The problem focused physical examination noted the man's slightly swollen right elbow, with marked pain on movement. No other problems were noted with his right upper extremity. The physician diagnosed the problem as elbow tendinitis and bursitis, recommended warm compresses, and gave the patient a prescription for an anti-inflammatory medication. The MDM complexity was straightforward.

    CPT Code: _____

    ICD-9-CM Codes: _____, _____

    (ICD-10-CM Codes: _____, _____)

3 A 72-year-old man was seen in the internal medicine clinic as an outpatient for medical clearance prior to the replacement of his right knee due to localized primary osteoarthritis. The patient had a history of essential hypertension and mild coronary artery disease. The internist noted, during the expanded problem focused history, that the patient had no complaints relative to his hypertension or heart disease. His blood pressure appeared to be controlled by his medication and low-salt diet. The patient denied any chest pain or discomfort either while working or at rest. In the physician's review, his cardiovascular and respiratory systems appeared to be negative. The physician performed an expanded problem focused physical examination of his head, neck, chest, and abdomen but found no major problems related to his cardiovascular or respiratory system. The internist confirmed the diagnoses previously established and made no changes in the management of either condition. The MDM complexity was straightforward.

    CPT Code: _____

    ICD-9-CM Code: _____ (ICD-10-CM Code: _____)

Continued

4 A 52-year-old patient was sent to a surgeon for an office consultation concerning bleeding internal hemorrhoids. A problem focused history and examination were performed. The consultant recommended treating with medication after a straightforward MDM.

    CPT Code: _____

    ICD-9-CM Code: _____ (ICD-10-CM Code: _____)

5 A 60-year-old man was seen in consultation by a cardiologist in the clinic for complaints of dyspnea, fatigue, and lightheadedness. His history included the insertion of a pacemaker 6 years earlier. He also had a history of mitral regurgitation. The cardiologist performed a comprehensive cardiology physical examination, including cardiac monitoring, pacemaker evaluation, and review of his associated respiratory status. Noted in the comprehensive history were a variety of complaints the patient had in addition to the past pacemaker insertion and current mitral valve regurgitation diagnosed by cardiac catheterization. The physician reviewed the patient's medical history, from the first signs of problems 6 years earlier until the present. His review of systems elicited positive findings in the cardiovascular, respiratory, gastrointestinal, genitourinary, musculoskeletal, and neurologic systems. The other systems had negative responses. The physician had multiple management options concerning the pacemaker function but also had to consider new valvular problems that might have been present as well as related gastrointestinal symptoms. Extensive tests that had been performed recently were reviewed, and additional testing was ordered. The MDM complexity was moderate.

    CPT Code: _____

    ICD-9-CM Codes: _____ (dyspnea), _____ (fatigue),

        _____ (dizziness), _____ (mitral insufficiency),

        _____ (V code for status, cardiac device, pacemaker)

    (ICD-10-CM Codes: _____, _____, _____,

        _____, _____)

6 A 65-year-old man had recently undergone a prostatectomy for prostate cancer. Since the surgery, his previously controlled atrial fibrillation had become a problem again. A cardiologist was called in for an inpatient consultation; he reviewed the patient's present status, including the duration and severity of his symptoms. The cardiologist's review of systems related strictly to the cardiovascular system during an expanded problem focused history. The expanded problem focused physical examination concentrated on the man's neck, chest, and abdomen and attempted to elicit all cardiovascular pathology. The consultant suggested that the atrial fibrillation could be controlled better with a different medication. The MDM complexity was straightforward.

    CPT Code: _____

    ICD-9-CM Code: _____ (ICD-10-CM Code: _____)

7 An internist requested an inpatient consultation from an orthopedic surgeon to evaluate and manage a 35-year-old female who had been in a motor vehicle accident. After reviewing the multiple x-ray reports and the documentation generated by the emergency department physicians, the paramedics' progress notes from the scene of the accident, and the history and physical examination produced by the internist, the orthopedist performed a complete review of systems; complete past, family, and social history; and extended details of the history of the present illness in a comprehensive history review. The comprehensive physical examination was a complete musculoskeletal and neurologic examination with a review of all other organ systems. Based on the patient's multiple fractures and internal injuries, the orthopedist concluded that the patient needed immediate surgery to repair and control the life-threatening conditions that existed. The MDM complexity was high. A neurosurgeon and a general surgeon were also asked to see the patient immediately and possibly to assist in surgery. (Code only the orthopedic consultation.)

    CPT Code: _____

8 A 55-year-old patient was injured at work when he fell from a house roof and struck his head. He was admitted for a right frontal parietal craniotomy with removal of a subdural hematoma. After 5 days of rapid recovery from this surgery, a consultation was requested regarding a drug reaction that produced a rash on his upper torso. The physician conducted a brief HPI during the expanded problem focused history, in addition to an ROS focused on the patient's condition. The expanded problem focused examination included three body areas and one organ system. The MDM complexity was straightforward.

CPT Code: _____

9 A 10-year-old was admitted 4 days ago for tympanotomy. Postsurgically, the child developed febrile seizures of unknown origin. A pediatric consultation was requested. The HPI was extended with a complete ROS. A complete PFSH was elicited from the mother as part of a comprehensive history. A comprehensive examination was conducted on all body areas and organ systems. The MDM complexity was high.

CPT Code: _____

ICD-9-CM Code: _____ (ICD-10-CM Code: _____)

10 A cardiologist was asked by a family practitioner to see an 80-year-old male inpatient a second time. One week prior, the patient, who had multiple other medical problems, had suffered an anterior wall myocardial infarction. Despite following the medical management suggested by the cardiologist, the patient continued to have angina and ventricular tachycardia. The cardiologist closely examined all of the documentation and test results that had been generated in the past week and performed a complete ROS and an extended HPI during the detailed interval history. The detailed physical examination performed was a complete cardiovascular system examination. Based on the subjective and objective findings, the cardiologist concluded that more aggressive medical management was in order. Given the patient's multiple problems coupled with the new threat of cardiorespiratory failure, the patient was immediately transferred to the intensive care unit. The MDM was of high complexity.

CPT Code: _____

ICD-9-CM Code: _____ (ICD-10-CM Code: _____)

11 The attending physician had requested an inpatient consultation on a 10-year-old admitted 7 days earlier for tympanotomy. Postsurgically, the patient developed fever and seizures. An initial consultation diagnosis was febrile seizure. Now, on day 7, the child's temperature had returned to normal but the child had had a recurrence of seizures of increased severity. A follow-up consultation was requested. The consultant performed a detailed history and physical examination. The MDM was of high complexity.

CPT Code: _____

ICD-9-CM Code: _____ (ICD-10-CM Code: _____)

12 Dr. Jones asked Dr. Williams to confirm the diagnosis of tetralogy of Fallot in a 6-day-old male infant prior to cardiovascular surgery. The patient was seen in the office, where Dr. Williams performed an initial comprehensive history and physical examination on the infant and reviewed the results of the extensive tests already performed. The consultant confirmed the diagnosis and concluded that the child's problem was of high severity and recommended immediate surgery. The MDM complexity was moderate.

CPT Code: _____

ICD-9-CM Code: _____ (ICD-10-CM Code: _____)

Continued

13 The 45-year-old female's insurance company required a second opinion regarding the degenerative disc disease of her lumbar spine. One orthopedic surgeon had recommended a laminectomy. A second orthopedic surgeon was consulted in the office and performed an expanded problem focused history and physical examination, particularly of her musculoskeletal and neurologic systems. Based on his findings and the conclusive findings of a recent myelogram, the second orthopedic surgeon was quick to conclude that the laminectomy was a reasonable course to follow. The MDM complexity was straightforward.

      CPT Code: _____

14 A third-party payer sought consultation for confirmation about a patient's ability to return to work after the removal of a subdural hematoma 2 months previously. The patient's primary physician had stated that the patient was not yet able to return to his employment, and the third-party payer wanted a second opinion. The patient stated that he continued to have severe and incapacitating headaches and was unable to return to work. A comprehensive history and physical examination were performed in the office. The MDM was of moderate complexity, based on physician findings.

      CPT Code: _____

Emergency Department Services

Emergency Department Services codes (99281-99288) are assigned for new or established patients when services are provided in an emergency department (ED) that is a part of a hospital and ED is available 24 hours a day. These patients are presenting for immediate attention. The codes are assigned for patients without appointments. Emergency Department Services codes are not assigned for patients at the hospital on observation status, even if the observation unit is located at or near the emergency department.

Codes 99281-99285 are based on the type of service the physician performs in terms of the history, the examination, and the complexity of the MDM. These codes require all three of the key components to be assigned. In addition to this information within each code, note that the paragraph at the end of each code that begins with "Usually, the presenting problem(s) are of…" identifies the immediacy of the care. For example, 99283 indicates that the presenting problem is of "moderate severity," whereas 99285 indicates that the presenting problem is of "high severity and poses an immediate significant threat to life…" Sometimes the patient's clinical condition poses an immediate threat to life, making it possible for the physician to use the higher level code even if it may not be possible to perform the required history and physical examination.

QUICK CHECK 10-9

1. What are the times associated with codes 99281-99285? _____
2. If a patient presents to the emergency department in a clinically life-threatening state that prevents the physician from performing a complete history or physical examination, could the code 99285 still be reported?

   Yes or No?

Critical care provided to a patient in the emergency department is reported using additional codes from the Critical Care Service code section, which we will discuss later in this chapter.

If a patient initially treated in the emergency department requires admittance to the hospital, the patient's attending physician would serve as the admitting physician.

Emergency department codes can be assigned to report the services not only of the ED physician, but also of any physician who cares for a patient in the ED. For example, if the patient's primary care physician (PCP) meets the patient at the ED or is called into the ED, and the PCP cares for the patient in the ED, not admitting the patient to the hospital, then the PCP reports the services using ED codes. Note that in this instance, the PCP was NOT a cunsultant but was serving as the patient physician in the emergency room location.

Also, ED physicians do not admit patients to a hospital. If a patient is seen in the ED and has to be admitted to the hospital, the patient's PCP or other designated physician will admit the patient. An example of a designated physician would be a hospitalist. A **hospitalist** is a hospital-based physician who only sees patients in the hospital and assumes the responsibility of the primary care physician for hospitalized patients. This is a relatively new approach to hospital coverage, but is fast gaining popularity.

Other Emergency Department Services.   The Other Emergency Department Services subheading is at the end of the Emergency Department Services subsection, and the code located there (99288) reports the services of a physician based at the hospital who provides two-way communication with the ambulance or rescue team. This physician provides direction and advice to the team as they attend the patient en route to the emergency department.

The subheading notes contain examples of the types of medical services the physician might direct. Be certain to read these notes so you understand the types of services the code refers to.

EXERCISE 10-13 *Emergency Department Services*

Use the information contained in the code descriptions in the Emergency Department Services subsection to answer the questions in this exercise.

1 The severity of the presenting problem for Code 99281 would usually be _____.

2 The severity of the presenting problem for Code 99284 would usually be _____.

3 The severity of the presenting problem for Code 99283 would usually be _____.

4 The severity of the presenting problem for Code 99282 would usually be _____.

Code the following:

5 A patient in the emergency department has extreme acute chest pains and goes into cardiac arrest. The emergency department physician is unable to obtain a history or perform a physical examination because the patient's condition is critical. The MDM is of high complexity.

   CPT Code: _____

   ICD-9-CM Code: _____ (ICD-10-CM Code: _____)

6 A patient in the emergency department has a temperature of 105° F and is in acute respiratory distress. Symptoms include shortness of breath, chest pain, cyanosis, and gasping. The physician is unable to obtain a history or perform a comprehensive physical examination because the patient's condition is critical. The MDM complexity is high.

   CPT Code: _____

   ICD-9-CM Code: _____ (ICD-10-CM Code: _____)

7 A child presents to the emergency department with his parents after being bitten by a dog. The child is in extreme pain and bleeding from a wound on the forearm. The animal has not been located to quarantine for rabies. An expanded problem focused history is obtained and an expanded problem focused physical examination is performed. The MDM complexity is moderate because of the possibility of rabies.

   CPT Code: _____

8 The physician directs the emergency medical technicians via two-way communications with an ambulance en route to the emergency department with a patient in apparent cardiac arrest.

   CPT Code: _____

Critical Care Services

Critical Care Services codes (99291, 99292) identify services that are provided during medical emergencies to patients over 24 months of age who are either critically ill or injured. These codes require the physician to be constantly available to the patient and providing services exclusively to that patient. For example, a patient who is in shock or cardiac arrest would require the physician to provide bedside critical care services. Critical care is often, but not required to be, provided in an acute care setting of a hospital. Acute care settings are intensive care units, coronary care units, emergency departments, and similar critical care units of a hospital. Codes in this subsection are listed according to the time the physician spends providing critical care to the patient. The time calculation is not just the face-to-face time the physician spends with the patient. The review of records and diagnostic results at the time of the encounter should also be counted in determining the time spent in providing critical care to the patient.

   The time the physician spends in providing other procedures must be deducted from the total critical care time. For example, if an adult patient is intubated during critical care, the time spent on the intubation (31500) is deducted from the total critical care time because the physician will report the intubation service separately.

The total critical care time, per day, the physician spends in care of the patient is stated in one amount of time, even if the time was not continuous. Code 99291 is reported only once a day for the first 30 to 74 minutes of critical care, and 99292 is reported for each additional 30 minutes beyond 74 minutes. If the critical care is less than 30 minutes, an E/M code would be assigned to report the service.

TOTAL DURATION OF CRITICAL CARE TIME	CPT CODES REPORTED
Less than 30 minutes	appropriate E/M code
30-74 minutes	99291 × 1
75-104 minutes	99291 × 1 and 99292 × 1
105-134 minutes	99291 × 1 and 99292 × 2
135-164 minutes	99291 × 1 and 99292 × 3
165-194 minutes	99291 × 1 and 99292 × 4
194 minutes or longer	99291 and 99292 as appropriate

As an example, if a physician sees a critical care patient for 74 minutes and then leaves and returns for 30 minutes of critical care at a later time in the same day, the coding would be for 104 minutes of care. The coding for 104 minutes would be:

99291 for the 74 minutes

99292 for the additional 30 minutes

CODING SHOT Most third-party payers will not pay for more than one physician at a time for critical care services.

There are service codes that are bundled into the Critical Care Services codes. These services are normally provided to stabilize the patient. An example of this bundling is as follows: A physician starts ventilation management (94002) while providing critical care services to a patient in the intensive care unit of a hospital. The ventilator management is not reported separately but, instead, is considered to be bundled into the Critical Care Services code. The notes preceding the critical care codes in the CPT manual list the services and procedures bundled into the codes. If the physician provided a service at the same time as critical care and that service is not bundled into the code, the service could be reported separately. Some third-party payers may require the use of modifier -25 with the critical care codes when reporting a service that is not bundled into the Critical Care Services. You will know what is bundled into the codes because this information is listed either in the extensive description of the code or in the notes preceding the code. Be certain to read these notes, as they contain many exclusions and inclusions for these codes.

If the patient is in a critical care unit but is stable, you report the services using codes from the Hospital Inpatient Services subsection, Subsequent Hospital Care subheading or from the Consultations subsection, Inpatient subheading.

QUICK CHECK 10-10

1. List two types of service and the CPT code for the service that are bundled into critical care services.

Such as: Gastric intubation (43752, 91105)

_____

_____

EXERCISE 10-14 *Critical Care Services*

Fill in the information for the following:

1 Critical care is provided to the patient for 70 minutes.

   🔗 CPT Code(s): _____

2 Can code 99292 be reported without code 99291? _____

3 A physician is called to the intensive care unit to provide care for a patient who has received second-degree burns over 50% of his body. The physician provides support for 2 hours. After leaving the unit, the physician returns later that day to provide an additional hour of critical care support to the patient.

   🔗 CPT Code(s): _____

   🔗 ICD-9-CM Code(s): _____   (🔗 ICD-10-CM Code(s): _____)

Nursing Facility Services

A **nursing facility** is not a hospital but does have inpatient beds and a professional health care staff that provides health care to persons who do not require the level of service provided in an acute care facility.

A **skilled nursing facility** (SNF) is one that has a professional staff that often includes physicians and nurses. The patients of a skilled nursing facility require less care than that given in an acute care hospital, but more care than that provided in a nursing home. Skilled nursing facilities are also called skilled nursing units, skilled nursing care, or extended care facilities. Professional and practical nursing services are available 24 hours a day. Rehabilitation services, such as occupational therapy, physical therapy, and speech therapy, are available on a daily basis. A skilled nursing facility was previously called an extended care facility. Patients may stay for several weeks in a skilled nursing facility before returning home or being transferred to an intermediate care facility for long-term care. Skilled nursing facilities provide care for individuals of all ages, even though the majority of services are provided to geriatric patients.

An **intermediate care facility** provides regular, basic health services to individuals who do not need the degree of care or treatment provided in a hospital or a skilled nursing facility. Residents, because of their mental or physical conditions, require assistance with their activities of daily living, such as bathing, dressing, eating, and ambulating. Intermediate care facilities generally provide long-term care, usually over several years. Professional and practical nursing services are available on a 24-hour basis. Activities, social services, and dietary and other therapies are available on a daily basis. The majority of residents of intermediate care facilities are geriatric individuals or individuals of any age with developmental disabilities.

The **long-term care facility** describes health and personal services provided to ill, aged, disabled, or mentally handicapped individuals for an extended period of time. Other types of facilities are better described as skilled or intermediate care facilities.

Four subheadings of nursing facility services are available: Initial Nursing Facility Care, Subsequent Nursing Facility Care, Nursing Facility Discharge Services, and Other Nursing Facility Services.

Initial Nursing Facility Care.   Initial Nursing Facility Care codes (99304-99306) do not distinguish between new and established patients. These codes report services provided by the physician at the time of admission or re-admission. Assessments by physicians play a central role in the development of the resident's individualized care plan. The care plan is developed by an interdisciplinary care team using the Resident Assessment Instrument (RAI) and the Minimum Data Set (MDS).

CHECK THIS OUT ☞   The MDS forms are located on the CMS website at www.cms.hhs.gov/NursingHomeQualityInits/Downloads/MDS20MDSAllForms.pdf

Subsequent Nursing Facility Care.   Subsequent Nursing Facility Care codes (99307-99310) do not distinguish between a new and an established patient. These codes reflect services provided by a physician on a periodic basis when a resident does not need a comprehensive assessment. Typically, such a resident has not had a major change in his or her condition since the previous physician visit but requires ongoing management of a chronic condition or treatment of an acute short-term problem. The higher level codes are assigned to patients with new problems or significant changes in existing problems.

Nursing Facility Discharge Services.   The Nursing Facility Discharge Services codes (99315, 99316) report the services the physician renders to the patient on the day of discharge. The codes are assigned based on the amount of time documented for discharge management. Code 99315 is assigned if 30 minutes or less or when no time is documented. Code 99316 is reported for documented time of greater than 30 minutes. The time spent need not be continuous or spent entirely with the patient but must be documented. The physician may conduct a final physical examination, give instructions to the patient's caregivers, and prepare all necessary discharge documentation, referral forms, and medication orders.

Other Nursing Facility Services.   Other Nursing Facility Services contains only one code, 99318, and reports the annual nursing facility assessment provided by the physician. By law, the nursing facility must conduct a comprehensive assessment of each resident at least once a year and determine if there is any significant change in the resident's physical or mental condition. As with many subheadings throughout the E/M section, if a patient is admitted to a nursing facility but the service was started elsewhere, such as a physician's office or emergency department, all the evaluation and management services provided to the patient in these other locations are considered part of the nursing facility code. For example, a patient was seen in the hospital emergency department, where a comprehensive history and examination were performed for a condition that required high MDM complexity (99285, Emergency Department Services). The physician made the decision to admit the patient to a nursing facility on the same day. Rather than reporting 99285 (Emergency Department Services), you would report the same level service from the subheading Initial Nursing Facility Care, 99306.

Nursing Facility Services codes are also assigned for services in a type of place you would not think would apply—psychiatric residential treatment centers. The center must be a stand-alone facility or a separate part of a facility that provides group living facilities and must have 24-hour staffing. Nursing Facility Services codes identify evaluation and management services. If a physician also provides medical psychotherapy, you would report those services separately.

When a patient has been in the hospital and is discharged from the hospital to a nursing facility, all on the same day, you can report the hospital discharge (99238-99239) and the nursing facility admission (99304-99306) separately. This is also true for same-day services for patients who are discharged from observation status (99217) and admitted to a nursing facility (99304-99306).

EXERCISE 10-15 *Nursing Facility Services*

Answer the following:

1 According to the code description for 99305, the usual level of severity of the problem(s) that

required admission to the nursing facility is: _____

2 A 72-year-old male patient is transferred to a nursing facility from a hospital after suffering a cerebrovascular accident (stroke) with cerebral infarction. The patient needs a comprehensive assessment before his active rehabilitation plan can be started. A comprehensive history is gathered by the internist, including the patient's chief complaint of paralysis and weakness, an extended HPI, and a complete ROS. Details of the patient's past, family, and social history add information to the care-planning process. The internist performs a comprehensive multisystem physical examination. After much deliberation with the multidisciplinary rehabilitation team, the physician determines that the patient is ready for active rehabilitation. The physician also writes orders to continue treatment of the patient's other medical conditions, including hypertension and diabetes. The MDM complexity is high.

    CPT Code: _____

    ICD-9-CM Codes: _____, _____, _____

    (ICD-10-CM Codes: _____, _____, _____)

Using the following information within the code descriptions in the Subsequent Nursing Facility Care subheading, match the medical decision making complexity in the description of the code with the code:

3 99307 _____   a. moderate

4 99308 _____   b. low

5 99309 _____   c. straightforward

Code the following:

6 Subsequent follow-up care is provided for a comatose patient transferred to a long-term care center from the hospital. The resident shows no signs of consciousness on examination but appears to have developed a minor upper respiratory tract infection with a fever and cough. The physician performs an expanded problem focused interval history (by way of nursing staff notes) and physical examination, including neurologic status, respiratory status, and status of related organ systems. Because the physician is concerned that the existing respiratory infection could progress to pneumonia, appropriate treatment is ordered. The MDM complexity is moderate.

    CPT Code: _____

    ICD-9-CM Codes: _____, _____

    (ICD-10-CM Codes: _____, _____)

Domiciliary, Rest Home (e.g., Boarding Home), or Custodial Care Services

These codes (99324-99337) are divided into subheadings based on the patients' status as new or established service provided. The codes are arranged in levels based on the documentation in the patient's medical record. Time estimates are established for codes in this category.

These codes are reported for the evaluation and management of residents who reside in a domiciliary, rest home, or custodial care center. Generally, health services are not available on site, nor are any medical services included in the codes. These facilities provide residential care, including lodging, meals, supervision, personal care, and leisure activities, to persons who, because of their physical, mental, or emotional condition, are not able to live independently. Such facilities might include alternative living residences, assisted living facilities, retirement centers, community-based living units, group homes, or residential treatment centers. These facilities provide custodial care for residents of all ages.

Domiciliary, Rest Home (e.g., Assisted Living Facility), or Home Care Plan Oversight Services

Codes 99339, 99340 apply to services provided to a patient who is being cared for at home and not enrolled with a home health care agency. These patients are being cared for by family members, health care professionals, and other types of caregivers. These codes are not reported if the patient is receiving his or her care from a home health agency, hospice program, or nursing facility. When reporting these codes the patient is not present, rather the physician is developing a care plan or overseeing the care of the patient. The physician's time may be reported if the time was over 15 minutes within a calendar month. Code 99339 reports 15-29 minutes, and 99340 reports 30 minutes or more. Again, these codes are only reported once for each calendar month.

Home Services

Health care services can also be provided to patients in their homes. Times have been established for this category of services. Note that there is a statement about typical time located under the code description in the paragraph that begins, "Usually, the presenting problem(s) is…" Never report a code based on time unless at least 50% of the time was spent on counseling or coordinating care. The codes (99341-99350) for these services are also divided into categories for new and for established patients.

From the Trenches

"I have found that there is definitely a sense of family among coders. Like all families, we don't always agree on everything, but we care about each other's thoughts and challenges . . . and know that there is always someone out there that can be there for you, whether it is a coding dilemma or a bigger, career-type decision."

JOAN

EXERCISE 10-16 *Home Services*

Code the following scenario:

1 A 64-year-old established female patient has diabetes mellitus and has been having problems adjusting her insulin doses. She has had an onset of dizziness and sensitivity to light. The physician makes a home visit during which he gathers a brief HPI and a problem-pertinent ROS during the problem focused history. The problem focused physical examination focuses on the body systems currently affected by the diabetes. The physician finds the patient's condition to be moderately severe and the MDM complexity is straightforward.

      CPT Code: _____

Prolonged Services

In the Prolonged Services subsection there are three subheadings:

- Prolonged Physician Service *With* Direct (Face-to-Face) Patient Contact
- Prolonged Physician Service *Without* Direct (Face-to-Face) Patient Contact
- Physician Standby Services

Prolonged Physician Services With or Without Direct Patient Contact. Prolonged Physician Services codes (99354-99359) are all add-on codes. Note the plus symbol (+) beside all codes in the 99354-99359 range. Because add-on codes can be reported only with another code, all Prolonged Physician Services codes are intended to be used only in addition to other codes to show an extension of some other service. The time is to be documented in the medical record to support the submission of the Prolonged Care code(s). The following example illustrates the use of these codes.

> **Example**
>
> An established patient with a history of COPD presents, in an office visit, with acute bronchospasm and moderate respiratory distress. The physician conducts a problem focused history followed by a problem focused examination, which shows a respiratory rate of 30, and labored breathing and wheezing are heard in all lung fields. Office treatment is initiated; it includes intermittent bronchial dilation and subcutaneous epinephrine. The service requires the physician to have intermittent face-to-face contact with the patient over a 2-hour period. The MDM complexity is low.

The office visit service would be reported using the office visit code 99212 (which has 10 minutes as the usual time); but the additional time the physician spent providing service to the patient over and above that which is indicated in code 99212 would have to be reported using a prolonged service code.

✋ **CAUTION** *If you hadn't carefully read the notes preceding the Prolonged Services codes, you would not know that there are many rules that govern the calculation of time when determining the codes.*

As the notes indicate, the first 30 minutes of prolonged services are not even counted but are considered part of the initial service. So you cannot use a prolonged services code until after the first 30 minutes of the prolonged services have been provided. The physician, therefore, has to spend 30 minutes with the patient in prolonged services before it is possible to report any prolonged service time.

The reporting on this service is as follows:

120 minutes spent with patient
−10 minutes for the usual time in 99212
110 minutes remaining

According to the grid before 99354, for 105 minutes or more you are to report 99354 × 1 and 99355 × 2.

The time the physician spends providing the prolonged services does not have to be continuous, as is the situation in this example; the physician monitored the patient on an intermittent basis, coming into the room to check on the patient and then leaving the room.

But let's change this case a bit and see how the coding changes. If the physician spent 70 minutes with the patient, you could code only the first hour at 99354. The additional 10 minutes beyond the first 60 are not coded separately. Remember that you would need at least 15 minutes beyond the first hour to code for the time beyond the first hour. For help in applying these codes, refer to the table preceding the codes; there you can locate the total time your physician spent with the patient and see an example of the correct coding.

The face-to-face Prolonged Physician Services codes describe services that require the physician to have **direct contact** with the patient; but the Prolonged Physician Services Without Direct (Face-to-Face) Patient Contact codes describe services during which the physician is not in direct contact with the patient. For example, a physician evaluates an established patient, a 70-year-old female with dementia, in an office visit. The physician then spends an extensive amount of time discussing the patient's condition, her treatment plan, and other recommendations with the daughter of the patient. The services would be reported by using an office visit code for the patient evaluation and the appropriate prolonged service without face-to-face contact code for the time spent with the daughter.

Prolonged Physician Services codes are most often reported with the higher level E/M codes, which themselves carry longer time frames. According to the CPT notes for Prolonged Physician Services, these codes are add-on codes and are reported in addition to another E/M code.

Prolonged Physician Services With Direct Patient Contact codes are divided on the basis of whether the services were provided to an outpatient or an inpatient.

Physician Standby Services. The code (99360) for Physician Standby Services is reported when a physician, at the request of another physician, is standing by in case his or her services are needed. The standby physician cannot be rendering services to another patient during this time. The standby code is reported in increments of 30 minutes. The 30-minute increments referred to here really mean from the first minute to the 30th minute and do not have any of the complicated rules for reporting time that exist for reporting prolonged services.

An important note concerning the standby code is that this code is reported only when **no service** is performed and there is **no face-to-face contact** with the patient. This code is not reported when a standby status ends, and the physician is providing a service to a patient. The service the physician provides is reported as any other service would be, even though it began as a physician standby service.

CODING SHOT — To report standby services, there must be a written request for standby services in the medical record.

Read the notes before Code 99360 before completing Exercise 10-17.

EXERCISE 10-17 *Prolonged and Physician Standby Services*

Using the notes in the subsections, answer the following:

1 Does the time the physician spends with the patient in prolonged, direct contact have to be continuous? _____

2 Can a code from the Prolonged Services subsection be reported alone? _____

3 If the prolonged contact with the patient lasts less than 30 minutes, is the time reported separately? _____

4 The codes in the Prolonged Physician Services With Direct Patient Contact subheading are based not only on the time the physician spends with the patient, but also on another factor. What is that other factor? _____

5 Are the codes in the subheading Prolonged Physician Services Without Direct Patient Contact categorized according to the place of service? _____

6 According to the notes in the Physician Standby Services subsection, can a physician report the time spent in proctoring (monitoring) another physician? _____

Case Management Services

The Case Management Services subsection (99363-99368) consists of codes used by physicians to report anticoagulant therapy and coordination of care services with other health care professionals.

Anticoagulant Management. The codes report anticoagulant services using Warfarin/Coumadin. Anticoagulants inhibit coagulation of the blood and are prescribed to patients with various thromboembolic disorders. Patients on this medication are monitored by means of blood tests and adjustments are then made in the blood thinner dosage if the physician determines the clotting levels are not ideal. Codes 99363 and 99364 report the monitoring services provided on an outpatient basis for the initial 90 days of therapy (with a minimum of eight assessments) and each subsequent 90 days of therapy (with at least three assessments). Any period less than 60 days is not reported.

Medical Team Conferences. The medical team must include at least three qualified health care professionals from different specialties. The team members must have all performed a face-to-face evaluation or treatment of the patient within the previous 60 days. Codes 99366-99368 are divided based on if the patient and/or family is/are present in the conference with the participation of the physician or a non-physician health care professional.

EXERCISE 10-18 *Case Management Services*

Complete the following:

1 What is the time component specified in the Medical Team Conference codes from the Case

Management Services subsection? _____

2 What are the three Medical Team Conferences codes? _____

Care Plan Oversight Services

At times, a physician is asked to manage a complex case that involves an individual such as a hospice patient or a patient who is homebound and receives the majority of his or her health care from visiting nurses. When regular communication is necessary between the nurses and the physician to discuss revising the care plan, coordinating the treatment plan with other professionals, or adjusting the therapies, codes from the Care Plan Oversight Services subsection (99374-99380) report these additional services. The codes are divided according to whether the physician is supervising a patient being cared for by home health workers or a patient in a hospice or nursing facility. The codes are also divided based on the length of time of the service—either 15 to 29 minutes or 30 minutes or more. Reporting is by time over a month-long period.

Preventive Medicine Services

Preventive Medicine Services codes (99381-99429) report the routine evaluation and management of a patient who is healthy and has no complaint. The codes in this subsection report a routine physical examination provided at the patient's request, such as a well-baby check-up. Preventive Medicine codes are intended to identify comprehensive services, not a single system review. The codes are reported for infants, children, adolescents, and adults; they differ according to the age of the patient and whether the patient is a new or an established patient.

CODING SHOT

If the physician should encounter a problem or abnormality during the course of a preventive service, and the problem or abnormality requires significant additional service, you can also code an office visit code with a modifier -25 added. The modifier -25 is added to indicate that a significant, separately identifiable E/M service was performed by the physician on the same day as the preventive medicine service. If you did not add the modifier -25, the third-party payer would think that you had made an error and were reporting both a preventive medicine service code and an office visit code for the same service. Only with the use of the modifier -25 can you convey that the services were indeed separate.

Note that in the code descriptions for both the New Patient and the Established Patient categories, the terms "comprehensive history" and "comprehensive examination" are used. These terms are not the same as the ones used with other E/M codes (99201-99350). Here, "comprehensive" means a complete history and a complete examination, as is conducted during an annual physical. The comprehensive examination performed as part of the preventive medicine E/M service is a multisystem examination, but the extent of the examination is determined by the age of the patient and the risk factors identified for that individual.

EXERCISE 10-19 *Preventive Medicine Services*

Complete the following:

1 According to the notes in the Preventive Medicine Services subsection, the extent and focus of the services provided, whether to a new or established patient, will depend largely upon what

   factor? _____

2 If, during the preventive medicine evaluation, a problem is encountered that requires the physician to perform a problem focused E/M service, what modifier would be appended to the

   code? _____

Counseling Risk Factor Reduction and Behavior Change Intervention. These codes (99401-99429) are for both new and established healthy patients. The services are based on whether individual or group counseling is provided to the patient and on the amount of time the service requires. Codes in this category report a physician's services to a patient for risk factor interventional counseling, such as a diet and exercise program, smoking cessation, or contraceptive management.

Non-Face-to-Face Physician Services

These codes are divided into Telephone Services (99441-99443) and On-Line Medical Evaluation (99444) assigned to report services provided by a physician. To report these same services provided by a non-physician, assign Medicine codes 98966-98969. The notes and the code descriptions for these codes indicate that the telephone or online service cannot originate from a related assessment that was provided within the previous seven days or result in an appointment within the next 24 hours or the soonest available appointment. The telephone services are reported based on the documented time, and the online service is per incident.

Although most payers and CMS do not currently reimburse for telephone services, some payers do, such as Workers' Compensation. Even if a payer does not reimburse, you should still submit all the codes necessary to completely explain the service. This type of historical data is used to analyze services provided and may, in the future, result in changes to reimbursement.

Special Evaluation and Management Services

The codes in this subsection (99450-99456) are used to report evaluations for life or disability insurance baseline information. The services can be performed in any setting for either a new or an established patient. The codes vary, based on whether the service is for an examination for life or disability insurance and whether the examination is done by the physician treating the patient's disability or by someone other than the treating physician.

EXERCISE 10-20   *Special Evaluation and Management Services*

Answer the following:

1 An insurance examination was conducted by the physician for a new patient for a term life insurance policy. From what subheading would you select a code to report this service?

_____

2 A 50-year-old man was referred for a disability examination. The patient had been injured at work when he slipped off a ladder and fell from a height of 10 feet, landing on his back. He has not returned to work since that time 6 months ago. The patient had been under the care of a physician from another state and was referred by the insurance company for the assessment of the patient's ability to return to work. His primary physician had stated that this patient will be unable to return to his previous work as a bricklayer. From what subheading would you select a code to report this

service? _____

3 What is the difference between the two codes in the Work Related or Medical Disability Evaluation

Services codes? _____

_____

_____

4 A 58-year-old man was seen by his private physician for an examination as part of his claim for long-term medical disability. The patient has chronic obstructive lung disease with severe emphysema and has been unable to work during the past year. The physician completed all the necessary documentation required by the insurance company, including his opinion that the patient would be unable to work in the future, as his pulmonary function is markedly impaired, in spite of continual respiratory and pharmacologic therapy.

CPT Code: _____

ICD-9-CM Codes: _____ (medical exam for insurance certification), _____

(COPD with emphysema) (ICD-10-CM Codes: _____, _____)

Newborn Care Services

Newborn Care Services codes (99460-99465) report services to normal newborns. Note that there are three history and examination codes; one is specifically for a newborn assessment and discharge from a hospital or birthing room on the same date (99463), one is for hospital or birthing room deliveries (99460), and one is for other than a hospital or birthing center (99461). The services are reported on a per day basis. Subsequent services are reported with 99462. If the physician provides a discharge service to a newborn discharged subsequent to the admission date, you would choose a code from the Hospital Inpatient Services subsection, Hospital Discharge Services subheading (99238, 99239).

Delivery/Birthing Room Attendance (99464, 99465) codes report the attendance of a physician, at the request of the delivering physician, to provide the initial stabilization of a newborn or for the resuscitation/ventilation of the newborn. The request for physician attendance must be documented in the patient's medical record.

Inpatient Neonatal Intensive Care and Pediatric and Neonatal Critical Care Services (99466-99480)

Pediatric Critical Care Patient Transport. These codes (99466, 99467) report physician face-to-face services provided to a pediatric patient (24 months of age or younger). During the provision of these services, the patient is being transported from one facility to another. The codes are time-based and report only face-to-face physician services provided to the critically ill pediatric patient during the interfacility transportation. If the physician is in physical attendance for less than 30 minutes, the service is not reported with these transportation codes. The codes are divided based on the first 30 to 74 minutes and each additional block of 30 minutes beyond 74.

CAUTION *Bundled into the codes are routine monitoring evaluations, such as heart rate and blood pressure. Other services provided by the physician before transport and nonroutine services provided during transport may be reported separately.*

Inpatient Neonatal and Pediatric Critical Care. Codes 99468-99476 report initial and subsequent critical care services to neonatal and pediatric patients. The codes are based on the age of the patient:

- Neonate, 28 days or younger
- Pediatric, 29 days through 24 months or 2 years to 5 years

The name of the intensive care unit does not matter in the assignment of these codes. The services can be provided in a pediatric intensive care unit, neonatal critical care unit, or any of the many other names that these types of intensive care units have. **Bundled** into the codes are many services you would anticipate would be used in the support of a critically ill neonate or pediatric patient (for example, arterial catheters, nasogastric tube placement, endotracheal intubation, and invasive electronic monitoring of vital signs). The notes preceding the codes list bundled services, descriptions, and codes for services (for example, blood transfusion, 36440). To ensure that you do not unbundle, you will need to refer back to these lists of bundled services. If the physician performed a service not listed in the bundle, you would report the service separately. Other notes indicating bundled services appear in the code descriptions. For example, cardiac and/or respiratory support is bundled into some of the codes.

Initial and Continuing Intensive Care Services. When a neonate or infant is **not** considered critically ill but still needs intensive observation and other intensive care services, the Initial and Continuing Intensive Care Services codes (99477-99480) are reported. These codes are not based on the age of the patient, but are based on weight.

- Very low birth weight (VLBW) is less than 1500 grams (less than 3.3 pounds)
- Low birth weight (LBW) is 1500-2500 grams (3.3-5.5 pounds)
- Normal birth weight is 2501-5000 grams (5.51-11.01 pounds)

The assignment of these codes changes when the neonate/infant weight changes. The codes from the subsection are reported only once in every 24-hour period (same day). There are no hourly service codes as there are in other critical care codes.

EXERCISE 10-21   *Newborn Care and Neonatal/Pediatric Critical Care Services*

Answer the following:

1 What does the abbreviation VLBW mean? _____

2 What code would you assign to report the face-to-face service provided by a physician during an interfacility transport of a critically ill patient who is 16 months of age? The service was for 60 minutes.

   CPT Code: _____

3 A normal newborn was admitted to the hospital on Saturday morning and was discharged Saturday evening. The physician provided evaluation and management services including the admission and the discharge. What code would you assign to report the physician service?

   CPT Code: _____

4 The physician provided a subsequent inpatient service to a 3-year-old critically ill patient.

   CPT Code: _____

5 The physician provided an intensive care service to an infant of very low birth weight on the patient's second day of the hospital stay.

   CPT Code: _____

Other Evaluation and Management Services

Other Evaluation and Management Services (99499) is the last subsection in the E/M section. Code 99499 is an unlisted code that is used to indicate that there is no other code that accurately represents the services provided to the patient. A special report would accompany the unlisted E/M service code.

Coding Practice

CONGRATULATIONS! Good job! You have been through all of the E/M codes and are now familiar with the basics of CPT code arrangement. Can you imagine how well you would know your favorite novel if you read it several times a month? Well, coders use their CPT manuals every day and become very familiar with the information in the guidelines, notes, and descriptions of the codes. Please be sure to locate the code in the CPT manual and read all notes, guidelines, and descriptions about each code you work with. In this way, you will build a solid knowledge foundation.

Now let's begin to do some coding that will require you to combine all the information you have learned as you begin to code patient cases.

EXERCISE 10-22 *Coding Practice*

Code the following:

1 A new patient is seen in the office for an earache (otalgia). The history and examination are problem focused and the MDM complexity is straightforward. The diagnosis was acute mastoiditis.

    CPT Code: _____

    ICD-9-CM Code: _____ (ICD-10-CM Code: _____)

2 An established patient is seen in the office of an ENT (ear-nose-throat) specialist with the chief complaint of otalgia. The physician completes a problem focused history and physical examination of the head, eyes, ears, nose, and throat. To the physician, this is a straightforward case of acute otitis media, and prescription medications are ordered. The MDM complexity is straightforward.

    CPT Code: _____

    ICD-9-CM Code: _____ (ICD-10-CM Code: _____)

3 An established patient is seen in the office for a blood pressure check, which is done by the physician's nurse.

    CPT Code: _____

4 Lilly Wilson, a new patient, is seen by the physician in the skilled nursing facility for an initial nursing facility assessment. Mrs. Wilson recently suffered a cerebral thrombosis with residual dysphagia and paresis of the left extremities. She was transferred from the acute care hospital to the skilled nursing facility for concentrated rehabilitation. Mrs. Wilson also has arteriosclerotic heart disease with a permanent pacemaker in place, rheumatoid arthritis, urinary incontinence, and macular degeneration in her right eye. The physician, who did not know Mrs. Wilson prior to her transfer, performs a comprehensive history and physical examination. Given the patient's multiple diagnoses and the moderate amount of data the physician has to review, the MDM is of a high level of complexity.

    CPT Code: _____

5 John Taylor is a 16-year-old outpatient who is a new patient to the office. John complains of severe pustule facial acne. The history and physical examination are expanded problem focused. The physician must consider related organ systems in addition to the integumentary system in order to treat the condition properly. With the minimal number of diagnoses to consider and the minimal amount of data to review, the physician's decision making is straightforward with regard to the plan of care.

    CPT Code: _____

    ICD-9-CM Code: _____ (ICD-10-CM Code: _____)

6 Jan Sharp, an established patient, has an office appointment because she needs a new dressing on the laceration on her arm. The physician's nurse changes the dressing.

    CPT Code: _____

7 Anna Rall is seen in the emergency department, complaining of pressure in her chest and the feeling that her heart is racing. After her vital signs are taken, an immediate electrocardiogram is performed, and her heart rate is found to be in excess of 160 beats per minute, with increased activity at the atrioventricular junction. After performing a comprehensive history and physical examination, the physician continues to evaluate the patient, who has been placed on continuous electrocardiographic monitoring. The emergency department physician documents the diagnosis of paroxysmal nodal tachycardia and calls a cardiologist for a consultation and possible admission of the patient to the hospital. Given the uncertainty of the diagnosis and the various other possible options, the physician's decision making is at a highly complex level. (Code only the emergency department physician's services.)

    CPT Code: _____

    ICD-9-CM Code: _____ (ICD-10-CM Code: _____)

8 A physician is called to the intensive care unit at the local hospital to care for Joe West, a patient in coronary crisis. The physician spends an hour at the patient's bedside, stabilizing him.

    CPT Code: _____

9 The physician is preparing to leave the hospital after seeing Joe West but is called back to the intensive care unit to see and stabilize another patient, Ted Keel. The service to the patient takes 1½ hours.

    CPT Codes: _____, _____

10 An established patient, Harriet Turner, comes into the office for a follow-up visit. She had been prescribed medication for her recent onset of depression, but since her last visit, when the dosage was increased, she has felt that the medication is making her sleepy and lethargic. Considering the other factors such as other medical problems and drug interactions, the physician spends 25 minutes with the patient performing a detailed history and physical examination. After reviewing the details as well as recent laboratory work, the physician concludes that a different medication should be prescribed. The physician's decision making is moderately complex, given the possible medical complications that could arise.

    CPT Code: _____

11 Dr. Welton calls Dr. Stouffer to perform a consultation on Carol Jones for advice on the management of her diabetes. Mrs. Jones is hospitalized for a hysterectomy, which had been an uncomplicated procedure, but is experiencing a slow recovery 4 days post op. Her abdominal wound does not appear to be healing well and her blood sugar has been fluctuating each day. Dr. Stouffer, who has never met Mrs. Jones before, performs a comprehensive, multisystem physical examination and completes a comprehensive history with a complete review of systems and extensive past medical history review. Dr. Stouffer recommends a new insulin regimen in addition to other medications to manage what might be a postoperative wound infection. Dr. Stouffer's medical decision making is of moderate complexity because he has to consider multiple diagnoses, a moderate amount of data, and the moderate risk of complications that Mrs. Jones could develop.

    CPT Code: _____

 CONGRATULATIONS! Now you're coding! Be sure to check your answers as you complete each activity. If you identify a code incorrectly, go back and read the CPT manual information again.

DOCUMENTATION GUIDELINES

Medicare recipients account for the majority of patients receiving services in the American health care system. Thus, any change by the third-party payer, Medicare, has dramatic effects on the health care system. One such change that currently is in development is the documentation necessary when submitting a claim for Evaluation and Management services provided to a Medicare patient. The Medicare program is the responsibility of the Centers for Medicare and Medicaid Services (CMS), formerly the Health Care Financing Administration (HCFA). Several years ago, CMS determined that there should be a nationally uniform requirement for documentation contained in the patient record when submitting charges for E/M services. The CMS developed a set of standards for documentation of E/M services. The standards are informational items that must be in the patient record to substantiate a given level of service. The standards are called the **Documentation Guidelines**. These guidelines apply only to E/M services and only to patients covered by Medicare and Medicaid. E/M services represent 50% of all services provided to these patients. The importance of the guidelines cannot be underestimated. Whatever guidelines the CMS institutes for patients have a dramatic effect on the systems in health care and will soon spread to other third-party payers, who will then begin to require the same or similar documentation.

History of the Development of Guidelines

The CMS published the first set of documentation guidelines in 1995, but did not require compliance for payment of claims. The 1995 Documentation Guidelines are posted on the Evolve website for this text (see Appendix A for free access information). The 1995 guidelines are easier to understand because they are not lengthy or complex. The documentation guidelines (DG) present information about what must be contained in the medical record for that information to "qualify" as documentation. For example, one DG states, "The CC, ROS and PFSH may be listed as separate elements of history, or they may be included in the description of the history of the present illness." This means that the location in the documentation of the chief complaint; review of systems; and past, family, or social history is not important, but what is important is that each of these items is documented in the record. Another example of the content of the 1995 guidelines is a DG for a general multisystem examination as: "The medical record for a general multisystem examination should include findings about 8 or more of the 12 organ systems." The documentation guidelines provide further clarification as to the documentation required to assign a level to the history, examination, and medical decision making as stated in the medial record.

A new set of guidelines was published in July 1997 for implementation January 1, 1998. The 1997 set of guidelines was intended to be the standard used when reviewing claims for payment and is also posted on the Evolve website for this text (see Appendix A for free access information). If the physician did not have the documentation required in the guidelines, payment would be adjusted based on what was actually in the medical record. The guidelines were so complex and required such extensive revision of medical record-keeping practices that the AMA (American Medical Association), on behalf of its physician members, requested an extension of the implementation date to allow time for education about the guidelines and for the CMS to meet with representatives of the AMA to reconsider the guidelines. Although the CMS rescinded the requirement for strict compliance with the guidelines, they continue random review of claims, based on whichever set of guidelines (1995 or 1997) the provider has elected to use.

The 1997 Documentation Guidelines specify the information that must be documented in the medical record for an E/M service to qualify for a given level of service. Fig. 10–8 illustrates the examination requirements

GENERAL MULTI-SYSTEM EXAMINATION

To qualify for a given level of multi-system examination, the following content and documentation requirements should be met:

- **Problem Focused Examination**—should include performance and documentation of one to five elements identified by a bullet (•) in one or more organ system(s) or body area(s).

- **Expanded Problem Focused Examination**—should include performance and documentation of at least six elements identified by a bullet (•) in one or more organ system(s) or body area(s).

- **Detailed Examination**—should include at least six organ systems or body areas. For each system/area selected, performance and documentation of at least two elements identified by a bullet (•) is expected. Alternatively, a detailed examination may include performance and documentation of at least twelve elements identified by a bullet (•) in two or more organ systems or body areas.

- **Comprehensive Examination**—should include at least nine organ systems or body areas. For each system/area selected, all elements of the examination identified by a bullet (•) should be performed, unless specific directions limit the content of the examination. For each area/system, documentation of at least two elements identified by a bullet is expected.

FIGURE 10-8 Documentation Guidelines for general multisystem examination requirements. (Courtesy U.S. Department of Health and Human Services, Centers for Medicare and Medicaid Services.)

for a general multisystem examination under the 1997 Documentation Guidelines. Note that for an examination to qualify as an expanded problem focused examination, the medical record must document that the physician performed at least six of the elements identified by a bullet (•) in Fig. 10–9. If the medical record documents that only five of the elements identified by a bullet were performed, the examination would have to be reported at the lower problem focused examination level.

A revised set of guidelines, published in 2000, took into consideration some of the suggestions put forth by the AMA. At the time of the publication of this text, the CMS and the AMA were still in discussions regarding which set of documentation guidelines would become the standard for documenting E/M services.

CHECK THIS OUT ☞ The CMS has its own website: www.cms.hhs.gov/ MLNEdWebGuide/25_EMDOC.asp#TopOfPage. You will find many articles regarding documentation guidelines for E/M services if you do a search of the CMS website.

Although the guidelines will continue to be revised, documentation guidelines will be a part of the standard for the medical record now and in the future for Medicare and Medicaid patients. You can anticipate that, as a coder, you will be required to learn about and follow these documentation guidelines.

General Multi-System Examination

System/Body Area	Elements of Examination
Constitutional	• Measurement of **any three of the following seven** vital signs: (1) sitting or standing blood pressure, (2) supine blood pressure, (3) pulse rate and regularity, (4) respiration, (5) temperature, (6) height, (7) weight (may be measured and recorded by ancillary staff) • General appearance of the patient (e.g., development, nutrition, body habitus, deformities, attention to grooming)
Eyes	• Inspection of conjunctivae and lids • Examination of pupils and irises (e.g., reaction to light and accommodation, size and symmetry) • Ophthalmoscopic examination of optic disks (e.g., size, C/D ratio, appearance) and posterior segments (e.g., vessel changes, exudates, hemorrhages)
Ears, Nose, Mouth, and Throat	• External inspection of ears and nose (e.g., overall appearance, scars, lesions, masses) • Otoscopic examination of external auditory canals and tympanic membranes • Assessment of hearing (e.g., whispered voice, finger rub, tuning fork) • Inspection of nasal mucosa, septum, and turbinates • Inspection of lips, teeth, and gums • Examination of oropharynx: oral mucosa, salivary glands, hard and soft palates, tongue, tonsils, and posterior pharynx
Neck	• Examination of neck (e.g., masses, overall appearance, symmetry, tracheal position, crepitus) • Examination of thyroid (e.g., enlargement, tenderness, mass)

FIGURE 10–9 1997 Documentation Guidelines of the general multisystem elements. (Courtesy U.S. Department of Health and Human Services, Centers for Medicare and Medicaid Services.)

CHAPTER REVIEW

CHAPTER 10, PART I, THEORY

Without using the CPT manual, complete the following:

1 Is examination of the back an organ system or body area examination?

_____

2 The four types of patient status are

_____, _____,

_____, and _____.

3 The first outpatient visit is called the

_____ visit, and the second visit is

called the _____ visit.

4 The first three factors a coder must consider

when coding are patient _____,

_____, and _____.

5 How many types of histories are there? _____

6 Which history is more complex: the problem focused history or the expanded problem

focused history? _____

7 The four types of examinations, in order of difficulty (from least difficult to most difficult), are as follows:

a _____

b _____

c _____

d _____

8 The examination that is limited to the affected

body area is the _____.

9 What does VLBW stand for?

_____

10 What medical decision making involves a situation in which the diagnosis and management options are minimal, data amount and complexity that must be reviewed are minimal/none, and there is a minimal risk to the patient of complications or death?

_____

11 What term is used to describe a patient who has been formally admitted to a hospital?

_____

CHAPTER 10, PART II, PRACTICAL

Using the CPT manual, identify the codes for the following cases:

12 The physician provides initial intensive care service for the evaluation and management of a critically ill newborn (5 days old) inpatient for one day.

CPT Code: _____

13 A 55-year-old man is seen by the dermatologist for the first time and complains of two cystic lesions on his back. Considering that the patient is otherwise healthy and has a primary care physician caring for him, the dermatologist focuses the history of the present illness on the skin lesions (problem focused history) and focuses the problem focused physical examination on the patient's trunk. The physician concludes with straightforward decision making that the lesions are sebaceous cysts. The physician advises the patient that the lesions should be monitored for any changes but that no surgical intervention is warranted at this time.

CPT Code: _____

ICD-9-CM Code: _____

(ICD-10-CM Code: _____)

14 A 68-year-old woman visits her internist again complaining of angina that seems to have worsened over the past 3 days. The patient had had an acute anterior wall myocardial infarction (MI) 2 months earlier. One month after the acute MI, she began to have angina pectoris. The patient also states that she thinks the medications are causing her to have gastrointestinal problems while not relieving her symptoms. She had refused a cardiac catheterization after her MI to evaluate the extent of her coronary artery disease. The physician performs a detailed history and a detailed physical examination of her cardiovascular, respiratory, and gastrointestinal systems. The physician indicates that the decision making process is moderately complex, given the number of conditions it is necessary to consider.

CPT Code: _____

15 A 22-year-old woman visits the gynecologist for the first time since relocating from another state last year. The patient wants a gynecologic examination and wants to discuss contraceptive options with the physician (think Preventive Medicine Services!). The physician collects pertinent past and social history related to the patient's reproductive system and performs a pertinent systems review extended to a limited number of additional systems. The physician completes the history with an extended history of her present physical state. A physical examination includes her cardiovascular and respiratory systems with an extended review of her genitourinary system. Given the patient's history of not tolerating certain types of oral contraceptives in the past, the physician's decision making involves a limited number of management options, all with low risk of morbidity to the patient.

CPT Code: _____

ICD-9-CM Codes: _____ (exam),

_____ (exam, gynecological, for contraceptive maintenance)

(ICD-10-CM Codes: _____,

_____)

16 An established patient is admitted on observation status for influenza symptoms and extreme nausea and vomiting. The patient is severely dehydrated and has been experiencing dizziness and mental confusion for the past 2 days. Prior to this episode the patient was well but became acutely ill overnight with these symptoms. Given the abrupt onset of these symptoms, the physician has to consider multiple possible causes and orders a variety of laboratory tests to be performed. The patient is at risk for a moderate number of complications. The MDM complexity is moderate. A comprehensive history is collected, and a comprehensive head-to-toe physical examination is performed.

CPT Code: _____

ICD-9-CM Codes: _____,

_____, _____

(ICD-10-CM Codes: _____,

_____, _____)

17 A physician visits another patient on observation status who has severe influenza. The decision is made to admit the patient, whose condition has worsened and who is not responding to the therapy initiated on the observation unit. The physician performs a detailed history and a detailed physical examination to reflect the patient's current status. The patient's problem is of low severity but requires ongoing active management, with possible surgical consultation. The MDM complexity is low.

CPT Code: _____

18 An 8-month-old infant, who is a new patient, is brought in by her mother for diaper rash. The physician focuses on the problem of the diaper rash for the problem focused history and examination. The MDM complexity is straightforward.

CPT Code: _____

ICD-9-CM Code: _____

(ICD-10-CM Code: _____)

19 A 33-year-old man is brought to his private physician's office by his wife. The man, who is an established patient, has been experiencing severe leg pain of 2 weeks' duration. In the past 2 days, the patient has experienced fainting spells, nausea, and vomiting. The patient has had multiple other vague complaints over the past month that he dismissed as unimportant, but his wife is not so sure, and she describes his general health as deteriorating. The physician performs a comprehensive multisystem physical examination after performing a complete review of systems and a complete past medical, family, and social history, with an extended history of the present illness (comprehensive history). The physician has to consider an extensive number of diagnoses, orders a variety of tests to be performed immediately, and indicates the MDM complexity to be high.

CPT Code: _____

ICD-9-CM Codes: _____ (leg pain), _____ (fainting), _____ (nausea with vomiting)

(ICD-10-CM Codes: _____, _____, _____)

20 A 42-year-old woman, who is an established patient, visits her family practitioner with the chief complaint of a self-discovered breast lump. She describes a feeling of fullness and tenderness over the mass that has become more pronounced in the past 2 weeks. Because the patient is otherwise healthy and has had a physical within the past 6 months, the physician focuses his attention on the breast lump during the taking of a problem focused history and the performance of a problem focused physical examination. The physician orders an immediate mammography to be performed and a follow-up appointment in 5 days. The physician has given the patient no other options and indicates that the MDM complexity is straightforward.

CPT Code: _____

ICD-9-CM Code: _____

(ICD-10-CM Code: _____)

21 Contusion of left knee and right elbow due to fall from roof. (Do not assign E codes.)

ICD-9-CM Codes: _____, _____

(ICD-10-CM Codes: _____, _____)

QUICK CHECK ANSWERS

QUICK CHECK 10-1
1. exceed, three

QUICK CHECK 10-2
1. True

QUICK CHECK 10-3
1. e. All of the above

QUICK CHECK 10-4
1. Yes

QUICK CHECK 10-5
1. outpatient

QUICK CHECK 10-6
1. Time

QUICK CHECK 10-7
1. Written or verbal request, report

QUICK CHECK 10-8
1. Yes

QUICK CHECK 10-9
1. None
2. Yes

QUICK CHECK 10-10
1. Any two of:
   - Interpretation of cardiac output measure (93561, 93562)
   - Chest x-rays (71010, 71015, 71020)
   - Pulse Oximetry (94760, 94761, 94762)
   - Blood gases and information data in computers (e.g., ECGs, blood pressures, hematologic data [99090])
   - Temporary transcutaneous pacing (92953)
   - Ventilation management (94002-94004, 94660, 94662)
   - Vascular access procedures (36000, 36410, 36415, 36591, 36600)

Why did you choose coding as a profession?

"I enjoy surgery and reading about the different approaches that it entails. Your profession should be something that you are passionate about."

Genieve R. Nottage, MBA, BSHA, CPC-I, CPC
Educator/Consultant
Chronicles Billing Inc.
Locust Grove, Georgia

Anesthesia

Chapter Topics

Types of Anesthesia

Anesthesia Section Format

Formula for Anesthesia Payment

Concurrent Modifiers

Unlisted Anesthesia Code

Other Reporting

Chapter Review

Quick Check Answers

Learning Objectives

After completing this chapter you should be able to

1 Define types of anesthesia.

2 Explain the format of the Anesthesia section and subsections.

3 Understand the anesthesia formula.

4 Identify other reporting issues.

5 Demonstrate ability to report anesthesia services.

Make sure to check

evolve
learning system
for the latest content updates

TYPES OF ANESTHESIA

The Anesthesia section is a specialized section that is used by an anesthesiologist, anesthetist, or other physician to report the provision of anesthesia services, usually during surgery. **Anesthesia** means induction or administration of a drug to obtain partial or complete loss of sensation. **Analgesia** (absence of pain) is achieved so that a patient may have surgery or a procedure performed without pain. Types of anesthesia may be general, regional, local, or moderate (conscious) sedation. Conscious sedation is not coded with anesthesia codes, but rather Medicine codes. Local anesthesia is usually administered by the surgeon.

The practice of anesthesiology is not limited to administration of anesthesia for the surgical patient. The American Society of Anesthesiologists (ASA) defines the practice of anesthesiology as follows:

- The management of procedures for rendering a patient insensible to pain and emotional stress during surgical, obstetrical, and other diagnostic and therapeutic procedures.
- The evaluation and management of essential physiologic functions under the stress of anesthetic and surgical manipulations.
- The clinical management of the patient unconscious from whatever cause.
- The evaluation and management of acute or chronic pain.
- The management of problems in cardiac and respiratory resuscitation.
- The application of specific methods of respiratory therapy.
- The clinical management of various fluid, electrolyte, and metabolic disturbances.*

Take a moment and consult a good medical dictionary under the entry "anesthesia." You will find that in addition to the definition of the term anesthesia, a wide variety of types of anesthesias are defined. Some types of anesthesia are named for the site of the anesthesia administration, such as sacral, lumbar, and caudal. Other types of anesthesia are named for the category of anesthesia, such as freezing (frost) for cryoanesthesia. Some of the more commonly used anesthesia terms are endotracheal, epidural, regional, and patient-controlled.

- **Endotracheal** anesthesia is accomplished by insertion of a tube into the nose or mouth, and passing the tube into the trachea for ventilation, as illustrated in Fig. 11-1.
- **Epidural** anesthesia is the injection of an anesthetic agent into the epidural spaces between the vertebrae, also known as peridural, epidural, or epidural block.
- **Spinal** or intraspinal anesthesia refers to anesthesia produced by an injection of local anesthetic into the subarachnoid space around the spinal cord.
- **General** anesthesia is a state of unconsciousness that is accomplished by the use of a drug administered intramuscularly, rectally, intravenously, or by inhalation.
- **Regional** anesthesia interrupts the sensory nerve conductivity in a region of the body and is produced by a field block (forming a wall of anesthesia around the site by means of local injections) or nerve block (injection of the area close to the site). Nerve block is also known as block, block anesthesia, or conduction anesthesia. Although not a type of anesthesia, a procedure used by anesthesiologists for treatment of a postdural puncture headache is a blood patch, also known as an epidural blood patch (EBP). A **blood patch** procedure is when

---

*Definitions excerpted from the *2009 Relative Value Guide,* American Society of Anesthesiologists, p. v. A copy of the full text can be obtained from ASA, 1501 M Street NW, Suite 300, Washington, DC 20005.

FIGURE 11–1   **A,** Placement of endotracheal tube for administration of anesthesia. **B,** General endotracheal anesthesia is a support system of major importance. (**B** from Stack RS, Roubin GS, O'Neill WW: *Interventional Cardiovascular Medicine: Principles and Practice,* ed 2, Philadelphia, 2002, Churchill Livingstone.)

a cerebrospinal fluid leak is closed by means of an injection of the patient's blood into the epidural space at or near the area of the dural puncture that was accessed during spinal anesthesia.

■ **Local** anesthesia can be accomplished by means of application of an anesthetic agent (such as lidocaine) placed directly on the area involved (**topical** anesthesia) or local infiltration through subcutaneous injection of an anesthetic agent. Lidocaine can be subcutaneously injected, as illustrated in Fig. 11–2.

Patient-controlled analgesia (PCA) is a system that allows the patient to administer an analgesic drug such as morphine to control pain.

A device is attached to a pump holding the drug and the patient can depress a handheld button to administer a dose of the drug (Fig. 11–3). In this way, the patient can control the amount of the drug and the frequency of administration. PCA is considered a hospital service and not generally reported by a physician. Refer to individual payer guidelines for instructions to report PCA management.

QUICK CHECK 11-1

1. In the index of the CPT, you would reference this main term and these two subterms to locate a blood patch code. _____

FIGURE 11–2   Administration of local anesthesia.

FIGURE 11–3   Patient-controlled sedation machine. (From Potter PA, Perry AG: *Basic Nursing: Essentials for Practice*, ed 6, St. Louis, 2007, Mosby.)

Each type of anesthesia will be covered in depth, but generally speaking, the types of anesthesia are:

- **Monitored Anesthesia Care** (MAC)
  MAC is provided by an anesthesiologist or CRNA. The patient is monitored, and if necessary, sedation is provided; even general anesthesia.

- **General anesthesia**
  Used for cases that require deep sedation, such as open heart surgery or complicated abdominal surgery. The patient is usually intubated. The patient is in a deep state of sedation and is not arousable or able to communicate or follow commands. Several different types of medication may be used during general anesthesia including drugs for analgesia (pain relief), sedation, amnesiacs (to lessen awareness), and paralytics for muscle relaxation to prevent movement or reflexive action by the patient during procedures.

- **Regional**
  Regional anesthesia uses injection to target the nerves of the area being treated.

- **Spinal and epidural anesthesia**
  Spinal anesthesia is administered into the cerebral spinal fluid or epidural area of the spine that corresponds with the area being treated. Spinals are generally used for procedures below the waist. Epidural catheters are often placed to facilitate administration of medication into the spinal region.

Moderate (Conscious) Sedation

Moderate or conscious sedation is a type of sedation that can be provided by a surgeon or the surgeon's staff while the surgeon is performing a procedure; it provides a decreased level of consciousness that does not put the patient completely to sleep. This level of consciousness allows the patient to breathe without assistance and to respond to stimulation and verbal commands. A trained observer must be present when moderate sedation services are provided by the same physician performing the therapeutic or diagnostic service in order to assist the physician in monitoring the patient. The codes to report conscious sedation are located in the Medicine section (99143-99150), not in the Anesthesia section. Codes 99143-99145 report the moderate sedation services when the service is provided by the same physician performing the diagnostic or therapeutic service and requires the presence of an independent trained observer. The codes are divided based on the patient's age of under or over 5 years of age and the duration of the service. Codes 99148-99150 report moderate sedation services when the anesthesia service is provided by a physician other than the health care professional performing the service. These codes are divided based on the patient's age of under or over 5 years of age and the duration of the service. Bundled into these codes is the assessment of the patient, establishment of intravenous access, administration of the sedation agent, sedation maintenance, monitoring of patient vital signs, and recovery from anesthesia.

The code descriptions for the Moderate (Conscious) Sedation codes include the term "intraservice time." **Intraservice** time begins with the administration of the sedation agent, and requires continuous face-to-face attendance by the physician and ends when the personal contact by the physician ends. The time the physician spends with the patient in assessment of the patient prior to administration of the sedation and the time in recovery is not included in the intraservice time.

CODING SHOT
Moderate (conscious) sedation codes are only reported when the physician performing the procedure administers the sedation and an independent trained observer assists.

Moderate or conscious sedation methods are much less invasive than anesthesia services that provide the complete loss of consciousness. For example, for a colonoscopy, a physician could administer an intravenous sedation, such as meperidine (Demerol), morphine, or diazepam (Valium). The patient would be monitored closely as the medication is administered so that the appropriate level of sedation is reached. After the procedure, the physician may administer a drug intravenously to reverse the effects of the sedation. The patient would have this procedure in an outpatient setting and be able to go home after the procedure. Moderate sedation is included in many CPT codes and, as such, is not reported separately. The bullseye (⊙) is displayed to the left of the codes in the CPT manual that include the moderate/conscious sedation bundled into the code. For example, the codes in the 33206-33208 range report insertion or replacement of pacemaker electrodes and include moderate sedation. Appendix G in the CPT manual lists the codes that include moderate sedation.

🖐 **CAUTION** *Do not confuse conscious sedation with monitored anesthesia care. Conscious sedation is administered by the surgeon or another physician; MAC is provided by an anesthesiologist or CRNA.*

ANESTHESIA SECTION FORMAT
Most anesthesia codes are divided first by anatomic site and then by specific type of procedure, as shown in Fig. 11-4.

FIGURE 11–4 Anatomic divisions in Anesthesia section.

The last four subsections in Anesthesia—Radiologic Procedures (01916-01936), Burn Excisions or Debridement (01951-01953), Obstetric (01958-01969), and Other Procedures (01990-01999)—are not organized by anatomic division. The CPT codes in the Radiologic Procedures subsection report anesthesia service when radiologic services are provided to the patient for diagnostic or therapeutic reasons.

Example

| Therapeutic reason: | 01925 | Anesthesia for therapeutic interventional radiological procedures involving the carotid and coronary |
| Diagnostic reason: | 01922 | Anesthesia for non-invasive imaging or radiation therapy |

Anesthesia providers may be a(n):

- Anesthesiologist
- Certified registered nurse anesthetist (CRNA)
- Anesthesiologist's assistant (who may not work without oversight of anesthesiologist)
- Resident (cannot bill if the case is performed without the participation of another anesthesia provider)
- Student registered nurse anesthetist (billing is based on specific rules for each payer depending on the payer's definition of medical direction)

EXERCISE 11-1 *Anesthesia Format*

Complete the following exercise:

1 Which subsections are *not* divided by anatomic site? _____

2 What is analgesia? _____

3 What is anesthesia? _____

4 Name three types of anesthesia: _____, _____, and _____.

5 What is the type of sedation that enables the patient to maintain breathing for himself/herself?

_____

6 In what section of the CPT are the sedation codes identified in Question 6 located?

_____

Wrong ? Ans.

FORMULA FOR ANESTHESIA PAYMENT

When an anesthesiologist provides an anesthesia service to a patient, the preoperative, intraoperative/intraservice (care during surgery), and postoperative care are all included in the CPT code. These services include the usual preoperative and postoperative visits (on day of surgery) to the patient by the anesthesiologist; the routine intraoperative care, such as administration of fluids and/or blood; and the usual monitoring services. The care also includes the patient's history taken by the anesthesiologist, ventilation establishment, and administration of preoperative and postoperative medications. Monitoring services include blood pressure, temperature, arterial oxygen levels (oximetry), exhalation of carbon dioxide (capnography), and spectrometry (blood analysis). The intraoperative care includes intubation to administer anesthesia. Postoperative care usually includes pain management. Some pain management is reported separately, e.g., spinal injection for significant postoperative pain. If the anesthesiologist provides care that is unusual or beyond that which would usually be provided, these services can be reported in addition to the basic anesthesia service. For example, if the patient requires intraoperative cardiac monitoring, the anesthesiologist may insert a Swan-Ganz catheter, as illustrated in Fig. 11–5.

FIGURE 11–5 Swan-Ganz catheter is the most commonly used central venous catheter.

A Swan-Ganz catheter is not a normal service provided during a surgery, so it could be reported using a code from the Medicine section for placement of a flow-directed catheter (93503). Some payers will require modifier -59 (distinct procedural service) be appended to the catheter code. The time necessary to insert the catheter is not counted in the anesthesia time because the service of the insertion is reported separately and is considered a surgical procedure. Reporting the insertion separately and also adding the insertion time to the anesthesia service would result in double payment for the insertion service.

QUICK CHECK 11-2

1. Where is the information regarding inclusive anesthesia service located within the CPT manual?

_____

What makes anesthesia coding different from any other coding is the way in which anesthesia services are billed. There is a standard formula for payment of anesthesia services that is, for the most part, nationally accepted. The formula is base units + time units + modifying units (B + T + M) × conversion factor. Let's look at each of these elements in more detail.

Another tool is the ASA CROSSWALK book from the American Society of Anesthesiologists and it provides anesthesia coders with a comprehensive list of CPT codes that are reported with anesthesia. This book also lists the base value of each anesthesia service. CPT codes are located in the crosswalk book enabling the anesthesia coder to select the service with the highest base value for submission. The book also lists alternative codes, allowing the anesthesia coder to make the most specific selection. The anesthesia crosswalk book is updated by the ASA annually.

B Is for Base Unit   The ASA publishes a *Relative Value Guide*™ (RVG), which contains codes for anesthesia services. The CPT manual also contains these anesthesia service codes in the Anesthesia section. Italicized comments appear in the American Society of Anesthesiologists' *Relative Value Guide*™ to clarify code assignment, as illustrated in Fig. 11–6. These italicized comments are not part of the CPT manual.

INTRATHORACIC		
00500	Anesthesia for all procedures on esophagus......................................	15 + TM
00520	Anesthesia for closed chest procedures; (including bronchoscopy) not otherwise specified.. *(For transvenous pacemaker insertion, report 00530.)*	6 + TM

FIGURE 11–6   The *Relative Value Guide* contains italicized comments that do not appear in the code description in the CPT. (Excerpted from 2009 Relative Value Guide, © 2008 of the American Society of Anesthesiologists. All Rights Reserved. *Relative Value Guide is a registered trademark of the American Society of Anesthesiologists.* A copy of the full text can be obtained from ASA, 520 N. Northwest Highway, Park Ridge, IL, 60068-2573.)

CODING SHOT   Anesthesia is paid based on:
- Base units +
- Time units +
- Modifying units (if allowed) × conversion factor

CMS's Base Units.   The RVG is not a fee schedule (a list of charges for services) but instead compares anesthesia services with each other. For example, anesthesia services provided for a biopsy of a sinus are less complicated than services provided for a radical sinus surgery. A team of physicians with expertise in anesthesiology developed the comparisons and assigned numerical values to each service, termed the **base unit value** (Fig. 11–7). Annually, CMS also publishes a list of the base unit values for the codes, as illustrated in Fig. 11–8.

The CMS's base unit value is accepted as the standard in the United States for most third-party payers.

One coding circumstance unique to anesthesia coding occurs when multiple surgical procedures are performed during the same session. In this case, only the procedure with the highest base unit value is assigned. For example, if during the same surgical procedure session a clavicle biopsy (base unit value of 3) and a radical mastectomy (base unit value of 5) are performed. The base unit value for both procedures becomes 5. The anesthesia service is then reported with only the code for the higher base unit value.

Base unit value

LOWER LEG (BELOW KNEE, INCLUDES ANKLE AND FOOT)
(For procedures on integumentary system, report code 00400.)

01462	Anesthesia for all closed procedures on lower leg, ankle, and foot	3 + TM
01464	Anesthesia for arthroscopic procedures of ankle and/or foot	3 + TM
01470	Anesthesia for procedures on nerves, muscles, tendons, and fascia of lower leg, ankle, and foot; not otherwise specified	3 + TM
01472	repair of ruptured Achilles tendon, with or without graft	5 + TM
01474	gastrocnemius recession (eg, Strayer procedure)	5 + TM

FIGURE 11–7   The ASA's *Relative Value Guide* lists the Base Unit value for the codes. (Excerpted from 2009 Relative Value Guide, © 2008 of the American Society of Anesthesiologists. All Rights Reserved. *Relative Value Guide is a registered trademark of the American Society of Anesthesiologists.* A copy of the full text can be obtained from ASA, 520 N. Northwest Highway, Park Ridge, IL, 60068-2573.)

Code	Base Unit Value
00100	5
00102	6
00103	5
00104	4
00120	5
00124	4
00126	4
00140	5
00142	4
00144	6
00145	6
00147	4
00148	4
00160	5
00162	7
00164	4
00170	5
00172	6
00174	6
00176	7
00190	5
00192	7
00210	11

FIGURE 11–8   CMS's annual list of base units. (Courtesy U.S. Department of Health and Human Services, Centers for Medicare and Medicaid Services.)

NCCI

For Medicare, anesthesia service involving multiple procedures is reported with the CPT anesthesia code for the procedure with the highest base unit value. The actual total time for all procedures is reported. Only one anesthesia code can be reported. There is an exception for the add-on codes for burn excision or debridement (01953) and obstetrics (01968, 01969).

The pricing for add-on anesthesia codes is different than other payers because only the base unit value of the add-on code is allowed and all anesthesia time is reported with the primary anesthesia code. There is an exception to this rule when reporting obstetrical anesthesia, as both the base unit value and time units for the primary and add-on, obstetrical codes are reported.

T Is for Time

Anesthesia services are provided based on the time during which the anesthesia was administered and calculated, in total minutes. The timing is started when the anesthesiologist begins preparing the patient to receive anesthesia and is in constant attendance with the patient, continues through the procedure, and ends when the patient is turned over to the post-anesthesia caregivers. The minutes during which anesthesia was administered are recorded in the patient record. Carriers independently determine the amount of time that is considered a unit. Often, 15 minutes equal a unit, but for some carriers, 1, 10, or 30 minutes equal a unit.

NCCI

For Medicare, time units are computed by dividing the reported actual anesthesia service time by 15 minutes and then rounding to one decimal place. No time units are reported for anesthesia CPT code 01996. Medicare reimburses for anesthesia services based on a combination of time and base units multiplied by a geographic-area-specific conversion factor. The start time on the anesthesia record should match the time reported on the claim form. The recorded time on all records must be the same:

- Anesthesia record
- CRNA anesthesiologist, or resident billing slip
- Time on all documents submitted to insurance company

When completing the Medicare claim, always record the actual time—that is, the time the anesthesia provider spent personally attending the patient. Many private payers also require actual time, so it is necessary to verify time submission requirements with each payer.

Private payers may or may not reimburse CRNA services, or they may require these services be reported under the supervising anesthesiologist's name and NPI (National Provider Identification) number. You must verify the method for submission for each payer.

When preparing the claim, always record the actual time that indicates the ending time of personal attendance. The time is illustrated in Fig. 11–9, *A*. The stop time is when the patient can be safely turned over to a non-anesthesia provider. This generally does not occur in the operating room.

The start time on the anesthesia record should match the time reported on the claim form and indicate the beginning time of the service. Note that Fig. 11–9, *B* illustrates the medical document that contains the pre-anesthesia evaluation that the provider completes prior to the start of surgery.

From the Trenches

"Continue to educate yourself. Don't second guess your initial thoughts, only code what is documented."

GENIEVE

M Is for Modifying Unit

As the name implies, modifying units reflect circumstances or conditions that change or modify the environment in which the anesthesia service is provided. There are two base modifying characteristics: qualifying circumstances and physical status modifiers.

Qualifying Circumstances. At times, anesthesia is provided in situations that make the administration of the anesthesia more difficult. These types of cases include those that are performed in emergency situations and those dealing with patients of extreme age. They also include services performed during the use of controlled hypotension or the use of hypothermia (refer to Fig. 11–10). The Qualifying Circumstances codes begin

AUTHORIZED FOR LOCAL REPRODUCTION

MEDICAL RECORD–ANESTHESIA

PROCEDURE

ITEM	START	STOP
Anesthesia		
Procedure		

DATE	OR NO.	PAGE OF	SURGEON(S)

PRE–PROCEDURE
- ☐ Identified ☐ ID Band ☐ Questioning
- ☐ Chart Review ☐ Permit Signed
- ☐ NPO Since ____
- Pre-anesthetic State: ☐ Calm
- ☐ Awake ☐ Asleep
- ☐ Apprehensive ☐ Confused
- ☐ Uncooperative ☐ Unresponsive

PATIENT SAFETY
- ☐ Anes. Machine # ____ Checked
- ☐ Safety Belt On ☐ Axillary Roll
- ☐ Arm Restraints ☐ Arms Tucked
- ☐ Pressure points checked and padded
- ☐ Eye Care: ☐ Ointment ☐ Saline
- ☐ Taped ☐ Pads ☐ Goggles

TIME:

MONITORS AND EQUIPMENT
- ☐ Steth ☐ Esoph ☐ Precord ☐ Other
- ☐ Non-Invasive B/P ☐ Nerve Stimulator
- ☐ Continuous EKG ☐ V Lead EKG
- ☐ Pulse Oximeter ☐ Oxygen Analyzer
- ☐ End Tidal CO_2 ☐ Resp Gas Anlyzr
- ☐ Temp ____ ☐ EEG
- ☐ Warming Blanket ☐ Fluid Warmer
- ☐ Airway Humidifier ☐ ____
- ☐ NG/OG Tube ☐ Foley Catheter
- ☐ Art Line ____
- ☐ CVP ____
- ☐ PA Line ____
- ☐ IV(s) ____
- ☐ ____

ANESTHETIC TECHNIQUES
- Method: ☐ General ☐ Spinal
- ☐ Epidural ☐ Caudal ☐ Brachial
- ☐ Bier Block ☐ Ankle Blk ☐ M.A.C.
- General: ☐ Pre-O_2 ☐ L.T.A.
- ☐ Rapid Sequence ☐ Cricoid Pressure
- ☐ Intravenous ☐ Inhalation
- ☐ Intramuscular ☐ Rectal
- Regional: ☐ Position ____
- ☐ Prep ____ ☐ Local ____
- ☐ Needle ____
- ☐ Drug(s) ____
- ☐ Dose ____ ☐ Attempts x ____
- ☐ Site ____ ☐ Level ____
- ☐ Catheter ____ ☐ See Remarks

AIRWAY MANAGEMENT
- ☐ Intubation ☐ Oral ☐ Nasal
- ☐ Direct Vision ☐ Magill's ☐ Blind
- ☐ Diff. see Rmks ☐ Fiber Op ☐ Stylet
- ☐ Attempts x ____ ☐ Blade ____
- ☐ Tube size ____ ☐ Endobronchial
- ☐ Regular ☐ RAE ☐ Armored ☐ Laser
- ☐ Cuffed ☐ Min. occ. pres. ☐ Air ☐ NS
- ☐ Uncuffed, leaks at ____ cm H_2O
- ☐ Secured at ____ ☐ ET CO_2 Present
- ☐ Breath Sounds ____
- ☐ Circuit: ☐ Circle ☐ Non-rebreathing
- ☐ Airway: ☐ Oral ☐ Nasal ☐ Natural
- ☐ Mask Case ☐ Via Tracheostomy
- ☐ Nasal Cannula ☐ Simple O_2 Mask

RECOVERY ROOM

Time	B/P		O_2 Sat.

- ☐ PACU P R T
- ☐ ICU ☐ L&D
- ☐ Awake ☐ Spont Resp ☐ Oral Airway
- ☐ Asleep ☐ Ventilator ☐ Nasal Airway
- ☐ Stable ☐ Extubated ☐ Face Shield O_2
- ☐ Unstable ☐ Intubated ☐ T-Piece O_2

CONTROLLED DRUGS

Drug	Used	Destroyed	Returned

Provider ____ Witness ____

AGENTS
- ☐ Hal ☐ Enf ☐ Iso (%)
- ☐ N_2O ☐ Air (L/min)
- Oxygen (L/min)
- ( )
- ( )
- ( )
- ( )
- ( )

TOTALS

FLUIDS

MONITORS
- Urine (ml)
- EBL (ml)
- EKG
- % O_2 Inspired (FIO_2)
- O_2 Saturation (SaO_2)
- End Tidal CO_2
- Temp: ☐ °C ☐ °F

VITAL SIGNS

Baseline Values

- 200
- 180
- 160
- 140
- B/P 120
- 100
- P 80
- 60
- 40
- R 20

SYMBOLS

- ✕ ANESTHESIA
- ⊙ OPERATION
- ∨∧ B/PCUFF PRESSURE
- ⊥T ARTERIAL LINE PRESSURE
- Δ MEAN ARTERIAL PRESSURE
- ● PULSE
- ○ SPONTANEOUS RESP
- ⊘ ASSISTED RESP
- ⊗ CONTROLLED RESP
- T TOURNIQUET

VENT
- Tidal Vol. (ml)
- Resp. Rate
- Peak Pres. (cm H_2O)
- PEEP (cm H_2O)

Symbols for Remarks

Position

ANESTHESIA PROVIDER(S)

REMARKS

PATIENT'S IDENTIFICATION
(For typed or written entries give: Name–last, first, middle: ID No. (SSN or other); hospital or medical facility.)

ANESTHESIA
Medical Record
OPTIONAL FORM 517 (7–95)
Prescribed by GSA/ICMR,
FPMR (41 CFR) 101–11.203(b)(10)

A

FIGURE 11–9A Anesthesia medical record. (Courtesy U.S. General Services Administration.)

PRE-ANESTHESIA EVALUATION

AGE	SEX ☐ M ☐ F	HEIGHT in./cm.	WEIGHT lb./kg.	PRE-PROCEDURE VITAL SIGNS
				B/P P R T

PROPOSED PROCEDURE

PREVIOUS ANESTHESIA/OPERATIONS (If none, check here ☐)	CURRENT MEDICATIONS (If none, check here ☐)

FAMILY HISTORY OF ANESTHESIA COMPLICATIONS (If none, check here ☐)	ALLERGIES (If NKDA, check here ☐)

AIRWAY/TEETH/HEAD AND NECK	HISTORY FROM ☐ PARENT/GUARDIAN ☐ POOR HISTORIAN ☐ CHART ☐ SIGNIFICANT OTHER ☐ PATIENT

SYSTEM	WNL	COMMENTS	PERTINENT STUDY RESULTS
RESPIRATORY Asthma Pneumonia Bronchitis Productive cough COPD Recent cold Dyspnea SOB Orthopnea Tuberculosis	☐	Tobacco Use: ☐ No ☐ Yes ____ Pack/Day for ____ Years	Chest X-ray Pulmonary Studies
CARDIOVASCULAR Angina MI Arrhythmia Murmur CHF MVP Exercise Tolerance Pacemaker Hypertension Rheumatic fever	☐		EKG
HEPATO/GASTROINTESTINAL Bowel obstruction Jaundice Cirrhosis N&V Hepatitis Reflux/heartburn Histal hernia Ulcers	☐	Ethanol Use: ☐ No ☐ Yes Frequency_____	
NEURO/MUSCULOSKELETAL Arthritis Paresthesia Back problems Syncope CVA/stroke Seizures DJD TIAs Headaches Weakness Loss of consciousness Neuromuscular disease Paralysis	☐		
RENAL/ENDOCRINE Diabetes Renal failure/Dialysis Thyroid disease Urinary retention Urinary tract infection Weight loss/gain	☐		
OTHER Anemia Bleeding tendencies Hemophilia Pregnancy Sickle cell trait Transfusion history			

PROBLEM LIST/DIAGNOSES	ASA PS	LAB STUDIES Hgb/HcT/CBC Electrolytes Urinalysis
	1	
	2	
PLANNED ANESTHESIA/SPECIAL MONITORS	3	Other
	4	
	5	
	E	**POST-ANESTHESIA NOTE**
PRE-ANESTHESIA MEDICATIONS ORDERED		
SIGNATURE OF EVALUATOR(S)		
		Signed Date Time

OPTIONAL FORM 517 BACK

B

FIGURE 11-9B   Anesthesia medical record, pre-anesthesia evaluation and post-anesthesia notes. (Courtesy U.S. General Services Administration.)

V. Qualifying Circumstances (more than one may be reported)

		Base Unit Value
+99100	Anesthesia for patient of extreme age, younger than 1 year and older than 70...	1
+99116	Anesthesia complicated by utilization of total body hypothermia..	5
+99135	Anesthesia complicated by utilization of controlled hypotension..	5
+99140	Anesthesia complicated by emergency conditions (specify)	2

(An emergency is defined as existing when delay in treatment of the patient would lead to a significant increase in the threat to life or body part.)

FIGURE 11-10   Qualifying Circumstances with relative value. (Excerpted from 2009 Relative Value Guide, © 2008 of the American Society of Anesthesiologists. All Rights Reserved. *Relative Value Guide is a registered trademark of the American Society of Anesthesiologists.* A copy of the full text can be obtained from ASA, 520 N. Northwest Highway, Park Ridge, IL, 60068-2573.)

with 99 and are considered **adjunct codes,** which means that the codes can never be reported alone but must be used in addition to another code to provide additional information. A Qualifying Circumstances code is reported in addition to the anesthesia procedure code. Qualifying Circumstances codes are located in two places in the CPT manual: the Medicine section and the Anesthesia section Guidelines. In both locations the plus symbol is located next to the codes (99100-99140), indicating their status as add-on codes.

STOP *You were just presented with some very important information about the use of certain codes in the CPT manual. The plus (+) symbol next to any CPT code—not just next to Qualifying Circumstances codes—indicates that that code cannot be used alone. Throughout the remaining sections of the CPT manual, the plus symbol will appear to caution you to use the code only as an adjunct code (with other codes).*

When used, the Qualifying Circumstances code is reported in addition to the primary anesthesia procedure code. For example, if anesthesia was provided for an 80-year-old patient during a corrective lens procedure, the reporting would be:

00142   Anesthesia for procedure on eye; lens surgery

99100   Anesthesia for 80-year-old patient

The RVG lists the Qualifying Circumstances along with the relative value for each code (see Fig. 11–10).

The CPT index lists the Qualifying Circumstances codes under Anesthesia, Special Circumstances.

Physical Status Modifiers.   The second type of modifying unit used in the Anesthesia section is the physical status modifier (refer to Fig. 11–11). These modifiers indicate the patient's condition at the time anesthesia was

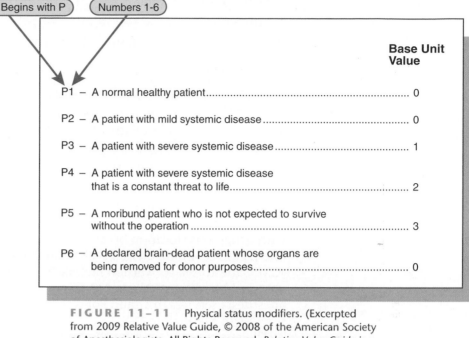

Begins with P   Numbers 1-6

Base Unit Value

P1 — A normal healthy patient... 0

P2 — A patient with mild systemic disease 0

P3 — A patient with severe systemic disease... 1

P4 — A patient with severe systemic disease
     that is a constant threat to life... 2

P5 — A moribund patient who is not expected to survive
     without the operation 3

P6 — A declared brain-dead patient whose organs are
     being removed for donor purposes.................................... 0

FIGURE 11–11 Physical status modifiers. (Excerpted from 2009 Relative Value Guide, © 2008 of the American Society of Anesthesiologists. All Rights Reserved. *Relative Value Guide is a registered trademark of the American Society of Anesthesiologists.* A copy of the full text can be obtained from ASA, 520 N. Northwest Highway, Park Ridge, IL, 60068-2573.)

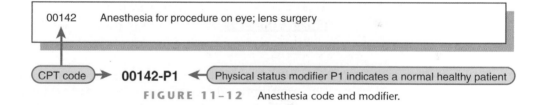

00142   Anesthesia for procedure on eye; lens surgery

CPT code → **00142-P1** ← Physical status modifier P1 indicates a normal healthy patient

FIGURE 11–12 Anesthesia code and modifier.

administered and identify the level of complexity of the services provided to the patient. For instance, anesthesia service to a gravely ill patient is much more complex than the same type of service to a normal, healthy patient. The physical status modifier is not assigned by the coder but is determined by the anesthesiologist and documented in the anesthesia record. The physical status modifier begins with the letter "P" and contains a number from 1 to 6 (see Fig. 11–11).

Note that the relative value for P1, P2, and P6 is zero because these conditions are considered not to affect the service provided. A physical status modifier is used after the five-digit CPT code and is illustrated in Fig. 11–12.

Summing It Up!

Most health care facilities have software that automatically performs the conversion calculations based on the various conversion factors and unit designations. However, you still need to understand the process used to convert the anesthesia formula into the anesthesia payment. Let's put the elements of the equation to practical use by applying the equation $(B + T + M)$ to a case.

An 84-year-old female (qualifying circumstance for extreme age, value 1) with severe hypertension (value of 1) has a 4-cm malignant lesion removed from her right knee (base value of 3). The total time of anesthesia service was 60 minutes and the carrier indicates a unit is 15 minutes (4 units). The anesthesiologist recorded that the patient's physical status at the time of the procedure was P3 for a severe systemic disease (relative value of 1).

3	base procedure value
4	time units
2	modifiers: physical status = 1; extreme age = 1
9	total units

The coding that identifies all elements of this case would be:

00400-P3	Anesthesia for procedure of integumentary system of knee for a patient with severe systemic disease (severe hypertension)
99100	Anesthesia for an 84-year-old patient
9	Units at the third-party payer established rate per unit

Conversion Factors. A conversion factor is the dollar value of each unit. Each third-party payer issues a list of conversion factors. The lists vary with geographic location because the cost of practicing medicine varies from one region to another. Fig. 11–13 shows an example of a third-party payer's (CMS) anesthesia conversion factors. Note that North Dakota is $19.71 per unit and Manhattan, NY, is $22.65 per unit, as it is less expensive to provide anesthesia services in Grand Forks, ND, than it is to provide the same services in Manhattan, NY.

The conversion factor for the locale is multiplied by the number of units in the procedure. For example, the previous case had 9 units. If the anesthesiologist was located in Manhattan, NY, and the conversion factor is $22.65, the total for the procedure would be $203.85 (9 × $22.65). If the same services were provided in North Dakota, with the conversion factor of $19.71, the total for the procedure would be $177.39 (9 × $19.71).

CHECK THIS OUT ☞ The CMS website posts the anesthesiology base unit values and conversion factors at www.cms.hhs.gov/center/anesth.asp

Multiple Procedures

- When multiple surgical procedures are performed during a single anesthetic administration, the anesthesia code that represents the highest base value unit procedure is reported. The time reported is the combined total for all procedures.
- Assign the code for procedure of highest base value unit
- Indicate cumulative start/stop time for all surgical procedures performed

Anesthesia time for a medically necessary surgical procedure performed during the same intra-operative session as a cosmetic procedure should be split and reported separately.

Locality Name	Anesthesia Conversion Factor
Manhattan, NY	22.65
NYC suburbs/Long I., NY	22.74
Queens, NY	22.28
Rest of New York	19.91
North Carolina	20.23
North Dakota	19.70

FIGURE 11–13 2009 CMS Anesthesia Conversion Factors.

CODING SHOT

According to Medicare rules, modifier -50 would not be used on anesthesia CPT codes. It would be used on anesthesia surgical procedures, such as femoral continuous block for pain management for bilateral knee replacement (64448-59-50), in addition to the ASA code or anesthesia CPT code.

EXERCISE 11-2 *Modifiers and Time in Anesthesia*

Complete the following:

1 If the anesthesia service was provided to a patient who had mild systemic disease, what would the physical status modifier be likely to be? _____

2 If the same service was provided to a patient who had severe systemic disease, what would the physical status modifier be likely to be? _____

3 Anesthesia complicated by utilization of total body hypothermia

   Code(s): _____

4 When filling out the claim, always record the _____ time, which indicates the ending time of the time spent personally attending to the patient for anesthesia services.

5 _____ time is that time when the anesthesia care of the patient can be safely turned over to a non-anesthesia provider. This generally never happens in the operating room.

6 The _____ time on the anesthesia record should match the time reported on the claim form and indicates the beginning time of the anesthesia service.

CONCURRENT MODIFIERS

Some third-party payers require additional modifiers to indicate how many cases an anesthesiologist was performing or supervising at one time. Certified registered nurse anesthetists (CRNAs) may administer anesthesia to patients under the direction of a licensed physician, or they may work independently. An anesthesiologist may medically direct up to four cases at the same time (concurrently). If a physician directs more than four cases, it is referred to as medical supervision. Medical direction means the directing anesthesiologist is present at the induction and emergence from anesthesia, for all key portions of the procedure, and is immediately available in case of an emergency. The CRNA would be with the patient the entire time.

NCCI

When medical direction occurs, certain documentation must be submitted for services for Medicare patients. The documentation supports that certain services were personally performed by the physician. These include:
1. Pre-anesthesia examination and evaluation
2. Prescription of an anesthesia plan
3. Personally participates in the most demanding procedures in the anesthesia plan, including induction and emergence
4. Ensures that any procedures in the anesthesia plan that he or she does not perform are performed by a qualified anesthetist
5. Monitors the course of anesthesia administration at frequent intervals

Continued

6. Remains physically present and available for immediate diagnosis and treatment of emergencies
7. Provides indicated post-anesthesia care

Additional modifiers that define the types of providers involved in anesthesia are:

AA Anesthesia services performed personally by an anesthesiologist

AD Medical supervision by a physician; more than 4 concurrent anesthesia procedures

G8 Monitored anesthesia care (MAC) for deep, complex, complicated, or markedly invasive surgical procedure

G9 Monitored anesthesia care for patient who has a history of severe cardiopulmonary condition

QK Medical direction of two, three, or four concurrent anesthesia procedures involving qualified individuals

QS Monitored anesthesia care service

QX Certified registered nurse anesthetist (CRNA) service, with medical direction by a physician

QY Medical direction of one certified registered nurse anesthetist by an anesthesiologist

QZ CRNA service, without medical direction by a physician

These modifiers are not CPT modifiers but HCPCS modifiers and further define the anesthesia services provided. Anesthesia modifiers are always placed first after the CPT anesthesia code. These anesthesia modifiers are pricing modifiers and are listed first to assure correct reimbursement.

QUICK CHECK 11-3

1. What is the difference between modifiers QX and QY? _____

_____

_____

_____

EXERCISE 11-3 *Modifiers*

Using Appendix A of the CPT manual, identify the following CPT modifiers:

1 Increased Procedural Services _____

2 Unusual Anesthesia _____

Using the descriptions for the preceding HCPCS modifiers, answer the following questions. Which modifier would be used to identify:

3 Medical supervision by a physician of more than 4 concurrent anesthesia procedures?

_____

4 Monitored anesthesia care service? _____

5 Medical direction by a physician of a CRNA? _____

UNLISTED ANESTHESIA CODE

In the Anesthesia section, an unlisted procedure code is available and is located under the Other Procedures subsection in the Anesthesia section. When there is no CPT code to indicate the anesthesia services, the unlisted Anesthesia code (01999) may be reported.

EXERCISE 11-4 *Anesthesia Codes*

Complete the following:

1 What is the unlisted anesthesia procedure code?

Code: _01999_

Locate anesthesia procedures in the CPT manual index under the entry "Anesthesia" and then subtermed by the anatomic site. Write the CPT index location on the line provided (e.g., Anesthesia, Thyroid). Then locate the code(s) identified in the Anesthesia section of the CPT manual. Choose the correct code(s) and write the code(s) on the line provided.

2 Needle biopsy of the thyroid (neck)

Index location: _Neck_

Code: _00322_

3 Cesarean section, delivery only

Index location: _OB_

Code: _01961_

4 Transurethral resection of the prostate

Index location: _Perineum_

Code: _00914_

5 Repair of cleft palate

Index location: _Head_

Code: _00172_

6 Repair of ruptured Achilles tendon without graft

Index location: _Lower leg_

Code: _01472_

Using the following information and the B + T + M formula, calculate the payment for the anesthesia services.

For the following questions a time unit will be 15 minutes. Base unit value for each case is provided within the questions. Refer to Fig. 11–13 for the conversion factors used in these questions; to Fig. 11–10 for the value of the Qualifying Circumstances; and to Fig. 11–11 for the value of the Physical Status Modifiers.

7 A needle biopsy lasting 15 minutes was conducted in North Dakota on a normal, healthy 75-year-old patient. The base unit value for the service is 3.

Anesthesia payment: _____

Continued

8 A patient with diabetes mellitus, controlled by diet and exercise, undergoes a 60-minute anesthesia period for a transurethral resection of the prostate (base unit value of 5). Calculate the anesthesia rate if the procedure were performed in the following locales:

a Manhattan _____

b North Carolina _____

9 A cesarean section was conducted in Alfred, NY, on a patient with preeclampsia (1 modifying unit). The base unit value for the service is 7. Calculate the anesthesia rates for procedures lasting two different lengths of time (refer to Fig. 11–13 for conversion rates):

a 30-minute procedure _____

b 45-minute procedure _____

OTHER REPORTING

Return to Operating Room

If a patient is returned to the operating room on the same day for the same or a related procedure, and the same physician is performing the second procedure, report the service with modifier -76. For example, the anesthesiologist provides the service for an upper gastrointestinal endoscopic procedure and reports the service 00740-AA. Later that day, the patient is returned for a lower intestinal endoscopic procedure. The second service would be reported 00810-76-AA. If that second procedure was performed by another anesthesiologist, the second service would be reported 00810-77-AA.

Pre-Anesthetic Examination

If the pre-anesthetic examination was provided by an anesthesiologist to a patient who did not undergo surgery, the service would be reported for consideration for reimbursement.

TOOLBOX

The patient presents for transabdominal repair of a diaphragmatic hernia. The patient has severe diabetes, but the surgeon indicates the patient is stable and able to undergo the procedure. The anesthesiologist provides medical direction to the CRNA.

QUESTIONS

1. What modifier identifies the medical direction? _____

2. What code reports anesthesia services for a transabdominal repair of a diaphragmatic hernia?

_____

3. What would be the physical status modifier documented in the medical record? _____

ANSWERS 1. -QY 2. 00756 3. P3

CHAPTER REVIEW

CHAPTER 11, PART I, THEORY

Complete the following:

1 Anesthesia services are based on

_____ time the patient is under
the anesthesiologist's care. Calculation of units
of time is determined by the third-party payer.

2 Anesthesia time begins when the

anesthesiologist _____,

_____

continues _____

_____

the procedure, and ends when

_____

_____.

3 According to the Anesthesia Guidelines, what is
the one modifier that is not used with

anesthesia procedures? _____

4 "P1" is an example of what type of modifier?

_____

5 What word means "in a dying state"?

_____

6 What word means "affecting the body as a

whole"? _____

7 The letter "P" in combination with what
number indicates a brain-dead patient?

_____

8 What type of circumstance identifies a
component of anesthesia service that
affects the character of the service?

_____

9 Anesthesia procedures are divided by what type

of site? _____

10 According to the Anesthesia Guidelines, the
Separate or Multiple Procedures section, when
multiple surgical procedures are performed
during a single anesthetic administration,
the anesthesia code representing the most

_____ procedure is reported and

the time reported is the _____

_____ for all procedures.

11 Is it true that a physician who personally
administers the anesthesia to the patient upon
whom he or she is operating cannot bill the

third-party payer? _____

12 What is the name of the guide that is published
by the American Society of Anesthesiologists
and provides the weights of various anesthesia

services? _____

CHAPTER 11, PART II, PRACTICAL

Using your CPT manual, identify the modifier for the following descriptions:

13 Anesthesia for tendon repair of the shoulder, normal, healthy patient

Anesthesia Code: _____

14 Anesthesia for a cesarean hysterectomy following neuraxial labor anesthesia, normal, healthy patient

Anesthesia Code: _____

15 Anesthesia for a missed abortion procedure in which the mother is in grave danger of death

Anesthesia Code: _____

16 Cranioplasty for a depressed skull fracture, simple, extradural, for a patient with mild diabetes, well-controlled

Anesthesia Code: _____

17 Total hip replacement in a 75-year-old patient with hypertension that is well controlled with medication

Anesthesia Codes: _____ ,

_____

18 Burn excision of 5% of the total body surface with skin grafting of the abdomen. Patient is 9 months old and in stable condition.

Anesthesia Codes: _____ ,

_____

19 Hospital management of a continuous epidural drug delivery system for 5 days

Anesthesia Code(s): _____

20 Arthroscopic total wrist replacement in a normal, healthy patient

Anesthesia Code(s): _____

QUICK CHECK ANSWERS

QUICK CHECK 11-1
1. In the CPT index, locate the main term "Injection," subterm "Spinal Cord," then subterm "Blood" for code 62273 OR main term "Spinal Cord," subterm "Injection," then subterm "Blood."

QUICK CHECK 11-2
1. Anesthesia Guidelines

QUICK CHECK 11-3
1. QX: Indicates medical direction of a CRNA by a physician and is appended to the CRNA portion of the charge.
   QY: Indicates medical direction by an anesthesiologist of one CRNA and is appended to the physician portion of the charge.

"Learn conflict resolution skills that use a 'win-win' approach and creates the proper atmosphere for resolving differences and working together as a team. Maintain a positive sense of self-esteem."

Robert H. Ekvall, PhD, CCS, CPC-H, CPMA, CPC

Radiation Oncology Coding/ Billing Specialist

Scripps Green Hospital

LaJolla, California

Surgery Guidelines and General Surgery

Chapter Topics

Introduction to the Surgery Section

Notes and Guidelines

Unlisted Procedures

Special Reports

Separate Procedure

Surgical Package

General Subsection

Chapter Review

Quick Check Answers

Learning Objectives

After completing this chapter you should be able to

1 Understand the Surgery section format.

2 Locate notes and Guidelines in the Surgery section.

3 State the use of the unlisted procedure codes.

4 Interpret elements of a special report.

5 Examine the separate procedure designation.

6 Analyze the contents of a surgical package.

7 Determine the contents of the General Subsection.

Make sure to check **evolve** learning system **for the latest content updates**

INTRODUCTION TO THE SURGERY SECTION

The Surgery section is the largest in the CPT manual. The codes range from 10021 to 69990. Surgery is divided into subsections. Most Surgery subsections are defined according to medical specialty or body system (e.g., integumentary or respiratory). Take a moment to review the Surgery subsections of the CPT manual so you have an understanding of the content of this important section.

Within the Surgery section, some of the more complex subsections are the Integumentary, Musculoskeletal, Respiratory, Cardiovascular, Digestive, and Female Genital subsections. Before we get into the details of the subsections, let's look at the general information that is pertinent to the entire Surgery section.

NOTES AND GUIDELINES

Guidelines are found at the beginning of each of the CPT sections. The section Guidelines define terms that are necessary to know for appropriately interpreting and reporting the procedures and services contained in the section. The following is an example of the type of information located in the Surgery Guidelines:

- Physicians' Services: A reference explaining how to assign E/M codes
- CPT Surgical Package Definition: Defines what is included in the surgical procedure
- Follow-up Care for Diagnostic Procedures: Defines follow-up care for diagnostic services
- Follow-up Care for Therapeutic Surgical Procedures: Defines follow-up care for therapeutic services
- Materials Supplied by Physician: Describes how and when to report supplies
- Reporting More Than One Procedure/Service: Identifies situations in which it may be appropriate to use modifiers for multiple services provided on the same day
- Separate Procedure: How to assign codes with this designation
- Subsection Information: Lists subsections that have instructional notes
- Unlisted Service or Procedure: Unlisted service codes from the Surgery section
- Special Reports: What to include in and when to submit a special report
- Surgical Destruction: Clarifies that destruction can be accomplished by any method, and that there are limited exceptions when the method is coded separately

QUICK CHECK 12-1

1. A listing of subsections that have instructional notes is not included in the Surgical section Guidelines.
   True or False?

The **Guidelines** contain information that you will need to know in order to correctly code in the section, and most of the information is not repeated elsewhere in the section. So always review the Guidelines before coding in the section. Remember that with each new edition of the CPT manual, you will need to review the Guidelines for any changes. The changes are indicated by the "New or Revised Text" symbols used throughout the CPT manual (Fig. 12–1).

Reporting More Than One Procedure/Service

▶ When a physician performs more than one procedure/service on the same date, during the same session, or during a postoperative period (subject to the "surgical package" concept), several CPT modifiers may apply. (See Appendix A for definition.) ◀

New or revised text symbol

FIGURE 12-1   New or revised text symbol.

Note that the content of the figures is only for illustration and the current year CPT may not display the information as stated in these text figures.

Common throughout the CPT manual are notes. Notes may appear before subsections (Fig. 12–2), subheadings (Fig. 12–3), categories (Fig. 12–4), and subcategories (Fig. 12–5).

The information in the notes indicates the special instructions unique to particular codes or groups of codes. The notes are extremely important

Subsection

Musculoskeletal System

Cast and strapping procedures appear at the end of this section.

The services listed below include the application and removal of the first cast or traction device only. Subsequent replacement of cast and/or traction device may require an additional listing.

Definitions

The terms "closed treatment," "open treatment," and "percutaneous skeletal fixation" have been carefully chosen to accurately reflect current orthopaedic procedural treatments.

Notes

FIGURE 12-2   Subsection notes.

Spine (Vertebral Column)

Cervical, thoracic, and lumbar spine

Within the Spine section, bone grafting procedures are reported separately and in addition to arthrodesis. For bone grafts in other Musculoskeletal sections, see specific code(s), descriptor(s), and/or accompanying guidelines.

Subheading

Notes

FIGURE 12-3   Subheading notes.

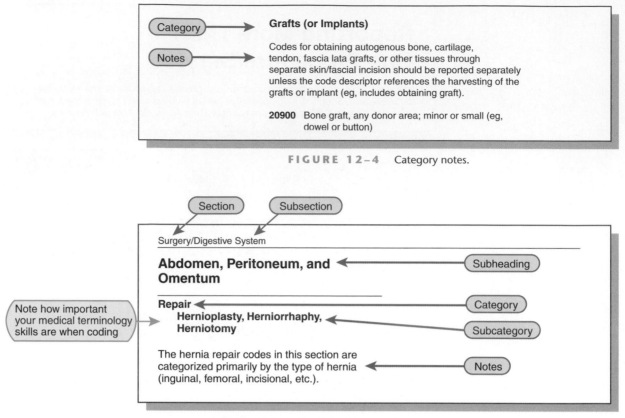

FIGURE 12-4   Category notes.

FIGURE 12-5   Subcategory notes.

because the information contained in them is not usually available in the section Guidelines. Always make it a practice to read any notes available before coding. If notes are present, they must be followed if the coding is to be accurate. Make it a practice to write in your coding manuals. Highlight important points, make notes in the margins, and personalize your coding manual. You will find these personal annotations are very helpful as you code.

Additional information is enclosed in parentheses, called parenthetical phrases or expressions. They sometimes follow the code or group of codes, and provide further information about codes that may be applicable. For example, 42120, Resection of the palate or extensive resection of a lesion, is followed by information about codes you would assign if reconstruction of the palate followed the resection (Fig. 12-6).

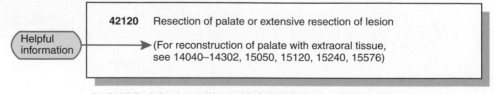

FIGURE 12-6   Additional helpful information in parentheses.

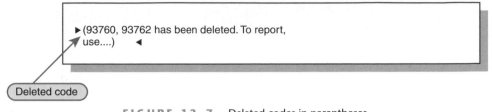

▶(93760, 93762 has been deleted. To report, use....) ◀

Deleted code

FIGURE 12-7 Deleted codes in parentheses.

Deleted codes are also indicated in the CPT manual, enclosed in parentheses. Often the code that is to be used in place of the deleted code will be listed (Fig. 12–7). Appendix B of the CPT manual has a summary of code additions, deletions, and revisions for the current year.

Also note in Fig. 12–7 that the arrows at the beginning and end of the information indicate that the information is new or has been revised for the current edition.

UNLISTED PROCEDURES

The Surgery Guidelines contain many unlisted procedure codes, presented by anatomic site. These unlisted codes are presented in alphabetical order by their location in the Surgery section Guidelines and in the subsections by body system. For example, the unlisted procedure code for procedures of the forearm or wrist, 25999, is located in the Surgery Guidelines and also at the end of the subheading Forearm and Wrist. The unlisted codes identify procedures or services throughout the Surgery section for which there is no CPT code. If a Category III code is available for the unlisted service you are reporting, you must use the Category III code, not the unlisted Category I code. Reimbursement for Category III codes will vary by payer.

QUICK CHECK 12-2

1. Before you can assign an unlisted code, you must first be certain there is no more specific code and that there is not a Category _____ code available.

From the Trenches

"Understand all the different types of devices/tools and what they are generally used for so you can learn which CPT codes were involved in the surgery."

ROBERT

EXERCISE 12-1 *Unlisted Procedures*

Using the CPT manual, locate the unlisted procedure codes in the Surgical Guidelines, and identify the unlisted procedure codes for the following anatomic areas:

1 Musculoskeletal system, general

Code: _____

2 Inner ear

Code: _____

3 Skin, mucous membranes, and subcutaneous tissue

Code: _____

4 Leg or ankle

Code: _____

5 Nervous system

Code: _____

6 Eyelids

Code: _____

SPECIAL REPORTS

When using an unlisted procedure code to report a surgical service, a special report describing the procedure must accompany the claim. According to the CPT manual, "Pertinent information *[in the special report]* should include an adequate definition or description of the **nature, extent,** and **need** for the procedure, and the **time, effort,** and **equipment** necessary to provide the service."

✋ **CAUTION** *Unlisted codes are assigned only after thorough research fails to reveal a more specific code.*

Example

When the first total disc arthroplasty (artificial disc) was performed there was no code to report the service, so a special report would have been submitted. The report contained a detailed description of the procedure, why it was being performed, the extent of the procedure, the length of time the procedure required, and the equipment necessary. There was a Category III code to describe this procedure (0090T). Later, 0090T was deleted and a Category I code was created (22856).

Medical supplier representatives may be of assistance to you in obtaining the information necessary to support the use of the new technique used during the procedure.

SEPARATE PROCEDURE

Some procedure codes will have the words "separate procedure" after the descriptor. The term, "separate procedure," does not mean that the procedure was the only procedure that was performed; rather, it is an indication of how the code can be assigned. Locate code 19100 in the CPT manual. The breast biopsy code 19100 has the words "(separate procedure)" after the description. Procedures followed by the words "separate procedure" (in parentheses) are considered **minor** procedures that are reported only when they are the only services performed or when they are performed with another major procedure but at a different site or unrelated to the major procedure. When the minor procedure is performed in conjunction with a related major procedure, the minor procedure is considered incidental and is bundled into the code for the major procedure.

Example

Separate procedure bundled into the major procedure: Breast biopsy (19100) has "separate procedure" after it. If a breast biopsy was performed in conjunction with a modified radical mastectomy (19307), only the mastectomy would be reported. Because the breast biopsy and the mastectomy were conducted on the same body area, the breast biopsy would be considered a minor procedure that was incidental and would be bundled into the major procedure of the mastectomy. Exception: As an example, a patient has a breast biopsy (19120) performed and then is brought back to the operating room for more extensive tissue removal (19304) the same day. The second procedure would have modifier -58 (Staged or related procedure or service by the same physician during the postoperative period) appended to the code (19304-58).

Example

Two separate procedures: If a breast biopsy (19100 a separate procedure) was performed in conjunction with an esophagoscopy (43200), both the breast biopsy and the esophagoscopy would be reported. The breast biopsy and the esophagoscopy were performed on different body areas and as such, the breast biopsy would not be bundled into the esophagoscopy procedure.

Example

Separate procedure bundled into the major procedure. Salpingo-oophorectomy (58720—removal of tubes and ovaries) has "separate procedure" after it. If a salpingo-oophorectomy was performed in conjunction with an abdominal hysterectomy (removal of the uterus, 58150), only the hysterectomy would be reported. Because the salpingo-oophorectomy and the abdominal hysterectomy were conducted on the same body area, the salpingo-oophorectomy would be bundled into the more major procedure of the hysterectomy.

Example

Two separate procedures: If a salpingo-oophorectomy (58720—separate procedure) was performed in conjunction with an esophagoscopy (43200), both the salpingo-oophorectomy and the esophagoscopy would be reported. Because the salpingo-oophorectomy and the esophagoscopy were conducted on different body areas, the salpingo-oophorectomy is considered a separate procedure, not a minor procedure incidental to a major procedure.

From the Trenches

"Learn how to read and abstract a medical report to know which CPT codes apply to what occurred in the operation, surgery, or medical procedure. Doctors don't often use the words that the CPT code describes."

ROBERT

QUICK CHECK 12-3

1. When a minor procedure is performed with a more major procedure of the same area, you would report both the minor and major procedure. True or False?

SURGICAL PACKAGE

Often, the time, effort, and services rendered when accomplishing a procedure are bundled together to form a surgical package. Payment is made for a package of services and not for each individual service provided within the package. The CPT manual describes the surgical package as including the operation itself, local anesthesia, and "typical postoperative follow-up care," one related E/M encounter prior to the procedure, and immediate follow-up care, including written orders. Read the information regarding the surgical package in the Surgery Guidelines and highlight the "included" elements because you will be referring back to this information as you report surgical services.

The surgical package contains the components of:

- Preoperative visits
- Intraoperative services
- Complications following surgery
- Post-operative visits
- Supplies
- Miscellaneous service—dressing changes, catheter removal, etc.

Local anesthesia is defined as local infiltration, metacarpal/digital block, or topical anesthesia. Follow-up care for complications, exacerbations (a worsening), recurrence, and the presence of other diseases that require additional services is not included in the surgical package. General anesthesia for surgical procedures is not part of the surgical package; general anesthesia services are reported separately by the anesthesiologist.

Third-party payers have varying definitions of what constitutes a surgical package and varying policies about what is included in the surgical package. Surgical packages also define the services for which you can or cannot submit additional charges because the rules of the surgical package define what is and is not included with the surgical procedure. Included in the definition of the surgical package are routine preoperative and postoperative care—including usual complications—and up to a predefined number of days before and after the surgery. Reimbursement policies vary from payer to payer because of the way each payer defines each surgical bundle. For instance, Medicare states that they averaged the costs associated with additional services for complications and added payments for those services into the initial surgical payment. Other commercial payers determine the reimbursement based on services associated only with performing the surgery and choose to let costs for services for complications be reported separately. The period of time following each surgery that is included in the surgery package is established by the third-party payer and is referred to as the **global (postoperative) surgery** period. The global period is usually **90** days for major surgery and **10** days for minor surgery.

Fig. 12–8 shows CPT codes 10080 and 10081 for incision and drainage of a pilonidal cyst. The third-party payer may indicate that code 10080 has zero days for the global surgical package, so you would charge for any additional services that were provided in addition to the 10080 incision and drainage itself. The payer may indicate that 10081 has 10 days for the global surgical package that would include routine follow-up care and services (such as removal of sutures) at no charge. You must know the number of days in the global service for a code to correctly bill for the services that are not included in the bundle and to be certain not to bill for services that were included in the bundle.

CHECK THIS OUT ☞ The Physician's Fee Schedule Relative Value Files are located on the CMS website at www.cms.hhs.gov/PhysicianFeeSched/ PFSRVF/list.asp#TopOfPage. It is within these files that the global days for each surgical procedure is located.

One last coding guideline that you have to know before you begin to code surgical procedures pertains to materials and supply codes. When **materials** or **supplies** over and above those usually used in an office visit have been used, you code and charge for these materials and supplies in addition to charging for the office visit or procedure. For example, when a physician does a wound repair during an office visit and uses a surgical tray, the surgical tray may be identified by CPT code 99070. Code 99070 is listed in the Medicine section, Special Services, Procedures, and Reports subsection, Miscellaneous subheading.

NCCI

HCPCS code A4550 also reports the use of a surgical tray. Third-party payers who pay separately for a surgical tray usually want the HCPCS "A" code to report the tray. Many third-party payers do not pay separately for a surgical tray. Medicare, however, does pay separately for a surgical tray for a limited number of surgical procedures.

This code would typically not include the office visit

Incision and Drainage

10080   Incision and drainage of pilonidal cyst; simple

10081   complicated

This code would typically include the office visit

FIGURE 12-8 Surgery package.

The following examples recap two major guidelines concerning surgical packages:

1. Surgical packages for procedures usually include the preoperative service, the procedure (intraoperative), related services, and routine postoperative services. Payers vary in their interpretation of the global surgical package. Although most follow the CPT guidelines, some payers, such as Medicare, expand the services that are included in the surgical package to include treatment of complications by the same physician.

Example

An established patient, Mary Smith is referred to a surgeon for excessive menstrual bleeding. The surgeon decides a hysterectomy is necessary and schedules the surgical procedure for 2 weeks later. The surgeon plans to recheck Mary in the office the day before surgery. The initial visit, at which the decision is made to perform surgery, is billable, but the preoperative visit on the day before surgery is bundled into the surgical package, as is the procedure itself and any routine follow-up.

2. Complications are usually added on a service-by-service basis.

NCCI

Medicare includes care for complications related to the surgical procedure in the global reimbursement and does not reimburse separately for the complications. If the complication requires a return to the operating room, the procedure is separately reported with modifier -78 (Unplanned return to the operating/procedure room by the same physician following initial procedure for a related procedure during the postoperative period) and the initial surgery global period continues. Most private payers follow the Medicare rules.

Even though the routine follow-up care is at no charge, the service is still coded to indicate that the service was provided. CPT code 99024 (Postoperative follow-up visit, included in global service) alerts the third-party payer that the services were rendered but the services were included in a surgical package and not charged for.

From the Trenches

"We see the importance of networking and assisting each other as we seek answers/ solutions to complex coding scenarios . . . . There are so many complexities to coding where there are no easy answers as we seek to code correctly and ethically."
ROBERT

Example

A patient undergoes a wound repair that is coded 12014 (the third-party payer indicated that there was a 10-day surgical package for this code) and 5 days afterwards sees the physician for routine follow-up care of the wound. The fee statement for the office visit at which the routine follow-up care is provided would be:

99024   Postoperative follow-up visit   No charge

However, if the patient returned during the global period because of a breakdown in the skin around the surgical wound (dehiscence) but with no signs of infection, and the patient was returned to the operating room at which time the physician trimmed the skin margins around the wound and resutured the wound, you would report and charge for this complication during the global period with:

12020-78   Dehiscence, simple closure $xx.xx

If a patient undergoes the repair of a 7.9-cm wound that is coded 12004 (the third-party payer indicated that there was no surgical package for this code) and sees the physician a few days later for routine follow-up care, the service is coded and charged for.

12004	Wound repair, 7.9 cm	$xx.xx
99070	Surgical tray	$xx.xx
99212-25	Office visit	$xx.xx

NCCI   Medicare assigns 12004 a 10-day global period. Medicare does not reimburse separately for supplies.

Inclusion or exclusion of a procedure in the CPT manual does not imply any health insurance coverage or reimbursement policy. Although the CPT manual includes guidelines on usage, third-party payers may interpret and accept the use of CPT codes and the guidelines in any manner they choose.

EXERCISE 12-2 *Surgical Package*

Answer the following:

1 What are the three parts of a surgery bundled into a surgical package?

   a _____

   b _____

   c _____

2 Is general anesthesia included in the surgical package? _____

3 Do all third-party payers follow the same reimbursement guidelines for the global packages? _____

GENERAL SUBSECTION

The General subsection contains codes for fine needle aspirations (10021, 10022), excluding bone marrow aspirations (see code 38220). The codes are divided based on whether **imaging guidance** was used during the aspiration. A **fine needle biopsy** is used to withdraw fluid that contains individual cells, as illustrated in Fig. 12–9. The needle is inserted into the area being biopsied and moved several times to take multiple samples without withdrawing the needle. The aspirated cells are then examined by a pathologist using a microscope (88172 or 88173). This type of biopsy is not to be confused with a needle core biopsy, such as that identified by 19100, percutaneous breast biopsy using a **needle core,** in which a core of suspicious tissue is removed for examination or the biopsy represented in 19101, breast biopsy using an open incision, which reports a procedure in which the biopsy site is exposed to the surgeon's view and a sample of the lesion is removed. Notes following codes 10021-10022 indicate several other codes that are used to report percutaneous needle biopsies based on what was biopsied.

EXERCISE 12-3   *General Subsection*

Using the CPT manual, report the services for the following:

1 The physician palpates a cyst on the right breast and performs a fine needle aspiration in the office.

   Code: _____

2 A patient presents to the outpatient surgical center at the clinic for a fine needle aspiration of the thyroid. Ultrasound guidance is utilized during the aspiration.

   Code aspiration: _____

   Code ultrasound guidance: _____

FIGURE 12–9   Fine needle biopsy. (From Forbes CD, Jackson WF: *Color Atlas and Text of Clinical Medicine,* ed 3, 2003, Mosby.)

CHAPTER REVIEW

CHAPTER 12, PART I, THEORY

Now is an excellent time to put all your newly learned coding skills to work by completing a Chapter Review.

1 What is the largest section of the six CPT manual sections? _____

2 Does Medicare reimburse for a surgical tray?

   Yes   No

3 The subsections in the Surgery section are usually divided according to _____.

4 These are found at the beginning of each section and contain information specific to the section.

   _____

5 This symbol indicates new or revised text within the current edition of the CPT manual.

   _____

6 Information within parentheses is referred to as _____ expression or phrase.

7 Before assigning this type of code, you must be certain that a more specific Category I or a Category III code is not available. _____

8 This report contains the nature, extent, need, time, effort, and at times equipment necessary to provide a service. _____

9 This designation within the CPT manual indicates a procedure that is only reported when it is performed as the only procedure or when another procedure performed at the same time is unrelated to this procedure. This is a _____ procedure.

10 When time, effort, and services are bundled together, they form a _____ package.

11 _____ anesthesia is defined as local infiltration, metacarpal/digital block, or topical anesthesia.

12 According to Medicare guidelines, _____ complications of a surgical procedure are usually included in the reimbursement for a major surgical procedure.

13 Code _____ is a CPT code that can be assigned to report a surgical tray.

14 Code _____ is a HCPCS code that can be assigned to report a surgical tray.

15 This code reports a postoperative follow-up visit that is included in the global service.

   _____

CHAPTER 12, PART II, PRACTICAL

With the use of the CPT manual Surgery Guidelines, answer the following:

16 _____ destruction is a part of a surgical procedure and different methods of destruction are not ordinarily listed separately.

17 Care of the condition for which a diagnostic procedure was performed or of other _____ conditions is not included and may be listed separately.

18 There are "Notes" in Burns, _____ Treatment subsection.

19 The only code in the Operating Microscope subsection is _____.

20 Follow-up care for therapeutic surgical procedures includes only that care which is usually part of the _____ _____.

According to the parenthetical information that follows code 10022:

21 The four codes for radiological supervision and interpretation are _____, _____, _____, and _____.

22 For evaluation of fine needle aspirate, see _____, _____.

QUICK CHECK ANSWERS

QUICK CHECK 12-1
1. False

QUICK CHECK 12-2
1. III

QUICK CHECK 12-3
1. False

CHAPTER 73

"Get to know what your doctors are doing—how they do procedures and how they document . . . . You can get all the codes correct up front. It sets the stage for anything you have to do with the insurance companies later."

Christopher P. Galeziewski, CPC
Coding Compliance Specialist
Coding Compliance Department
Kelsey-Seybold Clinic
Houston, Texas

Integumentary System

Chapter Topics

Integumentary System

Format

Skin, Subcutaneous, and Accessory Structures

Nails

Repair (Closure)

Burns

Destruction

Breast Procedures

Chapter Review

Quick Check Answers

Learning Objectives

After completing this chapter you should be able to

1 Describe the format of the Integumentary System in the CPT manual.

2 Identify the elements of coding Skin, Subcutaneous, and Accessory Structures services.

3 Review the main services in Nails.

4 Identify the major factors in Repair.

5 State the important coding considerations in destruction and breast procedures.

6 Demonstrate the ability to code integumentary services and procedures.

Make sure to check
evolve
learning system
for the latest
content updates

INTEGUMENTARY SYSTEM

The Integumentary System subsection includes codes assigned by many different physician specialties. There is no restriction on who reports the codes from this or any other subsection. You may find a family practitioner using the incision and drainage, debridement, or repair codes; a dermatologist using excision and destruction codes; a plastic surgeon using skin graft codes; or a surgeon using breast procedure codes.

You will learn about the Integumentary System subsection by first reviewing the subsection format and then learning about coding the services and procedures in the subsection.

QUICK CHECK 13-1

1. Dermatologists are the only providers who utilize the codes in the Integumentary System subsection of CPT manual.
   True or False?

FORMAT

The subsection is formatted on the basis of anatomic site and category of procedure. For example, an anatomic site is "Neck" and a category of procedure is "Repair."

The subsection Integumentary contains the subheadings:

- Skin, Subcutaneous, and Accessory Structures
- Nails
- Pilonidal Cyst
- Introduction
- Repair (Closure)
- Destruction
- Breast

Each subheading is further divided by category. For example, the subheading Skin, Subcutaneous and Accessory Structures is divided into the following categories:

- Incision and Drainage
- Excision—Debridement
- Paring or Cutting
- Biopsy
- Removal of Skin Tags
- Shaving of Epidermal or Dermal Lesions
- Excision—Benign Lesions
- Excision—Malignant Lesions

From the Trenches

"[Documentation] comes down to semantics. Certain words mean certain things . . . . That's what insurance companies look for to describe what type of test or work effort was done to determine the patient's illness."

CHRIS

SKIN, SUBCUTANEOUS, AND ACCESSORY STRUCTURES

Incision and Drainage

Incision and Drainage (I&D) codes (10040-10180) are divided according to the condition for which the I&D is being performed. Acne surgery, abscess, carbuncle, boil, cyst, hematoma, and wound infection are just some of the conditions for which a physician uses I&D (Fig. 13–1). The physician opens the lesion to allow drainage. Also included under this heading is a **puncture aspiration** code (10160), which describes inserting a needle into a lesion and withdrawing the fluid (aspiration). Whichever method is used—incision or aspiration—the contents of the lesion are drained. Packing material may be inserted into the opening or the wound may be left to drain freely. A tube or strip of gauze, which acts as a wick, may be inserted into the wound to facilitate drainage.

The I&D codes are first divided according to the condition and then according to whether the procedure was simple/single or complicated/multiple. The medical record would indicate the condition and complexity of the I&D. Verify the body area where the incision and drainage was performed for any specific CPT code that could be assigned outside of the range 10040-10180. For example, a simple finger abscess would be reported with an incision and drainage code (26010, 26011) from the Musculoskeletal System subsection, Hand and Finger, Incision codes. When you reference the index of the CPT manual, under the main term "Abscess" and subterm "Finger," you are directed to the Musculoskeletal System codes. Those codes are the most specific codes to report the incision and drainage of a finger abscess and you are to always assign the most specific code you can locate. Note that in the index of the CPT manual again under the main term "Abscess" and subterm "Skin," you are directed to the Integumentary codes. You should always reference the specific location of the abscess to receive direction to the most correct code(s) and only reference the skin subterm when there is no more specific location provided.

Debridement

Debridement is the removal of infected, contaminated, damaged, devitalized, necrotic, or foreign tissue from a wound. Debridement promotes wound healing by reducing sources of infection and other mechanical impediments to healing. The goal of debridement is to cleanse the wound, reduce bacterial contamination, and provide an optimal environment for wound healing or possible surgical intervention. The usual end point of debridement is removal of pathological tissue and/or foreign material until healthy tissue is exposed. Debridement techniques include, among others, sharp and blunt dissection, curettement, scrubbing, and forceful irrigation. Surgical

FIGURE 13–1 Massive staphylococcal carbuncle. (From Forbes CD, Jackson WF: *Color Atlas and Text of Clinical Medicine,* ed 3, 2003, Mosby.)

instruments may include a scrub brush, irrigation device, electrocautery, laser, sharp curette, forceps, scissors, burr, or scalpel. Prior to debridement, determination of the extent of an ulcer/wound may be aided by the use of probes to determine the depth and to disclose abscess and sinus tracts.

These debridement codes do not apply to debridement of burned surfaces. For debridement of burned surfaces, CPT codes 16000-16036 are reported.

Excision—Debridement

Codes in this category (11000-11044) describe services of debridement based on depth, body surface, condition, and for 11004-11006 by location. The first debridement codes (11000 and 11001) are reported for eczematous debridement. **Eczema** is a skin condition that blisters and weeps, as illustrated in Fig. 13–2.

The dead tissue may have to be cut away with a scalpel or scissors or, in less severe cases, washed with a saline solution. Code 11000 reports debridement of 10% of the body surface or less, and add-on code 11001 reports each additional 10% or part thereof.

> ### Example
>
> A patient presents for a debridement of 30% of the body surface. The service is reported: 11000, 11001 × 2. Code 11000 reports the first 10% and 11001 × 2 reports the remaining 20%.

Some codes in this category are based on the extent of the cleansing to the skin, subcutaneous tissue, muscle fascia, muscle, or bone.

CODING SHOT

Some surgical procedure codes include debridement as a part of the service. You may report a debridement as a separate service when the medical record indicates that a greater than usual debridement was provided. For example, if an extensive debridement was performed when usually a simple debridement would be performed, you report the additional service using a debridement code from the 11040-11044 range.

FIGURE 13–2   Eczematous dermatitis. (From Kumar V, et al: *Robbins & Cotran: Pathologic Basis of Disease,* ed 7, Philadelphia, 2005, Saunders.)

NCCI

According to Medicare Memorandum B-01-07, the following is considered when reporting debridement:

1. The care of minor wounds, either postoperative, traumatic, or otherwise, is incidental to other covered services. Many claims for debridement are essentially dressing changes and are not separately payable.
2. When the only service provided is the non-surgical cleansing of the wound or ulcer with or without the application of a surgical dressing, the provider should bill this service with an appropriate evaluation and management (E/M) code and not the debridement code(s).
3. The CPT code selected should report the level of debrided tissue, (e.g., partial-thickness skin, full-thickness skin, subcutaneous, muscle, bone), not the extent, depth, or grade of the ulcer or wound. For example, use CPT code 11042 if an ulcer extends to bone (grade 4) but only necrotic skin and subcutaneous tissue are debrided.
4. Select the most specific ICD-9-CM code that describes the primary reason for the service, at its highest level of specificity, as the diagnosis on the claim. Failure to do so will result in claim denial.
5. When the patient has required five or more debridement services per wound, the claim form must also include as secondary diagnoses ICD-9-CM codes reflecting neuropathic, vascular, metabolic, or other comorbid conditions that have resulted in excessive frequency of service.
6. Use of CPT codes 11000-11044 is not appropriate for the following services: washing bacterial or fungal debris from feet, paring or cutting of corns or calluses, incision and drainage of abscess including paronychia, trimming or debridement of nails, avulsion of nail plates, acne surgery, destruction of warts, or burn debridement. Report these procedures, when they represent covered, reasonable and necessary services, using the CPT or HCPCS code that most closely describes the service rendered.
7. An evaluation and management (E/M) service may be billed on the same day as the procedure if the E/M service represents a significant separately identifiable service. Modifier -25 must be appended to the E/M visit. Evaluation of the effect of a prior injection is not considered a "separately identifiable service."
8. Local infiltration, metacarpal/digital block, or topical anesthesia are included in the reimbursement for debridement services and are not separately payable.
9. Anesthesia administered by or incident to the physician or surgeon performing the debridement procedure is not separately payable.
10. A claim submitted without a valid ICD-9-CM diagnosis code will be returned as an incomplete claim under section 1833(e) of the Social Security Act.

Introduction to Lesions

Before you learn about coding the various methods of lesion destruction and excision, you need to review a few rules that apply broadly to this commonly performed procedure. After you have learned the general lesion information, you will review each of the destruction and excision methods.

Lesion Excision and Destruction. There are many types of lesions of the skin (Fig. 13–3) and many types of treatment for lesions. Types of treatment include **paring** (peeling or scraping), **shaving** (slicing), **excision** (cutting removal), and **destruction** (ablation). To code these procedures properly, you must know the **site, number,** and **size** of the excised lesion(s), as well as whether the lesion is malignant or benign.

Prior to excision, the greatest diameter of the lesion is measured. The measurement includes the margin (extra tissue taken from around the lesion) at its narrowest part. Fig. 13–4 illustrates calculations of a 2.0 cm lesion. The size of the margin necessary to completely remove the lesion is based on the physician's judgment. The pathology report is used to identify

MACULE
Flat area of color change; no elevation or depression

PAPULE
Solid elevation; less than 0.5 cm in diameter

NODULE
Solid elevation 0.5 to 1 cm in diameter; extends deeper into dermis than papule

TUMOR
Solid mass; larger than 1 cm

PLAQUE
Flat elevated surface found where papules, nodules, or tumors cluster

WHEAL
Type of plaque; result is transient edema in dermis

VESICLE
Small blister; fluid within or under epidermis

BULLA
Larger blister; greater than 0.5 cm

SCALES
Flakes of cornified skin layer

CRUST
Dried exudate on skin

FISSURE
Cracks in skin

EROSION
Loss of epidermis that does not extend into dermis

ULCER
Area of destruction of entire epidermis

SCAR
Excess collagen production following injury

ATROPHY
Loss of some portion of the skin

FIGURE 13-3   Lesions of the skin.

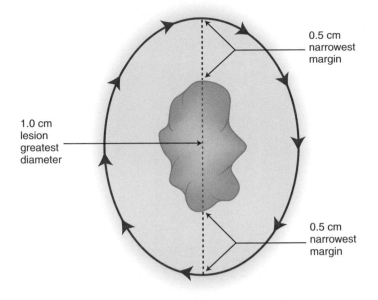

0.5 cm
narrowest
margin

1.0 cm
lesion
greatest
diameter

0.5 cm
narrowest
margin

FIGURE 13-4   Calculations of a 2.0 cm lesion.

the size of the lesion only if no other record of the size can be documented because the solution the lesion is stored in shrinks the lesion.

All lesions excised will have a pathology report for diagnosing the removed tissue as malignant or benign; since the codes are divided based on whether the excised lesion is malignant or benign, the billing for the excision is not submitted to the third-party payer until the pathology report has been completed.

> **CAUTION** *Destruction of lesions destroys the lesion, leaving available tissue for biopsy; therefore, there will be no pathology report for lesions that have been destroyed by laser, chemicals, electrocautery, or other methods. In these cases you will have to take the type of lesion from the physician's notes only, as there is no pathology report.*

Codes in the Integumentary System subsection differ greatly in their descriptions. Some codes indicate only one lesion per code, others are for the second and third lesions only, and still others indicate a certain number of lesions (e.g., up to 15 lesions). When reporting multiple lesions, you must read the description carefully to prevent incorrect coding.

If multiple lesions are treated, code the **most complex lesion procedure first followed by the others using modifier -51** to indicate that multiple procedures were performed. Remember that the third-party payer will usually reduce the payment for the services identified with modifier -51; so you want to be certain that you place the service with the highest dollar amount first, without the modifier. If the code description includes multiple lesions (a stated number of lesions), modifier -51 is not necessary. For example, if the code states "2 to 4 lesions" or "more than 4 lesions," modifier -51 is not required.

Closure of Excision Sites.   Included in the codes for lesion excision is the direct, primary, or simple closure of the operative site. A **simple excision** is a full thickness (through the dermis) excision and a **simple closure** is nonlayered closure (Fig. 13–5).

FIGURE 13–5 **A** and **B,** Simple subcuticular closure. (**B** courtesy Mary Garden.)

Closures can also be **intermediate** (layered; Fig. 13–6) or **complex** (greater than layered). The local anesthesia is included in the excision codes. Any closure other than a simple closure can be reported separately.

Three final notes on treatment of lesions:

1. The shaving of lesions requires no closure because no incision has been made.

2. Excision includes simple closure but may require more complex closure. If more complex closure is required, follow the notes in the CPT manual to appropriately code for these services.

3. Destruction may be by any method, including freezing, burning, chemicals, etc.

Paring or Cutting

Paring or Cutting codes (11055-11057) report the services when a physician removes a benign hyperkeratotic skin lesion such as a callus or corn (Fig. 13–7). Paring codes include removal by peeling or scraping. A

FIGURE 13–6 Intermediate two-layer closure. (**C** from Roberts JR, Hedges JR, eds: *Clinical Procedures in Emergency Medicine,* ed 4, Philadelphia, 2004, Saunders.)

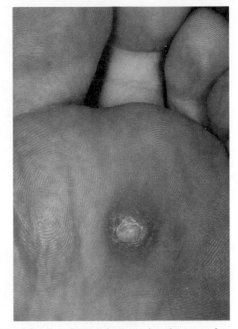

FIGURE 13–7 Corns (clavi) on the plantar surface. (From Habif TP: *Clinical Dermatology: A Color Guide to Diagnosis and Therapy,* ed 4, Philadelphia, 2004, Mosby.)

small ring-shaped instrument (curette), blade, or similar sharp instrument is used for paring. Bleeding is usually controlled by a chemical that is applied to the surface after removal of the lesion. The codes are divided based on the number of lesions removed.

Biopsy

"Biopsy" is a term applied to the procedure of removing some or all of the tissue of a lesion for histopathology (study of microscopic tissue changes). Removing a tissue sample of a lesion may be by needle aspiration, incisional biopsy (open, sharp, and partial removal), or by excisional biopsy (complete removal). You would not report **both** a biopsy and an excision performed at the same time as the biopsy is bundled into the excision service. In a biopsy, only a portion of the lesion and some of the surrounding tissue is removed. The section of surrounding tissue (margin) is included so the pathologist can compare the normal tissue to the lesion tissue and note the differences.

CODING SHOT Included in the Biopsy codes are codes for biopsies of mucous membranes. A mucous membrane is tissue that covers a variety of body parts, such as the tongue and the nasal cavities.

Many methods are used to obtain biopsies; the method chosen is determined by the size and type of the lesion and the physician's preference. Common biopsy methods are scraping, cutting, and the punch. A punch biopsy is illustrated in Fig. 13–8 and is used to excise a disc of tissue. A punch can also be used in the excision of the entire lesion, so just because the medical record refers to the use of a punch, it does not mean that a biopsy was performed.

Biopsy sites do not necessarily have to be closed; some are so small that they will close readily. Other sites are large enough that closure is required, and simple closure is bundled into the biopsy codes. If closure of the biopsy

FIGURE 13–8   Punch biopsy.

site is more than a simple closure, you would report the more extensive closure separately. You will learn more about closure later in this chapter.

On the CMS-1500 claim form, report the number of lesions treated in column 24G., Days or Units, as illustrated in Fig. 13–9.

✋ **CAUTION** *Do not assign modifier -51 with these biopsy codes, as 11100 reports a single lesion, and 11101 reports two or more lesions. The correct coding for three lesions would be 11100 for lesion one and 11101 × 2 for lesions two and three.*

Skin Tags   Skin tags are flaps of skin (benign lesions) that can appear anywhere, but most often appear on the neck or trunk, especially in older people (Fig. 13–10, *A*). Skin tags are removed in a variety of ways—scissors, blades, ligatures, electrosurgery, or chemicals. **Scissors removal** of a skin tag is illustrated in Fig. 13–10, *B*. Scissoring is often used for tissue column lesions. The forceps grasps the column, and the physician snips the lesion off at its base. Closure is achieved by using sutures or an aluminum chloride solution. In **ligature strangulation,** a thread is tied at the base of the lesion and left there until the tissue dies. The lesion then drops off. Whatever method

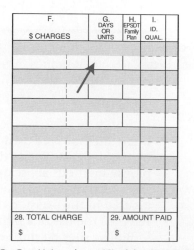

FIGURE 13–9   Units column (G) of the CMS-1500. (Courtesy U.S. Department of Health and Human Services, Centers for Medicare and Medicaid Services.)

FIGURE 13–10 **A,** Skin tag. **B,** Scissors removal. (**A** from Habif TP: *Clinical Dermatology: A Color Guide to Diagnosis and Therapy,* ed 4, Philadelphia, 2004, Mosby.)

of removal is used, simple closure is included in the skin tag codes, as is any local anesthesia that is used. Also, note that the codes (11200, 11201) are based on the first 15 lesions and then on each additional 10 lesions (or part thereof) after the first 15. On the CMS-1500 claim form, report the number of lesions treated in 24G., Days or Units (see Fig. 13–9).

CODING SHOT Do not use modifier -51 (multiple procedure) with skin tag codes, as the codes are based on the number of lesions removed.

Shaving of Epidermal or Dermal Lesions

The **shaving** of a lesion (11300-11313) can be performed by using a scalpel blade or other sharp instrument. The shaving of a lesion is illustrated in Fig. 13–11.

The blade is held horizontal to the skin and an epidermal or dermal lesion is sliced off. Anesthesia and cauterization (electrocautery or chemical cautery) to control bleeding are included in the lesion-shaving codes.

FIGURE 13–11 Shaving of a lesion.

Electrocautery is sometimes used to finish the edges of the shaving, but if electrocautery is the main method by which the lesion was removed, you would assign codes from the Destruction, Benign or Premalignant Lesions category (17000-17250), not from the Shaving category. Electrosurgery used in shaving a superficial lesion burns (destroys) the lesion, so the destruction code would be reported.

The Shaving codes are further defined according to the **location** of the lesion—trunk, neck, nose—and the **size** of the lesion. If more than one lesion was removed, you would add modifier -51 (multiple procedures) to any codes after the first code. For example, if one 2.0-cm lesion was removed from the trunk, and a 1.0-cm lesion was removed from the hand, you list the 2.0-cm lesion first with no modifier and the 1.0-cm lesion second, with modifier -51 added. Many third-party payers reimburse 100% for the first lesion and 50% for the second lesion, so by placing the more intensive procedure first, you optimize reimbursement.

Excision—Benign Lesions

The CPT manual divides the category of excision of lesions on the basis of whether a lesion is benign or malignant. Although at the time of excision it is not known for certain whether the lesion is benign or malignant, the physician makes an assessment of the lesion's status and usually plans the extent of the excision based on that assessment. The codes in the Excision—Benign Lesions category (11400-11471) are assigned for all benign lesions except skin tags, which you learned about earlier.

The codes include local anesthesia, so do not report local anesthesia separately, as that would be unbundling. The excision codes also include simple closure (see Fig. 13–5) of the excision site. If the closure is noted in the medical record as being more than simple (intermediate or complex), you would code the more complicated closure using a separate code from Repair subheading (12031-13160).

CODING SHOT You are not to assign the shaving codes if the shaving penetrated through the dermis (full thickness). Full-thickness shavings are to be reported with the excision codes found in the Excision—Benign Lesions or Excision—Malignant Lesions categories.

The codes in the Excision—Benign Lesions category are based on the **location** of the excision (e.g., trunk, scalp, ears, etc.) and the **size** of the lesion (e.g., 0.6-1.0 cm, 1.1-2.0 cm).

CODING SHOT In excision of either benign or malignant tissue, focus on the dimension of the normal tissue margin excised with the lesion. This normal tissue margin is the determining factor in selecting the correct CPT code.

There are several codes at the end of the category (11450-11471) for excision of the skin and subcutaneous tissue in cases of **hidradenitis** (Fig. 13–12), which is the chronic abscessing and subsequent infection of a sweat gland. The abscess is excised and the wound left open to heal. The hidradenitis codes are based on the abscess location (axillary, inguinal, perianal, perineal,

FIGURE 13-12 A hallmark of hidradenitis is the double and triple comedone, a blackhead with two or sometimes several surface openings that communicate under the skin. (From Habif TP: *Clinical Dermatology: A Color Guide to Diagnosis and Therapy,* ed 4, Philadelphia, 2004, Mosby.)

or umbilical) and the complexity of the repair (simple, intermediate, or complex).

Excision—Malignant Lesions

Codes in the Excision—Malignant Lesions subheading (11600-11646) are assigned for malignant lesions and include local anesthesia and simple closure (Fig. 13-13). As with the benign lesion codes, these codes refer to each lesion removed and are divided according to the **location** and **size** of the lesion. If you are coding a lesion removal that has been performed by a method other than excision (e.g., electrosurgery), the notes preceding the Excision codes direct you to the Destruction codes (17260-17286). If the closure is more than simple you would also use a repair code.

CODING SHOT If the excision is of a malignant lesion on the eyelid, and if the excision involves more than the skin of the eyelid (lid margin, tarsus, or conjunctiva), do **not** use malignant lesion excision codes. Instead, you would use a surgery code from the subsection Eye and Ocular Adnexa, Excision category (67800-67850).

From the Trenches

Would you recommend coding as a profession?

"I would for people who are meticulous and have a mind for detail . . . . People who take pride in their work. Someone who will say, 'I can find things out. I can learn things, and I can make it worthwhile for the physician to employ me.'"

CHRIS

FIGURE 13-13 Excision biopsy technique. (From Burkitt HG, Quick CRG: *Essential Surgery,* ed 3, 2002, Churchill Livingstone.

NAILS   Within the Nails category (11719-11765) are codes for the trimming of fingernails and toenails, debridement of nails, removal of nails, drainage of hematomas, biopsies of nails, repair of nails, reconstruction of nails, and excision of cysts of the nails. **Podiatrists** are physicians who specialize in the care of the foot; as such, these physicians use this category of codes extensively. However, all physicians can and do use these codes when providing nail care services to the feet and the hands.

The first code in the Nails category is 11719, which reports the trimming of nails that are not defective. This is a minimal service and the code reports trimming one fingernail/toenail or many fingernails/toenails. **Debridement** (11720) is a more complex service—the manual cleaning of up to five nails—and it includes the use of various tools, cleaning materials/solutions, and files. You would not report the supplies used for a nail debridement service separately, as these supplies are included in the codes. The two debridement codes are divided according to the number of nails attended to during the service. If the payer requires HCPCS codes, report G0127.

TOOLBOX

Mary presents to the physician for cleaning and trimming of 10 toenails. Mary is handicapped and lives alone and has not had anyone to help her with care of her toenails.

QUESTIONS

1. Which of the following correctly reports the service provided to Mary?

    a. 11720 × 10

    b. 11719 × 10

    c. 11732

    d. 11719

2. Why are you certain this is the correct answer? _____

ANSWERS 1. d 2. Because the code reports one or many toenail(s)

Avulsion is the separation and removal of the nail plate (11730, 11732), preserving the root so the nail will grow back. An anesthetic is administered, the nail is lifted away from the nail bed, and a portion or all of the nail plate is removed.

Place the number of nails treated in the units column (G) of the CMS-1500 form.

CODING SHOT

Do not use modifier -51 (multiple procedures) with nail removal codes, as there are two codes available: one for a single nail and one for each additional nail. For example, if three nails were removed, you would report: 11730 (for the first nail) and 11732 × 2 (for the second and third nails). Often, third-party payers require the use of HCPCS modifiers (F1-FA to indicate the finger and T1-TA to indicate the toe; Fig. 13–14) and the separate reporting of each digit treated.

A subungual hematoma (blood trapped under the nail) is evacuated by puncturing the nail with an electrocautery needle (11740). The trapped blood and fluid are drained by applying pressure to the top of the nail.

F1	Left hand, second digit	T1	Left foot, second digit
F2	Left hand, third digit	T2	Left foot, third digit
F3	Left hand, fourth digit	T3	Left foot, fourth digit
F4	Left hand, fifth digit	T4	Left foot, fifth digit
F5	Right hand, thumb	T5	Right foot, great toe
F6	Right hand, second digit	T6	Right foot, second digit
F7	Right hand, third digit	T7	Right foot, third digit
F8	Right hand, fourth digit	T8	Right foot, fourth digit
F9	Right hand, fifth digit	T9	Right foot, fifth digit
FA	Left hand, thumb	TA	Left foot, great toe

FIGURE 13–14 HCPCS modifiers used to indicate digits of hands and feet. (Modified from Buck CJ: *2009 HCPCS Level II Professional Edition,* St. Louis, 2009, Saunders.)

Onychocryptosis (ingrown toenail) is the most common condition of the great toe, as illustrated in Fig. 13–15. The nail grows down and into the soft tissue of the nail fold, causing extreme pain and often infection. Treatment for severe cases is a partial onychectomy (removal of the nail plate and root). The toe is anesthetized and a portion of the nail plate and root is removed (11750-11752). The nail will not grow back where the base has been removed.

CODING SHOT

Use of HCPCS modifiers is very important. For example, nail biopsies (11755) were performed on the left third finger (F2) and the left fourth finger (F3), in addition to the right fourth digit (F8). The reporting would be 11755-F2, 11755-F3, 11755-F8.

Pilonidal Cyst

The codes for the excision of a pilonidal cyst or sinus are 11770-11772. A pilonidal cyst is located in the sacral area and is most often caused by an ingrown hair. The codes are divided according to the complexity of the excision—simple, extensive, or complicated. For a simple cyst, the physician would excise the cyst and suture the skin together. A cyst larger than 2 cm is considered complicated and requires more extensive excision and closure. A complicated excision is very extensive and usually requires reconstructive surgical repair.

Introduction

Within the Introduction category of codes (11900-11983) are lesion injection, tattooing, tissue expansion, contraceptive capsule insertion/ removal, and hormone implantation services. Lesions are injected with medication to treat conditions such as acne, keloids (scar tissue), and psoriasis (autoimmune disorder that results in scaly patches). Lesion injection codes are divided according to the number of lesions injected (1-7 or 8+).

FIGURE 13–15 Removal of ingrown toenail. (From Rakel RE: *Saunders Manual of Medical Practice*, ed 2, Philadelphia, 2000, Saunders.)

CODING SHOT Lesion injection code 11901 is not an add-on code! You report 11900 for lesion injections numbering one through seven, and 11901 to report injections eight and more. For example, if seven lesions are injected, the service is reported with 11900. If eight lesions are injected, the service is reported with 11901.

Tattooing codes (11920-11922) are also located in the Introduction category. Tattooing is reported on the basis of square centimeters covered. Sometimes physicians use tattooing to disguise birthmarks or scars.

Codes for subcutaneous injection of filling material (11950-11954) are located in the Introduction category and are reported for services such as collagen or silicone injections (injectable dermal implants) used as a wrinkle treatment. The codes are based on the amount of material injected. The procedure is usually repeated at 2 to 3 week intervals until the results are those desired.

Tissue-expander codes (11960-11971) are also located in the Introduction category and report tissue expanders. A tissue expander is an elastic material formed into a sac that is then filled with fluid or air so it expands like a balloon. The expander is placed under the skin and is filled, stretching the skin. Expanders are most often used to prepare a site for a permanent implant. Expanders are also used to assist in the repair of scars and the removal of tattoos by stretching the skin, removing the expander, removing the scar or tattoo, and suturing the skin edges together. The codes are divided according to whether the service is an insertion, a removal, or an expander removal with replacement of a prosthesis.

CODING SHOT Do not report an expander code from the Introduction category after a mastectomy in which a temporary expander has been inserted. Code 19357 from the reconstruction section of the Integumentary subsection is a combination of the mastectomy and insertion of an expander. If at a later date the expander was replaced with a permanent prosthesis, you would report replacement of tissue expander with permanent prosthesis with 19342.

You will also find insertion of **implantable contraceptive capsules** in the Introduction category. Implantable contraceptive capsules such as Norplant are inserted under the skin by means of a small incision on the upper arm. A capsule is effective for a number of years; at the end of that time, it must be removed. Read the descriptions in the implantable contraceptive capsule codes (11975-11977) carefully, as there are codes for insertion, removal, and removal with insertion.

In addition to reporting the service of the introduction of the implantable contraceptive capsule, you report the supply of the contraceptive system with HCPCS code J7307.

Subcutaneous hormone pellet implantation is commonly used for the insertion of a hormone in a time-release capsule into the buttocks of women requiring hormone replacement therapy after menopause. The code for this implantation is in the Introduction category (11980). The implantation area is anesthetized and the pellet is inserted through a tube. The pellet is completely absorbed into the system and does not need to be removed, as does a contraceptive capsule. However, a new pellet must be inserted every 6 to 9 months (11980), and each reinsertion is reported separately.

EXERCISE 13-1 *Skin, Subcutaneous, and Accessory Structures*

Apply the information about lesion procedures by coding the following:

1 Paring of three common warts

    CPT Code: _____

    ICD-9-CM Code: _____

2 Removal of 15 skin tags

    CPT Code: _____

    ICD-9-CM Code: _____

3 Shaving of 1-cm dermal lesion of face

    CPT Code: _____

    ICD-9-CM Code: _____

REPAIR (CLOSURE)

Repair Factors

When reporting wound repair, the following three factors must be considered:

1. Length of the wound in centimeters
2. Complexity of the repair
3. Site of the wound repair

Remember **length, complexity,** and **site.** Fig. 13–16 illustrates an example from the CPT manual of these three factors in the wound repair codes.

Complexity of repair

Site of repair

REPAIR-SIMPLE
Sum of length of repairs for each group of anatomic sites.
12001 Simple repair of superficial wounds of scalp, neck, axillae, external genitalia, trunk, and/or extremities (including hands and feet); 2.5 cm or less

Length of repair

FIGURE 13–16 Wound repair. Note that metric measure is used throughout the CPT manual.

There are many different types of wounds (Fig. 13–17). Wound repair is classified by the type of repair necessary to repair the wound. There are three types of repair:

1. **Simple:** Superficial wound repair (12001-12021) that involves epidermis, dermis, and subcutaneous tissue (Fig. 13–18) and requires only simple, one-layer suturing. If the simple wound repair is accomplished with tape or adhesive strips, the charge for the closure is included in the E/M service code and would not be reported separately with a repair code. The repair codes are for suture closure.

2. **Intermediate:** Requires closure of one or more layers of subcutaneous tissue and superficial (non-muscle) fascia, in addition to the skin closure. You can report intermediate closure (12031-12057) when the wound has to be extensively cleaned, even if the closure was a single-layer (simple) closure.

3. **Complex:** Involves complicated wound closure including revision, debridement, extensive undermining, stents or retention sutures, and more than layered closure (13100-13160).

From the Trenches

"[It's my job] to make sure physicians are saying [everything] into their microrecorder, or writing it down. You would be surprised how many physicians [diagnose a patient] mentally, as an automatic thing as part of their evaluation of the patient's condition—then they do the medical decision making on how to treat the patient. Sometimes a third of it doesn't even get put down, and the coder can only count that third of information, until it's in the record .... I've told doctors 'You dictated this, and this is all you're going to get' so they can see the consequences."

CHRIS

FIGURE 13–17 Types of wounds. **A** and **B,** Laceration. **C** and **D,** Puncture. **E** and **F,** Abrasion. **G** and **H,** Avulsion. **I,** Incision. (**B** and **D** from Henry MC, Stapleton ER: *EMT Prehospital Care,* ed 3, St. Louis, 2004, MosbyJems. **F** and **H** from McCance KL, Huether SE: *Pathophysiology: The Biologic Basis for Disease in Adults and Children,* St. Louis, 2006, Mosby.)

FIGURE 13–18 Skin cross-section. (From deWit SC: *Fundamental Concepts and Skills for Nursing,* ed 2, Philadelphia, 2005, Saunders.)

CODING SHOT

HCPCS code **G0168** reports skin closures using adhesives (such as Dermabond, a special glue that is put into the wound, the edges are closed together; a bandage is placed over the wound). Most other third-party payers use the simple repair code to report skin closures using adhesives.

The lengths of wounds are totaled together by complexity (simple, intermediate, complex) and anatomic site (that is, all the simple wounds of the same site grouping are reported together; all the intermediate wounds of the same site grouping are reported together; and all the complex wounds of the same site grouping are reported together). The codes group together sites that require similar techniques to repair. For example, 12001 groups superficial scalp, neck, axillae, external genitalia, trunk, and extremities. When there is more than one repair type, the **most complex** type is listed as the first (primary) procedure. The secondary procedure is then reported using modifier -51 (multiple procedure). Remember that the placement of the -51 indicates a discounted service to the payer.

🖐 **CAUTION** *For repairs:*
- *Group together the same anatomic* **sites,** *such as face and hand.*
- *Group together the same* **classification,** *such as simple or intermediate.*

The CPT manual notes located under the subheading Repair (Closure) include extensive definitions of each level of repair. These notes must be read carefully before you code repairs.

Repair Component

Three things are considered components (parts) of wound repair:

1. Simple **ligation** (tying) of small vessels is considered part of the wound repair and is not reported separately. Simple ligation of medium or major arteries in a wound is, however, reported separately.
2. Simple **exploration** of surrounding tissue, nerves, vessels, and tendons is considered part of the wound repair process and is not listed separately.
3. Normal **debridement** (cleaning and removing skin or tissue from the wound until normal, healthy tissue is exposed) is not listed separately.

If the wound is grossly contaminated and requires extensive debridement, a separate debridement procedure may be assigned (11000-11044 for extensive debridement). Fig. 13–19 illustrates a surgical type of debridement.

Tissue Transfers, Grafts, and Flaps

There are many types of grafting procedures that can be performed to correct a defect (e.g., adjacent tissue transfers or rearrangements, skin replacement surgery and skin substitutes, flaps). To understand skin grafting, you must know that the **recipient site** is the area of defect that receives the graft, and the **donor site** is the area from which the healthy skin has been taken for grafting. (If a skin graft is required to close the donor site, the closure is reported as an additional procedure.) A brief description follows of some different types of skin grafting and coding guidelines specific to their assignment.

FIGURE 13–19 Surgical debridement for the removal of periwound nonmigratory tissue using a pair of scissors and forceps. (From Robinson JK, Sengelmann RD, Hanke CW, Siegel DM, editors: *Surgery of the Skin: Procedural Dermatology,* Edinburgh, 2005, Mosby.)

Adjacent Tissue Transfer or Rearrangement. There are many types of adjacent tissue transfers (14000-14350). Some of them are Z-plasty (Fig. 13–20), W-plasty, V-Y plasty, rotation flaps (Fig. 13–21), and advancement flaps. These procedures are various methods of moving a segment of skin from one area to an adjacent area, while leaving at least one side of the flap (moved skin) intact to retain some measure of blood supply to the graft. Incisions are made, and the skin is undermined and moved over to cover the defective area, leaving the base (connected portion) intact. The flap is then sutured into place.

Adjacent tissue transfers are reported according to the size of the **recipient site.** The size is measured in square centimeters (1 inch equals 2.54 cm). Simple repair of the donor site is included in the tissue transfer code and is not reported separately. If there is a complex closure, or grafting of the donor site, this could be reported separately. Adjacent Tissue Transfer or Rearrangement (14000-14350) in the CPT manual is divided based on the **location** of the defect (trunk or arm) and the **size** of the defect. In addition, there are codes at the end of the category for coding defects that are extremely complicated. Both the primary defect (results from the excision) and the secondary defect (results from the flap design) are added together to determine code selection.

FIGURE 13–20 Z-plasty is named for the shape of the incision.

FIGURE 13–21 **A,** Sacral ulcer. **B,** Closure by a large rotation flap based superiorly. **C** and **D,** Outline of flap and rotation downward and medially. (**A** and **B** from McCarthy, JG, ed: *Plastic Surgery,* vol 6, Philadelphia, 1990, WB Saunders. **C** and **D** from Converse JM, ed: *Reconstructive Plastic Surgery: Principles and Procedures in Correction, Reconstruction and Transplantation,* vol 5, Philadelphia, 1964, WB Saunders.)

Any excision of a lesion that is repaired by adjacent tissue transfer is included in the tissue transfer code. If you reported the excision in addition to the transfer, it would be considered unbundling.

Adjacent tissue transfer codes can be located in the CPT manual index under the main term Skin and subterm Adjacent Tissue Transfer.

Skin Replacement Surgery and Skin Substitutes (15002-15431).

These codes report site preparation using a variety of grafting materials and repair methods using skin or skin substitutes. The site of the defect (recipient) site may require surgical preparation before repair, and these repairs are reported with 15002-15005 based on the size of repair and site. Free skin grafts (such as 15100/15101 and 15120/15121) are pieces of skin that are either **split thickness** (epidermis and part of the dermis) or **full thickness** (epidermis and all of the dermis) as illustrated in Fig. 13–22. The grafts are completely freed from the donor site and placed over the recipient site. There is no connection left between the graft and the donor site (Fig. 13–23). Free skin grafts are reported by recipient **site, size** of defect, and **type** of repair. The size is measured in square centimeters.

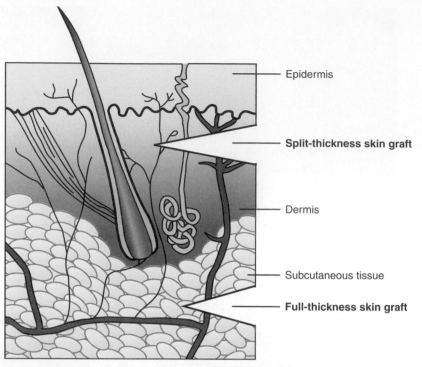

FIGURE 13–22   Split-thickness skin graft and full-thickness skin graft.

FIGURE 13–23   A, Small, localized, full-thickness burn of the first web space. **B,** Immediate postoperative results, after a dorsal metacarpal artery flap was transposed into the defect. (From Achauer BM, et al, eds: *Plastic Surgery: Indications, Operations, and Outcomes,* vol 4, St. Louis, 2000, Mosby.)

Many of the code definitions in the Skin Replacement Surgery and Skin Substitutes category refer to a measurement in square centimeters and a percentage of body area. The square centimeters measurement is applied to adults and children over 10 years of age and the percentage of body area is applied to infants and children under the age of 10.

A **pinch graft** (15050) is a small, split-thickness repair. Often a split-thickness graft is referred to in the patient record as STSG, and a full-thickness skin graft as FTSG.

Autografts are grafts that are taken from the patient's body (Fig. 13–24), whereas **allografts** (homografts) are grafts that are taken from a human donor. Epidermal autografts (15110-15116) and dermal autografts

FIGURE 13–24 Appearance during application of meshed autograft. (From Ignatavicius DD, Workman ML: *Medical-Surgical Nursing: Critical Thinking for Collaborative Care,* ed 5, St. Louis, 2006, Saunders.)

(15130-15136) are reported based on graft depth, location, and size. Tissue cultured epidermal autografts (15150-15157) are grafts that are cultured (grown) from the patient's own skin cells, thereby reducing the chances of rejection. **Acellular** dermal replacement (15170-15176) is the use of skin replacement products based on the location and size of repair. **Temporary** allografts are reported with 15300-15321 based on the location and size of repair. Temporary grafts are used to protect defect sites while healing is taking place (Figs. 13–25 and 13–26). A **permanent** graft may be placed over the site at a later date to complete the repair process.

Allograft/Tissue Cultured Allogeneic Skin Substitutes (15300-15366) are grafts obtained from a donor genetically different, but of the same species, which include healthy cadaveric donors. Xenografts (15400-15431) are grafts taken from a different species (cross species, such as pigskin grafts). Xenografts are also known as heterografts.

FIGURE 13–25 Three sheets of cultured epithelial autograft are in place on the left anterior thigh, which 3 weeks before was excised to muscle fascia and covered with cadaver allograft. (From Gallico GG, O'Connor NE: Cultured epithelium as a skin substitute. *Clin Plast Surg* 12:155, 1985.)

FIGURE 13–26 The same area of left anterior thigh in Fig. 13–25, 1 month after grafting. (From Gallico GG, O'Connor NE: Cultured epithelium as a skin substitute. *Clin Plast Surg* 12:155, 1985.)

Flaps.   A physician may develop a donor site at a location far away from the recipient site. The graft may have to be accomplished in stages. The graft code can be assigned more than once when the surgery is performed in stages. Notes specific to this group of codes state that when reporting transfer flaps (in several stages), report the **donor site** when a tube graft (Fig. 13–27) is formed for later use or when a delayed flap is formed before it is transferred (Fig. 13–28). The **recipient site** is reported when the graft is attached to its final site.

FIGURE 13–27   A, Correction of a radical mastectomy defect with a tube flap, created from the abdominal pannus. **B,** Intermediate inset of the tube flap following separation from its abdominal blood supply. This process of "waltzing" a tube-flap from the abdomen to the chest was used by Halsted and Billroth. **C,** Final inset into the sternum before shaping. **D,** The lateral half of the tube flap was then detached laterally and inset into the upper sternum to create the breast shape. This type of reconstruction usually took more than a year to complete, with more than a dozen procedures. (From Bland KI, Copeland EM: *The Breast: Comprehensive Management of Benign and Malignant Disorders,* ed 3, St. Louis, 2004, Saunders.)

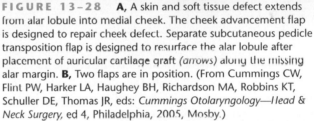

FIGURE 13-28 **A,** A skin and soft tissue defect extends from alar lobule into medial cheek. The cheek advancement flap is designed to repair cheek defect. Separate subcutaneous pedicle transposition flap is designed to resurface the alar lobule after placement of auricular cartilage graft *(arrows)* along the missing alar margin. **B,** Two flaps are in position. (From Cummings CW, Flint PW, Harker LA, Haughey BH, Richardson MA, Robbins KT, Schuller DE, Thomas JR, eds: *Cummings Otolaryngology—Head & Neck Surgery,* ed 4, Philadelphia, 2005, Mosby.)

In a **delayed graft,** a portion of the skin is lifted and separated from the tissue below, but it stays connected to blood vessels at one end. This keeps the skin viable while it is being moved from one area to another, and at the same time, it allows the graft to get used to living on a small supply of blood. It is hoped that living on a small blood supply will give the graft a better chance of survival when inserted into the recipient site.

There are two categories of codes for flaps. The first category, Flaps (Skin and/or Deep Tissues) (15570-15738), is subdivided based on the type of flap (i.e., pedicle, cross finger, delayed, or muscle flaps) and then by the location of the flap (scalp, trunk, or lips). The codes do not include any extensive immobilization that may be necessary, such as a large plaster cast. Extensive immobilization would be reported in addition to the flap procedure. Also not included in the flap procedure codes is the closure of a donor site, which would be reported in addition to the flap procedure.

The second category, Other Flaps and Grafts (15740-15776), is subdivided based on the type of flap (free muscle, free skin, fascial, or hair transplant).

Within the flap codes (15740-15750) the flap (donor site and recipient site remain connected for a period of time) can be an island pedicle or a neurovascular pedicle. The pedicle is the end of the flap that remains connected to the donor area. An **island pedicle flap** contains an artery and vein, and a **neurovascular pedicle flap** contains an artery, vein, and nerve. The term island refers to the removal of the fat and subcutaneous tissue prior to implantation into the recipient site. The neurovascular pedicle flap is used when the area of defect requires restoration of sensation in the area; for example, the end of a finger that has sustained damage that destroyed the sensation on the tip of the finger. A neurovascular graft from an adjacent finger could restore sensation to the defective area. A flap from the donor area is freed up and grafted into the recipient area. The connection between the donor and the recipient sites remains in place until the graft has satisfactorily healed, at which time the connection is severed. The donor area may require a separate skin graft and that graft would be reported separately.

QUICK CHECK 13-2

There are three types of measurements utilized in the Integumentary System subsection of the CPT manual. Match the procedure with the type of measurement.

a. length in cm
b. area in square cm
c. diameter in cm

1. Skin Grafts/Flaps _____

2. Lesion Removal _____

3. Wound Repair _____

Other Procedures

The Other Procedures codes (15780-15879) report a wide variety of repair services, such as abrasion, chemical peel, and blepharoplasty (surgical reconstruction of the eyelid). The codes are often divided based on the site or extent of repair.

Dermabrasion is used to treat acne, wrinkles, or general keratoses (horny growth) (Fig. 13–29). The skin area is anesthetized by a chemical that freezes the area (a cryogen), and the area is sanded down using a motorized brush. The facial dermabrasion codes (15780-15783) are divided according to the surface area of the face treated (total, segmental, regional).

A tattoo can be removed by dermabrasion. The process involves the use of a high-speed mechanical wheel to remove the epidermis and part of the papillary dermis. The service is reported with code 15783.

The **abrasion** codes (15786, 15787) report the use of abrasion to remove a lesion, such as scar tissue, a wart, or a callus. This technique is often used to remove areas of sun-damaged skin. The first abraded lesion is reported with 15786, and each additional four or fewer lesions are reported with 15787.

Chemical peels, also known as chemexfoliation, are treatments in which a chemical is applied to the skin and then removed (Fig. 13–30). The skin surface will then shed its outer layer, much as it does after a sunburn. The treatment is used for cosmetic purposes, such as smoothing the wrinkles around the mouth or removing liver spots (lentigines) (Fig. 13–31). The chemical peel codes (15788-15793) are divided according to whether the peel is on the face or not on the face, in addition to the depth of the peel (epidermal or dermal).

Cervicoplasty, 15819, is a surgical procedure in which the physician removes excess skin from the neck, usually for cosmetic reasons. **Blepharoplasty** (15820-15823), also performed predominantly for cosmetic purposes, is the removal of excess skin and to support the muscles of the upper eyelid. Rhytidectomy is the removal of wrinkles by pulling the skin tight and removing the excess. **Rhytidectomy** codes (15824-15829) report these cosmetic services. Excision of excess skin and subcutaneous tissue of other parts of the body (e.g., abdomen, thigh, buttock, and arm) most commonly due to bariatric surgery is reported

FIGURE 13–29 Large and disfiguring seborrheic keratosis reveals evidence of horn pearls. (From James WD, Berger TG, Elston DM: *Andrew's Diseases of the Skin: Clinical Dermatology,* ed 10, London, 2000, WB Saunders.)

FIGURE 13–30 Chemical peel. (From Cummings CW, Flint PW, Harker LA, Haughey BH, Richardson MA, Robbins KT, Schuller DE, Thomas JR, eds: *Cummings Otolaryngology—Head & Neck Surgery,* ed 4, Philadelphia, 2005, Mosby.)

FIGURE 13–31 Lentigines of the hand. (From Regezi JA, Sciubba JJ, Jordan RCK: *Oral Pathology: Clinical Pathologic Correlations,* ed 5, St. Louis, 2008, Saunders.)

with codes in the 15830-15839 range. To report abdominoplasty with panniculectomy (excision of the hanging tissue in the abdominal region [Fig. 13–32]), report 15830 with add-on code 15847.

Grafts for facial nerve paralysis (15840-15845) are procedures in which the physician harvests a graft from some location on the body and places the graft over the area damaged by facial paralysis.

There are also codes in the Other Procedures category for the removal of sutures and for dressing changes (15850-15852) performed under anesthesia.

Lipectomy (liposuction) codes (15876-15879) are divided according to the body area being treated—head, trunk, upper extremities, and lower extremity. If the procedure is performed bilaterally, add modifier -50 to the procedure code.

Pressure Ulcers

Pressure ulcers are also known as decubitus ulcers or bedsores (Fig. 13–33, A). Pressure ulcers are located on areas of the body that have bony projections, such as the hips and the area above the tailbone. Pressure on these areas causes decreased blood flow, and sores form. With continued pressure, the sores ulcerate, and deeper layers of tissue, such as fascia, muscle, and bone, may be affected. As illustrated in Fig. 13–33, B, the depth of the ulcer is referred to in stages—I, II, III, IV. Pressure ulcers commonly occur in patients who are unable to change position or have devices that prevent mobility (splints, casts).

Although a pressure ulcer can be seen, the depth to which the ulceration has penetrated cannot be seen. The ulcer may involve only superficial skin or may affect deeper layers. The treatment for a pressure ulcer (15920-15999) is excision of the ulcerated area to the depth of unaffected tissue, fascia, or muscle.

CODING SHOT

Only an adjacent tissue transfer is bundled into the pressure ulcer codes. If the medical record indicates a myocutaneous flap closure, or a muscle flap, report codes from both the Pressure Ulcer category (15920-15999) and from the Flaps (Skin and/or Deep Tissue) category (15570-15738). Also, if a free skin graft is used to close the ulcer, that closure would be reported separately with a code from the Other Flaps and Grafts category.

Before   After

FIGURE 13–32   Panniculectomy.

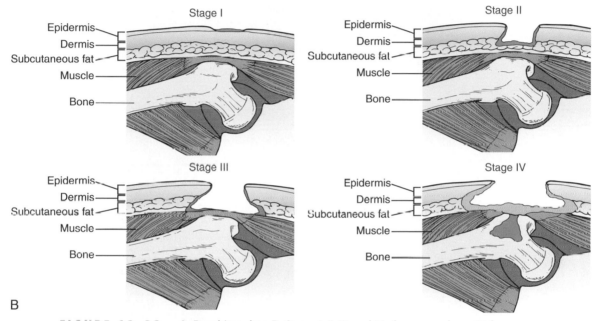

FIGURE 13–33   **A,** Decubitus ulcer. **B,** Stages I, II, III, and IV of pressure ulcers. (**A** from Callen J, Greer K, Hood A, et al: *Color Atlas of Dermatology,* Philadelphia, 1993, Saunders.)

You will note that many of the Pressure Ulcer codes have "with ostectomy" as the indented code. An **ostectomy** is the removal of the bone that underlies the ulcer area. The bony prominences are chiseled or filed down to alleviate future pressure. The operative report will indicate if the bone was removed.

Read the code descriptions carefully when coding from the ulcer repair category, as the codes are divided based on the location, type, and extent of closure required.

BURNS   Fig. 13–34 illustrates the Rule of Nines, which is used to calculate the percentage of body area in adults. Fig. 13–35 illustrates the Lund-Browder classification of burns, which is often used to calculate the percentage of body area in infants. Although the Lund-Browder approach is similar to the Rule of Nines, adjustments are made in the percentages because an infant's head is larger in proportion to the rest of his or her body. On the job, the medical coder is not required to calculate the percentage, as the physician

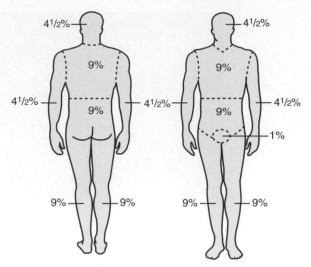

FIGURE 13-34 Rule of nines, adults.

Anterior **Posterior**

Relative percentage of body surface areas (% BSA) affected by growth

	0 yr	1 yr	5 yr	10 yr	15 yr
a – 1/2 of head	9 1/2	8 1/2	6 1/2	5 1/2	4 1/2
b – 1/2 of 1 thigh	2 3/4	3 1/4	4	4 1/4	4 1/2
c – 1/2 of lower leg	2 1/2	2 1/2	2 3/4	3	3 1/4

FIGURE 13-35 Lund-Browder chart for estimating the extent of burns on children.

is to indicate the percentages in the medical record. If the donor site for the graft requires repair by grafting, an additional graft code is used. Simple repair (closure) of the donor site is included in the graft code.

Burns are classified as first, second, or third degree based on the depth of the burn. If the medical documentation indicated a burn of the epidermis, that is a first degree burn, a dermal burn is a second degree, and a subcutaneous level burn is third degree (Fig. 13–36). The documentation should indicate the degree of burn at each location and the physician should be queried if the degree is not stated.

Burn treatment is unique in that it is common for a patient to undergo multiple dressing changes or debridements (Fig. 13–37) during the healing

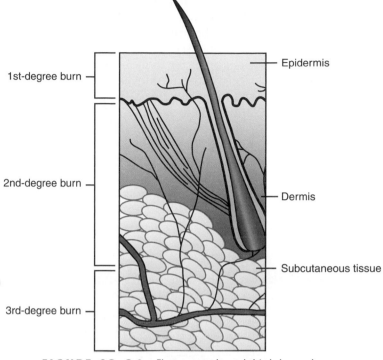

FIGURE 13-36   First-, second-, and third-degree burns.

FIGURE 13-37   Burn debridement. (From Converse JM, ed: *Reconstructive Plastic Surgery: Principles and Procedures in Correction, Reconstruction and Transplantation,* vol 1, Philadelphia, 1964, WB Saunders.)

period. Dressing and debridement codes report either initial or subsequent treatments. Burn dressing and/or debridement codes (16020-16030) are divided based on whether the dressing or debridement is of a small, medium, or large area. The definition of small is less than 5% of the total body surface area, medium is the whole face or an extremity equalling 5% to 10% of the total body surface area, and large is more than one extremity or greater than 10% of the total body area.

Bundled into codes 16000-16036 is the application of dressing, such as temporary skin replacement. The notes in the Burn, Local Treatment category refer to Biobrane® as one of the bundled materials. Biobrane® is a biosynthetic skin substitute that is constructed of a silicone film with a nylon fabric embedded into the film. Collagen is then embedded into the film and fabric. There are small pores on the skin substitute to make the covering permeable to allow for the application of topical antibiotics during healing.

The Burn category contains codes for **escharotomy** (16035, 16036), a procedure in which the physician cuts through the dead skin that covers the surface when there is a full-thickness burn. The crust covers the surface and diminishes blood flow and healing.

CODING SHOT

Some third-party payers allow you to submit charges for burn care using the first date of service to the last date of service. This allows you to indicate multiples of the same service (e.g., ×5 or ×3). Other payers require you to list each date of service and to report each service separately. For example, if the patient received five burn debridements on five separate days, you would report the CPT code five separate times, once for each day of service.

EXERCISE 13-2 *Repair (Closure) and Burns*

The patient record states: **"simple wound repair 12-cm wound, left hand."**

To locate the code for the repair in the CPT manual Index using the condition method, you first locate the main term **Wound,** and then the subterm **Repair.** Wound is the condition and Repair is the procedure. You then identify the type of repair (i.e., complex, simple).

To locate the code using the service or procedure method, you would first locate the main term, **Repair.** Repair is the service or procedure. The subterm **Wound** is located next, and finally the type (i.e., complex, simple). These are just two of the ways to locate this service in the Index.

From the main term Wound, subterms Repair, Simple, you are directed to a range of codes, 12001-12021. Locate this range in the CPT manual. The notes under the subheading, Repair (Closure), are "must" reading. Also, read the description of the first code in the category (12001). The description specifies that the code includes the term hands, which is what you are looking for. Now locate the correct length (12 cm), and you will have the correct code—12004.

Now you code the following:

The patient record states: complex wound repair on hand, 3.1 cm.

1 What are the correct codes?

CPT Code: _____13132 – Correct for 2010_____

ICD-9-CM Code: _____882.0_____

2 After an assault with a knife, a patient requires simple repair of a 3-cm laceration of the neck, simple repair of a 4-cm laceration of the back, simple repair of a 5-cm laceration of the forearm, and complex repair of a 3-cm laceration of the abdomen. (Note: Remember to use modifier -51 with the least intensive repair.)

CPT Codes: _____13101_____, _____12004-51_____

simple 3cm neck
12cm 4cm back
5cm forearm
comp 3cm Abd

3 Harry Torgerson, a 42-year-old construction worker, is injured at work when a box containing wood scraps and shingles falls from a second story scaffolding and strikes him on the left forearm, causing multiple lacerations. Forearm repairs: a 5.1-cm repair of the subcutaneous tissues and a 5.6-cm laceration, with particles of shingles and wood materials deeply embedded, both requiring intermediate closure. There is also a superficial wound of the scalp of 3.1 cm that requires simple closure.

CPT Codes: _12034_ , _12002-51_

10.7 forearm subcq c̄ particles

4 A patient with multiple healed scars requests they be removed and repaired for cosmetic reasons. The defects include a 100-cm² scar of the right cheek and a 200-cm² defect of the left upper chest. Several split-thickness skin grafts totaling 300 cm² are harvested from the left and right thighs. The scar tissue is cut away, and the sites are prepared for grafting.

Cheek graft: _15120_

Upper chest graft: _15100-51 15101_

Harvest *15040 X3* ?

Site prep, cheek, 100 cm²: _15004-51_

Site prep, chest, 200 cm²: _15002-51_ , _15003_

5 The patient had a 20-cm² defect of the right cheek that was repaired with a rotation flap (adjacent tissue transfer).

CPT Code: _14041_

6 The patient had a 10-cm² malignant neoplasm removed from the forehead. Z-plasty was used to repair this site. How would the excision and repair be coded?

CPT Code: _14040_

7 A patient has had a portion of his mandible removed due to excision of a malignant tumor. Repair of the site is now performed by use of a myocutaneous flap graft.

CPT Code: _15732_ *Myocutaneous flap*

8 A patient incurs second- and third-degree burns of the abdomen and thigh (10%) when she pulls a pan of boiling water off the stove. She requires daily debridements or dressing changes for the first week (Monday through Friday, ×5). She is in severe pain and requires anesthesia during these treatments. During the following 2 weeks she will be receiving dressing changes every other day (Monday, Wednesday, Friday, ×6), and it is expected that enough healing will have taken place that anesthesia will not be necessary. What codes would be reported for services during the 3-week treatment period?

Week 1 CPT Code: _16025 X5_

Weeks 2 and 3 CPT Code: _16025 X6_

DESTRUCTION The next subheading in the subsection of the Integumentary System is Destruction. The codes report destruction of lesions by means **other than excision.** Codes 17000-17286 are for benign, premalignant, or malignant lesions destroyed by means of electrosurgery (use of various forms of electrical current to destroy the lesion), cryosurgery (use of extreme cold), laser (Light Amplification by Stimulated Emissieon of Radiation), or chemicals (acids). Read the notes under the Destruction subsection heading because they contain a list of types of lesions. Destruction codes state "any method" and are divided according to type of lesion (benign or malignant). Further divisions are based on the number of lesions destroyed or the size of the area destroyed. The malignant lesions are divided based on location (nose, ear, and so forth) and size (0.6-1.0 cm, and so forth), regardless of the method used.

Codes 17000-17004 report destruction of lesions by the number treated. For example, a patient goes to his or her physician to have 20 lesions removed using cryosurgery reported with 17004. If the patient had six lesions removed, the first one would be reported with 17000 and lesions two through six are reported with 17003 × 5. Careful reading of the coding guidelines is a must for proper reporting of destruction codes.

Mohs Micrographic Surgery

One sophisticated procedure is Mohs micrographic surgery (17311-17315). The method is named after the physician who pioneered the basic microscopic technique, Frederic Mohs, MD. The microscope is used during the surgical procedure to view the lesion and assess its pathology by a single physician acting in two separate and distinct capacities—surgeon and pathologist. If another physician is delegated the role of pathologist, these codes should not be reported. If the lesion is malignant, it is immediately removed. Mohs micrographic surgery is especially useful in cases of large tumors. The procedure involves mapping the exact contour of the tumor and removing tissue down to the level at which cancerous cells are no longer found. The process involves stages in which the surgeon removes a layer of skin and examines it under a microscope for cancerous cells, then returns to the lesion to remove another layer of skin, again examining it under a microscope (Fig. 13–38). This process is continued until cancerous cells are no longer identified in the layers being removed. The surgeon acts as both the pathologist and the surgeon.

From the Trenches

"Find a subspecialty you like . . . [and] if it's a surgical subspecialty, get as many operative reports as you can. Read them. Compare the codes in the book to what's on the operative report. See if you can get into the operating room with the doctors . . . [and] know your sterile field techniques so you know what NOT to touch!"

CHRIS

The codes in the category include the removal of the lesion(s) and pathologic evaluation of the lesion(s). These codes are also divided based on the stage (e.g., first, second) of the surgery and the number of tissue blocks the surgeon takes during the surgery for pathologic examination.

FIGURE 13-38 Mohs micrographic surgical technique.

A new patient presents to the dermatologist with a lesion and the dermatologist performs a biopsy that he then examines in the office using a microscope. His determination is that the lesion is basil cell carcinoma and he advises the patient to have the lesion removed the same day using Mohs microscopic technique. The patient consents to this and the dermatologist makes arrangements to remove the lesion later that day. According to the notes before 17311, if a biopsy of a suspected skin cancer is "performed on the same day as Mohs surgery because there was no prior pathology confirmation of a diagnosis, then report diagnostic skin biopsy (11100, 11101) and frozen section pathology (88331) with modifier 59 to distinguish from the subsequent definitive surgical procedure of Mohs surgery." This means that you would report either 11100-59 or 11101-59 (biopsy service) and 88331-59 (pathology service) because the primary procedure is the Mohs surgery (17311).

QUICK CHECK 13-3

1. The Mohs notes before 17311-17315 indicate repairs are:
   a. bundled
   b. reported separately

EXERCISE 13-3 *Destruction*

1 Electrosurgical destruction of a herpetic lesion

   CPT Code: _____

2 Cryosurgical destruction of 14 actinic keratoses

   CPT Codes: _____, _____ × _____

   ICD-9-CM Code: _____

3 Mohs micrographic surgery by a single physician removing and examining three specimens, first stage of the neck

   CPT Code(s): _____

BREAST PROCEDURES

Breast procedures (19000-19499) are divided according to category of procedure (e.g., incision, excision, introduction, repair and/or reconstruction). You must read the documentation to identify the procedure used, such as incisional versus excisional biopsies. In an **incisional biopsy**, an incision is made into the lesion and a small portion of the lesion is taken out. In an **excisional biopsy**, the entire lesion is removed for biopsy. In some cases it may be necessary to mark the lesion preoperatively by placing a thin wire (radiologic marker) down to the lesion to identify its exact location (Fig. 13–39). The placement of the wire is coded 19290, and the excision of the lesion identified by the marker is coded separately.

Wire marker

FIGURE 13–39   Wire marker used to mark breast lesion. **A,** Mammography is used to place a preoperative needle used to mark a lesion. **B,** The wire marker serves as a guide for the surgeon to perform the biopsy. (Modified from Bland Kl, Copeland EM, eds: *The Breast: Comprehensive Management of Benign and Malignant Disorders,* ed 3, St. Louis, 2004, Saunders.)

Code 19295 is an add-on code that reports the placement of a metallic localization clip. The clip is placed to allow the physician to precisely identify the depth and position of the needle placement to obtain a breast tissue biopsy. After the biopsy, the clip is left in place to identify the biopsied area on subsequent mammography. The biopsy service is reported with 19102 or 19103 depending on the technique used to obtain the specimen.

There are many mastectomy codes and you need to carefully review the operative report to confirm whether pectoral muscles, axillary lymph nodes, or internal mammary lymph nodes were also removed. This information will be necessary to determine the correct mastectomy code.

A **partial** mastectomy (19301) is one in which only a portion of the breast tissue is removed. If an axillary lymphadenectomy is performed with a partial mastectomy, report the service with 19302. A partial mastectomy is also known as a lumpectomy, segmentectomy, or tylectomy. Fig. 13–40 illustrates the quadrants and axillary tail of the breast. Fig. 13–41 illustrates the simple, modified radical, radical, and partial mastectomies.

A **simple** or **complete** mastectomy (19303) is one in which all of the subcutaneous breast tissue is removed and the nipple and skin may or may not be removed. A **subcutaneous** mastectomy (19304) is one in which the skin and muscle is left but all the breast tissue is removed.

A **modified radical** mastectomy is one in which the breast is removed in addition to the axillary lymph nodes and the pectoralis minor muscle may or may not be removed. The pectoralis major muscle is not removed in the modified radical mastectomy.

A **radical** mastectomy (19305) is one in which the entire breast is removed in addition to the pectoral muscles and axillary lymph nodes (Fig. 13–42). Code 19306 reports another type of radical mastectomy that includes the internal mammary lymph nodes and is also known as an Urban type operation.

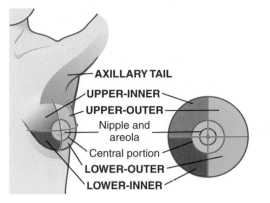

FIGURE 13–40 Female breast quadrants and axillary tail. (From Buck CJ: *2010 ICD-9-CM, Volumes 1, 2, & 3, Professional Edition,* St. Louis, 2009, Saunders.)

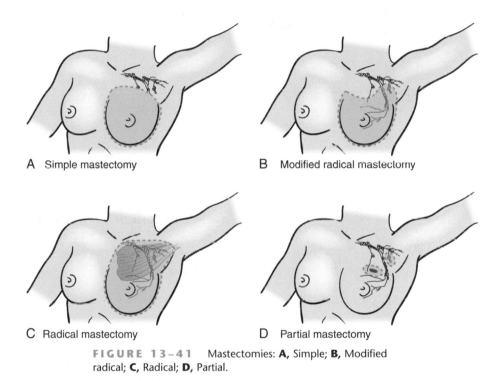

A Simple mastectomy

B Modified radical mastectomy

C Radical mastectomy

D Partial mastectomy

FIGURE 13–41 Mastectomies: **A,** Simple; **B,** Modified radical; **C,** Radical; **D,** Partial.

A breast lesion is often identified as a result of a screening mammogram, and a breast biopsy is then scheduled. During the biopsy, a specimen is obtained and sent to the pathologist for analysis. This biopsy is reported separately and is not bundled into the screening mammogram or any subsequent procedure. However, if a biopsy is obtained in the operating room and based on the results of the biopsy, a mastectomy is performed, the biopsy is bundled into the mastectomy.

The Repair and/or Reconstruction codes 19316-19396 include codes to report breast reduction (19318), augmentation (breast enlargement, 19324), and breast reconstruction (19357). The reconstruction includes the insertion of a tissue expander and the subsequent expansion. The tissue expander is placed to stretch the skin overlying the breast to allow for insertion of a permanent prosthesis.

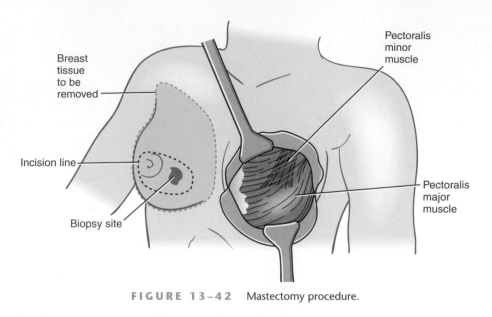

Breast tissue to be removed

Incision line

Biopsy site

Pectoralis minor muscle

Pectoralis major muscle

FIGURE 13-42   Mastectomy procedure.

CODING SHOT Any breast procedure performed on **both** breasts must be reported as a bilateral procedure (modifier -50).

EXERCISE 13-4   *Breast Procedures*

Locate the correct code for the following procedures. Be sure to read all notes in the CPT manual and the description of the code before applying the code.

1 Aspiration of one cyst, breast

   CPT Code: _____

2 Simple, complete bilateral mastectomies

   CPT Code(s): _____

3 Right modified radical mastectomy, including axillary lymph nodes without any muscles

   CPT Code: _____

4 Preoperative placement of one breast wire, left breast

   CPT Code: _____

5 Reconstruction of nipple/areola, right breast

   CPT Code: _____

 CONGRATULATIONS! You made it through the entire Integumentary System subsection! The subsection is quite complicated and you have done a great job if you understand the basics of these codes. As you use these codes here and on the job, your knowledge will continue to grow.

CHAPTER REVIEW

CHAPTER 13, PART I, THEORY

What are the three things that are considered components of wound repair?

1 _____

2 _____

3 _____

Wound repair codes are determined by what three criteria?

4 _____

5 _____

6 _____

What are the three classifications of wound repair?

7 _____

8 _____

9 _____

10 Modifier -51 indicates what?

_____

11 What is the title for the information that precedes each section? _____

12 _____ is the cleansing of an area or wound.

13 A(n) _____ biopsy may be performed to excise a disc of tissue.

14 What is the term for the elastic material formed into a sac that is then filled with fluid or air?

_____ _____

15 What is the name of the graft that is taken from the patient's body? _____

16 The major distinction in coding destruction of lesions is whether the lesion is

_____ or _____.

17 The division of malignant lesion excision is based on _____ and

_____.

18 What is the procedure used to treat acne or wrinkles by means of sanding?

_____

19 In order to report Mohs' surgery, the physician would act as the surgeon and the

_____.

20 In a(n) _____ biopsy, the entire lesion is removed for biopsy.

CHAPTER 13, PART II, PRACTICAL

Code the following cases for the surgical procedures and office visits only. Do not code the radiology services or laboratory work that may be included.

21 Margaret Wilson, a 26-year-old mother of three (new patient), has routine screening mammography of both breasts. (You do not need to code the mammography.) A shadow is visualized in the right breast. The physician performs a biopsy (needle core). The biopsy indicates malignancy. The patient agrees to and has a mastectomy (simple, complete) 1 week later.

There is no global period on this procedure. Pathology report indicated a primary malignant neoplasm.

CPT Codes: _19100___ _19303_,

_____

ICD-9-CM Code: _____

22 Shirley Peters, age 80, an established patient, presents to the office for removal of 12 skin tags.

CPT Code: _____

ICD-9-CM Code: _____

23 Removal of 180-cm² strawberry nevus of left cheek, autograft with split-thickness skin graft of 180 cm²

CPT Codes: _____,

_____, _____,

_____

ICD-9-CM Code: _____

24 Nipple reconstruction

CPT Code: _____

25 Destruction of 0.4-cm malignant lesion of the neck

CPT Code: _____

26 Simple repair of a superficial wound of the genitalia; 2.4 cm

CPT Code: _____

27 Adjacent tissue transfer of chin defect; 9 cm²

CPT Code: _____

QUICK CHECK ANSWERS

QUICK CHECK 13-1
1. False

QUICK CHECK 13-2
1. b
2. c
3. a

QUICK CHECK 13-3
1. b. reported separately

"Be the individual always willing to step in and help. Be the one to recognize issues and have solutions to those issues."

Martha Tracy, CPC, CPC-I
Coding & Compliance Manager
Mid-America Cardiology
Kansas City, Kansas

Musculoskeletal System

Chapter Topics

Format

Fractures and Dislocations

General

Application of Casts and Strapping

Endoscopy/Arthroscopy

Chapter Review

Quick Check Answers

Learning Objectives

After completing this chapter you should be able to

1 Differentiate among fracture and dislocation treatment types.

2 Understand types of traction.

3 Identify services/procedures included in the General subheading.

4 Analyze cast application and strapping procedures.

5 Understand elements of arthroscopic procedures.

6 Demonstrate the ability to code musculoskeletal services and procedures.

Make sure to check
evolve
learning system
for the latest
content updates

FORMAT   The Musculoskeletal System subsection is formatted by anatomic site, such as General, Head, and Neck.

The first subheading in this subsection is General and it contains procedures that are applicable to many different anatomic sites. The other subheadings are further divided by anatomic site, procedure type, condition, and description. They usually include:

- Incision
- Excision
- Introduction or Removal
- Repair, Revision, and/or Reconstruction
- Fracture and/or Dislocation
- Arthrodesis
- Amputation

Any or all of these categories of procedures may be located under each subheading.

The codes in the Musculoskeletal System subsection are reported extensively by orthopedic surgeons to describe the services provided to restore and preserve the function of the skeletal system. There are many codes, however, that are used frequently by a wide variety of primary care and family practice physicians, such as the splinting, casting, and fracture codes. Your study of the Musculoskeletal subsection of the CPT will focus on the format of the subsection, fracture types and repair, application of casts and strapping, the General subheading, and endoscopic procedures.

Thorough review of the medical record will help you to identify key information necessary for coding. The following tips will help you to choose the most correct code from this subsection:

1. Identify whether the procedure is being performed on soft tissue or bone.

2. Determine whether treatment is for a traumatic injury (acute) or a medical condition (chronic). The ICD-9-CM diagnosis codes indicating acute or chronic must match the treatment codes. E-codes from ICD-9-CM should also be assigned to describe accidents and injuries.

3. Identify the most specific anatomic site. For example, when coding vertebral procedures, it is necessary to know whether the procedure was for cervical, thoracic, or lumbar vertebrae.

4. Determine whether the code description includes grafting or fixation. If grafting or fixation is not listed within the major procedure code description, each may be reported as an additional procedure.

5. Read the code carefully to determine whether it describes a procedure that was on a single site (e.g., each finger). If the same procedure is performed on multiple sites (e.g., multiple fingers), you must indicate the number of units (such as 26060 × 2) or list the code multiple times. HCPCS modifiers are used to identify the digit treated, such as F6 for right hand, second digit.

6. Check any medical terms you do not understand in a medical dictionary or in the Glossary at the back of the book.

From the Trenches

"Be willing to constantly learn and research questions. Network with other coders, have fun and passion for your job!"

MARTHA

FRACTURES AND DISLOCATIONS

Fractures

Fractures are coded by treatment—open, closed, or percutaneous. **Open treatment** of a fracture is made when a surgery is performed in which the fracture is exposed by an incision made over the fracture and the fractured bone is visualized. **Closed treatment** is performed when the physician repairs the fracture without directly visualizing the fracture. The treatment method used—open or closed—depends on the type and severity of the fracture. A closed fracture (Fig. 14–1) may receive either closed, open, or percutaneous fixation, whereas a more complicated compound fracture usually requires an open treatment to provide internal fixation (e.g., wires, pins, screws). Fractures are coded to the specific anatomic site and then according to whether manipulation was performed. All fractures and dislocations are reported based on the reason for the treatment. For instance, if a hip replacement (arthroplasty) is performed for medical reasons, such as **osteoarthritis,** it is reported with 27130, located under the subheading

Greenstick

Avulsion

Comminuted

Simple (closed)

Impacted

Spiral

Oblique

Compound (open)

Transverse

Colles'

FIGURE 14–1 Types of fractures.

Pelvis and Hip Joint, category Repair, Revision, and/or Reconstruction. The osteoarthritis that caused the breakdown of the bone of the hip requiring repair was the reason for the treatment. If the hip replacement was performed for a **fracture,** it is reported with 27236, located under the subheading Pelvis and Hip Joint, category Fracture and/or Dislocation. The fracture, which is not a progressive, degenerative disease, was the reason for the treatment.

The CPT manual defines closed, open, and percutaneous treatments as follows:

Closed Treatment: This terminology is used to describe procedures that treat fractures by one of three methods: (1) without manipulation, (2) with manipulation, or (3) with or without traction.

Manipulation is attempted reduction, which is an attempt to maneuver the bone back into proper alignment. The physician may bend, rotate, pull, or guide the bone back into position.

Closed treatment without manipulation is a procedure in which the physician immobilizes the bone with a splint, cast, or other device but without having to manipulate the fracture into alignment. Code 25500 describes a closed treatment of a radial shaft fracture without manipulation. This code is correctly reported when a patient has a broken but stable radial shaft that is not displaced and the physician only applies a cast. Initial casting or splinting services are included in the fracture care, but the supplies used are not. Initial splinting or casting of fractures performed by another physician as the only service can be reported by that physician (i.e., an emergency department physician). If the cast needs to be removed and reapplied during the global period, the surgeon that charged the global fee may report the cast/splint application with 29000-29799 and append modifier -58 (staged or related procedure/service). Only charge for cast removal without reapplication if the physician or physician group is not assuming care for the fracture.

Closed treatment with manipulation is a procedure in which the physician has to reduce (put back in place) a fracture. Code 21320 describes a closed treatment of a nasal bone fracture with stabilization, as illustrated in Fig. 14–2. This code is correctly reported when a patient has a displaced nose that requires manipulation to return it to the normal position. The physician would then apply external and/or internal splints to immobilize the nose.

Open treatment is used when the fracture is opened (exposed to the external environment). In this instance, the fracture (bone) is open to

FIGURE 14–2   Realignment and support of nasal fracture.

view and internal fixation (pins, screws, etc.) may be used. For example, 23630, open treatment of greater humeral tuberosity fracture, includes internal fixation when performed. The physician opens the site, reduces the fracture, and applies internal fixation, as needed to maintain anatomic position of the fracture.

Open treatment can also mean that a remote site (not directly over the fracture) is opened to place a nail (intramedullary) across the fracture site.

Fracture is defined as open or closed fracture within the ICD-9-CM.

Open means the fracture has broken through the bone cortex or the bone has been exposed to air (elements).

Closed means the fracture does not penetrate bone cortex or the bone is not exposed to air.

QUICK CHECK 14-1

1. Which code would be reported for a repair of a femoral shaft fracture using an intramedullary rod?

   a. 27506
   b. 27507

Percutaneous skeletal fixation describes fracture treatment that is neither open nor closed. In this procedure, the fracture is not open to view, but fixation (e.g., pin, screw) is placed across the fracture site, usually under x-ray imaging. For example, percutaneous skeletal fixation of a fracture of the great toe, phalanx, or phalanges (28496). This procedure is performed entirely percutaneously.

Areas of bones, as Fig. 14–3 illustrates areas of the tibia, are important to know when identifying the location of a fracture. For example, there may be an open treatment of a proximal fibula fracture (27784), proximal being closer to the body, or of a distal fibula fracture (27792), distal being further from the body.

CODING SHOT

If the physician attempts a reduction of a fracture but is unable to align the fracture successfully, you still report a reduction service. List the attempted reduction service code and then list the more involved fracture care (i.e., open, endoscopic) the physician successfully performed to reduce the fracture with modifier -58 (staged or related procedure/service) appended.

Traction definitions are as follows:

Traction is the application of pulling force to hold a bone in alignment (Fig. 14–4).

Skeletal traction is the use of internal devices, such as pins, screws, or wires. The devices are inserted into the bone through the skin, with ends of the pins, screws, or wires sticking out through the skin, so traction devices can be attached (Fig. 14–5).

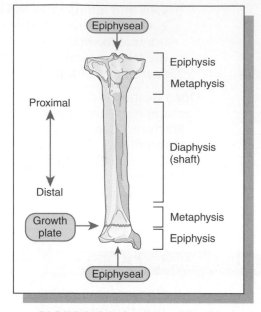

FIGURE 14-3   Areas of the tibia.

FIGURE 14-4   Traction is the application of a pulling force to hold a bone in alignment.

FIGURE 14-5   Skeletal traction uses the patient's bones to secure internal devices to which traction is attached.

TOOLBOX

Jerry broke his arm when he fell from a tree that he was trimming in his backyard.

QUESTIONS

What two E codes do you assign?_____ (fall = cause) and _____ (accident = place)

ANSWERS   **E884.9** (Fall, from, tree); **E849.0** (Accident, house)
ICD-10-CM: W14.XXXA (Fall, from, tree, initial encounter), **Y92.017** (Accident, house)

Skin traction involves strapping, elastic wrap, or tape that is fastened to the skin or wrapped around the limb. Weights are then attached to apply force to the fracture (Fig. 14–6).

Dislocations

Dislocation is the displacement of a bone from its normal location in a joint (Fig. 14–7), and the treatment of the dislocation injury is to return the bone to its normal location (anatomic alignment) by a variety of methods. For example, if a finger was dislocated and the bone did not protrude through the skin, the physician may administer a digital block (Fig. 14–8) and apply gentle traction until the finger realigns. A splint would then be applied to keep the finger immobile for about 3 weeks. If the shoulder was dislocated, the physician might elevate the arm and rotate the humerus while applying pressure to the head of the humerus. Or the patient might lie facedown on a table with the arm hanging off the edge while a weight is attached to the hand; the weight is sufficient to pull the arm back into place (Fig. 14–9). If external measures such as those just described do not relocate the joint, surgical reduction might be indicated.

FIGURE 14–6 Skin traction utilizes strapping, wraps, or tape to which traction is attached.

Vertebral dislocation   Subglenoid dislocation

FIGURE 14–7 Vertebral and subglenoid dislocations. (From *Dorland's Illustrated Medical Dictionary,* ed 31, Philadelphia, 2007, Saunders.)

Digital
nerves

FIGURE 14–8   Digital nerve block.

FIGURE 14–9   External technique for relocation of a
shoulder (Stimson technique). (From Rakel RE: *Saunders Manual of
Medical Practice,* ed 2, Philadelphia, 2000, Saunders.)

QUICK CHECK 14-2

1. According to the Musculoskeletal System notes before 20000, does
   the type of fracture/dislocation (i.e., open, closed) determine the
   type of treatment (e.g., open, closed)?

   Yes or No?

EXERCISE 14-1   *Fractures and Dislocations*

Using the CPT and/or ICD-9-CM manuals, provide the codes for the following:

1 Nasal bone fracture, closed treatment

CPT Code: _21310_

2 Uncomplicated, closed treatment of one fractured rib

CPT Code: _21800_

3 Interphalangeal joint dislocation of toe, open treatment with internal fixation

CPT Code: _28675_

4 Open distal fibula fracture repair with internal fixation

CPT Code: _27792_

5 Femoral shaft fracture repair using closed treatment

CPT Code: _27500_

6 Percutaneous skeletal fixation of impact fracture of proximal end, femoral neck

CPT Code: _27235_

7 Open treatment of shoulder dislocation with closed fracture of the greater humeral tuberosity, non-displaced

CPT Code: _23670_   Fx + Disloc of same loc.
Code only fx

ICD-9-CM Code: _812.03_ (ICD-10-CM Code: _____)

8 Closed treatment of closed mandibular fracture, including interdental fixation

CPT Code: _21453_

ICD-9-CM Code: _802.20_ (ICD-10-CM Code: _____)

9 Percutaneous skeletal fixation of a closed distal radius fracture

CPT Code: _25606_   813.81 - NO

ICD-9-CM Code: _813.42_ (ICD-10-CM Code: _____)

10 Closed ankle dislocation, closed treatment

CPT Code: _27840_

ICD-9-CM Code: _837.0_ (ICD-10-CM Code: _____)

GENERAL	The first subheading in the Musculoskeletal subsection is General. As the name implies, this subheading includes miscellaneous procedures that are not specific to an anatomic site.
Incisions	The first codes 20000 and 20005 are for the incision of a **soft tissue abscess** that is superficial or deep. There are codes in the Integumentary System for incisions that are for skin only. What makes the 20000/20005 codes different from those in the Integumentary System is that 20000 and 20005 are reported when the abscess is associated with the deep tissue and possibly even down to the bone that underlies the area of abscess. The physician would make an incision into the abscess, explore and clean the abscess, and debride it (remove dead tissue). This procedure is very different from the procedures you report with Integumentary System codes for incision of an abscess.

Wound Exploration

The Wound Exploration codes (20100-20103) report traumatic wounds that result from a penetrating trauma (e.g., gunshot, knife wound). Wound Exploration codes include basic exploration and repair of the area of trauma. These codes are used specifically when the repair requires enlargement of the existing wound for exploration, cleaning, and repair. Included in the Wound Exploration codes are not only the exploration and enlargement of the wound but also debridement, removal of any foreign body(ies), ligation of minor blood vessel(s), and repair of subcutaneous tissues, muscle fascia, and muscle, as would be necessary to repair the wound (Fig. 14–10).

If the wound does not require enlargement, you would report a code from the Integumentary System, Skin Repair codes. If, however, the wound is more severe than a Wound Exploration code would indicate, the repair code would come from the specific repair by anatomic site codes. For example, for a bullet wound to the chest with suspicion of cardiac injury, the treatment will be thoracotomy of any approach, as illustrated in Fig. 14–11, with control of the hemorrhage and repair of any injured intrathoracic organ. The thoracotomy code is located in the subsection Respiratory System under the subheading Lungs. As you can see from this example, you have to assess the extent of the procedure carefully, reading the medical record to ensure you are in the correct area so you can choose the correct code. In the case of the bullet wound to the chest, the wound exploration is included in the thoracotomy and would not be reported separately.

FIGURE 14–10   Gunshot wound requiring exploration. (From Swan KG, Swan RC: Principles of ballistics applicable to the treatment of gunshot wounds. *Surg Clin North Am* 71:221-239, 1991.)

FIGURE 14–11   Median sternotomy was performed because of the position of the entrance wound and the suspicion of cardiac injury. Palpation of the left hemidiaphragm revealed a defect and indicated laparotomy. (From Swan, KG, Swan RC: *Gunshot Wounds: Pathophysiology and Management,* ed 2, Chicago, Year Book Medical Publishers, Inc.)

QUICK CHECK 14-3

1. Penetrating wound exploration may be coded from the Musculoskeletal System, Integumentary System, or the appropriate _____ site.

Excision

The Excision category (20150-20251) codes are for the biopsies of muscle and bone. The codes are divided based on the type of biopsy (muscle, bone), the depth of the biopsy (superficial, deep), and, in some codes, the method of obtaining the biopsy (e.g., percutaneous needle).

The procedure for a muscle or bone biopsy typically includes the administration of local anesthetic into the biopsy area, an incision into the area allowing exposure of the muscle or bone, removal of tissue for biopsy, and suturing of the area. A **percutaneous biopsy**, as represented in 20206, differs in that the area is not opened to the physician's view. A trocar (hollow needle) or needle is placed into the muscle or bone by passing the needle through the skin and into the muscle or bone and withdrawing a sample. When the percutaneous method is used to obtain a biopsy, the area does not require suturing. If the biopsy is extremely complicated, the surgeon may request the assistance of ultrasound to be able to view the biopsy area during the procedure and receive guidance as to the placement of the needle. Notice the guideline in the CPT following 20206 directs you to the radiology codes if imaging guidance is utilized during the procedure.

Biopsy codes in the Excision category of the General subheading are not to be reported for the excision of tumors of muscle. If the medical record indicates excision of a muscle tumor, you would have to choose a code from the correct Musculoskeletal subsection. For example, 24071 reports excision of a tumor from the soft tissue of the upper arm or elbow.

Biopsy codes do not include the pathology workup that is performed on the sample.

General Introduction or Removal

Within the Introduction or Removal category there is a wide variety of injection, aspiration, insertion, application, removal, and adjustment codes. Because the category is within the General subheading of the Musculoskeletal subsection, the codes also have a wide application in coding services.

Therapeutic **sinus tract injection** procedure codes are within this category. You may initially think of the nasal sinuses, but these are not the sinuses that are being injected here. The term "sinus" refers to a cyst or abscess inside the body with a tract (known as a fistula) connecting to another surface—internal (to the gut) or external (to the skin). The infection is treated by injecting an antibiotic or other substance into the sinus by way of the sinus tract. With certain sinus injections, a radiologist provides guidance to ensure the correct placement of the needle and the guidance is reported separately. For example, an interstitial abscess located perirectally develops a sinus tract opening perianally may be treated by instilling a caustic substance to stimulate healing. Other methods that may be used in treatment of the sinus tract are the incision or opening of the tract (fistulotomy) to promote healing or by means of excision (fistulectomy).

Removal codes located in the Introduction or Removal category (20520-20525) report the removal of foreign bodies that are lodged in muscle. Recall that the Integumentary System removal codes describe foreign bodies lodged in the skin. **Injection** codes in this category report injections made into a tendon, ligament, or ganglion cyst (cystic tumor). An example of the use of these injection codes would be a corticosteroid injection as a ganglion cyst treatment.

CODING SHOT

You must read the codes carefully. For most injection codes (i.e., 20550, 20551, 20553) the code description states "Injection(s)." This means that one or more injections can be reported with the same code with no modifier.

Arthrocentesis is aspiration of a joint (Fig. 14–12), and the codes to report such a service are in the range of 20600-20610. Arthrocentesis is a procedure commonly used in the treatment of joint conditions. The area over the involved joint is injected with anesthetic, a needle is inserted into the joint, and fluid is withdrawn.

Code 20612 reports an aspiration and/or injection of a ganglion cyst, which is a rubbery swelling that may occur anywhere on the body but usually occurs over a joint or tendon of the wrist or foot. The treatment of a ganglion cyst is surgical removal, aspiration, or aspiration with injection of a corticosteroid steroid. Often, ganglion cysts will appear in a cluster and if multiple cysts are treated, report the service with 20612 with modifier -59 appended.

CODING SHOT

The code descriptions for arthrocentesis indicate that the codes can be used for an aspiration, an injection, or both an aspiration and an injection. You would not report the performance of both an aspiration and an injection at the same session by using multiple codes, as that would be unbundling. You would instead report both services using a single code.

The arthrocentesis codes are divided according to whether the joint is small (finger, toe), intermediate (ankle, elbow), or major (shoulder, hip). Note that while the shoulder is a major joint, the acromioclavicular joint, which

FIGURE 14–12 Arthrocentesis of a joint.

is a part of the shoulder, is only an intermediate joint. This often leads to incorrectly coding the acromioclavicular joint as a major joint rather than as an intermediate joint.

Lidocaine, Marcaine, and so forth, when used as anesthetics, are not reported separately. Any injected therapeutic drug such as a steroid is reported separately using a HCPCS J code (drug code).

Insertion of wires or pins to repair a bone (20650) is a procedure often used by orthopedic physicians. The procedure is performed using a local or general anesthetic. The bone is drilled through with a power drill and pins and/or wires are placed through the holes in the bone and allowed to emerge through the skin on each side of the bone. A traction device is then attached to the pins or wires to hold the bone immobile while healing takes place (refer to Fig. 14–5). This may sound painful, but actually, the procedure is used to allow well-aligned healing, as well as alleviate pain.

CODING SHOT The removal of the external skeletal wires or pins is included in the reimbursement for fixation; but for internal fixation removal, report separately using 20670, 20680.

The codes to report the **application** of many of the devices used for fixation of the bones of the body during the healing process—cranial tong, cranial halo, pelvic halo, femoral halo, caliper, stereotactic frame—are located in this category. Each of the applications includes the removal of the device, unless the device is removed by another physician (20665). When the application of these devices is performed through an open surgical procedure, the procedure is referred to as an open reduction with internal fixation **(ORIF)** and uses pins, wires, and screws to stabilize a fracture.

Implant removal codes (20670, 20680) are available for reporting the services of removal of buried wires, pins, rods, etc., previously implanted. If, for example, there is a complication, such as pain, the hardware may be removed. Diagnosis coding must support the necessity of removal of the deep hardware as a complication. If removed during the global period, report the service with modifier -58 (staged) appended to the procedure code. The implant removal codes are divided according to whether the implants are superficial or deep.

External fixation is the application of a device that holds a bone in place, but unlike internal fixation, the device is placed on the outside of the body and pins or wires are placed into the bone from the outside (Fig. 14–13). These wires and pins, when fastened to the bone, hold the device or system immobile. This type of fixation is commonly used with comminuted fractures (fragmented) that are difficult to hold in place. External fixation is used primarily in cases of limb fracture, major pelvic disruption, osteotomy, arthrodesis, bone infection, and bone lengthening.

Codes 20690 and 20692 report whether the device or system is placed on one surface (uniplane) or several surfaces (multiplane). With the uniplane device, two or more pins are inserted above the fracture site and two or more pins are inserted below the fracture site. Multiplane devices are more complicated and are usually reserved for highly complex fractures (see Fig. 14–13).

FIGURE 14–13 **A,** External fixation (Ilizarov multiplane). **B,** Example of an external fixation device on the right leg. The left leg is in a splint. (**B** from McCance KL, Huether SE: *Pathophysiology: The Biologic Basis for Disease in Adults and Children,* St. Louis, 2006, Mosby.)

CODING SHOT

The fixation devices codes are reported in addition to the code for the treatment of the fracture, unless the application code specifically states that fracture repair is included. For example, see code 25545: "Open treatment of ulnar shaft fracture includes internal fixation, when performed." This code specifies both the treatment of the fracture and the fixation. External fixation, if performed, would be reported separately.

Note also that the codes in the Introduction or Removal categories are for **unilateral** services, so if a procedure is bilateral you would assign modifier -50.

If the device is **adjusted,** the service is reported separately (20693). **Removal** of external fixation devices or systems is usually accomplished under anesthesia and is reported separately from the application (20694). However, if the removal does not require return to the operating room, you would not report the service separately but would consider the removal as being bundled into the application code. If the removal was performed outside the global period, some payers may reimburse the removal as an E/M service.

EXERCISE 14-2   *General*

Using the CPT and/or ICD-9-CM manual(s), provide the codes for the following:

1 Exploration of a penetrating wound of the left leg

  CPT Code: _____

2 Replantation of right foot after a complete, traumatic amputation

  CPT Code: _____

3 Radical resection of malignant neoplasm of cheek, less than 2 cm

  CPT Code: _____

4 Nonoperative, electrical stimulation of nonhealing femur fracture

  CPT Code: _____

5 Percutaneous needle biopsy of muscle of upper arm in a patient with congenital myotonic muscular dystrophy

  CPT Code: _____

  ICD-9-CM Code: _____ (ICD-10-CM Code: _____)

6 Intra-articular aspiration and injection of finger joint for arthritis

  CPT Code: _____

  ICD-9-CM Code: _____ (ICD-10-CM Code: _____)

Grafts (or Implants)

Codes 20900-20938 report the harvesting of bone, cartilage, fascia lata, tendon, or tissue through an incision separate from that used to implant the graft. Graft material is used in a wide variety of repair procedures. For example, if a tibial fracture has failed to heal in 20 weeks, the surgeon may decide that the fracture requires bone grafting to achieve healing. Bone grafting is also used in cases of large defects (>6 cm). Some types of fractures commonly heal with difficulty, so after debridement the surgeon may decide to allow a 5- to 7-day healing period before the bone grafting procedure is performed. The grafts are obtained from the patient or a donor. Donors can be either living or deceased (cadaver). The pieces of bone are shaped into bars or pegs and then used to repair the defect.

Fascia lata grafts are taken from the lower thigh area because the fascia is thickest in this area. Fascia is the fibrous tissue that serves as connective tissue; it may be shaved off with an instrument called a stripper or it may be incised (cut) away. The fascia lata is then used in the repair procedure. Codes for obtaining the fascia lata graft are based on whether a stripper (20920) was used to remove the fascia or whether a more complex removal procedure (20922) was required to obtain the graft material.

Tissue grafts include obtaining of the fat, dermis, paratenon (fatty tissue from the tendon compartment), and other tissue types. **Spine surgery** codes 20930-20938 report the obtaining and shaping of the tissue, whether from the patient (autograft) or from a donor (allograft). The obtaining and shaping of the spine graft material is reported in addition to reporting the implantation procedure, which is the primary procedure (definitive procedure), unless the description of the major procedure includes a graft.

Other Procedures

Other Procedure codes (20950-20999) report monitoring muscles, bone grafting with microvascular technique, free osteocutaneous flaps with microvascular technique, electronic/ultrasound stimulation, and computer-assisted navigation procedures. **Monitoring of interstitial fluid pressure** (20950) is a procedure in which the physician inserts a device into the muscle to measure the pressure within the muscle. Increased pressure in the muscle indicates that the tissue is not receiving a sufficient supply of blood due to accumulation of fluid.

Bone grafts (20955-20962) are identified by the site from which the graft is obtained. When the bone grafts are removed, the small blood vessels remain attached to the graft. The graft is then inserted and the blood vessels are attached to vessels in the area of implant, using an operating microscope. The use of the operating microscope (69990) is included in the code descriptions for 20955-20962. As a reminder, there is a parenthetical statement following 20962 that states, "(Do not report 69990 in addition to codes 20955-20962)."

Free osteocutaneous flaps (20969-20973) are bone grafts that include the skin and tissue that overlie the bone. The flap has an arterial pedicle that is attached (anastomosed) to an artery on the recipient site. The surgeon then utilizes the skin, tissue, and bone to reconstruct the defect, using an operating microscope. The codes are divided based on which part of the body the flap is taken from.

Codes 20955-20962 are vascularized bone grafts that are used where there are large defects, usually in long bones, where a standard iliac bone graft or other types of nonvascularized bone grafts are not likely to heal.

Electrical or ultrasound stimulation (20974-20979) is used to promote healing. Low-voltage electricity or ultrasound is applied to the skin, and both are often used in the treatment of fractures.

Computer-assisted surgical navigation (20985) is use of navigational assistance in musculoskeletal procedures. The code is listed in addition to the code for the primary procedure.

From the Trenches

"The most rewarding part of my job is helping others understand a coding or billing issue, whether they are a patient, employee, physician, or student. I enjoy teaching and mentoring others."

MARTHA

Spinal Instrumentation and Fixation

Within the subheading Spine (Vertebral Column) (22010-22899), services are often based on the cervical (C1-C7), lumbar (L1-L5), and thoracic (T1-T12) spinal areas. For example, codes in the range 22210-22216 identify osteotomy of the cervical, lumbar, or thoracic spinal area. Codes are often further divided based on the exact spinal location. For example, codes in the range 22590-22600 identify arthrodesis of three different cervical areas: occiput-C2, C1-C2, or cervical below the C2 segment. Of special note in the CPT manual is that the C1 is often referred to as the **atlas** and C2 is referred to as the **axis.**

Arthrodesis can be performed with another surgical procedure, such as fracture care or a laminectomy. If arthrodesis is performed with a more major procedure, use modifier -51 on the arthrodesis code to indicate multiple procedures were performed. An exception to this rule is when the code is an add-on code, which is exempt from use with modifier -51. For example, 22614 is used to report an arthrodesis of multiple vertebral segments. A code from the 22600-22612 range reports the first segment, and 22614 is reported for each additional vertebral segment. Modifier -51 is, therefore, not required.

CODING SHOT

When choosing codes for spine procedures, verify whether the code is describing a vertebral segment, the actual bony segment, versus an interspace (the space between two vertebral segments). If reporting a procedure performed at L4-L5, you would choose the primary code to represent L4 and the add-on code to represent L5. If the procedure code description was by interspace, only one code would be assigned.

Spinal instrumentation is used to stabilize the spinal column in some repair procedures. **Segmental instrumentation** is the attachment of a fixative device at each end of the area being repaired and at least one other attachment in the spinal area being repaired (Fig. 14–14). For example, if the repair was at T10 and T11 (thoracic vertebral bodies 10 and 11) and a rod was attached to T7 and L1, the repair rod may also be attached at T8, T9, T10, T11, and T12. **Nonsegmental instrumentation** is the application of the fixative device at each end of the area being repaired, as illustrated in Fig. 14–15. For example, if the repair was of T10, the rod may be attached at T7 and T12.

Many of the instrumentation codes are add-on codes (22840-22848 and 22851) and are reported in addition to the major procedure.

FIGURE 14–14 Decompensated lumbar curve after fusion of thoracic curve only. (From Canale ST, Beaty JH: *Campbell's Operative Orthopaedics,* ed 11, Philadelphia, 2007, Mosby.)

FIGURE 14–15 Fixation at each end of the area to be repaired (nonsegmental spinal instrumentation).

Foot and Toe Repairs

A common procedure performed on the toe is a hallux valgus correction (bunion surgery). Hallux is the great toe and valgus is the angulation of the toe away from the midline, as illustrated in Fig. 14–16.

A variety of procedures are performed to correct the defect, as represented by codes in the range 28290-28299. For example, the Keller type of procedure is reported with 28292 and describes a procedure in which a wire is inserted through the bones of a toe to hold the bones in correct alignment. Each code description indicates the procedure type that is included, many of which include specific eponyms (names of individuals for whom the procedures are named), so careful reading is necessary to choose the correct bunion repair code.

APPLICATION OF CASTS AND STRAPPING

Application of Casts and Strapping codes (29000-29799) are used for subsequent treatment of fractures of the extremities, ligament sprains/tears, and overuse injuries. They may also be reported for the initial stabilization of an injury until definitive restorative treatment can be provided. Because each injury is unique, each cast is unique in terms of size and position. The cast immobilizes the fracture with materials such as plaster, fiberglass, or thermoplastics. Each physician has a preference for the types of cast materials used.

Strapping is the taping of a body part, as illustrated in Fig. 14–17. Strapping is used to exert pressure on a body part to give it more stability, and is used in the treatment of sprains, strains, and dislocations. **Splints** are made of wood, cloth, metal, or plastic, as illustrated in Fig. 14–18, and are used to immobilize, support, or protect a body part, thereby allowing rest and healing. The **removal** of the cast, strapping, or splint is included in each of the Application of Casts and Strapping codes.

CODING SHOT

If a cast, strapping, or splint is applied as a part of a surgical procedure, you do not report codes from the Application of Casts and Strapping subheading because the musculoskeletal surgical procedure codes include the first cast, strapping, or splint as well as its later removal. The surgery, application, and removal are all bundled into the surgical code.

FIGURE 14–16 **A** and **B,** Hallux valgus, or bunion, is a bursa usually found along the medial aspect of the big toe. Most commonly, it is attributed to heredity or to poorly fitting shoes. (**A** from Seidel HM, et al: *Mosby's Guide to Physical Examination,* ed 6, St. Louis, 2006, Mosby.)

FIGURE 14–17 Types of strapping.

— Plaster splint

Cotton padding —

Elastic wrap

FIGURE 14–18 Splint used to immobilize a joint or bone.

If the cast, strapping, or splint is applied as a part of a **fracture repair,** the application service is not reported separately. The application service is bundled into all fracture repair codes, as is the removal. If a subsequent cast, strapping, or splint is applied within the follow-up period for either the surgical procedure or the fracture repair, you can bill the application with modifier -58 and also bill for the materials (A4580-A4590). You can bill for a separate office visit during which a second cast, strapping, or splint is applied only if the patient is provided some additional, separate and significant service. Modifier -25 would be appended to the E/M code.

QUICK CHECK 14-4

1. A replacement cast during the global period of fracture care may require which modifier? _____

You can report the Application of Casts and Strapping codes only when the physician:

- Applies an initial cast, strapping, or splint for stabilization prior to definitive treatment by another provider
- Applies a subsequent cast, strapping, or splint
- Treats a sprain and does not expect to provide any other type of restorative treatment

The subheading Application of Casts and Strapping is divided into three major categories:

- Body and Upper Extremity
- Lower Extremity
- Removal or Repair (provided by a physician other than the one who initially applied it)

The subcategories of Body/Upper Extremity and Lower Extremity are:

- Casts
- Splints
- Strapping—Any Age

The codes in all subcategories are divided primarily according to the **location** of the cast, splint, or strapping on the body—head, hand, extremity—and often on the **type**—Minerva, Velpeau, static (nonmovable), dynamic (movable).

EXERCISE 14-3 *Application of Casts and Strapping*

Using the CPT and HCPCS manuals, provide the codes for the following:

1 Replacement of fiberglass shoulder-to-hand (long-arm) cast for a 54-year-old patient

   CPT Codes: _____, _____

2 Initial application of a walking-type short leg cast for a sprain

   CPT Code: _____

3 Removal of a full leg cast by a physician who did not apply the cast

   CPT Code: _____

4 Strapping of a 46-year-old patient's knee

   CPT Code: _____

5 Replacement of a thigh-to-toes cast on the right leg of a 35-year-old female patient

   CPT Codes: _____, _____

ENDOSCOPY/ ARTHROSCOPY

Arthroscopy is often the treatment of choice for many orthopedic surgical procedures. The incisions are smaller, which decreases the risk of infection and speeds recovery time. Several small incisions are made through which lights, mirrors, and instruments are inserted, as illustrated in Fig. 14–19.

The arthroscopy codes are located at the end of the Musculoskeletal subsection. If multiple procedures are performed through a scope, they are reported with modifier -51. Bundled into all surgical arthroscopic procedure codes is the diagnostic arthroscopy. You must not unbundle and report a diagnostic arthroscopy and a surgical arthroscopy if both were performed during the same encounter. Do not report separately services performed during a procedure that are considered part of the procedure, such as shaving, removing, evacuating, casting, splinting, or strapping.

A note preceding the Endoscopy/Arthroscopy codes (29800-29999) states, "When arthroscopy is performed in conjunction with arthrotomy, add modifier -51." This note indicates that if a surgeon performs an arthroscopy and during the procedure extends the procedure to an arthrotomy, both services are reported. For example, a physician performs an arthroscopic shaving of the articular cartilage and also performs an open capsulotomy (posterior capsular release) of the knee. Both the arthroscopic shaving (29877) and the capsulotomy (27435) would be reported, and to the least expensive procedure add modifier -51 (multiple procedures).

In arthroscopic procedures, it is also correct to report multiple procedures in different compartments in the joint area. For example, in the knee, there are three compartments, the medial, lateral, and patellofemoral. If a meniscectomy (29881) is performed in the medial compartment, and a shaving (29877) is performed in the patellofemoral compartment, these procedures are both reported.

CODING SHOT When coding arthroscopic procedures of the knee, note the use of **basket forceps,** which indicates a meniscectomy (meniscus removal) rather than a shaving and debridement.

Monitor with view from arthroscope

FIGURE 14–19 Arthroscopy of knee.

The codes in the Arthroscopy subheading are divided according to body area—elbow, shoulder, knee—and then according to the type and extent of procedure performed. An example of type of service is as follows: 29805 reports an arthroscopy of the shoulder for **diagnostic** purposes, whereas code 29806 is an arthroscopy of the shoulder for a **surgical** repair procedure. Not only are there two different codes for surgical and diagnostic arthroscopic procedures, but also the reimbursement for the surgical procedures is higher than the diagnostic procedure. So great care must be taken to select the code that correctly describes the services supported in the medical record and in code placement. If the procedure began as a diagnostic procedure, which is often the case, and converts to a surgical procedure, only the surgical procedure is reported. The reimbursement for the surgical procedure is higher than the reimbursement for the diagnostic procedure. For example, one payer's reimbursement was $424.86 for the diagnostic procedure (29805) and $979.21 for the surgical procedure (29806).

CODING SHOT A diagnostic arthroscopy is always included in a surgical arthroscopy.

Note the description for code 29805: "Arthroscopy, shoulder, diagnostic, with or without synovial biopsy (separate procedure)." You will find the statement "separate procedure" several times in the Endoscopy/Arthroscopy subheading because often a minor arthroscopic procedure is part of a more major procedure. You cannot report the service of the minor procedure unless it has been performed as an independent service, addressing a distinctly separate problem. Also note that the parenthetical information indicates the codes "(23065-23066, 23100-23101)" are to be reported if the procedure was done as an open (incisional) procedure rather than as an endoscopic procedure.

EXERCISE 14-4 *Endoscopy/Arthroscopy*

Using the CPT manual, provide the codes for the following:

1 Surgical arthroscopy of ankle, which included extensive debridement

   CPT Code: _____

2 Diagnostic knee arthroscopy with a synovial biopsy

   CPT Code: _____

3 Diagnostic shoulder arthroscopy

   CPT Code: _____

4 Arthroscopic repair of tuberosity fracture of knee with manipulation

   CPT Code: _____

5 Surgical arthroscopy of ankle, including drilling and excision of tibial defect

   CPT Code: _____

CHAPTER REVIEW

CHAPTER 14, PART I, THEORY

Without the use of reference material, complete the following:

1 The Musculoskeletal System subsection is formatted according to what type of sites?

_____

2 Which physician subspecialty can report the codes from the Musculoskeletal System subsection?

_____

3 List the three types of fracture treatments and briefly describe each:

_____

_____

_____

_____

4 It is the _____ of the fracture that determines the method of treatment.

5 _____ is the application of pulling force to hold a bone in place.

6 What is the term that describes the physician's actions of bending, rotating, pulling, or guiding the bone back into place? _____

7 What term is used to mean "put the bone back in place"? _____

8 What term describes a bone that is not in its normal location? _____

9 What term describes the cleaning of a wound?

_____

10 This is a hollow needle that is often used to withdraw samples of fluid from a joint:

_____

11 Would a biopsy code usually include the administration of any necessary local anesthesia? _____

CHAPTER 14, PART II, PRACTICAL

With the use of the CPT and ICD-9-CM manuals, complete the following:

12 Incision of a superficial soft tissue abscess, secondary to osteomyelitis

CPT Code: _____

13 Radical resection of a 2.7 cm malignant neoplasm of the soft tissue of the upper back

CPT Code: _____

14 Closed treatment of three vertebral process fractures

CPT Code: _____

15 Under general anesthesia, manipulation of a right shoulder joint with external fixation

CPT Code: _____

16 Lengthening of four tendons of elbow

🔵 CPT Code(s): _____

17 Incision and drainage of bursa of elbow

🔵 CPT Code(s): _____

18 Open treatment of a carpal scaphoid fracture with internal fixation applied

🔵 CPT Code(s): _____

19 Arthroplasty of two metacarpophalangeal joints

🔵 CPT Code(s): _____

20 Tenotomy of two flexor tendons of a finger using an open procedure

🔵 CPT Code(s): _____

21 Amputation, lower arm, using Krukenberg procedure

🔵 CPT Code(s): _____

22 Open treatment of radial and ulnar shaft fractures with internal fixation of both radius and ulna

🔵 CPT Code(s): _____

23 Osteoplasty for shortening of both of radius and ulna for adult Kienböck's disease

🔵 CPT Code(s): _____

ICD-9-CM Code: _____

(ICD-10-CM Code: _____)

24 Percutaneous lateral tenotomy for tennis elbow (lateral epicondylitis)

🔵 CPT Code(s): _____

ICD-9-CM Code: _____

(ICD-10-CM Code: _____)

25 Replantation of right arm, including the neck of the humerus through the elbow joint, following a complete traumatic amputation

🔵 CPT Code(s): _____

ICD-9-CM Code: _____

(ICD-10-CM Code: _____)

QUICK CHECK ANSWERS ✓

QUICK CHECK 14-1
1. a. 27506

QUICK CHECK 14-2
1. no

QUICK CHECK 14-3
1. anatomic

QUICK CHECK 14-4
1. -58

CHAPTER 75

"I really like how my work contributes to higher reimbursement rates and less denials for the physicians. That in turn always improves quality of patient care because we have the resources to provide that based on reimbursement and fewer denials."

Lynda Kross, CPC
Certified Reimbursement Assistant
University Physicians—University of Missouri Health Care
Columbia, Missouri

Respiratory System

Chapter Topics

Format

Endoscopy

Nose

Accessory Sinuses

Larynx

Trachea/Bronchi

Lungs and Pleura

Chapter Review

Quick Check Answers

Learning Objectives

After completing this chapter you should be able to

1 Differentiate between services reported with codes from the Respiratory subsection and those reported with codes from other subsections.

2 Explain the effects of extent and approach when reporting endoscopy respiratory procedures.

3 Identify highlights of nasal procedure coding.

4 Analyze the codes to report services to the accessory sinuses.

5 Categorize the codes in the Larynx subheading.

6 Explain the structure of the trachea/bronchi codes.

7 Distinguish the difference amongst the codes assigned to report lungs and pleura services and procedures.

8 Demonstrate the ability to code respiratory services and procedures.

Make sure to check
evolve
learning system
for the latest content updates

FORMAT The Respiratory System subsection is arranged by anatomic site (e.g., nose, accessory sinus, larynx) and then by procedure (e.g., incision, excision, introduction). Your knowledge of respiratory terminology is important (Fig. 15–1), as you assign codes from the Respiratory System subsection.

In the Musculoskeletal System section, arthroscopy codes are placed at the end of the subsection, but in the Respiratory System subsection, the **endoscopy** codes are listed throughout, according to anatomic site. **Fracture repair**, such as that of the nose or sternum, is listed in the Musculoskeletal System subsection, not in the Respiratory System subsection. Procedures that are performed on the **throat** or **mouth** are not located in the Respiratory System subsection, but instead are located in the Digestive System subsection.

The Respiratory System subsection contains some codes that may be considered **cosmetic**. It is important to note each of the components performed during the procedure because there are many services bundled into some of these codes. For example, under the subheading Nose and the category Repair, there is code 30400 for rhinoplasty. The rhinoplasty may be performed either through external skin incisions (open) or through intranasal incisions (closed), and both approaches can be reported with 30400. The extent of the procedure varies based on the desired outcome, but a rhinoplasty can include fracturing a deformed septum, repositioning the septum, reshaping and/or augmenting the nasal cartilage, removing fat from the area, performing a layered closure, and applying a splint or cast. If all of these components of a rhinoplasty were performed, they would be bundled into 30420. You have to read all of the notes and the code information carefully to ensure that you do not code components of the procedure separately if there is one code that includes all the components.

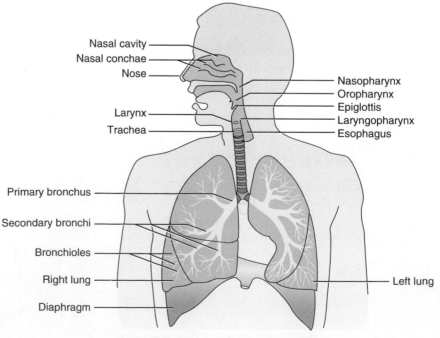

FIGURE 15–1 Respiratory system.

QUICK CHECK 15-1

1. Rhinoplasty can be performed either _____, through external skin incisions, or closed, through _____ incisions.

ENDOSCOPY

During endoscopic procedures, a scope is placed through an existing body orifice (opening), or a small incision is made into a cavity for scope placement.

When sinus endoscopies are performed, a scope is placed through the nose into the nasal cavity. Codes for sinuses (31231-31294) report unilateral (on one side) procedures except in the case of a diagnostic nasal endoscopy, which is unilateral or bilateral. Multiple procedures may be performed within different sinuses (frontal, maxillary, and ethmoid sinuses) during the same operative session. The CPT manual has combined into a single code some multiple sinus procedures commonly performed at the same operative session.

Example

31276   Nasal/sinus endoscopy, surgical with frontal sinus exploration, with or without removal of tissue from frontal sinus

🤚 **CAUTION** *Code to the full **extent** of the procedure.*

Endoscopic procedures may start at one site (such as the nose) and follow through to another site (such as the larynx or bronchial tubes). It is important to choose the code that most appropriately reflects the furthest extent of the procedure. For example, if a direct laryngoscopy is performed, and the scope is progressed past the larynx and includes examination of the trachea the service is reported with 31515 because the code description states either with or without tracheoscopy. However, if it is necessary to continue the procedure to the bronchial tubes, service would be reported with 31622 (bronchoscopy). The larynx and trachea must be passed to get to the farthest point (bronchial tubes). In these instances, it is the full extent of the procedure that determines the code assignment.

🤚 **CAUTION** *Code the correct **approach** for the procedure.*

The same surgical procedure may be performed using different approaches. For example, code 32141 describes a **thoracotomy** with "excision-plication (removal/shortening) of bullae (blisters); with or without any pleural procedure." Code 32655 describes a surgical **thoracoscopy** with excision-plication of bullae, including any pleural procedures. Code 32655 describes the same procedure as 32141, except that 32655 is a procedure performed through very minute incisions utilizing a thoracoscope, whereas code 32141 describes an open incision through the thorax, opening the full operative site to the surgeon. In these instances, it is the approach utilized to perform the procedure that determines the code assignment.

Multiple endoscopic procedures may be performed through the same scope during the operative session. When this occurs, each procedure should be reported with modifier -51 (multiple procedures) placed on subsequent procedure(s). For example, a bronchoscopy with biopsy is performed as well as a bronchoscopy with removal of a foreign body. Not only would you report a bronchoscopy with biopsy, but you would also report the removal of a foreign body. The multiple procedure modifier -51 would be placed after the lower priced (least resource-intensive) procedure. The exception to this occurs when the CPT manual offers a code for which the description includes all the separate elements of the procedure bundled into one code.

> **CAUTION** *Do not confuse nasal/sinus endoscopic procedures with intranasal procedures. Intranasal procedures may require that surgical instruments be placed into the nose but do not require the use of an endoscope. When an endoscope is used in a nasal/sinus procedure, assign a nasal/sinus endoscopy code.*

Remember that a diagnostic endoscopy is always bundled into a surgical endoscopy. For example, if a physician began a diagnostic endoscopic nasal procedure and continued on to complete a surgical procedure, you report only for the surgical procedure. To report both a diagnostic and a surgical nasal endoscopy is unbundling if the diagnostic and surgical procedures are performed on the same nasal space. However, if a diagnostic sinus endoscopy is performed on the right maxillary sinus and a surgical endoscopic maxillectomy on the left, both procedures are reported with appropriate -LT and -RT modifiers because two different procedures were performed.

When reporting laryngoscopic procedures, note that the terms "indirect" and "direct" are often stated in the code description. For example, locate codes 31505, indirect, and 31515, direct in the CPT manual. **Indirect** in 31505 means that the physician used a tongue depressor to hold the tongue down and view the epiglottis (the lid that covers the larynx) with a mirror. The patient vocalizes (says "ah") and the physician can then view the vocal cords. **Direct** in 31515 means that the endoscope is passed into the larynx and the physician looks directly at the larynx through the endoscope. The operative report will indicate whether the procedure was indirect or direct.

Locating Endoscopy Codes. Endoscopy codes can be located in the CPT manual index under Endoscopy and then under the anatomic subterm of the site. You can also locate an endoscopic procedure by the anatomic endoscopy title. For example, a bronchial biopsy using endoscopy is listed under Bronchoscopy and then under the subterm Biopsy.

EXERCISE 15-1 *Radiology Terminology*

Using the CPT manual, complete the following:

1 Endoscopic maxillary antrostomy

CPT Code: ___31256___

31256 - 31267

2 Direct laryngoscopy for removal of fish bone

CPT Code: ___31530___

31515 - 31571

3 After the airway is sufficiently anesthetized, a flexible bronchoscope is inserted through the mouth and advanced to the bronchus, where a transbronchial biopsy of one lobe is obtained.

CPT Code: ___31628___   *31625 - 29   31632-33*

4 Diagnostic thoracoscopy of the mediastinal space is accomplished with the use of a flexible endoscope that is inserted through a small incision on the chest.

CPT Code: ___32605___   *32601 - 6*

5 Segmental resection of the right lung using a flexible endoscope (surgical thoracoscopy)

CPT Code: ___32657___ *32663 Segmental*

NOSE Many of the codes in the Nose subheading are reported by physicians who specialize in treating conditions of the nose (otorhinolaryngologist; ear, nose, and throat specialists), but there are also many codes in the subheading that are more widely used. For example, it is in the Nose subheading that you will locate codes for commonly performed office procedures, such as control of nosebleeds, incision of abscesses, removal of foreign objects from the nose (think children!), and removal of nasal cysts and lesions.

Incision Codes for incision of a nasal abscess (30000, 30020) are divided on whether the abscess is on the nasal mucosa or the septal mucosa. If a nasal abscess is approached from the outside of the nose **(external approach),** you would assign a code from the Integumentary System subsection; but if the approach is from the inside of the nose **(internal approach),** you would assign a code from the Respiratory System subsection. The medical record will describe the approach to the procedure.

After an abscess has been penetrated, the physician may close the area immediately or place a tube in the incision to ensure that the pus continues to drain from the abscess area. After the drain is removed, the abscess may be packed with gauze, with one end of the packing material left outside the surface to act as a wick, as illustrated in Fig. 15–2, *A-C.*

The insertion and removal of the tube and/or gauze and any required sutures and/or anesthesia are bundled into the code, so you should not report these services separately. You should report any additional supplies over and above those usually used for the procedure by using the Medicine section code for supplies, 99070, or a HCPCS code, as directed by the third-party payer.

FIGURE 15–2 **A,** Nasal mucosal abscess. **B,** Incision of abscess. **C,** Gauze packed into abscess with end extended outside the abscess, acting as a wick.

Excision   Within the Nose subheading, the Excision category (30100-30160) contains a wide range of procedures that describe removal of tissue from the nose—for example, biopsy, polyp excision, and cyst excision—as well as resection of the turbinate bone.

 CODING SHOT   When two procedures are completed during the same surgical session, the most complex procedure is sequenced first.

From the Trenches

"When someone expresses an interest in coding, I explain not only what I do day to day, but also why coding is so important. Many people don't realize that selecting proper codes is in the patient's best interest as they can give a detailed picture of the patient's medical condition and history."

LYNDA

The **biopsy** code (30100) reports a biopsy that is performed intranasally; but if the procedure was for a biopsy of the skin outside of the nose, you assign the biopsy code 11100 from the Integumentary System.

Nasal polyps develop and mature, causing nasal obstruction (Fig. 15–3, *A*). The physician removes the polyps, usually with a snare, as illustrated in Fig. 15–3, *B*.

The excision of **nasal polyps** is reported with one of two codes (30110 and 30115). The difference between the codes is the extent of the excision. Code 30110 reports a simple polyp excision that would usually be performed in the office, whereas 30115 reports a more extensive polyp excision that would usually be performed in a hospital setting.

 CODING SHOT   Modifier -50 (bilateral) is assigned when the polyps are removed from the left and right sides of the nose.

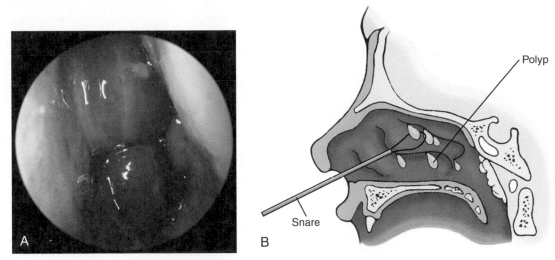

FIGURE 15–3 **A,** Nasal polyp. **B,** A nasal snare is used to remove nasal polyps. The nose is anesthetized, a snare is slipped around the polyp, which is transected, and a forceps is used to remove the polyp. (**A** from Zitelli BJ, Davis HW: *Atlas of Pediatric Physical Diagnosis,* ed 5, Philadelphia, 2007, Mosby. **B** from Monahan FD et al: *Phipps' Medical-Surgical Nursing: Health and Illness Perspectives,* ed 8, St. Louis, 2007, Mosby.)

The codes for excision or destruction of **lesions** inside the nose are divided based on the approach—internal or external. Usually, if the approach to the procedure is external, you are referred to the Integumentary System subsection to locate the correct code; but the nasal lesion excision/ destruction codes can be assigned for either an external or an internal approach to a lesion.

You have to read the code descriptions carefully to ensure that you understand all of the circumstances that surround assignment of the code, and you have to identify codes such as the lesion excision/destruction that are exceptions to the usual rules.

All methods of lesion destruction, including laser, are included in the Excision codes. Usually, if laser was used in the destruction of a lesion, you would be referred to a separate set of codes just for laser destruction; but with the lesion destruction codes in the Nose category, laser is included as one of the destruction methods.

Turbinates are the bones on the inside of the nose. These bones are shaped like a spiral shell and humidify, warm, and filter the air. These bones are referred to as the nasal concha. The turbinates are divided into three sections—inferior, middle, and superior (Fig. 15–4). Portions of or all of a turbinate bone may be removed because of chronic congestion or neoplastic growth. Because third-party payers usually do not pay for cosmetic surgical procedures, you must document the medical necessity for noncosmetic procedures carefully to ensure appropriate reimbursement. Watch for and read the extensive notes inside the parentheses throughout this category.

Introduction

Introduction codes (30200-30220) include injection, displacement therapy, and insertion. **Injections** into the turbinates (30200) are therapeutic injections usually performed to shrink the nasal tissue to improve breathing. For example, if a patient has inflamed nasal passages due to an allergic reaction or a deviated septum, the patient may benefit from a steroid injection into the turbinates. **Displacement therapy** (30210) is a procedure in which the physician flushes saline solution into the sinuses to remove mucus or pus. The insertion of a **nasal button**

FIGURE 15–4   Superior, inferior, and middle nasal turbinates.

(30220) (as illustrated in Fig. 15–5) is a technique used for a patient who has a perforated septum. The physician places the button into the opening and fastens the button in place with sutures. The button is usually made of silicone or rubber. This technique is used as a method of repairing the septum without surgical grafting.

Removal of a Foreign Body   A variety of objects are inserted into the various orifices (openings) of the body, and the nose is a common place into which these foreign objects are placed. The code to report an office procedure for the removal of a foreign body from the nose is 30300. Codes for more extensive procedures are also available for removal of foreign objects from the nose, such as those requiring general anesthesia (30310) and a more invasive surgical procedure.

Repair   Within the Repair category (30400-30630) are the plastic procedures—rhinoplasty, septoplasty, and septal dermatoplasty. **Rhinoplasty** is a procedure to reshape the nose internally, externally, or both. The codes are divided based on the extent (minor, intermediate, major), on whether the septum

FIGURE 15–5   Insertion of nasal button.

was also repaired (septoplasty), and on whether the procedure was an initial or secondary procedure. **Secondary** procedures are those that are performed after an initial procedure. For example, if a rhinoplasty was performed and the results were not as successful as the patient desired, the surgeon could perform a second procedure (secondary) to improve the result.

Septoplasty is rearrangement of the nasal septum. This procedure is commonly performed due to a deviated septum.

> ✋ **CAUTION** *Do not use a septoplasty code if the operative report indicates that only a resection of the inferior turbinate(s) was performed. The resection of the inferior turbinate(s) is reported with 30140 and is not a procedure performed on the septum. The septoplasty code, 30520, is reported when the nasal septum is resected. There is a note enclosed in parentheses following both codes—30140 and 30520—that cautions you to use the correct code, depending on whether the turbinate or the septum was resected.*

Destruction

Destruction can be accomplished by use of ablation. **Ablation** is removal, usually by cutting. Ablation or cauterization is performed to remove excess nasal mucosa or to reduce inflammation. The destruction codes (30801, 30802) are divided according to the extent of the procedure—superficial or intramural. **Intramural** is ablation of the deeper mucosa, as compared to **superficial** ablation, which involves only the outer layer of mucosa.

Other Procedures

Codes (30901-30999) for the control of nasal hemorrhage are located in the Other Procedures category and are often reported. The physician may use anterior or posterior pressure to control the hemorrhage. Anterior nasal packing (Fig. 15–6) is the application of pressure using packing to the anterior aspect of the nasal cavity and posterior nasal packing is the application of pressure to the posterior aspect of the nasal cavity. The nasal pack is inserted via the nasal opening. A balloon may be inserted and inflated to further control bleeding (Fig. 15–7). The codes are divided according to the type and extent of control required.

> **CODING SHOT** ✏️ The key to correctly coding nasal hemorrhage is to know the type of control (anterior/posterior) and the level of complexity (simple/ complex) utilized by the physician to control the hemorrhage.

There are times when neither cauterization nor packing will control a nasal hemorrhage, and ligation of the bleeding artery is required. Ligation of ethmoidal arteries involves opening the upper side of the nose and locating and tying the ethmoid artery (Fig. 15–8). Ligation of the internal maxillary artery is performed to gain control of nasal hemorrhage by locating and ligating the maxillary artery (Fig. 15–9).

A **therapeutic fracture** of the nasal turbinate is a procedure in which the physician fractures the turbinate bone and then repositions it, under local anesthetic. Repositioning the turbinate(s) often alleviates obstructed airflow caused by a previous fracture that has healed out of alignment and resulted in a deviation of the nose.

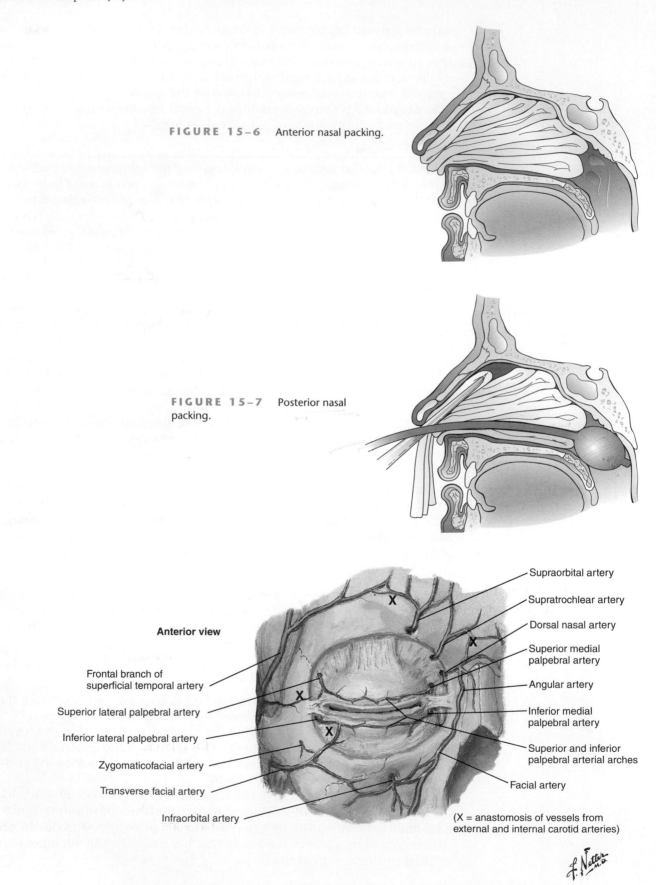

FIGURE 15–6 Anterior nasal packing.

FIGURE 15–7 Posterior nasal packing.

Anterior view

Supraorbital artery

Supratrochlear artery

Dorsal nasal artery

Superior medial palpebral artery

Angular artery

Inferior medial palpebral artery

Superior and inferior palpebral arterial arches

Facial artery

Frontal branch of superficial temporal artery

Superior lateral palpebral artery

Inferior lateral palpebral artery

Zygomaticofacial artery

Transverse facial artery

Infraorbital artery

(X = anastomosis of vessels from external and internal carotid arteries)

FIGURE 15–8 Arteries of the eye. (From Netter FH: *Atlas of Human Anatomy,* ed 4, Philadelphia, 2006, Saunders.)

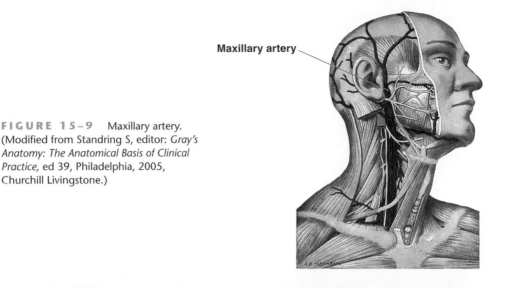

Maxillary artery

FIGURE 15-9 Maxillary artery. (Modified from Standring S, editor: *Gray's Anatomy: The Anatomical Basis of Clinical Practice,* ed 39, Philadelphia, 2005, Churchill Livingstone.)

EXERCISE 15-2 *Nose*

Using the CPT manual, complete the following:

1 Biopsy of an intranasal lesion

CPT Code: _____30100_____

ICD-9-CM Code: _____478.19_____ (ICD-10-CM Code: _____)

2 Primary rhinoplasty including major septal repair due to deviated nasal septum, acquired

CPT Code: _____30420_____   30400-30420

ICD-9-CM Code: _____470_____ (ICD-10-CM Code: _____)

3 Anterior control of nasal hemorrhage by means of limited chemical cauterization and simple packing

CPT Code: _____30901_____

ICD-9-CM Code: _____784.7_____ (ICD-10-CM Code: _____)

4 Septoplasty with contouring and grafting

CPT Code: _____30520_____

5 Removal of crayon from nose of 5-year-old boy, conducted as an office procedure

CPT Code: _____30300_____

ACCESSORY SINUSES

Incision

Within the Incision category are codes for services that you would not think of as being incisional. For example, the nasal sinuses can be washed (lavage) with a saline solution introduced through a canula (hollow tube) to remove infection. The Incision category code 31000 describes lavage of the maxillary sinus. Lavage can be performed on both the maxillary and the sphenoid sinuses (Fig. 15–10). If the lavage is of the sphenoid sinus, you report 31002.

CODING SHOT Use modifier -50 (bilateral) when the lavage is performed on both the left and right maxillary sinuses.

FIGURE 15–10   Paranasal sinuses.

Many of the codes in the Incision category are for sinusotomies. A **sinusotomy** is a procedure in which the physician enlarges the passage or creates a new passage from the nasal cavity into a sinus. This procedure is usually performed due to chronic sinus infection; the procedure improves sinus drainage. The codes are divided according to the extent of the procedure.

EXERCISE 15-3   *Accessory Sinuses*

Using the CPT manual, complete the following:

1 Lavage of the maxillary sinus, bilateral

CPT Codes: ___31000___ , ___31000-50___ > payor specified

2 Simple frontal sinusotomy using an external approach

CPT Code: ___31070___

3 Unilateral sinusotomy of frontal, ethmoid, and sphenoid

CPT Code: ___31090___

4 Radical sinusotomy

CPT Code: ___31030___

5 Pterygomaxillary fossa surgery, transfacial approach, due to chronic antritis of maxillary sinus

CPT Code: ___31040___

ICD-9-CM Code: ___473.0___ (ICD-10-CM Code: _____)

LARYNX   The procedures reported with codes in the Larynx subheading (31300-31599) include a wide range of surgical procedures, such as laryngectomy, plastic repair, and nerve destruction.

Excision   **Laryngotomy** is an incision that is made over the larynx (thyrotomy) to expose the larynx to view. With the larynx exposed, the surgeon can remove a tumor, a laryngocele (air-filled space), or a vocal cord (cordectomy). A laryngotomy can also be performed for diagnostic purposes, without a surgical procedure being performed.

Be careful not to get the codes from the Laryngotomy category confused with the tracheostomy codes located in the Trachea and Bronchi subheading, Incision category, which you will learn more about later in this chapter. The codes from the two categories differ, depending on the **purpose** of the procedure. The Laryngotomy category codes describe procedures in which the surgeon performs a thyrotomy (incision of the larynx through the thyroid cartilage) for the purpose of exposing the larynx. The codes in the Trachea and Bronchi subheading, Incision category describe a procedure in which the surgeon performs only the tracheostomy, usually to establish airflow, and no procedure or exposure of the larynx is planned or is involved.

Radical neck dissection, as referred to in the codes for laryngectomy, is the removal not only of the larynx but also of lymph glands and/or other surrounding tissue. Many of the codes in the Larynx subheading, Excision category are divided according to whether radical neck dissection was or was not performed. The operative report would indicate the extent of the dissection by referring to excision of lymph nodes in a radical procedure.

Introduction   **Intubation** is the establishment of an airway. The intubation represented in 31500 is provided on an emergency basis at such time as the patient experiences respiratory failure or the occurrence of an inadequate airway. Fig. 15–11 illustrates endotracheal intubation. The other Introduction code (31502) is for the replacement of a previously inserted tracheostomy tube.

Repair   Within the Repair category are several plastic procedures. A laryngoplasty for a **laryngeal web** is a surgical procedure, usually performed in two stages, for the repair of congenital webbing between the vocal cords. The surgeon removes the webbing and places a spacer between the vocal cords. At a later time, the surgeon will again expose the vocal cords, using the same tracheostomy incision made on the initial procedure, and remove the spacer.

FIGURE 15–11   Endotracheal intubation.

EXERCISE 15-4 *Larynx*

Using the CPT manual, complete the following:

1 Diagnostic laryngotomy

CPT Code: ___31320___

2 Laryngoplasty, two stages, for repair of congenital laryngeal web, removal of spacer

CPT Code: ___31580___

3 Emergency establishment of positive airway by means of endotracheal intubation

CPT Code: ___31500___

4 Subtotal supraglottic laryngectomy with removal of adjacent lymph nodes and tissue due to a primary malignant neoplasm of glossoepiglottic folds

CPT Code: ___31368___

ICD-9-CM Code: ___146.4___ (ICD-10-CM Code: _____)

5 Pharyngolaryngectomy with radical neck dissection for a primary malignant neoplasm of pharyngeal region

CPT Code: ___31390___

ICD-9-CM Code: ___149.0___ (ICD-10-CM Code: _____)

TRACHEA/BRONCHI

Procedures in the Trachea and Bronchi subheading (31600-31899) include incisions, introductions, and repairs, in addition to the endoscopic procedures.

Incision

Tracheostomy is the most common procedure reported with codes from the Incision category. A tracheostomy can be planned or performed as an emergency procedure. A planned tracheostomy is usually performed when there is a need for prolonged ventilation support, beyond the level of support that can be provided by endotracheal intubation, or when a patient cannot tolerate an endotracheal tube.

Code 31603 is assigned for an emergency **transtracheal** tracheostomy, and 31605 is assigned for an emergency **cricothyroid** tracheostomy. These codes represent two different approaches to establishing an airway. Fig. 15–12 illustrates the transverse (across) incision used in a transtracheal approach; it is made between the cricoid cartilage and the sternal notch. Fig. 15–13 illustrates entry into the trachea using the transtracheal approach. Fig. 15–14 illustrates the vertical incision made for a cricothyroid tracheostomy. Fig. 15–15 shows the entry into the trachea using the cricothyroid approach.

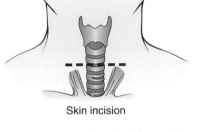

Skin incision

FIGURE 15–12 Transverse incision used in a transtracheal approach.

FIGURE 15–13 Transtracheal entry into the trachea using the transtracheal approach.

Skin incision

FIGURE 15–14 Vertical incision made for a cricothyroid tracheostomy.

Cricothyroid membrane

FIGURE 15–15 Cricothyroid entry into the trachea.

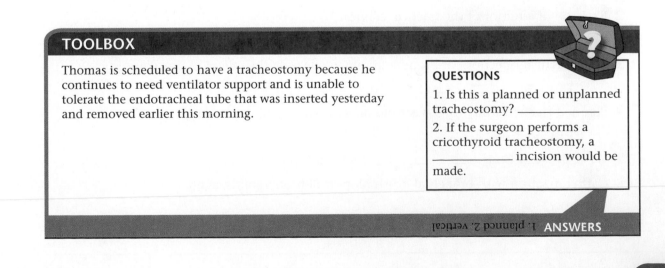

TOOLBOX

Thomas is scheduled to have a tracheostomy because he continues to need ventilator support and is unable to tolerate the endotracheal tube that was inserted yesterday and removed earlier this morning.

QUESTIONS

1. Is this a planned or unplanned tracheostomy? _____

2. If the surgeon performs a cricothyroid tracheostomy, a _____ incision would be made.

ANSWERS 1. planned 2. vertical

Introduction

Codes in the Introduction category (31715-31730) report catheterization, instillation, injection, and aspiration of the trachea and the placement of tubes into the trachea.

Some of the Introduction codes represent the instillation of contrast material into the larynx to improve viewing during bronchographic procedures. The contrast material is suspended in a gas that the patient inhales. The gas contains radiant energy that appears darker on the x-ray if there is an obstruction in the area, such as a tumor. Codes from the Radiology section are reported in conjunction with injection of contrast material. For example, if a physician provided the service of a unilateral bronchography with contrast material injection, you would assign 31715 for the service of injecting the contrast material into the trachea, and 71040 for the supervision and interpretation of the unilateral bronchography. The injection of contrast material is not bundled into the radiology service for a bronchography, so you would have to report each part (component) of the service separately.

Excision, Repair

Excision, Repair procedures (31750-31830) in the Trachea and Bronchi subheading include plastic repairs, such as tracheoplasty and bronchoplasty, in addition to the excision of stenosis or of tumors, the suturing of tracheal wounds, and scar revision.

Tracheoplasty involves the surgical repair of a damaged trachea. The repair may involve reconstruction of the trachea by the use of grafts or splints formed from cartilage taken from other areas of the body or by the use of prostheses. The codes are divided according to the approach used (cervical or thoracic) and the extent and type of repair.

Bronchoplasty is repair of the bronchus and often involves the use of grafting repair or stents. A chest tube may be left in the area as a drain after the procedure and is not reported separately because it is bundled into the code to report the procedure. A grafting procedure is not bundled into the bronchoplasty code 31770 and is reported separately.

EXERCISE 15-5 *Trachea and Bronchi*

Using the CPT manual, complete the following:

1 Emergency tracheostomy, cricothyroid approach

  CPT Code: _____31605_____

2 Excision of a tumor of the trachea, cervical

  CPT Code: _____31785_____

3 Transtracheal injection for bronchography (code only the injection procedure)

  CPT Code: _____31715_____

4 Planned tracheostomy in 47-year-old patient with acute respiratory failure

  CPT Code: _____31600_____

  ICD-9-CM Code: _____518.81_____ (ICD-10-CM Code: _____)

5 Catheterization with bronchial brush biopsy for bronchiolitis, acute

  CPT Code: _____31717_____

  ICD-9-CM Code: _____466.19_____ (ICD-10-CM Code: _____)

LUNGS AND PLEURA

The Lungs and Pleura subheading (32035-32999) includes a wide range of codes to report procedures such as thoracentesis, thoracotomy, and pneumonostomy, in addition to lung transplants and plastic procedures.

Incision

Thoracotomy involves making a surgical incision into the chest wall and opening the area to the view of the surgeon. This is a major surgical procedure during which the patient is under general anesthesia. The codes are divided according to the reason for the procedure, such as biopsy, control of bleeding, cyst removal, foreign body removal, or cardiac massage. Again, the surgeon may insert a chest tube that is bundled into the thoracotomy code.

Excision

The Excision category contains codes for pleurectomy, biopsy, pneumonocentesis, removal, and reconstructive lung procedures.

Pleurectomy is a procedure in which the physician opens the chest cavity to full view. With the chest open and the ribs spread apart by a rib spreader, the parietal pleura is removed. The parietal pleura lines the mediastinum and body walls as illustrated in Fig. 15–16. If a pleurectomy is performed as part of another, more major procedure such as the removal of a lung (pneumonectomy), you would not report the pleurectomy separately. Note that after code 32310, pleurectomy, parietal "separate procedure" warns you not to report a pleurectomy if the pleurectomy was performed as a part of a more major procedure.

Percutaneous needle lung or mediastinum **biopsy** is often performed under radiologic guidance so that correct placement of the needle can be ensured. As with the bronchography procedure described earlier, in the discussion of the Trachea and Bronchi subheading, if radiologic guidance was used, you report the service with a code from the Radiology section. There is a note following code 32405 (biopsy) that directs you to the Surgery section, General subsection, code 10022, when a fine-needle aspiration is performed which differs from a tissue biopsy. A fine-needle aspiration is a procedure in which fluid is withdrawn for examination.

Removal

Pneumonocentesis is the withdrawal of fluid from the lung by means of an aspirating needle. Air or gas in the pleural cavity is known as pneumothorax and occurs when the lung is traumatically ruptured or an emphysematous bulla ruptures. When the thoracic cavity (intrathoracic) air pressure increases, the pressure on the lung can result in collapse of the lung. The surgeon withdraws the fluid to allow the lung to reinflate.

Parietal pleura

Visceral pleura

FIGURE 15–16 Parietal and visceral pleura.

The codes for the removal of the lung are based on how much of the lung is removed—segmentectomy for one segment, lobectomy for one lobe, bilobectomy for two lobes, total pneumonectomy for an entire lung—as well as on the extent of the procedure and the approach.

CODING SHOT If a part of the bronchus was removed or repaired at the same time as the lobectomy or segmentectomy, report the service with add-on code 32501.

The preferred method of accomplishing a **thoracentesis** is by having the patient sit with arms supported, as illustrated in Fig. 15–17; local anesthesia is administered, a needle is inserted (Fig. 15–18) between the ribs, and fluid is withdrawn. Thoracentesis is performed to withdraw fluid from the pleural space that has accumulated as a result of a variety of conditions, such as congestive heart failure, pneumonia, tuberculosis, or carcinoma.

Thoracentesis may also be performed to insert a **chest tube** as an indwelling method of draining the accumulated fluid in the pleural space (pleural effusion), as illustrated in Fig. 15–19. Local anesthesia is administered, and a small incision is made through the skin, fat, and muscle. The hole is then enlarged by using an instrument, and the tube is inserted into the pleural space. A suture is placed through the skin and tied to the tube. The tube is then secured with tape. The fluid is withdrawn by means of a suction device called a multichamber water-seal suction tube. This therapeutic procedure may be performed when the patient's pleural space contains air or gas (pneumothorax), blood (hemothorax), or a large amount of fluid (pleural effusion). These conditions can be due to trauma, secondary to another disease process, or occur spontaneously.

From the Trenches

"Certification has made a huge difference in my career. It has allowed me to move up from the follow-up world of payments and denials to the front-end world of reviewing documentation and coding."

LYNDA

FIGURE 15–17 Patient position for a thoracentesis.

Point of access

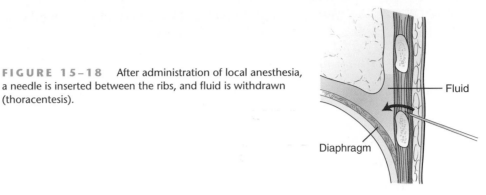

FIGURE 15–18 After administration of local anesthesia, a needle is inserted between the ribs, and fluid is withdrawn (thoracentesis).

Fluid

Diaphragm

FIGURE 15–19 A chest tube may be inserted after thoracentesis to allow for further fluid draining.

Surgical Collapse Therapy; Thoracoplasty

Thoracoplasty is a procedure in which a portion of the internal skeletal support is removed to treat a condition in which pus chronically collects in the chest cavity (chronic thoracic empyema). The procedure is major and requires extensive resecting of the membrane that lines the chest cavity. Gauze is left in the cavity and after several days is removed. Note that code 32905, thoracoplasty, refers to "all stages." The subsequent stages are for the removal of the packing and are bundled into the surgical code.

Pneumonolysis is a procedure that is performed to separate the inside of the chest cavity from the lung to permit the lung to collapse. This procedure was originally used as a treatment for tuberculosis but is now used in the evaluation of pleural diseases, debridement of chronic emphysema, and as a treatment for emphysematous blebs, in addition to other therapeutic treatments.

Pneumothorax injection (32960) is a therapeutic procedure in which the surgeon inserts a needle into the pleural cavity and injects air into the pleural cavity. The pressure in the thoracic cavity is increased and the lung partially collapses. This procedure is sometimes performed to treat tuberculosis. A chest tube may be inserted into the space for further injections of air. You would not report the insertion of the chest tube separately, as the insertion is bundled into the procedure code.

EXERCISE 15-6 *Radiology Terminology*

Using the CPT manual, complete the following:

1 Limited thoracotomy for lung biopsy

CPT Code: ___32095___

2 Percutaneous needle lung biopsy

CPT Code: ___32405___

3 Lobectomy and bronchoplasty performed at same surgical session

CPT Codes: ___32480___, ___+ 32501___

4 Resection of an apical lung neoplasm

CPT Code: ___32503___ — malig not indicated

ICD-9-CM Code: ___239.1___ (ICD-10-CM Code: _____)

5 Pneumonostomy with open drainage of abscess (pulmonary necrosis)

CPT Code: ___32200___

ICD-9-CM Code: ___513.0___ (ICD-10-CM Code: _____)

CHAPTER REVIEW

CHAPTER 15, PART I, THEORY

Without the use of reference material, complete the following:

1 The Respiratory System subsection is arranged by ___anatomical___ site.

2 The procedure in which a scope is placed through a small incision and into a body cavity is called a(n) ___endoscopy___.

3 When coding endoscopic procedures you must be certain to code to the fullest ___extent___ of the procedure and to code the correct approach for the procedure.

4 If more than one distinct procedure was performed during an endoscopic procedure, what modifier would you add to the lesser-priced service? ___-51___

5 What type of endoscopy is always bundled into a surgical endoscopy? ___diagnostic___

6 A(n) ___indirect___ laryngoscopy is performed when a physician uses a tongue depressor to hold the tongue down and view the epiglottis with a mirror.

7 A(n) ___direct___ laryngoscopy is performed when the endoscope is passed into the larynx and the physician can look at the larynx through a scope.

8 An otorhinolaryngologist is a physician who specializes in treating conditions of the ___ear___, ___nose___, and ___throat___.

9 When coding a nasal abscess or a nasal biopsy of the skin using the external approach, you use codes from the ___Integumentary___ System subsection.

10 When coding a nasal abscess or a nasal biopsy using the internal approach, you use codes from the ___Respiratory___ System subsection.

11 What are the three sections of turbinates?

_____,

_____, and

_____

12 What is the name of the therapy in which the physician flushes saline solution into the sinuses to remove mucus or pus?

_____

CHAPTER 15, PART II, PRACTICAL

With the use of the CPT and ICD-9-CM manuals, code the following procedures. Code only the physician services in this exercise; do not code the laboratory or radiology services.

13 A unilateral, total lung lavage following smoke inhalation

CPT Code: _____

ICD-9-CM Code: _____

(ICD-10-CM Code: _____)

14 Performed as a separate procedure, a parietal pleurectomy for pleurisy with bacterial, nontuberculous

CPT Code: _____

ICD-9-CM Code: _____

(ICD-10-CM Code: _____)

15 Resection of apical lung tumor, secondary site malignant neoplasm, with chest wall resection and reconstruction, unknown primary site

CPT Code: _____

ICD-9-CM Codes: _____,

_____

(ICD-10-CM Codes: _____,

_____)

16 Removal of a crayon lodged inside nasal passage, office procedure

CPT Code: _____

ICD-9-CM Code: _____

(ICD-10-CM Code: _____)

17 Surgical nasal cavity endoscopy with polypectomy for nasal polyps

CPT Code: _____

ICD-9-CM Code: _____

(ICD-10-CM Code: _____)

18 Direct, operative laryngoscopy for removal of button lodged in 2-year-old child's larynx

CPT Code: _____

ICD-9-CM Code: _____

(ICD-10-CM Code: _____)

19 Indirect laryngoscopy with biopsy of nodule

CPT Code(s): _____

ICD-9-CM Code(s): _____

(ICD-10-CM Code(s): _____)

20 Internal approach used to drain nasal septum hematoma

CPT Code(s): _____

ICD-9-CM Code(s): _____

(ICD-10-CM Code(s): _____)

21 External, simple, frontal sinusotomy for chronic frontal sinusitis

CPT Code(s): _____

ICD-9-CM Code(s): _____

(ICD-10-CM Code(s): _____)

22 Surgical sinus endoscopy with sphenoidotomy for acute sphenoidal sinusitis

CPT Code(s): _____

ICD-9-CM Code(s): _____

(ICD-10-CM Code(s): _____)

23 Submucous resection of nose with scoring of cartilage and contouring for an overdevelopment of nasal bones, acquired

CPT Code(s): _____

ICD-9-CM Code(s): _____

(ICD-10-CM Code(s): _____)

24 Jack Rogers developed chest pain and difficulty breathing. He has also been coughing up thick, blood-tinged sputum. A chest radiograph shows an ill-defined mass. A diagnostic bronchoscopy of one lung is performed and a specimen of the mass is taken. The pathology report comes back positive for primary cancer of upper lobe. One week later, a lobectomy is performed.

CPT Code(s): _31625, 32480-58_

ICD-9-CM Code(s): _____

(ICD-10-CM Code(s): _____)

25 James Wilson has been having difficulty breathing and has had continual chronic ethmoidal sinusitis. Dr. Adams takes James to the operating room to perform a sinus endoscopy with anterior and posterior ethmoidectomy and removal of polyps.

🌑 CPT Code(s): _____

🌑 ICD-9-CM Code(s): _____

(🌑 ICD-10-CM Code(s): _____)

26 Mary Bronson has a nosebleed that won't stop. She goes to the emergency department, where anterior packing is done to control the anterior nasal hemorrhage. She also has documented benign hypertension.

🌑 CPT Code(s): _____

🌑 ICD-9-CM Code(s): _____

(🌑 ICD-10-CM Code(s): _____)

QUICK CHECK ANSWERS

QUICK CHECK 15-1
1. open, intranasal

"The world of coding is wide open; coders should explore all available opportunities and find what most interests them."

Letitia Patterson, MPA, CPC, CCS-P

Director of Clinical Operations— Department of Ophthalmology

University of Chicago Medical Center

Chicago, Illinois

Cardiovascular System

Chapter Topics

Coding Highlights

Cardiovascular Coding in the Surgery Section

Cardiovascular Coding in the Medicine Section

Cardiovascular Coding in the Radiology Section

Chapter Review

Quick Check Answers

Learning Objectives

After completing this chapter you should be able to

1 Understand cardiovascular services reported with codes from the Surgery, Medicine, and Radiology sections.

2 Review cardiovascular coding terminology.

3 Recognize the major differences in the subheadings of the Cardiovascular subsection.

4 Define rules of coding cardiovascular services when using codes from the Medicine section.

5 Identify the major rules of coding cardiovascular services using the Radiology section codes.

6 Demonstrate ability to code Cardiovascular services.

Make sure to check
evolve
learning system
for the latest
content updates

CODING HIGHLIGHTS

Cardiology is one of the largest subspecialties in medicine, and numerous modern techniques are used to diagnose and treat cardiac conditions. A **cardiologist** is an internal medicine physician who is specialized in the diagnosis and treatment of conditions of the heart. A cardiologist can further specialize in cardiovascular surgical procedures or other treatment and diagnostic specialties. In a smaller practice a cardiologist may do many of these procedures himself/herself, whereas in a larger practice a cardiologist may be more specialized and provide a more limited number of services.

Coding from Three Sections

When you are reporting cardiology services you will often be using codes from three sections: Surgery, Medicine, and Radiology.

- The Surgery section contains codes for cardiovascular surgical procedures.
- The Medicine section contains codes for nonsurgical cardiovascular services.
- The Radiology section contains diagnostic study or radiologic visualization codes.

Fig. 16–1 is a list of the section information that is most often used when reporting cardiovascular services. The confusion in coding cardiology usually comes from not understanding the components (parts) of coding cardiovascular services, the various locations of these codes in the CPT manual, and the terminology associated with cardiovascular services. To clarify cardiology coding, let's begin by reviewing the definitions of invasive, noninvasive, electrophysiology, and angiography as they relate to cardiovascular coding.

Invasive

Invasive is entering the body—breaking the skin—to make a correction or for examination. An example of an invasive cardiac procedure is the removal of a tumor from the heart. The chest is opened, the ribs spread apart, the heart fully exposed to the view of the surgeon, and the tumor removed. Another example is the removal of a clot from a vessel. The surgeon usually enters the body percutaneously (through the skin) by means of a catheter that is threaded through the vessel to the location of the clot. The clot can then be pulled out of the vessel through the catheter or can be injected with a substance that dissolves it. Although an open surgical procedure was not used, the body was entered—an invasive procedure. Invasive cardiology procedures are also called **interventional** procedures; some codes are located in the Surgery section for the surgical technique, and others are located in the Radiology section for the radiologic supervision and guidance and both codes are reported for the one procedure. Sometimes,

SURGERY SECTION	MEDICINE SECTION	RADIOLOGY SECTION
Cardiovascular System (33010-37799)	Cardiovascular System (92950-93799)	Diagnostic Radiology (75557-75791)
Heart and Pericardium	Therapeutic Services	Heart
Endoscopy	Cardiography	Aorta and Arteries
Arteries and Veins	Echocardiography	Diagnostic Ultrasound (various)
Adjuvant Techniques	Cardiac Catheterization	Ultrasonic Guidance Procedures
	Intracardiac Electrophysiological Procedures	Radiologic Guidance (77001-77032)
	Peripheral Arterial Disease Rehabilitation	Nuclear Medicine (78414-78499)
	Other Vascular Studies	Cardiovascular System
	Other Procedures	

FIGURE 16–1 A list of the section information that is most often used when reporting cardiovascular services.

one physician provides both components of the procedure and in other instances, two physicians will provide the components.

From the Trenches

What qualities best describe a medical coder?

"Detail oriented, investigative and research oriented, patient, and excellent analytical skills."

LETITIA

Noninvasive

Noninvasive services and procedures—not breaking the skin—are usually performed for diagnostic purposes. Usually, performing these procedures does not require entering the body; rather, they are diagnostic tests that can be performed from outside the body, for example, echocardiography (93303-93350) or cardiography (93000-93278) from the Medicine section.

CODING SHOT To choose the correct cardiology code, first determine whether the procedure or service was invasive (interventional, open, percutaneous) or noninvasive.

Electrophysiology

Electrophysiology (EP) is the study of the electrical system of the heart and includes the study of arrhythmias. Diagnostic procedures include procedures such as recordings from inside the heart by placing an electrical catheter into the heart percutaneously and by means of an electrogram, recording the electrical activity within the heart. The codes for these invasive diagnostic procedures are located in the Medicine section (93600-93662).

As a treatment for abnormal electrical activity in the heart, more invasive treatments can be performed, such as the placement of a pacemaker, cardioverter-defibrillator, or other devices to regulate the rhythm of the heart. These invasive treatments are surgical procedures and the codes are located in the Surgery section, Cardiology subsection, Pacemaker or Pacing Cardioverter-Defibrillator (33202-33249). There are also Surgery codes for operative procedures to correct electrophysiologic problems of the heart (33250-33266), when the electrical problems are corrected surgically by incision, excision, or ablation. For example, code 33250 reports an operative ablation performed for patients with conduction disorders such as Wolff-Parkinson-White syndrome, in which there is a short circuit between the atria and ventricles. This is a congenital defect that results in rapid heartbeats due to a muscle fiber that remains after the heart developed. This fiber would usually not be present in the normally developed heart and when it is present it interrupts normal conduction. The surgeon ablates the fibers by means of a small wire that destroys the fibers and restores normal heart rhythm. You will be learning more about the electrical conduction system of the heart later in this chapter.

Angiography

Nuclear cardiology is a diagnostic specialty that plays a very important role in modern cardiology. A physician who specializes in nuclear cardiology uses radioactive radiologic procedures to aid in the diagnosis of cardiologic conditions. For example, during angiography of peripheral vessels, a nuclear cardiologist may inject a radioactive dye into the bloodstream to improve the detail of the study. The code for the angiography comes from the Radiology section (Heart, 75557-75574; Aorta and Arteries, 75600-75791; Veins and Lymphatics, 75801-75893), and the code for the injection procedure comes from the Medicine section. For example, 75600 reports the radiological portion of an aortography and 93544 reports the injection portion of the procedure. There is a directional note following 75600 in the CPT manual that directs the coder to assign 93544 to report the injection procedure.

EXERCISE 16-1 *Coding Highlights*

Complete the following:

1 This term means entering the body. _____

2 A cardiologist is a(n) _____ medicine physician who has chosen to specialize in the diagnosis and treatment of conditions of the heart.

3 What three sections of the CPT will you often use to code cardiology services? _____, _____, and _____

4 What type of cardiology enters the body—breaks the skin—to make a correction or for examination? _____

5 What is the term that describes the study of the electrical system of the heart and includes the study of arrhythmias? _____

6 _____ is an x-ray examination that enables the study of the patient's blood vessels and organs by injecting contrast media into the blood vessels and viewing the results on x-ray film.

Now that you are familiar with some of the basic terms and coding of the cardiovascular services and procedures, let's look at the three sections where you will locate the components (parts) of cardiovascular coding: Surgery, Medicine, and Radiology.

CARDIOVASCULAR CODING IN THE SURGERY SECTION

The Cardiovascular System subsection (33010-37799) of the Surgery section contains diagnostic and therapeutic procedure codes that are divided on the basis of whether the procedure was performed on the heart/pericardium or on arteries/veins. The Heart and Pericardium subheading (33010-33999) contains codes for procedures that involve the repair of the heart and coronary vessels, such as placement of pacemakers, repair of valve disorders, and graft/bypass procedures. In the Arteries and Veins subheading (34001-37799) are the same types of procedures, but for noncoronary (nonheart) vessels. For example, a thromboendarterectomy is the removal of a thrombus (stationary obstruction) and a portion of the lining of an artery. When a thromboendarterectomy is performed on a coronary artery, you would assign a code from the Heart and Pericardium subheading; but if the procedure was performed on a noncoronary artery, you would assign a code from the Arteries and Veins subheading.

CODING SHOT The location of the procedure—coronary or noncoronary—is the first step in selecting the correct cardiovascular surgical code, because the CPT codes are divided on the basis of whether a procedure involved coronary or noncoronary vessels.

Heart and Pericardium

The Surgery section, Cardiovascular System subsection, Heart and Pericardium subheading (33010-33999) contains procedures that are performed both percutaneously and through open surgical sites. There are always many revisions and additions in this subheading each year to reflect the many advances in this important specialty. Numerous notes are located throughout the subheading, and they must be read prior to coding. Codes in the Heart and Pericardium subheading are for services provided to repair the heart (Fig. 16–2), pericardium, or coronary vessels (Fig. 16–3). Pericardium codes 33010 and 33011 are divided based on initial or subsequent service.

Veins b w/o oxy
aorty b = oxy
pulm. art b w/o oxy
pulm vein b w/ oxy

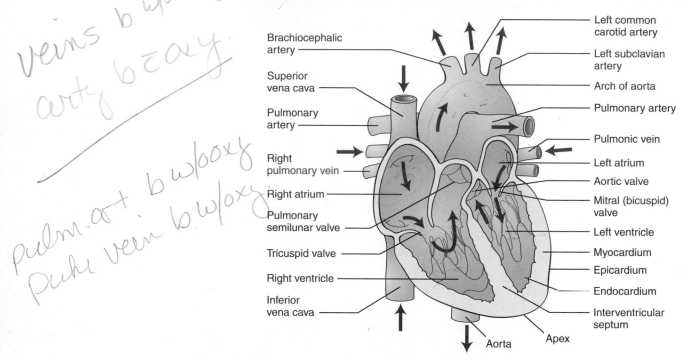

FIGURE 16-2 Internal view of heart.

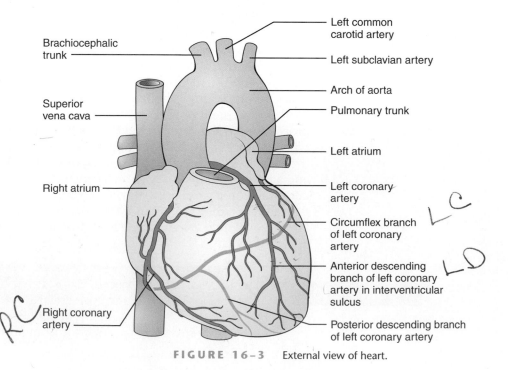

LC
LD
RC

FIGURE 16-3 External view of heart.

QUICK CHECK 16-1

1. Using Fig. 16–3, name the coronary arteries:

_____

Pericardium

Pericardiocentesis (33010, 33011) is a procedure in which the surgeon withdraws fluid from the pericardial space by means of a needle inserted percutaneously into the space as illustrated in Fig. 16–4. The insertion can be performed using radiologic (ultrasound) guidance—the use of which would be reported with a separate code from the Radiology section. There is a note following the pericardiocentesis codes that states: "(For radiological supervision and interpretation, use 76930)"; that is, ultrasonic guidance for pericardiocentesis, imaging supervision, and interpretation. Watch for these directional features throughout the Cardiovascular System subsection.

The fluid withdrawn during a pericardiocentesis is then examined for microbial agents (such as tuberculosis), neoplasia, or autoimmune diseases (such as lupus or rheumatoid arthritis). The pericardiocentesis codes are divided on the basis of whether the service was initial or subsequent.

A tube pericardiostomy (33015) uses the same procedure described above, but a catheter is left in the pericardium leading to the outside of the body to allow for continued drainage.

The remaining procedures in the Pericardium category (33020-33050) are open surgical procedures for the removal of clots, foreign bodies, tumors, cysts, a portion of the pericardium, or to create a window to allow pericardial fluid to drain into the pleural space.

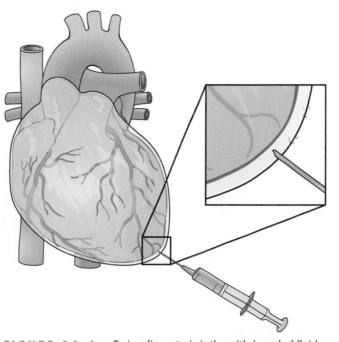

FIGURE 16–4   Pericardiocentesis is the withdrawal of fluid from the pericardium by means of aspiration.

Cardiac Tumor

A procedure performed to remove a tumor of the pericardium is reported using a code from the Pericardium category (33010-33050), but if a tumor is removed from the heart, you would select a code from the category Cardiac Tumor (33120, 33130). There are only two tumor-removal codes in the Cardiac Tumor category, one for a tumor that is removed from inside the heart (intracardiac) and one for a tumor that is removed from outside the heart (external). Both procedures are open surgical procedures that involve opening the chest, spreading the ribs, and excising the tumor.

Transmyocardial Revascularization

Laser transmyocardial revascularization describes a procedure in which areas of cardiac ischemia (reversible muscle damage) are exposed to a laser beam to create holes in the surface of the heart. This procedure encourages new capillary growth, thereby revitalizing the damaged area by increasing the blood flow in the area. This procedure can be performed alone, as the only surgical procedure performed (33140) or at the time of another open cardiac procedure (add-on code 33141).

Pacemaker or Pacing Cardioverter-Defibrillator

A pacemaker and a cardioverter-defibrillator (33202-33249) are devices that are inserted into the body to electrically shock the heart into regular rhythm (as illustrated in Figs. 16–5 and 16–6). When a pacemaker is inserted, a pocket is made and a generator and lead(s) are placed inside the chest (Fig. 16–7). Sometimes, only components of the pacemaker are reinserted, repaired, or replaced. You need to know three things about the service provided to correctly code the pacemaker:

1. Where the electrode (lead) is placed: atrium, ventricle, or both ventricle and atrium
2. Whether the procedure involves initial placement, replacement, or repair of all components or separate components of the pacemaker
3. The approach used to place the pacemaker (epicardial or transvenous)

CODING SHOT

A single pacemaker has one lead (atrium or ventricle), a dual pacemaker has two leads (one lead in the right atrium and one in the right ventricle), and a biventricular pacemaker has three leads (one in the right atrium, one in the right ventricle, and one in the left ventricle via the coronary sinus vein.)

FIGURE 16–5 Permanent cardiac pacemaker unit. (From Forbes CD, Jackson WF: *Color Atlas and Text of Clinical Medicine,* ed 3, 2003, Mosby.)

FIGURE 16–6 Left ventricular pacing. (From Miller RD, ed, *Miller's Anesthesia,* ed 6, Philadelphia, 2005, Churchill Livingstone.)

Initial Perm.
Insertion
Elec + gen

Single
33207

33208

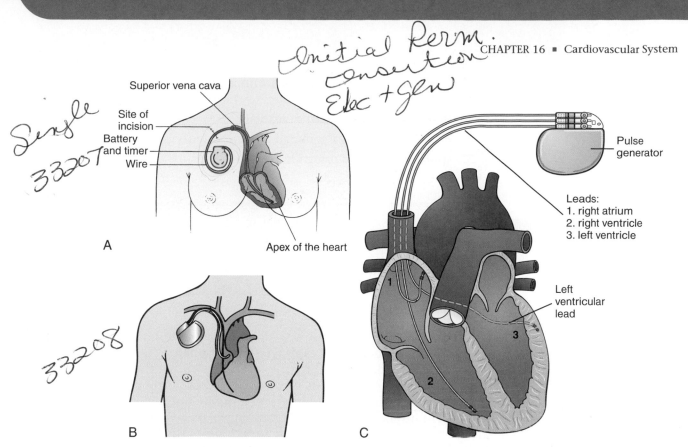

FIGURE 16-7   **A,** Single pacemaker insertion. **B,** Dual chamber pacemaker. **C,** Biventricular pacemaker. (**B** from Christensen Bl, Kockrow EO: *Adult Health Nursing,* ed 5, St. Louis, 2006, Mosby.)

Approaches.   The two approaches that are used when inserting a pacemaker are epicardial (on the heart) and transvenous (through a vein), and the codes are divided according to the surgical approach.

1. The **epicardial** approach involves opening the chest cavity and placing a lead on the epicardial sac of the heart. A pocket is formed in either the upper abdomen or under the clavicle, and the pacemaker generator is placed into the pocket. The wires are then connected to the pacemaker generator and the chest area is closed. Codes for the epicardial process are further divided based on the approach to the heart—thoracotomy, upper abdominal (xiphoid region), or endoscopic.

2. The **transvenous** approach involves accessing a vein (subclavian or jugular) and inserting an electrode (lead) into the vein. The pacemaker is affixed by creating a pocket into which the pacemaker generator is placed. The fluoroscopic (views the internal structure by means of x-rays) through the body portion of the procedure is reported separately with a radiology code (71090) because it is not bundled into the pacemaker codes. Transvenous codes are further divided based on the area of the heart into which the pacemaker is inserted. For example, 33207 (single-chamber pacemaker) is reported for transvenous placement of a pacemaker into the ventricle of the heart. If the pacemaker components were placed in both the atrium and ventricle, 33208 (dual-chamber pacemaker) is reported.

The documentation in the medical record will indicate whether a pacemaker or cardioverter-defibrillator was inserted or replaced.

The same set of criteria applies to choosing the correct cardioverter-defibrillator codes:

1. Revision or replacement of lead(s)
2. Replacement, repair, removal of components
3. Approach used for insertion or repair

CODING SHOT

A change of batteries in a pacemaker or cardioverter-defibrillator is a **removal** of the implanted generator and the **reimplantation** (insertion) of a new generator. Both the removal and the reimplantation are reported separately.

If electrophysiology (EP) is used to diagnose a condition that resulted in the insertion of a pacemaker or cardioverter-defibrillator, the EP is not included in the surgery code reported for the insertion. Rather, the EP is reported separately using the Medicine section codes 93600-93660.

Radiology supervision and interpretation are not included in the pacemaker implantation codes. If radiology supervision and interpretation are provided, you would report the service using the Radiology code 71090, Insertion of pacemaker, fluoroscopy, radiography, radiological supervision and interpretation.

Remember to use modifier -26 on a radiology service when only the professional portion of the service was provided and -TC when only the technical portion was provided.

CODING SHOT

If a patient with a pacemaker or other implantable device is seen by the physician within the 90-day follow-up (global) period for implantation but for a problem not related to the implantation, the service for the new problem can be billed. Documentation in the medical record must support the statement that the service is unrelated to the implantation. Append the E/M service code with modifier -24 (unrelated E/M service). If the patient is returned to the operating room for repositioning or replacement of the pacemaker or cardioverter-defibrillator during the global period by the same physician, modifier -78 would be appended to the code.

EXERCISE 16-2 *Pericardium, Cardiac Tumors, and Pacemakers*

Using the CPT and ICD-9-CM manuals, code the following:

1 Allen Jackson gets very tired walking up and down stairs. He has a hard time catching his breath and experiences instances when his heart feels as if it is beating fast. His physician has told him that he will require a pacemaker implantation. Allen goes to surgery and has a single-chamber pacemaker implanted with a ventricular lead.

CPT Code: _____33207_____

2 Five days after the pacemaker is implanted, Allen (from Question 1) feels very dizzy and his electrocardiogram is showing some abnormalities. His physician returns him to the operating room and discovers that the pacemaker lead is malfunctioning. The pacemaker lead is replaced, and Allen recovers nicely.

CPT Code: _____33216⁻⁷⁸, 33234 ?_____

3 Five years later, the battery in Allen's pacemaker is found to have become depleted. He is also having some other symptoms that his physician believes necessitate not only a replacement pacemaker but also an upgrade to a dual-chamber device.

CPT Code: _____33214_____

4 A new patient with a chief complaint of sharp, intermittent retrosternal pain that is reduced by sitting up or leaning forward is evaluated by a cardiologist. Chest films reveal acute pulmonary edema with acute pericardial effusion. The physician performs a pericardiocentesis. (Code only the procedure.)

CPT Code: _____33010_____

ICD-9-CM Codes: _____518.4_____, _____420.90_____

(ICD-10-CM Codes: _____, _____)

5 Resection of an endocardium primary malignant tumor in which cardiopulmonary bypass is required

CPT Code: _____33120_____

ICD-9-CM Code: _____164.1_____ (ICD-10-CM Code: _____)

Electrophysiologic Operative Procedures

Electrophysiology, as you learned earlier in this chapter, is the study of the electrical system of the heart, and most of the codes for the EP tests are in the Medicine section. The codes in the Surgery section (33250-33266) apply to the surgical repair of a defect that causes an abnormal rhythm. Cardiopulmonary bypass is usually required during these major operative procedures in which the chest is opened to expose the heart to the full view of the surgeon. Codes 33265 and 33266 are used to report endoscopic approach for EP procedures. The surgeon maps the locations of the electrodes of the heart and notes the source of the arrhythmia. The source of the arrhythmia is then ablated (separated). The codes are divided on the basis of the need for cardiopulmonary bypass, the reason for the procedure (atrial fibrillation, atrial flutter, etc.), and the approach. Percutaneous electrophysiology is discussed later in this chapter under the heading Intracardiac Electrophysiologic Procedures/Studies.

From the Trenches

"It is important to be a multi-tasker in the work environment. Also, be as flexible as possible. Learn the basics of the entire practice if the opportunity presents itself."

LETITIA

Patient-Activated Event Recorder

A patient-activated event recorder is also known as a cardiac event recorder or a loop recorder. Codes 33282 and 33284 involve surgical implantation into the subcutaneous tissue in the upper left quadrant, with leads running to the outside of the body. The recorder senses the heart's rhythms, and when the patient presses a button, the device records the electrical activity of the heart. The recording can assist the physician in making a diagnosis of a hard-to-detect rhythm problem. Codes are divided on the basis of whether the device was implanted or removed.

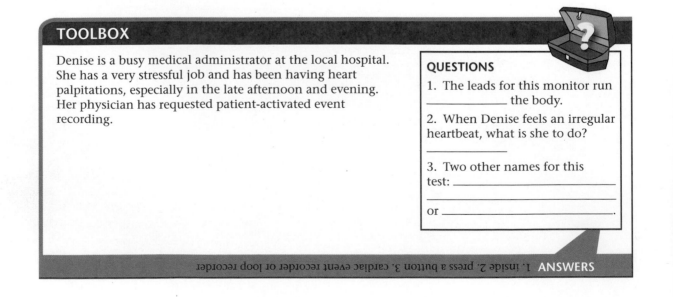

TOOLBOX

Denise is a busy medical administrator at the local hospital. She has a very stressful job and has been having heart palpitations, especially in the late afternoon and evening. Her physician has requested patient-activated event recording.

QUESTIONS

1. The leads for this monitor run _____ the body.

2. When Denise feels an irregular heartbeat, what is she to do? _____

3. Two other names for this test: _____
_____ or _____.

ANSWERS 1. inside 2. press a button 3. cardiac event recorder or loop recorder

Cardiac Valves

The category Cardiac Valves (33400-33496) has subcategory codes of aortic, mitral, tricuspid, and pulmonary valves. The procedures listed are similar for each valve; some are a little more extensive than others. Code descriptions vary depending on whether a cardiopulmonary bypass (heart-lung) machine was used during the procedure. The cardiopulmonary bypass is a resource-intensive procedure that requires a heart-lung machine to assume the patient's heart and lung functions during surgery.

The cardiac valve procedures are located in the CPT manual index under the valve type or under what was done, such as a repair or a replacement. For example, the replacement of an aortic valve is located in the CPT index under "Aorta," subterm "Valve," subterm "Replacement."

EXERCISE 16-3   *EP, Event Recorder, and Valves*

Using the CPT and ICD-9-CM manuals, code the following:

1 Mary Black's echocardiogram and cardiac catheterization show severe mitral stenosis with regurgitation. Her physician believes that because she is symptomatic, she should have her mitral valve replaced. The mitral valve replacement includes cardiopulmonary bypass

CPT Code: _____33430_____

2 Andrew Nelson has a loud heart murmur and, after study, is found to have severe aortic stenosis. He elects to have an aortic valve replacement. He is taken to the operating room and placed on a heart-lung machine. He then has his aortic valve replaced with a prosthetic valve.

CPT Code: _____33405_____

3 With the heart exposed through the sternum and the patient's functions supported by a cardiopulmonary bypass, the right atrium is opened and the bigeminal arrhythmia focuses are ablated by using electrical current. Bypass is discontinued and the atrium and sternum are closed in the usual fashion.

CPT Code: _____33251_____

ICD-9-CM Code: _____427.89_____ (ICD-10-CM Code: _____)

4 Implantation of a patient-activated cardiac loop device with programming for a diagnosis of palpitations and dizziness.

CPT Code: _____33282_____

ICD-9-CM Codes: _____785.1_____ , _____780.4_____

(ICD-10-CM Codes: _____ , _____)

Coronary Artery Anomalies

The Coronary Artery Anomalies category (33500-33507) contains codes to report the services of repair of the coronary artery by various methods, such as graft, ligation (tying off), and reconstruction. The codes include endarterectomy (removal of the inner lining of an artery) and angioplasty (blood vessel repair). Do not unbundle the codes and report the endarterectomy or angioplasty separately. Also, the procedures often require the use of cardiopulmonary bypass to allow the surgeon to repair the defect while the heart is without blood flow, which makes a difference in the choice of codes.

Coronary Artery Bypass

Arteries deliver oxygenated blood to all areas of the body, and veins return the blood that is full of waste products. The heart muscle is fed by coronary arteries that encircle the heart. When these arteries clog with plaque (atherosclerosis) (Fig. 16–8), the flow of blood lessens. Sometimes the arteries clog to the point that the heart muscle begins to perform at low levels due to lack of blood **(reversible ischemia)** or actually die **(irreversible ischemia).**

Reversible ischemia means that if the bloodflow is increased to the heart muscle, the heart muscle may again begin to function at normal or near-normal levels. **Coronary artery bypass grafting** is one way to increase the flow of blood (as illustrated in Fig. 16–9). The diseased portion of the artery is bypassed by attaching a healthy vessel above and below the diseased area and allowing the healthy vessel to then become the conduit of the blood, thus bypassing the blockage (Fig. 16–10). Blockage can also be pushed to the sides of the coronary arterial walls by a procedure in which a balloon is expanded inside the artery. This procedure is known as a **percutaneous transluminal coronary angioplasty (PTCA)** (Fig. 16–11).

Coronary Art.
Disease or
CAD
414.0

FIGURE 16–8 **A,** Atherosclerosis. **B,** Atherosclerotic vessel. (**B** from Damjanov I: *Pathology for the Health-Related Professions,* ed 3, St. Louis, 2006.)

FIGURE 16–9 Coronary artery bypass graft (CABG) surgery. (From Chabner DE: *The Language of Medicine,* ed 8, St. Louis, 2007, Saunders.)

FIGURE 16–10   Coronary artery bypass.

FIGURE 16–11   Percutaneous transluminal coronary angioplasty.

QUICK CHECK 16-2

1. What is the acronym commonly used for coronary artery bypass graft? _____

To correctly report coronary bypass grafts, you must know whether an artery (33533-33536), a vein (33510-33516), or both (33517-33523, plus 33533-33536) are being used as the bypass graft. You must also know how many bypass grafts are being performed. There may be more than one blockage to be bypassed and, therefore, more than one graft. If only a vein is used for the graft (most often the saphenous vein from the leg is harvested and used for this purpose; see Fig. 16–10), the code reflecting the number of grafts would be assigned from the category Venous Grafting Only for Coronary Artery Bypass (33510-33516).

The following exercise will help you understand the differences in coding for bypass grafts using arteries, veins, or both, and for coding anomalies.

EXERCISE 16-4   *Coronary Artery Bypass and Anomalies*

Using the CPT and ICD-9-CM manuals, code the following:

1   Two coronary bypass grafts using veins only

CPT Code: ___33511___

The code for Question 1 came from the category Venous Grafting Only for Coronary Artery Bypass because the bypass was accomplished using a venous graft. If the bypass had been accomplished using an arterial graft, the codes in the category Arterial Grafting for Coronary Artery Bypass would be used to report the service. If both veins and arteries were used to accomplish the bypass, you would report the service by reporting an artery bypass code and a code from the category Combined Arterial-Venous Grafting for Coronary Bypass. Because the title of the category contains the words "arterial-venous," you might think that the codes in the category report both the artery and the vein; but this is not the case. The category codes under "arterial-venous" are used only when a venous graft has been used in addition to an arterial graft and these arterial-venous codes are used only in combination with the arterial graft codes (33533-33536).

For example, a patient has had a **five-vessel** coronary artery bypass graft, for which two bypasses were accomplished using internal mammary arteries and three bypasses were accomplished using veins (reported with 2A and 2B):

2A   Coronary artery bypass using two arterial grafts

CPT Code: ___33534___

2B   Coronary artery bypass using three venous grafts in addition to the arterial grafts for coronary artery disease, native arteries, due to arteriosclerotic coronary heart disease

CPT Code: ___33519___

ICD-9-CM Code: ___414.01___ (ICD-10-CM Code: _____)

3   Coronary artery bypass of native arteries using one internal mammary artery graft and three venous grafts. Patient has documented arteriosclerotic coronary heart disease and hypertensive heart disease, benign.

Codes: ___33533___, ___33519___

ICD-9-CM Codes: ___414.01___, ___402.10___

(ICD-10-CM Codes: _____, _____)

CODING SHOT   Modifier -51 would not be assigned with the code for the venous grafts because codes 33517-33523 are add-on codes. Parenthetical notations with each code indicate the code is to be used in conjunction with 33533-33536. This means that the venous code is never reported alone, but always follows an arterial code.

Arteries and Veins   Code groupings for arteries and veins vary according to procedures such as thrombectomies, aneurysm repairs, bypass grafting, repairs, angioplasties, and all other procedures. Codes in the subheading Arteries and Veins (34001-37799) refer to all arteries and veins except the coronary arteries and veins (Figs. 16–12 and 16–13).

Basilar artery
Right common carotid artery
Vertebral artery
Subclavian (right) artery
Brachiocephalic trunk
Aortic arch
Ascending aorta
Abdominal aorta
Internal iliac artery
Deep femoral (profunda) artery
Femoral artery
Popliteal artery

Circle of Willis
Internal carotid artery
External carotid artery
Left common carotid artery
Vertebral artery
Subclavian (left) artery
Descending aorta
Axillary artery
Celiac trunk
Brachial artery
Radial artery
Ulnar artery
Anterior tibial artery
Posterior tibial artery

FIGURE 16–12   Arteries of the body.

Superior vena cava
Inferior vena cava
Common iliac vein
Deep femoral vein

Common iliac vein
Internal iliac vein
External iliac vein
Great saphenous vein
Femoral vein

FIGURE 16–13   Veins of the body.

Vascular Families— Selective or Nonselective Placement

A vascular family can be compared to a tree with branches. The tree has a main trunk from which large branches and then smaller branches grow. The same is true with vascular families. A main vessel is the main trunk, and other vessels branch off from the main vessel. Vessels connected in this manner are considered families.

Catheters, as shown in Fig. 16–14, may have to be placed in vessels for monitoring, removal of blood, injection of contrast materials, or infusion. When coding the placement of a catheter it is necessary to know where the catheter starts and where it ends.

Catheter placement is nonselective or selective. **Nonselective catheter placement** means the catheter or needle is placed directly into an artery or vein (and not manipulated farther along) or is placed only into the aorta from any approach. **Selective catheter placement** means the catheter must be moved, manipulated, or guided into a part of the arterial system other than the aorta or the vessel punctured (that is, into the branches), generally under fluoroscopic guidance. The following codes illustrate nonselective and selective placement:

Example

Nonselective: 36000 Introduction of needle or intracatheter, vein

Selective: 36012 Selective catheter placement, venous system; second order, or more selective, branch

---

Code 36000 describes the placement of a needle or catheter into a vein with no further manipulation or movement. Code 36012 describes the placement of a catheter into a vein and its manipulation or moving to a second-order vein or farther.

The first note in the Cardiovascular System subsection in the CPT manual (before code 33010) refers to selective placement. The note appears at the beginning of the section because it is very important and applies to the entire Cardiovascular System subsection. When coding selective placement for any procedure, you report the fullest extension into one vascular family, just as you would when coding a gastrointestinal endoscopic procedure, when you report to the farthest extent of the procedure. The same is true of selective placement into a vascular family: Code to the farthest extent of the placement within the vascular family.

The **first order** is the main artery in a vascular family, the **second order** is the branch off the main artery, the **third order** is the next

FIGURE 16–14   Catheters for arterial cannulation. (From Roberts JR, Hedges JR, eds: *Clinical Procedures in Emergency Medicine*, ed 4, Philadelphia, 2004, Saunders.)

branch off the second order, and so on. A vascular family can have more than one second-order, third-order, and so on, vessel, as illustrated in Fig. 16–15. Note that the first order in Fig. 16–15 is the brachiocephalic artery, the second order is the common carotid artery, and that there are two third order arteries. If the farthest extent of the placement was to the third order, only the third-order code would be reported. For example, if a catheter was placed into the first-order brachiocephalic artery and from there manipulated through the second-order artery (right common carotid), and finally into the third-order artery (right internal or external carotid), you would report only the third-order artery, with code 36217, which describes an initial third-order placement within the brachiocephalic family.

CODING SHOT
Appendix L of the CPT manual is a listing of the vascular families based on the starting point of the aorta.

If the catheter placement continued from one branch of the brachiocephalic family into another branch of the family, you would report the additional second order, third order, and beyond using an add-on code—36218. Oftentimes, a physician will investigate not only one branch of an artery but several others. Report all subsequent catheter placement to the farthest extent of each placement.

CODING SHOT
Code to the farthest extent of the vascular family using an initial code; then code any additional services of the second order, third order, or beyond by using an add-on code.

Catheter placement codes may vary according to the vascular family into which the catheter is placed. Look at the following two codes and note the difference in vascular families.

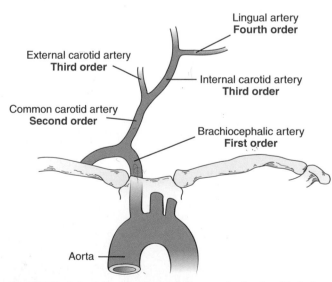

FIGURE 16–15 Brachiocephalic vascular family with first-, second-, third-, and fourth-order vessels.

Example

| 36215 | Selective catheter placement, arterial system; each first order **thoracic or brachiocephalic** branch, within a vascular family |
| 36245 | Selective catheter placement, arterial system; each first order **abdominal, pelvic, or lower extremity artery** branch, within a vascular family |

QUICK CHECK 16-3

1. Which CPT Appendix would be a helpful resource for selective vascular coding? _____

Embolectomy/Thrombectomy. An **embolus** is a mass of undissolved matter that is present in blood and is transported by the blood. A **thrombus** is a blood clot that occludes, or shuts off, a vessel. When a thrombus is dislodged, it becomes an embolus. Thrombectomies or embolectomies are performed to remove the unwanted debris, or clot, from the vessel and allow unrestricted bloodflow. A thrombus or embolus may be removed by opening the vessel and scraping out the debris or by percutaneously placing a balloon within the vessel to push the material to the sides and out of the vessel (see Fig. 16–11). A catheter may also be used to draw a thrombus or embolus out of the vessel, as illustrated in Fig. 16–16. Embolectomy/Thrombectomy codes (34001-34490) are divided based on the artery or vein in which the clot or thrombus is located (e.g., radial artery, femoropopliteal vein), with the site of incision for the catheter specified in the code description (e.g., by arm, by leg, by abdominal incision). You can locate these codes in the CPT manual index under embolectomy or thrombectomy, subdivided by arteries and veins (e.g., carotid artery, axillary vein).

When more involved procedures such as grafts are performed, inflow and outflow establishment is included in the major procedure codes. This means that if a thrombus is present and a bypass graft is performed, the removal of the thrombus is bundled into the grafting procedure if performed on the

FIGURE 16-16 Embolectomy.

same vessel. Also bundled into the aortic procedures is any sympathectomy (interruption of the sympathetic nervous system) or angiogram (radiographic view of the blood vessels).

EXERCISE 16-5 *Embolectomy/Thrombectomy*

Using the CPT and ICD-9-CM manuals, code the following:

1 Thrombectomy of the aortoiliac artery, by leg incision

   CPT Code: _____

2 Embolectomy, carotid artery, by neck incision

   CPT Code: _____

3 Thrombectomy of venous bypass graft, post-op complication

   CPT Code: _____

   ICD-9-CM Code: _____ (ICD-10-CM Code: _____)

Cardiovascular Repairs

The category Venous Reconstruction (34501-34530) contains codes for the various repairs made to the valves of the vena cava, saphenous vein, and femoral vein. The repair to heart valves is made by opening the site and clamping off the vessels that lead to the heart. The surgeon then tacks down excess material of the valve with sutures (plication). If there is a defect in the valve, the surgeon repairs the defect with a graft, usually harvested from elsewhere in the body. **Vein repairs** are performed by locating the defective vessel, clamping the vessel off, and bypassing or grafting the defect.

The category Direct Repair of Aneurysm or Excision (Partial or Total) and Graft Insertion for Aneurysm, Pseudoaneurysm, Ruptured Aneurysm, and Associated Occlusive Disease (35001-35152) contains **aneurysm repair** codes that are divided according to the type of aneurysm and the vessel the aneurysm is located in (subclavian artery, popliteal artery). The aneurysm is formed by the dilation of the wall of an artery, a vein, or the heart; it is filled with fluid or clotted blood. During repair, the aneurysm is located, and clamps are placed above and below it. The section containing the aneurysm is then removed or bypassed. The aneurysm codes often refer to a **pseudoaneurysm** (false aneurysm), which is an aneurysm in which the vessel is injured and the aneurysm is being contained by the tissue that surrounds the vessel.

Endovascular aneurysm repair (EVAR) is a technology that involves placing a stent graft, a fabric tube, inside the affected area of the blood vessel accessed through an artery. For example, abdominal aortic aneurysm repair by endovascular technique is reported with codes 34800-34834 and iliac aneurysm endovascular repair is reported with 34900.

Repair, Arteriovenous Fistula category codes (35180-35190) are reported for **fistula repair** and are divided on the basis of whether the fistula (abnormal passage) is congenital, acquired, or traumatic. An arteriovenous fistula occurs when blood flows between an artery and a vein. An example of an acquired arteriovenous fistula is the creation of an arteriovenous connection that is used for a hemodialysis site (Fig. 16–17). In repairing a fistula, the surgeon separates the artery and vein and then patches the area of separation with sutures or a graft.

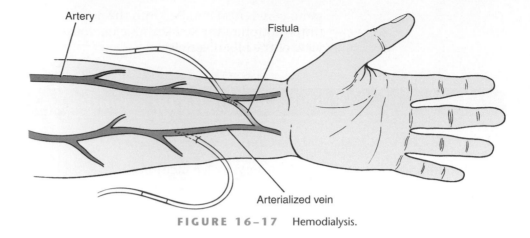

Artery

Fistula

Arterialized vein

FIGURE 16–17 Hemodialysis.

If an **angioscopy** of the vessel or graft area is performed during a therapeutic procedure, code 35400, Angioscopy (noncoronary vessels or grafts) during therapeutic intervention, is listed in addition to the procedure code. For example, the surgeon performed the repair of an acquired arteriovenous fistula of the neck (35188) and then placed a scope into the artery to determine visually whether the repair was complete. Code 35188 describes the primary therapeutic procedure of repair of the acquired arteriovenous fistula, and 35400 describes the use of the angioscope to accomplish the repair. Note that 35400 is an add-on code and cannot be reported alone, but only in conjunction with another procedure code.

A **transluminal angioplasty** is a procedure in which a vessel is punctured and a catheter is passed into the vessel for the purposes of stretching the vessel. The category codes 35450-35476 are divided on the basis of whether the catheter was passed into the vessel by incising the skin to expose the vessel (open) or by passing the catheter through the skin (percutaneous) into the vessel. Further divisions of the codes are based on the vessel into which the catheter is placed (e.g., iliac, aortic).

A **transluminal atherectomy** (35480-35495) is a procedure in which a vessel is punctured and a guidewire is threaded into the vessel. The surgeon then inserts a device called an atherectomy catheter into the vessel. This catheter contains a device that can destroy the materials clogging the vessel. This procedure can be performed by an open or a percutaneous method, and the codes are divided based on the method used and the vessel into which the catheter was passed.

Bypass Grafts, Veins

As with coronary artery bypass grafting (CABG), you must know the type of grafting material used for vascular bypass grafts (Bypass Grafts 35500-35671). Grafts can be vessels harvested from other areas of the body or they may be made of artificial materials. Codes are chosen on the basis of the type of graft and the specific vessel(s) that the graft is being bypassed from and to. For example, 35506 describes a graft that is placed to bypass a portion of the subclavian artery. During this procedure the surgeon sews a harvested vein to the side of the carotid artery and attach the other end of the vein to the subclavian artery below the damaged area, creating a bypass around the defect.

QUICK CHECK 16-4

1. According to the CPT manual notes for bypass grafts, which of the following procurements is bundled in the bypass?
   a. upper extremity graft
   b. composite graft(s)
   c. saphenous vein graft
   d. femoropopliteal vein graft

One way to locate the graft codes in the CPT manual index is to reference "Bypass Graft" and then the subterm type (e.g., carotid, subclavian, vertebral).

Vascular Access

Some treatments are administered through the blood by means of vascular access. For instance, in patients receiving hemodialysis, arteriovenous fistulas may be created for dialysis treatments (see Fig. 16–17). This means that an artificial connection is made between a vein and an artery, allowing blood to flow from the vein through the graft for dialysis (cleansing of waste products) and then be returned to the artery.

Vascular Injection Procedures

Bundled into the vascular injections (36000-36522) are the following items:

- Local anesthesia
- Introduction of needle or catheter
- Injection of contrast media
- Pre-injection care related to procedure
- Post-injection care related to procedure

Vascular injections bundles do not include the following items:

- Catheter
- Drugs
- Contrast media

For items not bundled into the injection procedure, report each item separately.

CAUTION *Just for a moment, think about what a difference a seemingly small fact—such as what is included in the vascular injection procedures— makes in the amount received for the procedure over the course of a year! It is your responsibility as the coder to know the rules of coding to ensure appropriate reimbursement for services provided by physicians. Details are important in the business of coding!*

Code 99070 (supplies and materials) from the Medicine section or HCPCS supply codes report items such as catheters, drugs, and contrast media if the procedure is performed in the clinic facility. If the procedure is performed in the hospital catheterization laboratory, the hospital-based coder would report the supply.

As previously discussed, knowledge of the vascular families is critical in coding vascular injection procedures because the initial placement and the extent of placement are usually the characteristics that determine the codes. You now know that the initial placement of the catheter is reported first and that add-on codes report any additional services. For example, review the following initial and additional third-order placement code descriptions in this example:

Example

36217	Selective catheter placement, arterial system; **initial** third order or more selective thoracic or brachiocephalic branch, with a vascular family
36218	Selective catheter placement, arterial system; **additional** second order, third order, and beyond, thoracic or brachiocephalic branch, within a vascular family

---

In the service described in 36217, the physician inserts a needle through the skin and into an artery. The needle has a guidewire attached to it, as illustrated in Fig. 16–18, and when the needle is withdrawn, the guidewire is left inside the artery. The guidewire can then be manipulated into the particular artery. Once the guidewire is in the correct artery, a catheter is threaded into place over the guidewire and into the first-order brachiocephalic artery. The catheter is manipulated through the second-order artery and arrives at the third-order artery, where contrast material is injected into the artery through the catheter and an arteriography is completed.

After the completion of the service described in 36217, the physician pulls the catheter back into the artery and then manipulates the catheter into another third-order artery (36218), where contrast material is again injected into the artery through the catheter and another arteriography is completed.

Figs. 16–19 and 16–20 illustrate vascular coding with a common femoral artery approach.

FIGURE 16–18   Catheter insertion.

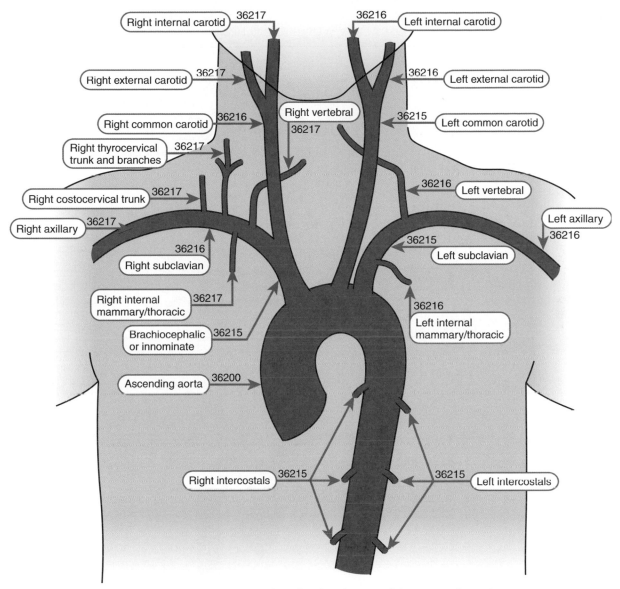

FIGURE 16–19   Arterial Head and Neck approach is common femoral.

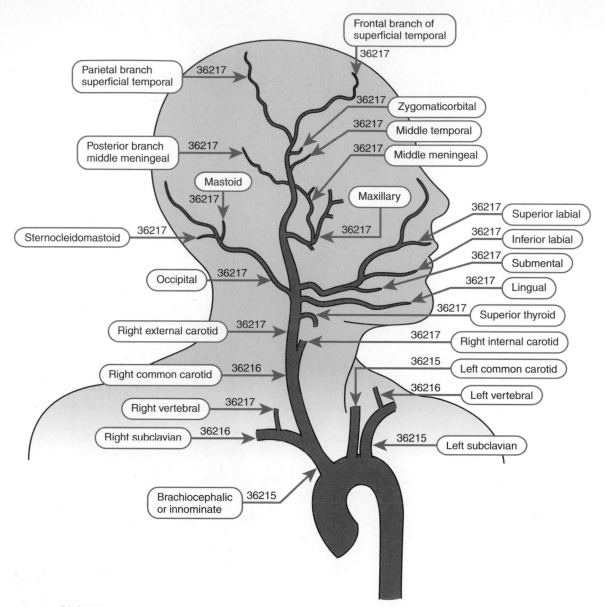

FIGURE 16-20 Arterial Head and Neck—right external carotid approach is the common femoral.

EXERCISE 16-6   *Repairs, Grafts, and Vascular Access*

Using the CPT and ICD-9-CM manuals, code the following:

1 Bypass graft, with vein; carotid-subclavian

CPT Code: _____

2 Bypass graft, with vein; femoral-popliteal

CPT Code: _____

3 Bypass graft, using Gore-Tex; axillary-axillary

CPT Code: _____

4 Excision, with application of a patch graft, for an aneurysm, common femoral artery

CPT Code: _____

ICD-9-CM Code: _____ (ICD-10-CM Code: _____)

5 From a right femoral artery approach, the catheter is placed in the abdominal aorta and is then threaded into the left external iliac artery where contrast material is injected and angiography is done. The surgeon then pulls back the catheter into the right internal iliac where contrast is injected and angiography is completed. The catheter is withdrawn. The patient was diagnosed as having peripheral vascular disease. *(Note: Report only the catheterization as radiographic guidance services would be reported separately.)*

CPT Codes: _____ -RT, _____ -59-LT, _____
(angiography)

ICD-9-CM Code: _____ (ICD-10-CM Code: _____)

CARDIOVASCULAR CODING IN THE MEDICINE SECTION

Services in the Cardiovascular subsection of the Medicine section (92950-93799) can be either invasive/noninvasive or diagnostic/therapeutic. The invasive treatments are not a matter of cutting open the body so the surgeon can view it, as was the case in the Cardiovascular subsection of the Surgery section, but are invasive in that there is an incision into or a puncture of the skin. Review the subheadings in the Cardiovascular subsection in the Medicine section of the CPT manual.

Therapeutic Services

It is within the Therapeutic Services and Procedures subheading that you locate many commonly assigned cardiovascular codes, such as cardioversion, infusions, thrombolysis, placement of catheters and stents, atherectomy, and angioplasty. Many of these services used to be performed as open operative procedures, but with the advent of modern techniques, many are now performed by means of percutaneous access. Division of the codes is based on **method** (balloon, blade), **location** (aorta or mitral valve), and **number** (single or multiple vessels).

Thrombolysis, as described in 92975, is a percutaneous procedure in which the physician inserts a catheter into a coronary vessel and injects contrast material into the vessel to further enhance the visualization of a blood clot. The clot is then destroyed by a drug that the physician injects through the catheter. The Medicine section code 92975 represents the total procedure when the thrombolysis is performed in a coronary vessel. If vessels other than the coronary vessels are treated, a code from the Surgery section, Cardiovascular subsection, would be assigned to report an infusion of a thrombus (37201).

Intravascular ultrasound of the coronary vessels can be reported using the two codes 92978 and 92979, depending on the number of vessels being diagnosed. A needle is inserted percutaneously into the vessel and a guidewire introduced, followed by an ultrasound probe. The probe allows a two-dimensional image of the inside of the vessel to be viewed on the ultrasound monitor. The physician can assess the vessel before and after treatment. The physician may reposition the probe to assess additional vessels, and 92979 is reported to indicate this subsequent placement. Note that both 92978 and 92979 are add-on codes intended to be reported only in conjunction with the primary procedure. For example, intravascular ultrasound with coronary stent placement would be reported as 92980 (placement of stent) and 92978 (intravascular ultrasound).

Intracoronary stent placement (92980, 92981) is performed using a catheter to reinforce a coronary vessel that has collapsed or is blocked. The placement of the stent is usually accomplished with radiographic guidance. The surgeon usually reports the stent placement, and the radiologist who provides the ultrasonic guidance reports the guidance. The codes are divided on the basis of whether more than one coronary vessel was cleared of obstruction and had a stent placed within it.

Fig. 16–21 illustrates an angioplasty/stent report in which the coronary artery is repaired by placement of a stent. Percutaneous transluminal coronary angioplasty (PTCA) is described in codes 92982 and 92984. The codes are divided on the basis of whether a single vessel or multiple vessels are treated during the procedure. Add-on code 92984 (PTCA for each additional vessel) is of interest because it can be assigned not only with 92982 but also with other codes in the category. For example, 92984 can be assigned with 92980, placement of a stent, when a stent is placed in one vessel and the PTCA is performed in a different vessel. If a patient had an intracoronary stent placed in one coronary vessel, report 92980, and if the physician also performed a PTCA on another coronary vessel, report 92984. This is the first time that you have used an add-on code with a code other than the one(s) that appears directly above it in the same group of codes,

---

Angioplasty/Stent

Patient: Marlene Castello   **Number:** 45900   **Room:** Cardiac Cath Lab 5F

DOB: 02/13/43   **Attending Physician:** Dr. Helen Palmer

DATE OF STUDY: 04/06/0X

PROCEDURE: Angioplasty/stent of 80 to 90 percent proximal/mid-right coronary artery stenosis.

INDICATIONS: Chest pain and abnormal Cardiolite stress test.

COMPLICATIONS: None

RESULTS: Successful angioplasty/stent of 80 to 90 percent proximal/mid-right coronary artery stenosis with no residual stenosis at the end of the procedure.

David H. Robinson, MD

David H. Robinson, MD

Cardiology Department

DHR/jkl

FIGURE 16-21   Angioplasty/stent report.

so be certain to read the code descriptions for each of the codes used in the example and pay special attention to the notes that follow 92984.

CODING SHOT There are HCPCS modifiers to identify the specific coronary arteries that are treated, such as **-RC,** right coronary; **-LC,** left circumflex; and **-LD,** left anterior descending.

Valvuloplasty can also be performed by inserting a catheter percutaneously. The procedure opens a blocked valve by using a balloon, which is inflated to clear the blockage. Codes 92986-92990 are divided based on the valve being repaired.

The balloon technique is also used to treat congenital heart defects such as vessels that are too narrow. A blade can also be deployed inside the coronary vessels. A special catheter that has a retractable blade is guided into the vessel and the surgeon manipulates the blade to enlarge the area, using ultrasound or fluoroscopic guidance.

Cardiography

This category (93000-93278) of the Cardiovascular System subsection contains frequently assigned codes, such as those for electrocardiograms and heart monitoring, which are certain to be used in most office practices, even if the practice does not include a cardiologist.

The Cardiography subheading codes report electrocardiographic procedures such as stress tests. **Stress tests** are performed to assess the adequacy of the amount of oxygen getting to the heart muscle (at rest and during exercise) and thus indicate the presence or absence of heart disease (Fig. 16–22). The top number on a blood pressure reading is systole (heart muscle is contracting); the bottom number is diastole (heart muscle is relaxing). The heart muscle is fed by three coronary arteries and their branches. If these arteries are clear, the amount of blood going to the muscle is adequate during rest and exercise. The heart muscle is fed only during diastole. Normal blood pressure is about 120/80 mm Hg, and the normal heart rate is about 60-100 beats per minute. During low blood pressure, little blood and oxygen get to the heart.

FIGURE 16-22 Stress test. (From Young AP, Proctor DB: *Kinn's The Medical Assistant,* ed 10, St. Louis, 2007, Saunders.)

As the heart beats faster, such as during exercise, the heart rate increases and diastolic pressure time decreases, meaning that there is less time to supply blood to the heart muscle. As the heart beats faster, more oxygen is required. With narrowing of coronary arteries and branches, too little blood may circulate to the heart muscle, supplying even less oxygen than during rest. Chest pain may result as an indication that heart muscle tissue is dying. Indications of heart disease during a stress test are chest pain and a depressed or elevated ST wave segment on the ECG, as illustrated in Fig. 16–23.

The **Holter** monitor, as illustrated in Fig. 16–24, is similar to an electrocardiogram (ECG), as illustrated in Fig. 16–25, in that leads are attached to the patient. There are portable Holter monitors that record the patient's ECG readings for 24 hours. Leads are attached to the chest and to a cassette machine. The monitor converts the ECG readings to sound, and the sound is converted back to an ECG reading when completed. The reading is then sped up to hundreds of times faster than normal by computers. Any reading that varies from a normal reading will be identified. The Q, R, and S waves are related to the contraction of the ventricles of the heart. The QRS waves and heartbeats can be monitored by Holter monitors. Cardiac arrhythmias can be identified using the Holter monitor process. An example of a Holter report is presented in Fig. 16–26.

FIGURE 16–23 Normal and abnormal ECG test results. **A,** Normal ECG reading. **B,** Abnormal ECG reading. The ST segment dips. QRS complex and T waves are related to the contraction of the ventricles. Indications of heart disease during a stress test are chest pain and lengthened ST segments.

FIGURE 16–24 Holter monitor. (From Forbes CD, Jackson WF: *Color Atlas and Text of Clinical Medicine*, ed 3, 2003, Mosby.)

FIGURE 16–25 **A** and **B,** Placement of the electrodes for a standard ECG. The ECG is a visual record of the electrical activity of the heart. (**A** from Young AP, Proctor DB: *Kinn's The Medical Assistant: An Applied Learning Approach,* ed 10, St. Louis, 2007, Saunders.)

Holter Report

INDICATIONS: Patient with atrial fibrillation on Lanoxin. Patient with known cardiomyopathy.

BASELINE DATA: 84-year-old gentleman with congestive heart failure on Elavil, Vasotec, Lanoxin, and Lasix.

The patient was monitored for 24 hours.

INTERPRETATION: 1. The predominant rhythm is atrial fibrillation. The average ventricular rate is 74 beats per minute, minimal 49 beats per minute, and maximum 114 beats per minute.
2. A total of 4948 ventricular ectopic beats were detected. There were 4 forms. There were 146 couplets with 1 triplet and 5 runs of bigeminy. There were 2 runs of ventricular tachycardia, the longest for 5 beats at a rate of 150 beats per minute. There was no ventricular fibrillation.
3. There were no prolonged pauses.

CONCLUSION: 1. Predominant rhythm is atrial fibrillation with well-controlled ventricular rate.
2. There are no prolonged pauses.
3. Asymptomatic, nonsustained ventricular tachycardia.

Raymond P. Price, MD

Raymond P. Price, MD

Cardiology Department

RPP/lpm

FIGURE 16–26 Holter report.

CODING SHOT Many CPT monitoring codes cannot be billed with modifiers -TC or -26, as there are individual codes for the professional and technical components.

An ECG is typically conducted by attaching 10 electrodes (leads) to the patient's chest to monitor 12 areas. The ECG provides a reading of the electrical currents of the heart and is a standard test conducted to detect suspected cardiac abnormalities, such as arrhythmias and conduction abnormalities. Codes report the tracing only (the technical component), the interpretation and report only (the professional component), or the entire procedure of tracing and interpretation (the technical and professional components). The medical record will indicate the components provided. Codes 93000-93010 are for the standard 12-lead ECG; the codes are divided on the basis of the component(s) provided.

Codes 93040-93278 report other various ECGs and are divided according to the type of recording and the component(s) provided. Only careful reading will reveal the often slight differences between codes.

Of special note is **signal-averaged electrocardiography (SAECG)** reported with 93278. SAECG is a type of electrocardiography that can help physicians predict certain tendencies to abnormalities such as ventricular tachycardia. The signal is recorded during nine periods, each lasting 10 to 20 minutes, and the computer manipulates the data produced and predicts certain tendencies. The SAECG is a more sophisticated ECG than the standard ECG and is used when a standard ECG is unable to demonstrate the suspected conductive abnormalities.

CODING SHOT

If only the interpretation and report are done with an SAECG, report 93278-26 to indicate that only the professional component was provided.

Telephonic transmission of an electrocardiogram is made possible by a device the patient wears that records irregular rhythms. The readings can then be sent to the physician by means of a telephone to transmit the information, which is subsequently printed for the physician's review. Third-party payers usually restrict the payment of telephonic transmissions to one every 30 days. The codes 93012 and 93014 are divided on the basis of the component(s) the physician provides.

A **cardiovascular stress test** is used to evaluate and diagnose chest pain, to screen for heart disease, to evaluate irregular heart rhythms, and to investigate many other cardiovascular abnormalities. The patient is placed on a treadmill or a stationary bicycle and ECG leads are attached. The patient then exercises until he or she reaches maximal (220 minus age) or submaximal (85% of maximal) heart rate. During certain intervals, the physician or technician records the ECG, heart rate, and blood pressure of the patient.

The codes for stress tests (93015-93018) are divided on the basis of the components provided. Code 93015 reports the global outpatient service, and 93016-93018 reports components (parts) of the service. The ECG is bundled into the stress test, so do not unbundle and report an ECG or any reading separately. Medication can be administered to mimic the stressing of the heart and is used when factors are present that limit a patient's ability to exercise, such as arthritis, morbid obesity, or stroke. Stress test codes are used for both stress-induced (exercise) and pharmacologically induced (drug) studies. Medications and radiology services may be reported separately.

Implantable and Wearable Cardiac Device Evaluations

Cardiovascular monitoring is a diagnostic service that may be performed in person or using technology to access cardiovascular data and these services are reported with codes in the 93279-93299 range. Codes 93279-93285 are reported per procedure, such as a single, dual, or multiple pacemaker or cardioverter-defibrillator. There are extensive notes before the subheading that are must reading before you begin to assign these codes.

Codes 93286 and 93287 report periprocedural (shortly before, during, or shortly after) evaluation of a device based on if the device is a pacemaker or cardioverter-defibrillator. The codes may be reported once before and once after surgery because they are the testing of the device to ensure it functions correctly.

Codes in the 93288-93292 range are reported per procedure and are in-person evaluations of a pacemaker or cardioverter-defibrillator system based on the type of device and the type of analysis performed.

Evaluation of a pacemaker by means of a telephone is reported once in a 90-day period with 93293. The service includes the written report of the data analysis. Face-to-face evaluations of the device are referred to as interrogation device evaluations and reported with 93294-93299. These codes are divided based on the type of device (pacemaker or cardioverter-defibrillator) and the time period. For example, 93297 reports remote interrogation evaluation(s) up to 30 days and 93294 reports remote interrogation evaluation(s) up to 90 days.

Echocardiography

Echocardiography is a noninvasive diagnostic method that uses ultrasonographic images to detect the presence of heart disease or valvular disease. A sliced image is used to detail the various walls of the heart. A **transducer** is placed on the outside of the chest wall, and it sends sound waves through the chest (Fig. 16–27).

As the sound reflects back from each organ wall, dots are recorded, indicating the point of reflection. When the heart is in systole, it is contracting, and the dots on the recording appear farther apart. When the heart is in diastole, it is relaxing, and the dots on the recording appear closer together.

Bundled into the complete echocardiography procedures (93303-93352) are the obtaining of the signal from the heart and great arteries by means of two-dimensional imaging and/or Doppler ultrasound, the interpretation,

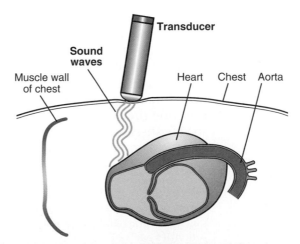

FIGURE 16-27 Echocardiography. A transducer is placed on the outside of the chest wall, and it sends sound waves through the chest. When the heart is in systole, the heart is contracting and the dots on the echocardiogram appear farther apart. When the heart is in diastole, it is relaxing and the dots on the echocardiogram appear closer together.

and the report. Modifiers -26, professional service only, and -TC, technical component, may be applied to these codes if only one component is provided. The codes are divided on the basis of whether it was a complete echocardiogram or a follow-up/limited study, the type of echocardiogram, and the approach used.

EXERCISE 16-7 *Therapeutic Services, Cardiography, and Echocardiography*

Using the CPT and ICD-9-CM manuals, code the following:

1 A physician provides CPR to a patient in cardiac arrest.

    CPT Code: _____

2 Cardiovascular stress test using submaximal bicycle exercise with continuous ECG; physician was in attendance for supervision and provided the interpretation and report.

    CPT Code: _____

3 Percutaneous transluminal coronary balloon angioplasty of the right coronary artery and two vessels of the left anterior descending.

    CPT Codes: _____, _____

4 SAECG with ECG, interpretation and report only. Diagnosis of unsustained ventricular tachycardia.

    CPT Code: _____

    ICD-9-CM Code: _____ (ICD-10-CM Code: _____)

Cardiac Catheterization

Catheterization (93501-93533) is an invasive diagnostic medical procedure in which the physician percutaneously inserts a catheter and manipulates the catheter into coronary vessels and/or the heart. Fig. 16–28 illustrates a percutaneous method of catheterization called the Seldinger technique, after the inventor of the method. This catheterization is at the right subclavian artery. Following insertion of the fine-gauge needle, a guidewire and then a catheter are inserted. The cardiac catheter measures pressure, oxygen, and blood gases, takes blood samples, and measures the output of the heart. A cardiac catheterization is a study of both the circulation and the movement of the blood of the heart; the physician may inject a dye into the vessel or heart and observe the movement of the dye by means of angiography. When injection of contrast material is used to improve visualization, additional injection procedure codes (such as 93540 or 93544) must be assigned to specify the site of the injection.

Example

During a cardiac catheterization procedure, contrast medium is injected into a bypass graft and into the coronary arteries. CPT codes would be assigned to identify each of the areas of injection as follows:

93540	injection into the bypass graft
93545	injection into selective coronary arteries

FIGURE 16–28 Percutaneous method of catheterization (Seldinger technique).

Each of these two codes would be reported in addition to the code for the type of cardiac catheterization (e.g., left and right heart catheterization, 93526). But you wouldn't be finished coding this one yet. If the cardiologist also supervises, interprets, and reports on the x-ray imaging of the angiography, codes 93555 and 93556 would be assigned to report the imaging services. This is a good example of component coding. Component coding requires you to examine services that were provided to the patient, identify each component, or part, of that service, identify who performed each component, and code each service provided. At this point, you are probably thinking there should be just one code that includes all the components of a cardiac catheterization into one code, which would make code assignment easier. In earlier editions of the CPT manual there were just such bundled codes, but as practice of medicine changed to have more specialists—each performing a component of a procedure—the codes changed to reflect these practice changes. Being able to identify each component makes the coding more specific.

If the private physician (such as the clinic physician) performs the catheterization procedure in the catheterization laboratory at the hospital, you would add modifier -26 to the imaging codes (93555, 93556) and the cardiac catheterization code (93526). The hospital would submit charges for the technical component of the procedure.

Access for cardiac catheterization can be made in several locations, depending on the patient's condition and the physician's preference—for example, the right femoral artery (access site).

From the Trenches

"Teamwork is important in this environment . . . . As a profession, we must be a resource to each other and the health care community as a whole."

LETITIA

Cardiac catheterization can indicate valve disorders, abnormal flow of blood, and a variety of cardiac output abnormalities. Often, a cardiac catheterization leads to a more definite treatment, such as a valvoplasty, stent placement, angioplasty, or bypass.

Bundled into the cardiac catheterization codes are the introduction, positioning, and repositioning of the catheter(s); the recording of pressures inside the heart or vessels; the taking of blood samples; rest/exercise studies; final evaluation; and final report.

There are three components in the coding of cardiac catheterization:

1. **Placement** of the catheter, using codes 93501-93533
2. **Injection** procedure, using codes 93539-93545
3. **Imaging** supervision, interpretation, and report on the injection procedure, using codes 93555, 93556

In the case of a complete cardiac catheterization, which is the usual procedure, you will find all the codes you need to fully report the service in the Medicine section, Cardiac Catheterization category. It is a good idea to make a notation of the code ranges for the three components of cardiac catheterization so you remember to look for the components when coding.

CODING SHOT Some cardiac catheterization codes (93539, 93540, 93544-93556) are modifier -51 exempt. The remainder of the codes (93501-93543) are subject to multiple procedure rules and reporting with modifier -51.

The Cardiac Catheterization injection codes (93539-93545) are not to be assigned unless the injection procedure is a part of a cardiac catheterization. The injection codes are professional only; therefore, would never require modifier -26.

There are several codes (93561-93572) in the category that are not a part of the usual three components of the cardiac catheterization. These codes are for the **indicator dilution studies,** which are already bundled into the cardiac catheterization codes and are to be reported only when the complete cardiac catheterization procedure was not performed. For example, if only the dye or thermal dilution study was performed, without a cardiac catheterization, an indicator dilution study code would be assigned to report the service.

EXERCISE 16-8 *Cardiac Catheterization*

Code the following using the CPT and ICD-9-CM manuals:

1 Right heart catheterization was performed by means of the introduction of a cardiac catheter into the venous system, with further manipulation into the right atrium, including injection into the right atrium of contrast material, multiple measurements, and sampling; image supervision was provided by the physician.

Code(s):

_____ Catheterization procedure

_____ Injection procedure

_____ Supervision, interpretation, and report for injection procedure

2 Retrograde left heart catheterization of left ventricle was performed, with cutdown entry into the brachiocephalic artery, and contrast medium was injected for left ventricular angiography, including supervision, interpretation, and report. Diagnosis of coronary artery disease, native and unstable angina.

Codes: _____, _____, _____

ICD-9-CM Codes: _____, _____ (ICD-10-CM Code: _____)

3 Indicator dilution studies when done with a cardiac catheterization are to be billed separately.

True   False

4 Bundled into the cardiac catheterization codes are the positioning and repositioning of the catheter(s).

True   False

5 Modifier -51 can be added to all codes in the Cardiac Catheterization subheading.

True   False

Intracoronary Brachytherapy

Intracoronary brachytherapy is the use of radioactive substances as a therapy for in-stent restenosis of a coronary vessel, as illustrated in Fig. 16–29. For example, a patient has a coronary artery stent placed to open a vessel that is blocked with plaque (stenosis). The stent reopens the vessel so blood can once again flow without obstruction. However, the stent can also become occluded with plaque and when this happens, the physician may

FIGURE 16–29 Brachytherapy delivery systems for coronary artery stent restenosis. **A,** The Novoste Transfer Device uses a saline-filled syringe to advance the radiation seeds to the treatment site. The same device is used to remove the seeds at the end of the brachytherapy treatment. **B,** The Novoste delivery catheter advances seeds to the site of angioplasty. (From Zipes DP, editor: *Braunwald's Heart Disease,* ed 7, Philadelphia, 2005, Saunders.)

use intracoronary brachytherapy in which a radioactive strip of material is inserted by means of a catheter into the area of blockage, where it is left for up to 45 minutes and then removed.

The procedure would usually be performed by an interventional cardiologist and a radiation oncologist. The interventional cardiologist would place the radioactive-element guidewire and report that service with 92974, which is the catheter placement code. The radiation oncologist would then place the radioactive elements and report the services with whichever codes applied to the service, such as planning (77261-77263), simulation (77280-77295), dosimetry (77300-77370), and/or clinical brachytherapy codes (77785-77787).

Intracardiac Electrophysiologic Procedures/Studies

As you learned earlier in this chapter, surgical electrophysiologic procedures (33250-33261) are those that repair the electrical system of the heart using invasive surgical procedures. In the Medicine section, the Intracardiac Electrophysiological Procedures/Studies category (93600-93662) contains codes that describe services that diagnose and treat the electrical system of the heart using less invasive procedures. Although the Medicine section procedures are invasive, they are percutaneous procedures, not open procedures.

Fig. 16–30 illustrates the electrical conduction system of the heart, which begins with the sinoatrial node (SA), known as the heart's pacemaker. The sinoatrial node sends impulses to the atrioventricular (AV) node, which in turn passes the impulses to the bundle of His, and finally on to the Purkinje fibers to stimulate the muscle tissues of the ventricles of the heart to contract. Lesions or diseases involving these structures along the electrical conduction pathway underlie many of the disturbances of cardiac rhythm.

To diagnose the origin of an electrophysiologic abnormality, the physician takes recordings at various sites along the pathway. The physician may also stimulate the heart to induce arrhythmia by means of a catheter attached to a pacing device that sends electrical impulses to various sites within the heart. A protocol (a set order) for the placement of the catheter is a **programmed stimulation.**

Pacing is the regulation of the heart rate. A cardiac pacemaker is a permanent pacer; but the pacing referred to in the EP codes is a temporary pacing done in an attempt to stabilize the beating of the heart. **Recording** is a record of the electrical activity of the heart taken by means of an ECG. Recording services are reported with codes in the range of 93600-93603, and pacing services are reported with codes 93610 and 93612. Combination codes that indicate both recording and pacing begin with 93619. These codes are not

FIGURE 16–30 Electrical conduction system of the heart.

used as much as they used to be when EP was a new technique and readings were commonly taken at just one site. Today, more complex EP studies are usually done, including multiple pacings and recordings in combinations based on established protocols using three or more catheters. These complex services are reported with codes in the 93619-93622 range. Carefully read the notes in parentheses following several of the combination codes, as the notes indicate when the use of the combination code is appropriate and even indicate the codes that are bundled into the one combination code.

> ✋ **CAUTION** *Most of the EP codes have many items bundled into them, so read the description of each code completely so as to avoid unbundling the services.*

Bundle of His recording is a reading taken inside the heart (intracardiac) at the tip of the bundle of His. The bundle of His is also known as the atrioventricular bundle or AV bundle and is the bundle of cardiac muscle fibers that conducts electrical impulses that regulate heartbeats. The physician percutaneously inserts into a vessel a special catheter that can sense electrical impulses. The catheter is advanced to the right heart. The femoral vein is the usual site of entry and fluoroscopic guidance is usually used for placement of the catheter into the heart.

Codes 93602 and 93603 describe a single **recording** based on the location—intra-arterial or right ventricle. Codes 93610 and 93612 describe single intra-arterial or intraventricular **pacing** in an atrial or a ventricular location.

Code 93631 reports **pacing** and **mapping** done during an open surgical procedure in which the surgeon opens the chest and exposes the heart. The EP physician performs the mapping (locating the origin of the arrhythmia and defining the pathway), and the surgeon then destroys the source of the arrhythmia. When reporting the services of both physicians for this procedure, use 93631 to report the mapping service and a surgery code from the range 33250-33261 to report the arrhythmia ablation. Make a notation next to the mapping code 93631 to report any surgical ablation (33250-33261) to remind yourself to code both procedures if required. If the mapping is not done intraoperatively (during surgery), report the service with 93609 or 93613.

Ablation can also be performed by using a catheter with a tip that emits electric current. When the tip is placed on tissue and activated, the tissue is destroyed. Sometimes physicians destroy certain sites along the conduction pathway as a treatment for slow (bradycardia) or fast (tachycardia) heart rhythms. Ablation procedures are reported with codes 93650-93652, according to whether they were at the AV node, above the ventricles (supraventricular), or in the ventricles.

There are two ways ablation can be performed. The first way does not require surgery. An area of the patient's upper thigh is numbed, but the patient is awake. Then the physician inserts a thin tube through a blood vessel (usually the femoral artery) and all the way up to the heart. At the tip of the tube is a small wire that can deliver **radiofrequency** energy to burn away the abnormal areas of the heart. Then the heart can beat normally again.

The second way ablation can be performed is by means of surgery. In the Maze procedure, the surgeon makes small **cuts** in the heart to direct healthy electrical rhythms. In **cryoablation,** a very cold substance is used to freeze the cells that are creating problems. In **endocardial resection,** the surgeon removes a section of the thin layer of the heart where the abnormal rhythms originate.

Peripheral Arterial Disease Rehabilitation

Peripheral arterial disease (PAD) rehabilitation sessions (93668) last 45 to 60 minutes; these are rehabilitative physical exercises done either on a motorized treadmill or on a track to build the patient's cardiovascular endurance. An exercise physiologist or nurse supervises the sessions. If a session produces symptoms of angina or other negative symptoms, the physician reviews the information and may determine to reevaluate the patient. The physician services are not included in the PAD codes, rather the physician services are reported with an additional Evaluation and Management (E/M) code.

Noninvasive Physiologic Studies and Procedures

If a patient has a pacemaker or defibrillator in place, periodic monitoring must occur to ensure that the device is functioning properly. Codes from the Noninvasive Physiologic Studies and Procedures (93701-93790) category and the Implantable and Wearable Cardiac Device Evaluations (93279-93299) category reflect these services. Codes are assigned according to the type of pacemaker (single- or dual-chamber) or cardioverter-defibrillator and whether reprogramming of an existing pacemaker or defibrillator was done.

Plethysmography (93720-93722) is a recording of the change in the size of a body part when blood passes through it and is used to determine vascular abnormalities. For example, respiratory function may be assessed using total body plethysmography. There are two components in a plethysmography process—the professional component and the technical component. There are codes for the total procedure, for only the technical component of tracing, and for only the professional component of interpretation and report.

Ambulatory blood pressure monitoring (93784-93790) is an outpatient procedure that is conducted over a 24-hour period by means of a portable device worn by the patient. There is a code for the total procedure—including recording, analysis, and interpretation/report—and there are codes for each of the individual components—recording only, analysis only, and interpretation/report only.

Other Procedures

The Other Procedures codes (93797-93799) report physician services that are provided for cardiac rehabilitation of outpatients, either with or without electrocardiographic monitoring.

EXERCISE 16-9 *EP and Vascular Studies*

Using the CPT and ICD-9-CM manuals, code the following:

1 Bundle of His recording

   CPT Code: _____

2 Comprehensive electrophysiologic evaluation was performed, including recording and pacing of the right atrium and right ventricle. Three electrodes were repositioned. Left ventricular recordings were also made, with pacing and induction of arrhythmia. Diagnosis of Vasovagal syncope.

   CPT Codes: _____, _____

   ICD-9-CM Code: _____ (ICD-10-CM Code: _____)

3 Total body plethysmography, including tracing, interpretation, and report

   CPT Code: _____

CARDIOVASCULAR CODING IN THE RADIOLOGY SECTION

The Radiology section of the CPT manual used to contain combination codes that included both the **professional** and **technical components** in one code. For example, 75659 existed to report the services of both the angiography (technical component) and the injection procedure (professional component) in a brachial angiography procedure. When the complete procedure code, 75659, was deleted, the injection procedure (professional component) was moved to the Surgery section and a code to report the technical component (angiography) remained in the Radiology section. Now, to report both the injection procedure and the angiography services (the complete procedure), the coder assigns a Surgery code to report the professional component and a Radiology code to report the technical component. The division of the technical and professional components makes it possible to specify the various parts of a procedure, which is important because some cardiologists perform both components of these cardiovascular procedures, and some cardiologists perform only the injection procedure and have a radiologist do the angiography portion of the procedure. Component coding allows for the flexibility necessary to report these various situations. Component coding also makes it easier to identify the various diagnostic tests used in cardiovascular conditions. For example, one cardiologist may prefer to use an ultrasonic procedure in the diagnosis of arterial stenosis and another may prefer angiography. Both procedures require the insertion of a catheter and, as such, the insertion code remains the same, but the diagnostic tools may change.

Radiology codes often contain the statement "supervision and interpretation." **Supervision** is the radiologist's overseeing of the technician who is performing the procedure or indicates that the radiologist is performing the procedure himself/herself. **Interpretation** is the summary of the findings, also known as the final report, and the radiologist or cardiologist may do this portion of the service. There are actually two components (parts) in a code with supervision and interpretation in the description—the professional and technical components. The technical component is the equipment and the technician who actually provides the service. The professional component is the interpretation of the results and the writing of a report about the results, as illustrated in Fig. 16–31. Both components are not necessarily done by the same organization. Let's take an x-ray as an example of a service and see how you report the components.

If a clinic owns its own x-ray equipment and employs a radiologist to interpret the x-rays and write the reports, and also employs the technician who, under the supervision of the radiologist, takes the x-rays, the clinic could report the x-ray service using the appropriate radiology code, with supervision and interpretation in the description and no modifier. The clinic provides the total service, also known as the **global service.**

Another clinic owns the equipment and employs the technician who takes the x-ray, but then the clinic sends the x-ray out to a radiologist at another clinic who reads the x-ray and writes the report. The radiologist would report the service with the appropriate radiology code and modifier -26 to indicate that he or she provided only the professional component of the service. The clinic that employs the technician and owns the equipment would report the same radiology code but would attach the HCPCS modifier -TC (technical component) to indicate that only the technical component of the service was provided.

A third clinic has no x-ray equipment, so the physicians in the clinic send patients to an outside radiologist who hires the technician who takes x-rays on equipment owned by the radiologist, the radiologist interprets the results, and writes the report. The outside radiologist would report the service using

Examination:	Chest
Clinical symptoms:	Aortic stenosis, abnormal cardiac stress test
Date ordered:	Today's date
Date Completed:	Today's date
Ordering Dr.:	Timothy Swenson, MD
Attending Dr.:	Timothy Swenson, MD
Date of Birth:	04/13/65 Record #: 456980
PA & Lateral chest:	Radiographic examination reveals no abnormality of the lungs, heart, mediastinum, or visualized bony structures.
Impression:	Radiographically normal chest.

Ronald A. Potts, MD

Ronald A. Potts, MD

Radiologist

RAP/rnf

FIGURE 16–31   The final radiology report contains the radiologist's interpretation of findings.

the global radiology code with no modifier, because both the professional component and the technical component were provided.

Contrast material is commonly used with radiology procedures to enhance the image. If the Radiology section code states "with contrast" or "with or without contrast," you will know that the injection of contrast material and the contrast material itself (the substance used for contrasting) are bundled into the code; therefore, you would not report the contrast material or injection separately. If, however, there is no indication of contrast in the code description, and the physician used contrast, you would code both the injection of the contrast material and the contrast material itself. Injection of contrast is usually included in the radiology code. If guidelines state that you should report injections separately, report with the appropriate code from the Surgery section—for example, 47500, Injection procedure for percutaneous transhepatic cholangiography, and 74320 for the radiology portion of the service. The contrast material is reported separately using code 99070 from the Medicine section or with a HCPCS code.

CODING SHOT   Not all contrast material can be reported separately! Oral or rectal contrast is considered a part of the procedure and is not reported separately. Intravenous, intra-arterial, or intrathecal (fluid-filled space between the layers of tissue covering the brain and spinal cord) injection of contrast material can be reported separately if the code description does not refer to inclusion of contrast material.

STOP *Now, don't get discouraged with all of these codes from all of these sections! Remember that only with repeated use of these codes can you master them. At first, it sounds so confusing that you might wonder if you can ever absorb all of this information and the variations. You can! But you must be patient with the process. To be a coder is to be able to concentrate on details and commit yourself to the process of learning the details through repeated use. Everyone starts at the same place. Now, let's get back to learning about component coding.*

Two physicians, a cardiologist and a radiologist from the same facility, perform an angiography of the brachiocephalic artery (first order) using contrast material. Access was the right femoral artery. The coding is as follows:

- Cardiologist placing the catheter: 36215, Surgery section
- Radiologist performing the angiography: 75710, Radiology section
- Supply of the contrast material: 99070, Medicine section, or HCPCS Level II code (such as A9521, Technetium Tc-99m)

Two physicians, a cardiologist and a radiologist from different facilities, perform an angiography of the brachiocephalic artery (first order) using contrast material. The coding for the cardiologist is as follows:

- Cardiologist placing the catheter: 36215, Surgery section

The coding for the radiologist is as follows:

- Radiologist performing the angiography: 75710, Radiology section
- Supply of the contrast material: 99070, Medicine section, or a HCPCS Level II code (such as A9521, Technetium Tc-99m)

CODING SHOT If the radiologist is at the same facility as the equipment, you report 75710 (angiography). If the angiography was performed at the hospital and the radiologist from a clinic read the angiography, the radiologist would report 75710-26 and the hospital would report 75710-TC.

Heart The Heart subsection (75557-75574) of the Radiology section contains codes that report cardiac magnetic resonance imaging (MRI) of the heart. An **MRI**, as illustrated in Fig. 16–32, *A* and *B*, is the use of radiation to show the body in a cross-sectional view. MRI may include the use of injectable dyes (radiographic contrast) to aid in imaging. Other MRI codes are located throughout the Radiology section according to body part being imaged, but the codes in the Heart subsection are just for cardiac MRIs.

Aorta and Arteries In Radiology, the Aorta and Arteries subsection (75600-75791) includes codes for aortography excluding the heart—thoracic, abdominal, cervicocerebral, brachial, external carotid, carotid, vertebral, spinal, extremity, renal, visceral, adrenal pelvic, pulmonary, and internal mammary.

The Aorta and Arteries subsection codes are often reported in coding components of cardiovascular services.

FIGURE 16–32   **A,** Preoperative MRI of a patient with an ascending aortic aneurysm. **B,** Post-operative MRI of the same ascending aortic area. (From Bennett JC, Plum F: *Cecil Textbook of Medicine,* ed 20, Philadelphia, 1996, WB Saunders.)

EXERCISE 16-10   *Heart, Aorta, and Arteries*

Using the CPT and ICD-9-CM manuals, code the following:

1 Code a selective catheter placement in the first-order brachiocephalic artery, with angiography, including contrast with Tc-99m, 24 millicuries done at the clinic catheterization laboratory.

CPT Codes: _____, _____, _____

2 A cardiologist performs a selective catheter placement into the left external carotid artery (first-order branch) via a direct puncture to the left common carotid artery; a radiologist performs an angiographic procedure without contrast.

CPT Codes: _____, _____

3 A cardiologist performs selective catheter placement via the femoral artery. The catheter is advanced into the aorta and then into the left common carotid artery, terminating in the left external carotid artery. The radiologist performs an angiographic procedure without contrast.

CPT Codes: _____, _____

4 Complete cardiac MRI for morphology and function without contrast followed by contrast along with four additional sequences and stress imaging. Diagnosis of congestive heart failure and premature ventricular contractions.

CPT Code: _____

ICD-9-CM Codes: _____, _____

(ICD-10-CM Codes: _____, _____)

CHAPTER REVIEW

CHAPTER 16, PART I, THEORY

Without the use of reference material, complete the following:

1 What are the two subheadings within the Cardiovascular System subsection?

_____,

_____

2 The subspecialty of internal medicine that is concerned with the diagnosis and treatment of the heart is _____.

3 In Chapter 16 you learned about coding from which three sections of the CPT?

_____, _____, and

_____

4 Procedures that break the skin for correction or examination are known as _____ procedures.

5 Procedures that do not break the skin are known as _____ procedures.

6 The study of the heart's electrical system is known as _____.

7 The use of radioactive radiologic procedures to aid in the diagnosis of cardiologic conditions is termed _____ _____ cardiology.

8 A catheter that is inserted into an artery and manipulated to a further order is termed _____ placement.

9 A catheter that is inserted into an artery and not manipulated to a further order is termed _____ placement.

10 Surgical procedures in the Heart and Pericardium subheading contain procedures that are performed through both open surgical sites and _____.

CHAPTER 16, PART II, PRACTICAL

Code the following cases for the surgical procedures, the office visits, and the cardiology-related Radiology and Medicine section codes and the diagnoses codes. Do not code the laboratory work.

11 Dennis Smith, a 42-year-old railroad employee (established patient), has a history of severe mitral stenosis with regurgitation, rheumatic. He is now symptomatic and his physician recommends a mitral valve replacement, to be done in 2 weeks. Dennis agrees to the surgery, and the physician does a comprehensive history and physical in preparation for surgery. The physician orders a general health panel blood workup and a urinalysis (automated). Two weeks later, the physician performs a mitral valve replacement. Dennis recovers uneventfully and is discharged from the hospital 5 days later.

CPT Codes: _____,

_____

ICD-9-CM Code: _____

(ICD-10-CM Code: _____)

12 Thrombectomy of arterial graft

CPT Code: _____

13 Direct repair of aneurysm and graft insertion for occlusive disease of the common femoral artery

CPT Code: _____

14 A surgical assistant (MD) assists in performing five venous grafts in a coronary artery bypass procedure for arteriosclerosis of native arteries.

CPT Code: _____

ICD-9-CM Code: _____

(ICD-10-CM Code: _____)

15 Open-heart repair of mitral valve with use of cardiopulmonary bypass

CPT Code: _____

16 Removal of a single-chamber pacing cardioverter-defibrillator pulse generator, subcutaneous

CPT Code: _____

17 Pericardiotomy for removal of clot

CPT Code: _____

18 Complete repair of tetralogy of Fallot is made with closure of a ventricular septal defect, and a conduit from the pulmonary artery to the right ventricle is constructed. A pulmonary graft valve is then secured.

CPT Code: _____

19 Shunting from subclavian to pulmonary artery using the Blalock-Taussig operation for Fallot's tetralogy

CPT Code: _____

ICD-9-CM Code: _____

(ICD-10-CM Code: _____)

20 Pulmonary endarterectomy with embolectomy requiring cardiopulmonary bypass

CPT Code: _____

21 Direct repair of aneurysm associated with occlusion of the vertebral artery

CPT Code: _____

ICD-9-CM Codes: _____,

_____

(ICD-10-CM Codes: _____,

_____)

22 Thromboendarterectomy with patch graft of iliac artery

CPT Code: _____

ICD-9-CM Code: _____

(ICD-10-CM Code: _____)

QUICK CHECK ANSWERS

QUICK CHECK 16-1
1. Left and right coronary arteries. The rest are branches (e.g., circumflex branch of the left coronary artery).

QUICK CHECK 16-2
1. CABG

QUICK CHECK 16-3
1. Appendix L

QUICK CHECK 16-4
1. c. saphenous vein graft

"One of the benefits of working in medical coding is to know you're making a positive impact on the health care industry . . . . I consider myself as taking care of the patient by looking out for their best interest, especially with accuracy in diagnostic coding."

Sharon J. Oliver, CPC, CPC-I, CPMA

Sr. Inpatient Coder
East Tennessee State University
Physicians & Associates
Johnson City, Tennessee

Hemic, Lymphatic, Mediastinum, and Diaphragm

Chapter Topics

Hemic and Lymphatic Systems

Mediastinum and Diaphragm

Chapter Review

Quick Check Answers

Learning Objectives

After completing this chapter you should be able to

1 Review the Hemic and Lymphatic Systems subsection format.

2 Understand the Hemic and Lymphatic Systems subheadings.

3 Demonstrate the ability to code Hemic and Lymphatic System services.

4 Review the format of the Mediastinum and Diaphragm subsection codes.

5 Understand the Mediastinum and Diaphragm information.

6 Demonstrate the ability to code Mediastinum and Diaphragm services.

Make sure to check
evolve
learning system
**for the latest
content updates**

HEMIC AND LYMPHATIC SYSTEMS

Format

The Hemic and Lymphatic Systems subsection (38100-38999) is divided into subheadings: Spleen, General, and Lymph Nodes/Lymphatic Channels (Fig. 17–1). Further division is based on type of procedure (i.e., excision, incision, repair). The codes for spleen and lymph nodes are located in the CPT manual index under main terms such as Spleen, Lymph Nodes, or Bone Marrow.

FIGURE 17-1 Lymph nodes and lymph channels.

Coding Highlights

Spleen.   The spleen is composed of lymph tissue and is located in the left upper quadrant of the abdomen. The spleen is easily ruptured and may result in massive hemorrhage. The spleen initiates an immune response, filters, removes bacteria from the bloodstream, and destroys worn out blood cells. A person can live without a spleen because the bone marrow, liver, and lymph nodes take over the work of the spleen after a total removal (splenectomy).

Codes in the subheading Spleen (38100-38200) are further divided into categories of excision, repair, laparoscopy, and introduction. Codes in the Excision category are based on the type of splenectomy: total, partial, or total for extensive disease. The splenectomy (total and partial) carries the designation "(separate procedure)" behind the code description (38100, 38101). This means that if the splenectomy is an integral part of another procedure, it is bundled into the primary procedure code and not reported separately.

CODING SHOT   If a repair of a ruptured spleen was performed and the surgeon removed only a portion of the spleen, you would report only the repair code (38115) because removal is bundled into primary repair code.

Laparoscopy.   The surgical laparoscopy codes (38120, 38129) always include a diagnostic laparoscopy if one is performed. Report a diagnostic laparoscopy with 49320, Laparoscopy, abdomen, peritoneum, and omentum, diagnostic, with or without collection of specimen(s) by brushing or washing (separate procedure).

Introduction.   A splenoportography is an x-ray of the portal and circulatory vessels of the spleen. Code 38200 reports the injection portion of the procedure. The physician makes an incision in the left axilla area and inserts a catheter into the spleen. Radiopaque dye is inserted and x-rays are taken. The physician then removes the catheter and closes the area. The radiological supervision and interpretation portion of the service is reported with 75810.

General.   A marrow or blood cell transplant is a treatment for some blood diseases, such as leukemia or lymphoma. During the procedure, the patient's marrow or blood cells are replaced with healthy marrow or blood cells from a donor. There are three sources for blood cell formation: bone marrow, bloodstream, and umbilical cord. Bone marrow is the inner core of bones that manufactures most blood cells. Immature blood cells, called stem cells, originate in the marrow of bones. Leukemia is a malignant disease of the bone marrow in which excessive white blood cells are produced. Treatment often includes total-body irradiation or aggressive chemotherapy followed by transplantation of normal bone marrow. **Bone marrow aspiration** (38220) is a procedure in which a sample of the bone marrow is taken by means of a needle that is inserted into the marrow cavity. Marrow is then aspirated (pulled) through the needle and into the syringe. Usually the marrow is taken from the iliac crest, pelvic bone, or sternum. **Bone marrow biopsy** (38221) is a procedure in which small pieces of the marrow are obtained by means of a needle or trocar. These small chips are then processed in the laboratory by dissolving the pieces in a decalcification solution. The resulting substance is then analyzed and the service is reported with a Pathology/Laboratory code (88305). **Bone marrow harvesting** (38230) is a procedure in which a larger amount of marrow is aspirated from a donor by means of a large aspiration needle. The marrow is then transplanted into the recipient patient. **Transplantation,** 38240-38242, is a procedure in which the donor bone marrow or stem cells are injected into the patient. The preparation and storage of the cells prior to transplantation or infusion are reported with 38207-38215. **Allogenic** bone marrow is from the same species (human), such as a cadaver, a close relative, or a non-related donor. Testing is performed to determine a close genetic match for the recipient. **Autologous** bone marrow is collected from the patient, processed, and later transplanted or reinfused into the patient. **Stem cell harvesting** is the collection of stem cells from the blood system through a process termed apheresis. A needle is placed into a vein in one arm of the donor and the blood is removed. The blood is then filtered to remove the stem cells. The blood, with the stem cells removed, is returned to the donor through the other arm. Usually this process takes 4-6 hours and is usually completed in two sessions. The harvesting and return of the blood to the donor (replantation) is reported with codes 38205-38206.

QUICK CHECK 17-1

1. According to the notes in the CPT, the Bone Marrow/Stem Cell Services (38207-38215) may be reported only once per day.
   True or False?

Lymph Nodes and Lymphatic Channels

The lymphatic system is a transportation system to take fluids, proteins, and fats through the lymphatic channels and back to the bloodstream. Stations along the lymphatic system are called lymph nodes. The nodes fight disease when lymphocytes from the nodes produce antibodies. The subheading of Lymph Nodes and Lymphatic Channels is divided on the basis of the various procedures (i.e., incision, excision, resection, and introduction). The majority of the Excision codes (38500-38555) are for biopsy or excision based on the method (open or needle) and the location (e.g., axillary or cervical). For the open procedures, the choice of codes depends on whether the procedure was superficial (38500) or deep (38510-38530).

Within the Lymph Node and Lymphatic Channels subheading are two categories of codes for lymphadenectomies that are based on whether the lymphadenectomy is limited or radical. A **limited** lymphadenectomy (38562-38564) is the removal of the lymph nodes only; a **radical** lymphadenectomy (38700-38780) is the removal of the lymph nodes, gland(s), and surrounding tissue. Sometimes, a limited lymphadenectomy will be bundled into a more major procedure, such as prostatectomy. If this is the case, you would not report the lymphadenectomy separately. Rather, you would report only the more major procedure.

The codes to report a laparoscopic lymph node biopsy or removal are located in the 38571-38589 range. The codes are divided based on the extent of the procedure:

- 38570 reports single or multiple biopsy
- 38571 reports a bilateral total pelvic lymphadenectomy
- 38572 also reports a bilateral total pelvic lymphadenectomy and includes the single or multiple biopsy of the periaortic lymph node

A surgical laparoscopy always includes a diagnostic laparoscopy and is, therefore, not unbundled and reported separately. If only a diagnostic laparoscopy is performed, you would report the Digestive System code 49320.

QUICK CHECK 17-2

1. Review the Radical Lymphadenectomy codes (38700-38780). According to the parenthetical statements, what modifier may be used under appropriate circumstances? _____

Regions of Neck Lymph Nodes. The lymph nodes of the neck are named based on the anatomical location:

- Submental and submandibular nodes are located at the chin area and above (superior to) the mandibular.
- Upper jugular nodes are divided in two groups and are located at the mandibular angle and the front of the sternocleidomastoid muscle.
- Middle jugular nodes are located between the hyoid bone and the cricoid cartilage.
- Lower jugular nodes are located between the cricoid cartilage and the clavicle.
- Posterior triangle nodes that are divided into two groups.
- Upper visceral nodes are located by the hyoid bone.
- Superior mediastinal nodes are located between the left and right common carotid arteries.

Refer to Fig. 17–2 for the lymph vessels and nodes of the head and neck.

The term complete neck dissection in code 38720 is the same as radical neck dissection. During a complete or radical neck dissection, the lymph nodes in all five regions are resected (removed). In addition, the internal jugular vein, spinal accessory nerve, and sternocleidomastoid muscle are removed. The code is a unilateral code, so modifier -50 is required if a bilateral procedure is reported. A modified radical neck dissection as reported with 38724 is the removal of all lymph nodes that are routinely removed by radical neck dissection; however, the internal jugular vein, spinal accessory nerve, and sternocleidomastoid muscle are preserved rather than removed. The code is a unilateral code, so modifier -50 is required if a bilateral procedure is reported. The **suprahyoid neck dissection** is a variation of the modified radical neck dissection and is reported with 38700.

A lymphangiogram (38790) is a procedure in which contrast medium is injected into lymph vessels in the foot, and x-rays are taken to image the lymph flow. This procedure is often performed for staging and diagnosis of lymphoma. **Staging** is determining the grade or level of a neoplasm based on a common grading system, such as the TNM (tumors, nodes, and metastases). A unilateral procedure is reported with 38790. The radiological supervision and interpretation portion of the service is reported with codes 75801-75807.

NCCI

Sentinel node biopsy may be indicated in breast carcinoma and is eligible for Medicare reimbursement when the following conditions are met:

1. Clinical Stage I and II carcinoma of the breast (primary tumor 2.0-5.0 cm in size with no palpable lymph nodes in the axilla)
2. Sentinel lymph node biopsy is negative and axillary lymphadenectomy is not planned

Examples of payable diagnosis codes: 172.0-172.9, 174.0-174.9, 175.0-175.9

Superficial parotid nodes
(deep parotid nodes
deep to and within
parotid gland)

Subparotid node

Facial nodes
Nasolabial
Buccinator

Mandibular
nodes

Submandibular
nodes

Submental
nodes

Suprahyoid node

Superior deep lateral cervical
(internal jugular) nodes

Superior thyroid nodes

Juguloomohyoid node

Anterior deep cervical
(pretracheal and thyroid) nodes
(deep to infrahyoid muscles)

Anterior superficial cervical
nodes (anterior jugular nodes)

Jugular trunk

Supraclavicular nodes*

Subclavian trunk and node

Occipital nodes

Mastoid nodes

Sternocleidomastoid
nodes

Superior lateral
superficial cervical
(external jugular)
node

Jugulodigastric node

Posterior lateral
superficial cervical
(spinal accessory)
nodes

Intercalated node

Inferior deep
lateral cervical
(scalene) node

Thoracic duct

Transverse
cervical
chain of
nodes

*The supraclavicular group of nodes (also
known as the lower deep cervical group),
especially on the left, are also sometimes
referred to as the signal or sentinel lymph
nodes of Virchow or Troisier, especially when
sufficiently enlarged and palpable. These
nodes (or a single node) are so termed because
they may be the first recognized presumptive
evidence of malignant disease in the viscera.

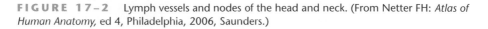

FIGURE 17–2 Lymph vessels and nodes of the head and neck. (From Netter FH: *Atlas of Human Anatomy*, ed 4, Philadelphia, 2006, Saunders.)

A sentinel lymph node biopsy is bundled into a planned lymphadenectomy and not paid separately. The injection of dye to visualize the sentinel node should be reported by the surgeon/physician who performs the injection with 38792. This code is reported only once for the injection of the dye regardless of the number of injections made around the lesion.

EXERCISE 17-1   *Hemic and Lymphatic Systems*

Using the CPT and ICD-9-CM manuals, code the following:

1 Excision of an axillary cystic hygroma, which the patient medical record indicates involved no deep neurovascular dissection

    CPT Code: ___38550___

    ICD-9-CM Code: ___228.1___ (ICD-10-CM Code: _____)

2 Total removal of the spleen due to Gaucher's splenomegaly

    CPT Code: ___38100___

    ICD-9-CM Code: ___272.7___ (ICD-10-CM Code: _____)

3 Injection procedure for a radiographic view of the portal vein of the spleen

    CPT Code: ___38200___

4 Bone marrow transplant, autologous

    CPT Code: ___38241___

MEDIASTINUM AND DIAPHRAGM

Mediastinum

The mediastinum is the area between the lungs (Fig. 17–3). The Mediastinum subheading of the Mediastinum and Diaphragm subsection (39000-39599) of the CPT manual is divided by procedures and includes incision, excision, and endoscopy.

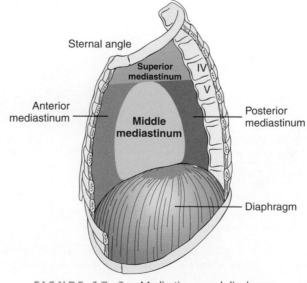

FIGURE 17–3   Mediastinum and diaphragm.

Incision. The difference between the mediastinotomy codes (39000, 39010) is the surgical approach. The approach can be either cervical (neck area), across the thoracic area (transthoracic), or sternum. A mediastinotomy is performed by making an incision next to the breastbone for the purposes of exploration, drainage, removal of a foreign body, or biopsy. You may think removal of a foreign body would be in the Excision codes, but the Excision codes are only reported for cysts or tumors.

Excision. Excision codes 39200 and 39220 are based on whether a cyst or tumor was excised. The surgical approach is one in which the surgeon makes the incision just below the nipple line and retracts the rib cage and muscles to expose the thoracic cavity. The cyst or tumor is removed and the incision closed.

If the thyroid gland is removed using an excision into the mediastinum, the procedure is reported with 60270 from the Endocrine System subsection and not with an excision code from the Mediastinum subcategory. Also, if the thymus gland is removed using a mediastinum approach, you would report the procedure with 60520.

Endoscopy. There is only one mediastinoscopy code (39400) and the procedure includes any biopsy performed during the procedure. The procedure is performed by making a small incision above the sternum. The scope is inserted through the incision for exploration (and/or biopsy) performed.

Diaphragm

The diaphragm is the wall of muscle that separates the thoracic and abdominal cavities. The codes in the Diaphragm subheading (39501-39599) are repair codes. Repairs are usually for a hernia or laceration. Diaphragm codes are located in the CPT manual index under "Diaphragm."

There is one code for imbrication of the diaphragm. An imbrication of the diaphragm may be performed for eventration, which is when the diaphragm moves up, usually because of the paralysis of the diaphragmatic nerve (phrenic nerve). In this case the surgeon sutures the diaphragm back into place.

EXERCISE 17-2 *Mediastinum and Diaphragm*

Using the CPT and ICD-9-CM manuals, code the following:

1 Repair of paraesophageal hiatus hernia, abdominal approach, with limited fundoplasty

CPT Code: _____43336_____

ICD-9-CM Code: _____553.3_____ (ICD-10-CM Code: _____)

2 Exploratory mediastinotomy with biopsy of mediastinal lesion accomplished with approach through the neck. Pathology report later indicated primary, malignant neoplasm.

CPT Code: _____39000_____

ICD-9-CM Code: _____164.9_____ (ICD-10-CM Code: _____)

3 Excision of benign tumor of the mediastinum

CPT Code: _____39220_____

ICD-9-CM Code: _____212.5_____ (ICD-10-CM Code: _____)

4 Repair of an esophageal hiatal hernia accomplished with approach across the thoracic area

CPT Code: _____43334_____

CHAPTER REVIEW

CHAPTER 17, PART I, THEORY

Complete the following:

1 The difference between the mediastinum incision codes is the surgical _____.

2 The spleen initiates an immune response, filters and removes _____ from the bloodstream and destroys worn out blood cells.

3 Total or partial splenectomy codes are designated in the CPT manual as _____ procedures.

4 A marrow or _____ _____ transplant is a treatment for patients with blood diseases, such as leukemia or lymphoma.

5 A bone marrow _____ is a procedure in which a sample of bone marrow is taken by means of a needle that is inserted into the marrow cavity.

6 A(n) _____ bone marrow comes from a close relative.

7 A(n) _____ bone marrow comes from the patient, is processed, and later transplanted or reinfused.

8 A(n) _____ lymphadenectomy is the removal of the lymph node only.

9 The Mediastinum category of codes is based on the _____ _____ taken to perform the mediastinotomy.

10 Another name for the diaphragmatic nerve is the _____ nerve.

CHAPTER 17, PART II, PRACTICAL

Code the following cases:

11 Using a cervical approach, ligation of the thoracic duct was accomplished.

CPT Code: _____

12 Surgical laparoscopy with bilateral total pelvic lymphadenectomy

CPT Code: _____

13 Superficial inguinofemoral lymphadenectomy with pelvic lymphadenectomy including the external iliac, hypogastric, and obturator nodes

CPT Code: _____

14 Diaphragmatic resection of a secondary, malignant lesion that included extensive use of prosthetic material. The primary malignancy was of the uterus, which has been previously removed, followed by a course of radiation and chemotherapy.

CPT Code: _____

ICD-9-CM Code: _____

(ICD-10-CM Code: _____)

15 Excisional biopsy of superficial lymph nodes of the neck by means of an open procedure for non-Hodgkin's lymphoma

CPT Code: _____

ICD-9-CM Code: _____

16 Dissection of the deep jugular nodes, diagnosis of thyroid gland primary cancer

CPT Code: _____

ICD-9-CM Code: _____

(ICD-10-CM Code: _____)

17 Excision of congenital cervical cystic hygroma with dissection of deep neurovascularity

CPT Code: _____

ICD-9-CM Code: _____

(ICD-10-CM Code: _____)

18 Limited lymphadenectomy for staging of para-aortic lymph nodes in malignant primary prostate cancer

CPT Code: _____

ICD-9-CM Code: _____

(ICD-10-CM Code: _____)

19 Bilateral injection procedure for lymphangiography of axillary node enlargement

CPT Code: _____

ICD-9-CM Code: _____

(ICD-10-CM Code: _____)

20 Mediastinoscopy with biopsy for mass

CPT Code: _____

ICD-9-CM Code: _____

(ICD-10-CM Code: _____)

QUICK CHECK ANSWERS

QUICK CHECK 17-1
1. True

QUICK CHECK 17-2
1. -50

CHAPTER *18*

"Continuing education is vital. Gain as much knowledge and experience in other specialties, fields, or branches of HIM as possible."

Cynthia Stahl, CPC, CCS-P, CPC-H
Reimbursement and Coding Specialist
Lebanon, Indiana

Digestive System

Chapter Topics

Format

Lips

Vestibule of Mouth

Tongue and Floor of Mouth

Dentoalveolar Structures

Palate and Uvula

Salivary Gland and Ducts

Pharynx, Adenoids, and Tonsils

Esophagus

Stomach

Intestines (Except Rectum)

Meckel's Diverticulum and the Mesentery

Appendix

Rectum

Anus

Liver

Biliary Tract

Pancreas

Abdomen, Peritoneum, and Omentum

Chapter Review

Quick Check Answers

Learning Objectives

After completing this chapter you should be able to

1 Understand the format of the Digestive System subsection.
2 Report procedures of the lips.
3 Report procedures of the vestibule of mouth.
4 Report procedures of the tongue and floor of mouth.
5 Report procedures of the dentoalveolar structures.
6 Report procedures of the palate and uvula.
7 Report procedures of the salivary gland and ducts.
8 Report procedures of the pharynx, adenoids, and tonsils.
9 Report procedures of the esophagus.
10 Report procedures of the stomach.
11 Report procedures of the intestines (except rectum).
12 Report procedures of the Meckel's diverticulum and mesentery.
13 Report procedures of the appendix.
14 Report procedures of the rectum.
15 Report procedures of the anus.
16 Report procedures of the liver.
17 Report procedures of the biliary tract.
18 Report procedures of the pancreas.
19 Report procedures of the abdomen, peritoneum, and omentum.

Make sure to check
evolve
learning system
for the latest content updates

FORMAT   The format of the Digestive System subsection (40490-49999) is divided according to anatomic site (Fig. 18–1) and procedure. Included in this subsection are codes for sites beginning with the mouth and ending with the anus. Also included are those internal organs that aid in the digestive process, including the pancreas, liver, and gallbladder.

This subsection includes codes for procedures of the abdomen, peritoneum, omentum, and hernia repairs. Endoscopic codes are located throughout the subsection on the basis of the anatomic site.

LIPS   Codes in the Lips subheading (40490-40799) include the categories of Excision, Repair (Cheiloplasty), and Other Procedures. If the procedure was performed on the skin of the lips, assign a code from the Integumentary System, not a Digestive System code.

A **vermilionectomy** (40500) is shaving of the lip. The vermilion zone is the red part of the lips (Fig. 18–2). The surgeon removes an area of tissue and repairs the defect by moving the mucosal surface to reconnect the lip, thereby forming a new vermilion border. If the area of defect is larger, a more extensive excisional procedure may be necessary (40510-40527). For example, during a **transverse wedge excision** (40510) a wedge of lip tissue is removed and tissue flaps are placed to repair the defect. Code 40525 describes a full-thickness lip excision with reconstruction with local flap.

FIGURE 18–1   Digestive system.

FIGURE 18-2 Vermilion border. (Modified from Liebgott B: *The Anatomical Basis of Dentistry,* ed 2, St. Louis, 2001, Mosby, Inc.)

There are many services bundled into 40525, such as:

- 11440-11444 and 11446 (benign lesion excision)
- 11640-11644 and 11646 (malignant lesion excision)
- 40500 (vermilionectomy with mucosal advancement)
- 40510 and 40520 (excision of lip)

The **Abbe-Estlander** (40527, also known as Abbe' flap or cross flap) is a reconstructive procedure in which a graft is taken from a portion of the lip and the non-defective area above the lip is used to repair the area of defect. For example, a patient had cancer of the lower lip due to smoking, as illustrated in Fig. 18–3, *A.* The surgeon removed the area of defect from the lower lip and identified a superior (above lip) flap. In Fig. 18–3, *B,* the superior flap was moved to cover the area of defect. Fig. 18–3, *C,* illustrates the results of the **reconstruction**. If more than one-fourth of the lip surface is removed, the procedure is considered a **resection** and is reported with 40530. If reconstruction of the lip is required to repair the defect that remains after the resection, the procedure is reported separately with a code from 13131-13153 (complex repair of lip and face). The reconstruction code is assigned based on location and size of the defect.

FIGURE 18-3 **A,** Abbe-Estlander flap for lip reconstruction with defective area excised and flap area outlined. **B,** Abbe-Estlander flap for lip reconstruction with flap moved down and positioned in defect area. **C,** Completed Abbe-Estlander flap. (From Kavanagh KT: Abbe-Estlander Flap for Lip Reconstruction in a Patient with Skin Cancer of the Lower Lip, Ear, Nose & Throat - U.S.A. (website): www.entusa.com/abbe_estlander.htm. Accessed January 25, 2008.)

QUICK CHECK 18-1

1. An Abbe-Estlander flap is also known as an Abbe' or _____ flap.

The codes for **cheiloplasty** (lip repair) are located in the Repair category. There are two types of Repair codes: those that report full-thickness repair of the lip (40650-40654) and those that report cleft lip repair (40700-40761). The full-thickness repairs are based on the extent of the repair, for example, vermilion only (40650), up to half of the vertical height of the lip (40652), and over one-half of the vertical height of the lip (40654, complex repair).

A **cleft lip** is a congenital defect in which the muscle and tissue of the lip did not close properly. Fig. 18–4, *A,* illustrates a unilateral defect and Fig. 18–4, *B,* illustrates a bilateral defect. Some of the cleft lip Repair codes report bilateral procedures (40701, 40702) and other codes report unilateral procedures (40700, 40720). If a bilateral procedure was performed and the code description does not indicate a bilateral procedure, add modifier -50.

A **rhinoplasty** may be required if a nasal deformity has occurred with the cleft lip defect. These defects occur when the muscle, rather than encircling the mouth, attaches to the nose and pulls the nose out of normal position. If a rhinoplasty is performed with a cleft lip repair, the rhinoplasty is reported separately with 30460 or 30462. **A cleft** palate may also be present with a cleft lip, and if repair of the palate is performed at the time of the lip repair, the palate repair is reported separately with codes from the 42200 series. For example, 42205 reports a palatoplasty for a cleft palate with closure of the soft tissue of the alveolar ridge.

VESTIBULE OF MOUTH

The vestibule of the mouth is also known as the buccal cavity and is part of the oral cavity. Codes for the Vestibule of Mouth (40800-40899) do not include codes for services of the Tongue and Floor of Mouth (41000-41599) or Dentoalveolar Structures (41800-41899). The categories included within the Vestibule of the Mouth subheading are incisions (e.g., abscess, cyst, or hematoma), excision/destruction (e.g., biopsy or lesion excision), and repair (e.g., closure or vestibuloplasty). The procedures are based on the complexity of the procedure (e.g., simple or complex), and whether the procedure is bilateral or unilateral.

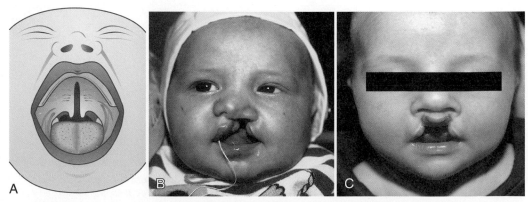

FIGURE 18–4 **A,** Cleft palate. **B,** Unilateral cleft lip. Note the nasal deformity in which the nose is out of normal position. **C,** Bilateral cleft lip. (**A** from Buck CJ: *2010 ICD-9-CM, Volumes 1, 2, & 3, Professional Edition,* St. Louis, 2010, Saunders. **B** and **C** from Zitelli BJ, Davis HW: *Atlas of Pediatric Physical Diagnosis,* ed 5, Philadelphia, 2007, Mosby.)

TONGUE AND FLOOR OF MOUTH

The Tongue and Floor of Mouth subheading (41000-41599) includes codes to report the incision and drainage of abscess, cyst, or hematoma of the tongue or floor of the mouth. These incision and drainage codes (41000-41009) are based on the location of the abscess, cyst, or hematoma, such as under the tongue **(sublingual)**, under the mandible **(submandibular)**, or within the space from the floor of the mouth to the hyoid bone **(masticator space)**. The sublingual codes are further based on whether the abscess, cyst, or hematoma is superficial or deep.

The **lingual frenum** is the flap of skin under the tongue. **Ankyloglossia** (tongue tie) is illustrated in Fig. 18–5 and is due to a tight lingual frenum. This condition is often diagnosed by the pediatrician during a newborn examination. Ankyloglossia occurs in 4.8% of the population and may interfere with feeding. The procedure in which an incision is made in this flap is a frenotomy. The incision procedure (41010) frees the tongue to allow greater motion. During a frenotomy, the lingual frenum is only incised, not excised. If a frenectomy (excision of the lingual frenum) is performed, the service is reported with 41115 from the Excision category. If the lingual frenum is surgically repaired (frenoplasty) the procedure is reported with 41520 from the Other Procedures category.

Extraoral incision and drainage (I&D) is performed on an abscess, cyst, or hematoma located outside the mouth or on the floor of the mouth. Code range 41015-41018 reports extraoral (outside the mouth) incision and drainage based on the location of sublingual, submental (under the chin), submandibular, or masticator space. The masticator space is a deep facial space, bounded by the superficial layer of deep cervical fascia and containing the four muscles of mastication, ramus, and posterior body of the mandible.

Excision codes (41100-41155) report oral biopsies, excision of oral lesions, and removal of all or part of the tongue (glossectomy). The biopsy codes (41100-41108) are reported based on the location from which the biopsy was obtained. The codes for excision of a lesion are also based on the location (such as floor of mouth, tongue, or lingual frenum). If a local tongue flap is required to repair the excisional defect, report the repair with 41114 in addition to the code for the primary excision procedure.

FIGURE 18–5 Ankyloglossia. (From Grosfeld JL, O'Neill JA, Coran AG, Fonkalsrud EW, Caldamone AA: *Pediatric Surgery,* ed 6, St. Louis, 2006, Mosby.)

Repair (41250-41252) of the tongue is reported based on the size of the repair:

- 2.5 cm or less
- Over 2.6 cm

In addition to the size, the tongue repair codes are also based on the location of the repair:

- Anterior two thirds
- Posterior one third or floor of mouth

If the length of the repair is stated in inches, the measurement must be converted to centimeters. One inch equals 2.54 cm and the formula for conversion is:

- Centimeters × 0.3937008 = inches
- Inches × 2.54 = centimeters

If the repair is stated in millimeters (mm) the conversion to centimeters is:

- 1 millimeter = 0.1 centimeters

For example, if the medical record indicated 15 millimeters, the calculation would be 15 × 0.1 = 1.5 centimeters.

DENTOALVEOLAR STRUCTURES

The dentoalveolar structures are the bone (osseous) and soft structures of the mouth that anchor the teeth (Fig. 18–6). Codes 41800-41899 report incision, excision/destruction, and other types of procedures performed on the dentoalveolar structures. Examples of these procedures include drainage of an abscess, cyst, or hematoma (41800) or excision of a lesion with simple repair (41826). Some of the codes are based on the quadrant in which the procedure is performed, such as excision of the gingiva (gingivectomy) reported with 41820 for each quadrant or, as another example, excision of the alveolar mucosa reported with 41828 for each quadrant.

The American Dental Association (ADA) publishes a dental claim form, as illustrated in Fig. 18–7, and this is the form that is most often used to report dental services.

FIGURE 18–6 Alveolar mucosa. (From Liebgott B: *The Anatomical Basis of Dentistry,* ed 2, St. Louis, 2001, Mosby, Inc.)

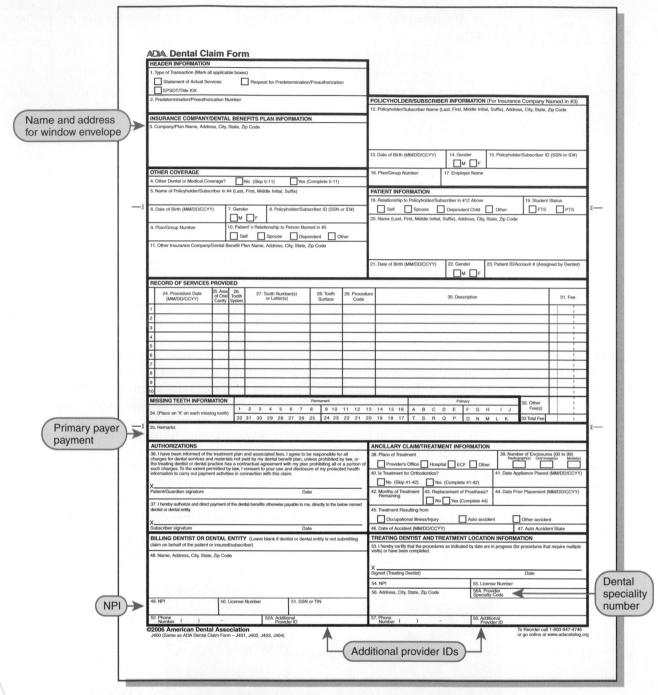

FIGURE 18–7 American Dental Association (ADA) dental claim form. (From American Dental Association: *ADA Dental Claim Form* (website): www.ada.org/prof/resources/topics/topics_claimform. pdf. Accessed February 27, 2009.) Copyright © American Dental Association. Used with permission. Unauthorized copying strictly prohibited.

NCCI

For current information on the dental coverage for Medicare patients refer to the Internet Only Manuals (IOM) (www.cms.hhs.gov/Manuals/IOM/list.asp) 100-01, Chapter 5, Section 70.2 and 100-02, Chapter 15, Section 150.

PALATE AND UVULA

Services to the palate (roof of mouth) and uvula (pendulous structure at the back of the throat) are reported with codes 42000-42299. This subheading contains the usual codes for incision, excision/destruction, and repair. If grafting is required to repair the area of defect after excision of a lesion, the grafting service is reported in addition to the excision code. The choice of grafting codes is based on whether a skin graft (14040-14302) or an oral mucosal graft (40818) was used for repair. Within the Repair codes you will also locate the codes to report repair procedures for cleft palate (42200-42225), as discussed previously.

Code 42145 describes a palatopharyngoplasty (palate and pharynx repair) procedure and has limited medically indicated reasons for the surgical procedure. One medically indicated reason for the procedure is obstructive sleep apnea (OSA) that is documented to be unresponsive to conservative measures, such as continuous positive airway pressure [CPAP], positional therapy, dental devices, and weight loss. OSA is characterized by frequent episodes of hypopnea (shallow breathing) or apnea during sleep.

SALIVARY GLAND AND DUCTS

There are three salivary glands as illustrated in Fig. 18–8 (parotid, submandibular, and sublingual). It is important to note the technique for performing biopsy procedures of the salivary glands. Code 42400 states the biopsy of the salivary gland using a needle technique, and 42405 uses an incisional approach. There is an injection procedure that is reported

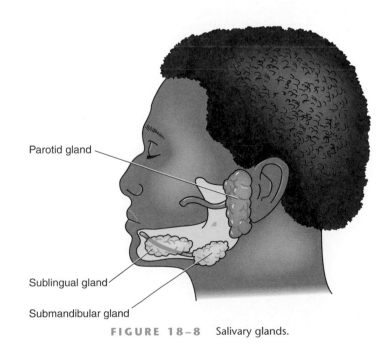

Parotid gland

Sublingual gland

Submandibular gland

FIGURE 18–8   Salivary glands.

with 42550 for a sialography (x-ray of salivary gland) and the radiological component of the procedure is reported with 70390. It is important to read all notes before or after a code description because the parenthetical statement in the CPT manual located after 42550 directs the coder to report the radiological supervision and interpretation with 70390. Imaging guidance may be used for salivary gland biopsy (42400) and is reported in addition to the biopsy service depending on the guidance type—77002 (fluoroscopic), 77012 (CT), 77021 (MRI), or 76942 (ultrasound).

The codes in this subheading (42300-42699) are often divided based on the gland. For example, excision of a tumor of the parotid gland is reported with 42410; of the submandibular gland, 42440; and of the sublingual gland, 42450. Other services are reported based on the number of glands involved. The parotid duct is a duct opening from the cheek into the vestibule of the mouth opposite the neck of the upper second molar tooth as illustrated in Fig. 18–9. The parotid duct is also known as the Steno's or Stensen's duct. When a gland is excised with the parotid duct diversion, the service for both the diversion and excision of one submandibular gland is reported with 42508. If the excision is of both submandibular glands, report the service with 42509.

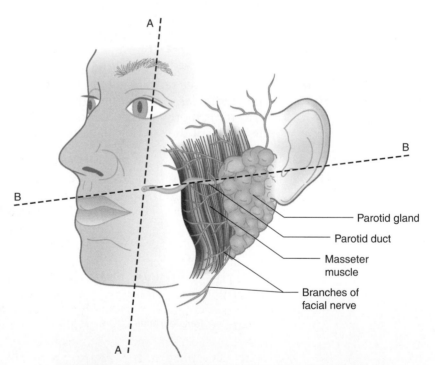

FIGURE 18–9 Parotid gland and duct (Stensen's) with the surrounding branches of the facial nerve. Line B approximates the course of the duct, which enters the mouth at the junction of lines A and B. (From Marx JA, ed: *Rosen's Emergency Medicine: Concepts and Clinical Practice*, ed 6, Philadelphia, 2006, Mosby.)

EXERCISE 18-1 *Lips, Vestibule of Mouth, Tongue, and Floor of Mouth, Dentoalverolar Structures, Palate, and Uvula, Salivary Gland and Ducts*

Using the CPT and ICD-9-CM manuals, complete the following:

1 A _____ is shaving of the lip.

2 In addition to the sites from the mouth to the anus, the Digestive System codes include codes for the pancreas, liver, and _____.

3 How many centimeters are there in 4 inches (round to the nearest tenth)? _____

4 An Abbe-Estlander reconstruction

   CPT Code: _____

   ICD-9-CM Code: _____ (ICD-10-CM Code: _____)

5 A complex, full-thickness repair of the vermilion after resection of buccal-mucosal squamous cell carcinoma

   CPT Code: _____

   ICD-9-CM Code: _____ (ICD-10-CM Code: _____)

6 Simple drainage of a hematoma of the vestibule of the mouth

   Code: _____

7 Repair of a laceration of the tongue, measuring 1.5 inches

   Code: _____

PHARYNX, ADENOIDS, AND TONSILS

It is within the 42700-42999 range of codes that you will locate the often reported codes for tonsillectomy and adenoidectomy. In addition there are codes for biopsies, excisions, and repair procedures.

The Incision category (42700-42725) codes report the drainage of an abscess. The codes are assigned based on the **location** (peritonsillar [behind the tonsil], retropharyngeal [behind the pharynx], parapharyngeal [adjacent to the pharynx]) of the abscess and the **approach** utilized (intraoral or external). Careful reading of the operative report is necessary to identify the location and approach to ensure correct code assignment.

Biopsy codes 42800-42806 include obtaining the biopsy sample but do not include the use of a scope to obtain the sample. If a laryngoscopic biopsy is performed, the service is reported with a code from the Respiratory System, not with a code from the Digestive System. For example, 31510 (indirect diagnostic, views through reflection with a mirror), 31535 (direct operative, views with a scope), or 31536 (direct operative, views direct with scope, plus operating microscope assistance).

A **branchial cleft** cyst is a congenital defect that appears as a gill located on the neck. Branchia is Greek for gills, which the cyst resembles. Reporting an excision of the branchial cleft cyst is based on the extent of the procedure. If the extent of the defect was confined to the skin and subcutaneous tissue, report the service with 42810. If the defect extended beneath the subcutaneous tissue and perhaps into the pharynx, report the service with 42815.

Tonsillectomy and **adenoidectomy** are commonly reported surgical procedures (42820-42836). The tonsils are two glands located at the back of the throat (Fig. 18–10, *A*), and the adenoids (Fig. 18–10, *B*) are located behind the nose and above the soft palate (roof of mouth) and cannot be visualized without a mirror or scope. The selection of the correct code is based on if:

■ Only the tonsils are removed
■ Only the adenoids are removed
■ Both the tonsils and adenoids are removed
■ The patient is under 12 years of age, age 12, over age 12

Many codes contain age descriptors or primary (initial removal) or secondary (subsequent removal of tissue that has grown back).

CODING SHOT

> The codes for tonsillectomy and/or adenoidectomy in the range 42820-42836 are performed bilaterally. If a procedure is reported with the -50 modifier, or with modifiers -RT and -LT, the third-party payer will usually not recognize the modifier(s) and will pay based on the amount for a single procedure. If only one side is removed, modifier -52 (Reduced service) must be appended to the CPT code.

A **pharyngoplasty** (42950) is the surgical repair of the pharynx and includes the use of flaps fashioned from the skin, tongue, and/or tissue located near the area of defect (regional cutaneous flaps) used in the repair procedure. If a pharyngeal flap is used, report the service with 42225, as directed in the parenthetical note.

A **pharyngostomy** (42955) is a procedure to create an opening for insertion of a long-term feeding tube. An incision is made below the jaw line on the skin and the incision is carried down to the pharynx. The opening is reinforced with sutures, and a long-term feeding tube is inserted through the opening into the pharynx. A nasogastric feeding tube (NGT, nose to stomach) is a more well-known method, but in some patients (i.e., severe facial trauma), pharyngostomy is the necessary approach.

Codes to report the control of oropharyngeal (between the soft palate and the epiglottis) or nasopharyngeal (above the soft palate) hemorrhage are located in the Other Procedures subheading (42955-42999). Codes 42960-42972 (esophagotomy or myotomy) are reported based on whether the procedure is a primary or secondary procedure and the level of complexity.

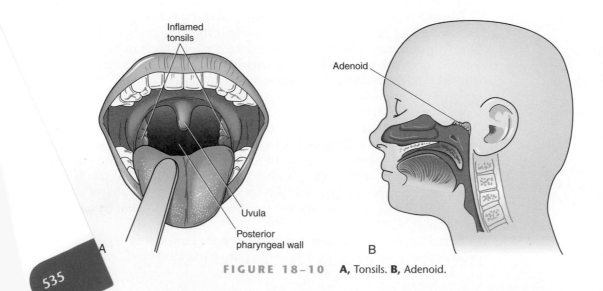

Inflamed tonsils

Adenoid

Uvula

Posterior pharyngeal wall

A

B

FIGURE 18–10 **A,** Tonsils. **B,** Adenoid.

ESOPHAGUS   Procedures of the esophagus are reported with codes in the 43020-43499 range and are performed by incision, excision, and endoscopy. The **approach** is the first step to determine selection of the correct code. For example, 43100 describes the excision of lesion, esophagus, with primary repair; cervical approach and 43101 describes the same procedure but with a thoracic or abdominal approach. Codes 43200-43228 report endoscopic services limited to the esophagus. The scope may be advanced into the stomach but does not advance to the pylorus (stricture at end of stomach).

The types of esophagus procedures are diagnostic endoscopy, injection, biopsy, removal of foreign body, insertion of plastic tube/stent, dilation, and hemorrhage control. Some codes, such as 43220 (balloon dilation), do not include imaging guidance (74360), whereas other codes include the guidance, such as 43231 (diagnostic esophagoscopy with endoscopic ultrasound examination). Note that many codes include conscious sedation as a part of the service as indicated by the bullseye symbol to the left of the code.

The Incision codes include both cervical approach (43020) and thoracic approach (43045) for removal of a foreign body as illustrated in Fig. 18–11. It is important to confirm the approach used when coding removal of a foreign body from the esophagus. The Excision codes (43100-43135) also include various approaches in the code description, such as cervical, thoracic, and abdominal.

If a lesion is removed from the esophagus, report the service with 43100 (cervical) or 43101 (thoracic or abdominal) depending on the approach used. If a partial, near total, or total removal (wide excision) of the esophagus is performed with total removal of the larynx, the service may or may not include extensive (radical) neck dissection. These removal services are reported with 43107, 43116 (with graft), 43124, or 31360 (total laryngectomy from the Respiratory System). Note that some of these codes also specify the approach. For example, 43116 indicates a cervical approach.

Code 43200 describes an esophagoscopy, by means of either a rigid or flexible scope. The procedure is diagnostic and may be with or without the collection of specimen(s). The specimens are collected by brushing or washing. Code 43200 is categorized as a separate procedure and is only reported if no other more major esophageal procedure was performed. The 43200 service is a diagnostic service and is always bundled into the surgical service.

Medical necessity for a diagnostic procedure must be documented in the medical record. For example, the signs and/or symptoms demonstrate the medical necessity of the service. If the service has 0 global days, this

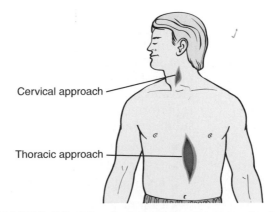

FIGURE 18–11   Cervical and thoracic approaches for removal of a foreign body.

means the procedure includes all preoperative and postoperative care related to performing the procedure on the day of the procedure; but before or after the day of the procedure any services related to the procedure are reported separately. The 43200 diagnostic esophagoscopy is bundled into all endoscopy procedures reported with 43201-43232 and 43234-43259.

Codes 43201-43232 describe therapeutic procedures on the esophagus. Code 43201 describes a rigid or flexible esophagoscopy with submucosal injections of any substance. You must report the substance injected. For example, botulinum toxin (J0585) to treat esophageal spasms.

Code 43202 describes an esophagoscopy (rigid or flexible) with biopsy (single or multiple). Report this code only once (one unit) no matter how many biopsies were taken because the code description indicates multiple biopsies. As with all codes, the diagnosis must support the medical necessity of the esophagoscopy. For example, some diagnoses that would support the medical necessity of the esophagoscopy would be 530.83, esophageal leukoplakia, 530.81, esophageal reflux, or 787.20, unspecified dysphagia.

Code 43215 reports a rigid or flexible esophagoscopy for removal of a foreign body. The medical necessity of this procedure would be demonstrated by a diagnosis code such as 935.1 (foreign body in esophagus). If radiology is used during the procedure, report the radiology service with 74235 (Removal of foreign body(s), esophageal, with use of balloon catheter, radiological supervision and interpretation).

The removal or ablation of esophageal polyp, tumor, or other lesion is reported with 43216 or 43217. The codes are divided based on technique (hot biopsy forceps, bipolar cautery, snare). Make a note in your CPT manual next to these two codes as a reminder the technique used for the removal determines the code selected.

The following dilation procedures may use fluoroscopy (74360) but do not include endoscopy:

- 43450, dilation of the esophagus, by unguided sound or bougie (cylinder), single or multiple passes
- 43453, dilation of the esophagus, over guidewire
- 43456, dilation of the esophagus, by balloon or dilator, retrograde (against the flow)
- 43458, dilation of the esophagus for condition of achalasia (difficulty swallowing due to the failure of the muscle ring at the upper end of the stomach to relax), with a balloon 30 mm diameter or larger
- 43460, esophagogastric tamponade, with balloon (Sengstaaken type) (A balloon is placed into the esophagus and inflated to stop bleeding.)

If an endoscopy is performed in addition to any of these dilation procedures, report the endoscopy service separately.

A submucosal injection is one that is performed to ease the removal of polyps. Fluid, usually saline, is injected around the polyp and the fluid elevates the polyp to allows for easier excision. When a submucosal injection is performed, report the service based on the delivery method. For example, submucosal injection by means of:

- Esophagoscopy, 43201
- EGD, 43236
- Sigmoidoscopy, 45335
- Colonoscopy, 45381

An **EGD** (esophagogastroduodenoscopy) is a procedure performed to examine the esophagus, stomach, duodenum, and sometimes the jejunum for signs of bleeding, tumors, erosion, ulcers, or other abnormalities.

The EGD is often performed in conjunction with another procedure. For example, code 43405 reports an EGD with suturing of the esophagogastric junction. During this procedure, a special suturing system is inserted through the scope, the physician then places a series of stitches in the esophagogastric junction, essentially pleating the sphincter to prevent the backflow of stomach acid into the esophagus. The medical necessity of the procedure would be demonstrated with a diagnosis code, such as 530.81, esophageal reflux [ICD-10-CM: K21.9].

CODING SHOT — EGD code 43259 is assigned when an endoscopic **ultrasound** examination is performed. The radiological supervision and interpretation is reported separately with 76975.

More than one procedure may be performed during the same operative session. For example, an EGD performed with **biopsy** and **dilation** of gastric outlet due to obstruction. The services are performed during the same endoscopic session and are reported as:

- **43245** (Upper gastrointestinal endoscopy including esophagus, stomach, and either the duodenum and/or jejunum as appropriate; with **dilation** of gastric outlet for obstruction, any method)

- **43239** (Upper gastrointestinal endoscopy; including esophagus, stomach, and either the duodenum and/or jejunum as appropriate; with **biopsy**, single or multiple)

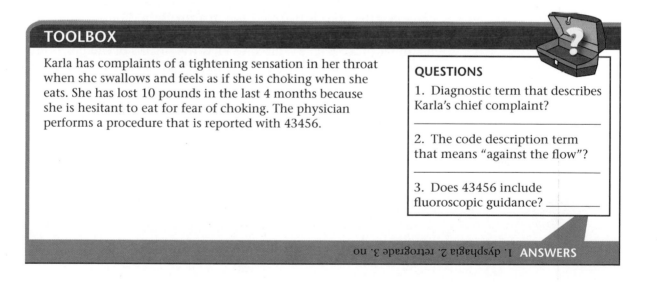

TOOLBOX

Karla has complaints of a tightening sensation in her throat when she swallows and feels as if she is choking when she eats. She has lost 10 pounds in the last 4 months because she is hesitant to eat for fear of choking. The physician performs a procedure that is reported with 43456.

QUESTIONS

1. Diagnostic term that describes Karla's chief complaint?

2. The code description term that means "against the flow"?

3. Does 43456 include fluoroscopic guidance? _____

ANSWERS 1. dysphagia 2. retrograde 3. no

An endoscopic retrograde cholangiopancreatography (**ERCP,** 43260-43272) is an endoscopic procedure of the pancreatic ducts, hepatic ducts, common bile ducts, duodenal papilla, and/or gallbladder (hepatobiliary system) and is performed primarily to diagnose and treat conditions of the bile ducts, including gallstones, inflammatory strictures (scars), leaks (due to trauma or surgery), and cancer. ERCP combines the use of x-rays and endoscope. Through the endoscope, the physician can visualize the inside of the stomach and duodenum, and injects dye into the ducts of the biliary tree and pancreas to be viewed on x-ray. The scope is advanced through the esophagus, into the stomach, to the duodenal papilla (papilla of Vater) and contrast is then injected to visualize the bile ducts and biliary tract, including the gallbladder. Assignment of these codes is based on purpose of the procedure as diagnostic or therapeutic. The codes do not include the radiological supervision and interpretation, so when performed, report:

- 74328 (biliary ductal system)
- 74329 (pancreatic ductal system)
- 74330 (biliary and pancreatic ductal systems)

When an ERCP is performed for a **diagnostic** purpose by means of an endoscopy, report the service with 43260. During the procedure, the physician may view the common bile duct or the entire biliary tract. The procedure may be with or without the collection of specimen(s) by brushing or washing, which is not reported separately because collection is included in the code description. If there is no definitive diagnosis documented in the medical record, assign code(s) for the documented signs and symptoms.

CODING SHOT There are times when the injection for visualization cannot be accomplished, due to a variety of factors. A failed ERCP is reported with 43260-52. Modifier -52 indicates a service that was reduced at the physician's discretion.

Laparoscopy (43279-43289). Surgical laparoscopy is a procedure to examine the organs of the abdominal cavity and always includes diagnostic laparoscopy. A laparoscope is a thin flexible tube containing a video camera. The scope is placed through a small incision in the abdomen (Fig. 18–12) and produces images that can be viewed on a computer screen. A similar procedure is utilized to view the organs of the pelvis (gynecologic laparoscopy or pelviscopy).

FIGURE 18-12 Location of incisions for insertion of laparoscope.

EXERCISE 18-2 *Pharynx, Adenoids, Tonsils, and Esophagus*

Using the CPT and ICD-9-CM manuals, code the following:

1 Tonsillectomy of an 18-year-old with chronic hypertrophic tonsillitis

   CPT Code: _____

   ICD-9-CM Code: _____ (ICD-10-CM Code: _____)

2 Suture of pharynx after injury

   CPT Code: _____

3 Esophagotomy using a thoracic approach for removal of a penny that was lodged in the child's throat

   CPT Code: _____

4 Thoracic approach was employed for excision of a lesion from the esophagus. The procedure included primary repair.

   CPT Code: _____

5 Fiberoptic dilation of the esophagus by means of a bougie with multiple passes.

   CPT Code: _____

STOMACH

The Stomach codes 43500-43999 include incisional procedures in which the stomach is exposed to the view of the surgeon, such as 43500 (gastrotomy with exploration or foreign body removal). Other procedures are performed by means of a scope, such as 43653 (laparoscopic gastrostomy). Be certain to identify the method used to perform the procedure before assigning a code.

Gastric bypass surgery is performed on patients who are morbidly obese with the outcome of decreasing the size of the stomach and/or intestines to aid with weight loss. There are many techniques used for gastric bypass procedures. A **Roux-en-Y** (RNY) is a Y-shaped surgical connection in which the intestine is detached from its original origin and reattached so as to bypass a part of the stomach and the entire duodenum (first part of the small intestine) as illustrated in Fig. 18–13. The Roux-en-Y term is used in several code descriptions, such as 43621 (total gastrectomy with Roux-en-Y reconstruction) and 43644 (laparoscopic gastric restriction, with gastric bypass and Roux-en-Y gastroenterostomy). For an open procedure, a 6- to 9-inch incision is made in the abdomen to gain access to the stomach and intestines. For a laparoscopic procedure about six access ports are established measuring about ¼ to ½ inch each in diameter through which the surgical instruments are inserted. The laparoscopic procedures are much less invasive and decrease the time the patient spends in the hospital, recovery time, and complications.

Bariatric Surgery codes 43770-43775 also report procedures performed for gastric restrictive procedures that are accomplished by placing a restrictive device around the stomach to decrease its functional size. Code 43770 reports "placement of adjustable gastric restrictive device (e.g., gastric band and subcutaneous port components)" (Fig. 18–14). The band is adjustable because the band is hollow and contains a tube that can be inflated with fluid. After surgery, fluid is gradually inserted into the tube through a subcutaneous port (just beneath the skin) with a syringe. The physician can adjust the amount of fluid in the tube and thereby adjust the amount of food that can pass through the banded area. The procedure may be performed on an outpatient basis and is reversable by removal of the banding apparatus.

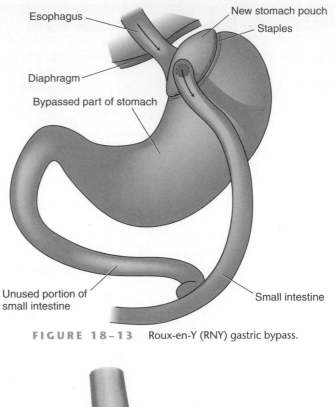

Esophagus

New stomach pouch

Staples

Diaphragm

Bypassed part of stomach

Unused portion of
small intestine

Small intestine

FIGURE 18-13 Roux-en-Y (RNY) gastric bypass.

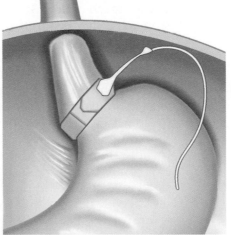

FIGURE 18-14 Adjustable gastric restrictive device.
Adjustable gastric restrictive device. (From Feldman M, Friedman
LS, Brandt LJ: *Sleisenger & Fordtran's Gastrointestinal and Liver
Disease,* ed 8, Philadelphia, 2006, Saunders.)

NCCI

Medicare has specific rules when billing bypass procedures.
Gastric bypass surgery, which is a variation of the
gastrojejunostomy, is performed to treat clinically severe obesity.
Gastric bypass surgery for extreme obesity is covered under the
Medicare program if the procedure is medically appropriate for
the individual and the surgery is to correct an illness, which
caused the obesity or was aggravated by the obesity. Severe or
morbid obesity is defined as a body mass index (BMI) of 35 kg/m^2
(weight in kilograms divided by the square of the height in
meters).

INTESTINES (EXCEPT RECTUM)

The large intestine is about 5 feet long with a wider diameter than the small intestine. The small intestine is about 30 feet long. The Intestine codes 44005-44799 exclude codes to report services for the anus and rectum.

Separate procedures are common in this subheading. Colostomies (creation of an artificial opening) are always bundled into a more major procedure unless the code specifically states to report the colostomy separately. For example, code 44141 is a partial colectomy and includes establishment of a colostomy.

Many intestinal procedures are performed through endoscopes (such as the gastroscopy in Fig. 18–15). Endoscope codes are available for procedures depending on how far down (through the mouth) or up (through the anus) the scope is passed. The code selection varies according to the procedure performed and includes the sites the scope passed through to accomplish the procedure. To choose the proper code, the extent of the procedure must be determined. For example, if a scope is passed to the esophagus only, the code would be chosen from the endoscopy codes 43200-43232. If the scoping

FIGURE 18–15   Illustration of endoscopy and endoscopic images of the gastroesophageal junction. **A,** Endoscopy. **B,** Esophageal constriction. **C,** Esophageal constriction after dilation. **D,** Esophageal cancer at the gastroesophageal junction. (**B, C,** and **D** from Drake RL, Vogl W, Mitchell AWM: *Gray's Anatomy for Students,* Philadelphia, 2005, Elsevier Inc.)

is continued through the esophagus to the stomach, duodenum, and/or jejunum, the code selection would be from the endoscopy codes 43235-43259 (upper GI). Once the anatomic site of the endoscope procedure is correctly identified, the surgical procedure(s) performed guides the selection of the code. A surgical endoscopy always includes a diagnostic endoscopy. Assign modifier -51 if more than one procedure is performed.

CODING SHOT To choose the correct endoscopy, identify the farthest **extent** to which the scope was passed and then the procedure(s) performed.

Resection of the intestine means taking out a portion of the intestine and either joining the remaining ends (anastomosis) directly or developing an artificial opening (exteriorizing) through the abdominal wall. Fig. 18–16 illustrates three types of anastomoses. The artificial opening (stoma) allows for the removal of body waste products (Fig. 18–17), as with the colostomy. The type of anastomosis or exteriorization depends on the medical condition of the patient and on the amount of intestine (large or small) that has to be removed. Some patients have temporary exteriorization for the length of time it takes the remaining intestine to heal and begin to perform the necessary functions. Other patients have permanent exteriorization because too much of the intestine has been removed to allow for adequate functioning. Openings to the outside of the body are named for the part of the intestine from which they are formed—colostomy is an artificial opening

Anastomoses

End to end

End to side

Side to side

FIGURE 18–16 Three types of anastomoses.

FIGURE 18–17 Stoma.

Sigmoid colostomy   Descending colostomy   Transverse (single B) colostomy

Ascending colostomy   Ileostomy

FIGURE 18-18   Various ostomies.

from the colon, ileostomy from the ileum, gastrostomy from the stomach, and so forth (Fig. 18–18). To assign the correct code, identify the correct anatomic site from which the ostomy originated, as well as the procedure used to establish the ostomy.

QUICK CHECK 18-2

1. The first step to choosing the correct GI endoscopic code is to determine the _____ to which the scope was passed.

Sometimes, a laparotomy is used as the approach in digestive system surgeries and the approach is never coded separately. An exploratory laparotomy may be performed to investigate the cause of a patient's illness. If only the exploratory laparotomy is performed, it is appropriate to report the service with an exploratory laparotomy code, such as 49000. However, if the exploratory procedure progressed to a more definitive surgical treatment (such as an appendectomy), only the definitive treatment (appendectomy) is reported.

MECKEL'S DIVERTICULUM AND THE MESENTERY

A Meckel's diverticulum is a fairly common congenital pouch on the wall of the small bowel that may contain pancreatic or stomach tissue and may require surgical removal (44800). Removal of the omphalomesenteric duct refers to the embryonic passage that connects an egg sac to the intestine and is included in the code description of 44800.

EXERCISE 18-3 *Stomach and Intestines (Except Rectum)*

Using your knowledge of medical terminology, identify the following surgical communications:

1 Coloproctostomy: from the _____ to the _____

2 Ileostomy: from the _____ to the _____ surface

3 Colostomy: from the _____ intestine to the _____ surface

4 Enteroenterostomy: between _____ of intestine

Using the CPT and ICD-9-CM manuals, code the following:

5 Partial bowel resection with colostomy for primary, malignant neoplasm

    CPT Code: _____

    ICD-9-CM Code: _____ (ICD-10-CM Code: _____)

6 Resection of small intestine, single resection, with anastomosis

    CPT Code: _____

APPENDIX   Surgical procedures of the appendix may be accomplished by means of

Open procedures:

- 44900, open I&D of abscess
- 44950, open surgical appendectomy

Percutaneous procedures:

- 44901, percutaneous I&D of abscess

Laparoscopic procedures:

- 44970, laparoscopic appendectomy

There are two other codes to report appendectomy procedures.

- 44955, appendectomy performed at the time of a major procedure for an indicated purpose
- 44960, appendectomy when appendix has ruptured or there is generalized peritonitis

The reporting of 44950 and 44955 need special attention because there are times when a surgeon will remove a healthy appendix during the course of another abdominal procedure. Because the abdomen is already open to the view of the surgeon, the incidental appendectomy (44950) does not add to the complexity of the procedure and is not reported separately. If, however, during another major abdominal procedure, the surgeon removes the appendix due to a medically necessary reason, the service is reported with 44955.

RECTUM   Rectum procedures are reported with codes from the 45000-45999 range. These procedures involve the rectum and employ techniques such as incision, excision, and destruction. Many of the codes are very complex.

For example:

- 45126, Pelvic exenteration for colorectal malignancy, with proctectomy (with or without colostomy), with removal of bladder and ureteral transplantations, and/or hysterectomy, or cervicectomy, with or without removal of tube(s), with or without removal of ovary(s), or any combination thereof

This complex code description contains many procedures that may or may not have been performed as indicated by the "with or without." For example, with or without colostomy or with or without removal of tubes and ovaries. If any of the listed procedures were performed, they are bundled in the main code (45126) and not reported separately. Complex codes such as 45126 increase the potential for unintentional unbundling.

Endoscopy (Proctosigmoidoscopy, Sigmoidoscopy, and Colonoscopy)

Rectal endoscopic procedures are frequently performed and include proctosigmoidoscopy, sigmoidoscopy, and colonoscopy (Fig. 18–19).

Proctosigmoidoscopy. Endoscopic examination of the rectum (proct/o = rectum) and the sigmoid colon (45300-45327). The scope is advanced 6-25 cm (2.4-9.8 in). Code 45300 describes a rigid proctosigmoidoscopy, diagnostic, with or without collection of specimen(s) by brushing or washing (separate procedure). Do not assign 45300 when reported with codes 45303-45327, because these codes report surgical procedures, so the diagnostic service of 45300 is bundled into the surgical procedure. If no definitive diagnosis is documented, report the documented signs/symptoms.

Sigmoidoscopy. Endoscopic examination of the sigmoid colon may include the descending colon (45330-45345). The scope is advanced 26-60 cm (10.2-23.6 in). A sigmoidoscopy is the examination of the entire rectum, sigmoid colon, and may include examination of a portion of the descending colon but stops before reaching the splenic flexure (the turn beneath the spleen that connects the descending to the transverse colon). Code 45330 describes a flexible diagnostic sigmoidoscopy that may or may not include the collection of specimen(s) by brushing or washing (separate procedure). Do not code 45330 when also reporting 45331-45345 because they are surgical procedures and the diagnostic procedure (45330) is always

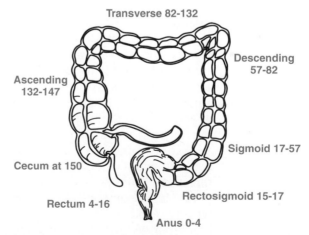

FIGURE 18–19 Colonoscopy measurements (cm). (Courtesy U.S. National Cancer Institute, Surveillance, Epidemiology, and End Results (SEER) Program.)

included in the surgical procedure. If a definitive diagnosis has not been documented, report the documented signs/symptoms.

Diagnostic Colonoscopy. Endoscopic examination of the colon from rectum to cecum is reported with codes from the 45355-45392 range. The scope is advanced more than 60 cm (more than 23.6 in).

The diagnostic colonoscopy codes are divided based on the extent and the purpose of the procedure. The diagnostic stand-alone codes 45300, 45330, and 45378 each have a list of indented procedure codes based on the purpose of the procedure (such as biopsy, foreign body removal, ablation, control of bleeding, etc.). Take a moment to locate these codes in the CPT manual and familiarize yourself with the types of procedures reported with the codes.

If the patient is fully prepared for the endoscopic procedure, and the procedure has begun but is not completed because of extenuating circumstances, use modifier -53 (Discontinued Procedure) appended to the endoscopic code. Some payers, such as Medicare, require the coder to report -53 for a procedure that could not be completed. These extenuating circumstances could be that the patient has become unstable, the bowel preparation for the surgery was not sufficient to continue the procedure, or an equipment failure occurred. Use either -52 or -53 and provide supporting documentation as to why the procedure was discontinued.

Colonoscopy. Codes 45378-45392 describe procedures in which the endoscope is advanced to the proximal (past) the splenic flexure or into a portion of the terminal ileum (most distant part of the small intestine).

To report colonoscopy procedures, first determine how the procedure was performed:

- Through a colostomy (44388-44397)
- Through a colotomy (45355)
- Through the rectum (45378-45392)

When the colon is examined through a colostomy (surgically created opening in the abdominal wall) the diagnostic or therapeutic service is reported with codes 44388-44397.

Report 45380 (colonoscopy with biopsy(ies)) when a "**cold biopsy**" is performed. A cold biopsy is generally accepted to mean the use of forceps to grasp and remove a small piece of tissue without the application of cautery. For example, one polyp was snared and three polyps were biopsied with cold biopsy forceps. The service would be reported with 45385 (colonoscopy with removal of tumor/polyp/lesion with by snare technique) and 45380 (colonoscopy with biopsy(ies)). During a snare procedure, a wire loop is placed around the lesion and the wire is then heated to shave off the lesion. Larger lesions may be removed with a single application of the snare or with several applications (called piecemeal). Remnants may also be cauterized or ablated to completely destroy the lesion. The assignment of the code is not dependent on the histology of the tissue obtained for analysis. Report only one technique for each lesion or polyp.

Colonoscopy with removal by snare technique (45385) should not be reported when describing the removal of a small polyp by biopsy or cold forceps technique.

A colonoscopy with biopsy and polypectomy in separate sites are reported with two codes. The biopsy may require modifier -59 to identify the service as a separate procedure from the polyp procedure.

Code 45378 describes a flexible diagnostic colonoscopy up to the splenic flexure and is bundled into the colonoscopy procedure codes 45379-45392. If no definitive diagnosis is documented assign diagnosis code(s) for signs/symptoms.

NCCI

When a covered colonoscopy is attempted but cannot be completed due to extenuating circumstances (e.g., the inability to extend beyond the splenic flexure), Medicare will usually pay for the interrupted colonoscopy at the rate of a flexible sigmoidoscopy.

Here are some endoscopic biopsy highlights:

- If a single lesion is biopsied, but not entirely removed, only a biopsy code would be assigned.
- If a biopsy is obtained and the lesion is also excised, only the excision of a lesion code would be reported.
- If a biopsy and excision were performed, it would be appropriate to report the biopsy if taken from a lesion other than the lesion that was excised. The CPT code for the excision will sometimes state "with or without biopsy," in which case you would not report the biopsy separately. If multiple biopsy specimens are obtained, whether from the same or different sites, and none of the lesions are excised, only one unit (×1) of the biopsy code is assigned.

Evaluation and Management Services Reported with a Diagnostic Colonoscopy. Reporting a minor procedure (10-day global period) with an office visit service can be problematic. The E/M service must be medically necessary and include work above and beyond what is required for the minor procedure. If the E/M service is medically necessary, the E/M code will require modifier -25, which reports a significantly separate E/M service that occurs on the same day as the procedure or service by the same provider. Check the documentation to determine if the E/M service was prompted by a complaint, symptom, condition, problem, or circumstance that was or was not related to the procedure or other service provided.

NCCI

HCPCS Level II Codes for Colorectal Cancer Screening
The following are the guidelines to report screening services for colorectal cancer for patients who are beneficiaries under the Medicare program. Screening means no presenting symptoms or disease is present.

A therapeutic examination is reported when a disease is identified, or additional procedures are performed via the scope (biopsy, ablation, etc.). The examination may begin as screening and changes to a therapeutic service if pathology is found or if additional procedures (biopsy, etc.) were performed. The diagnosis code(s) assigned would identifying the condition for which the service was provided and the screening code V76.51 would be assigned (Special screening for malignant neoplasms, colon), when appropriate [ICD-10-CM: Z12.11].

HCPCS code G0328 (immunoassay) reports fecal-occult blood tests, which examine the stool for blood. When the patient returns

Continued

the fecal sample cards, the laboratory performs one to three simultaneous determinations. This means that one to three of the cards will be tested for the presence of blood. Occult blood is that which cannot be seen but is present microscopically. The order for and the results of the test must be documented in the medical record. Usually this service is provided to patient 50 years of age and older once every year as a screening for colorectal cancer.

Coverage of G0104, a flexible sigmoidoscopy, is provided to patients who are at least 50 years of age and is covered once every 4 years. If a lesion is identified, removed, or biopsied during a screening flexible sigmoidoscopy, the procedure is reported as a diagnostic flexible sigmoidoscopy with biopsy or removal of lesion using 45331, 45332, 45333, 45338, 45339 (sigmoidoscopy with biopsy, removal or ablation). The first-listed diagnosis code would report the lesion (the finding).

Code G0105 reports a colonoscopy on a patient at high risk; which means the patient has a:

- Personal history of colorectal cancer (V10.05, V10.06) [ICD-10-CM: Z85.3, Z85.04]
- Personal history of adenomatous polyps (V12.72) [ICD-10-CM: Z86.010]
- Inflammatory bowel disease, including Crohn's disease, and ulcerative colitis
- A close relative (sibling, parent, or child) who has had colorectal cancer or an adenomatous polyposis (V16.0, V18.5X) [ICD-10-CM: Z80.0, Z83.7X]
- Family history of adenomatous polyposis (V18.5X) [ICD-10-CM: Z83.7X]
- Family history of nonpolyposis colorectal cancer (V16.0) [ICD-10-CM: Z80.0]

If during a screening colonoscopy, a lesion or growth is detected that results in a biopsy or removal of the growth, the appropriate diagnostic procedure is reported rather than the diagnostic code G0105.

Code 45378 describes a diagnostic, flexible colonoscopy of the proximal to splenic flexure. An appropriate screening diagnosis for this procedure would be V76.51 (Special screening for malignant neoplasms, colon) [ICD-10-CM: Z12.11]. This code is reported when there are no additional procedures performed by means of the scope.

These are the HCPCS colorectal screening codes:

- G0104 flexible sigmoidoscopy
- G0105 colonoscopy on individual at high risk
- G0106 alternative to G0104, screening sigmoidoscopy, barium enema
- G0120 alternative to G0105, screening colonoscopy, barium enema
- G0121 colonoscopy on individual not meeting criteria for high risk
- G0122 barium enema

A barium enema is a series of x-rays of the colon and rectum taken after the patient drinks a white, chalky solution that contains barium (a metallic element). The barium outlines the intestines on the x-rays. The barium enema (G0106, screening sigmoidoscopy, barium enema) may be performed as an alternative to a screening sigmoidoscopy (G0104, flexible sigmoidoscopy) based on documentation that the physician determined that the barium enema would be as good as or better than a flexible sigmoidoscopy or screening colonoscopy due to the patient's specific medical problem. There must be a written order from the physician for the procedure in the patient's medical record. G0104 may also be assigned as an alternative to G0106 for patients who are:

- At least 50 years old
- Not at high risk for colorectal cancer
- It has been at least 48 months since the last screening was performed

Code G0120 reports a screening colonoscopy with barium enema that is performed as an alternative to G0105 (colonoscopy on individual at high risk for colorectal cancer). The screening colonoscopy with barium enema is performed at least 24 months after a previously covered screening barium enema or screening colonoscopy was performed.

If the patient does not meet the criteria for a high-risk patient, G0121 is reported once every 10 years for patients over 50 years of age. The diagnosis code V76.51 (Screening for malignant neoplasm of the colon) [ICD-10-CM: Z12.11] is reported with submission of G0121.

CAUTION *When a biopsy is taken, the physician removes a tissue sample for pathological evaluation. Excision is the removal of the entire lesion and ablation destroys the entire lesion.*

Colonoscopy Injection. The injection service described in 45381 may be performed when the polyp is injected with saline to lift the polyp prior to removal by another technique. Other injection services include the placement of a tattoo with India ink for later identification of the area during a surgical procedure. When the purpose of an injection is to control spontaneous bleeding from conditions such as diverticulosis and angiodysplasia (AVM), report the service with 45382 (colonoscopy with control of bleeding, including injection) rather than 45381 (colonoscopy with submucosal injection). Code 45381 is reported as an additional service to another therapeutic service procedure, but it is not an add-on code. Bleeding caused by the procedure and controlled by any method is considered part of the therapeutic procedure and is not reported separately with codes 45382 or 45381.

Multiple Procedures. If multiple lesions are removed from the colon using the same technique (snare), use only one code to report the services because the colon is considered one anatomical location. If the procedure is prolonged or unusually extensive, report modifier -22 and include the time the procedure extended beyond the time usual for the procedure. The submission of modifier -22 requires documentation sent with the claim form that supports the assignment of the modifier.

Virtual Colonoscopy. A virtual colonoscopy (VC) utilizes x-rays and computer to produce a two- and three-dimensional image of the colon. The procedure is used to diagnose colon and bowel disease, including polyps, cancer, and diverticulosis. The VC can also be performed using computed tomography (CT) or magnetic resonance imagining (MRI), as illustrated in Fig. 18–20. The procedure is performed in a radiology department and does not require sedation. A tube is inserted into the rectum and air is pumped into the colon thereby inflating the colon, which allows for better visualization. The patient lies on a table that is moved into a scanner that produces the images by means of the computer. This process is repeated with the patient lying on his/her back and again, on the stomach.

Virtual colonoscopy may be performed when a colonoscopy cannot be successfully completed and is used as a technique for screening. Because colonoscopy can more accurately detect colon cancer, virtual colonoscopy may be medically necessary only when colonoscopy cannot be successfully performed or extended to the cecum.

NCCI

When reporting the VC service for Medicare patients, report:

- **74263** (Computed tomographic [CT] colonography [ie, virtual colonoscopy]; **screening**)
- **74261-74262** (Computed tomographic [CT] colonography [ie, virtual colonoscopy]; **diagnostic**)

FIGURE 18-20 The virtual colonoscopy.

EXERCISE 18-4 *Appendix and Rectum*

Using the CPT and ICD-9-CM manuals, code the following:

1 Appendectomy on a patient with ruptured appendix

   CPT Code: _____

   ICD-9-CM Code: _____ (ICD-10-CM Code: _____)

2 Flexible sigmoidoscopy with three biopsies

   CPT Code: _____

3 Colonoscopy with removal of polyp by a snare

   CPT Code: _____

4 The patient presents for removal of sigmoid and rectal polyps. The Pentax video sigmoidoscope was inserted and four polyps were seen scattered between the rectum and proximal sigmoid colon. The largest measured about 1.5 cm in diameter. The others were diminutive, about 4 or 5 mm in diameter. Biopsies were taken of two of these polyps. The pathology report indicated benign polyps.

   CPT Code: _____

ANUS Abscess is a common anal condition that is usually treated with incision and drainage; however, when I&D fails to satisfactorily treat the abscess, other methods may be used. Procedures on the anus are reported with 46020-46999 and include incision, excision, introduction, endoscopy, repair, destruction, and suture.

Several of the codes in the Anus subheading refer to a seton, such as 46020 (seton placement) or 46030 (seton removal). A seton is a treatment for anal fistula (abnormal passage between anus and skin), which is usually the result of a previous abscess that has drained but not completely healed. A nonabsorbable suture is threaded through the fistula, out through the anus, and the two ends of the suture are tied together, as illustrated in Fig. 18–21. The seton is left in place until healing has occurred. Scar tissue forms around the suture and the ends of the seton are eventually cut away. Usually the seton can be placed during an office procedure that does not require anesthesia. If the fistula is more complex and requires opening of the fistula track the service would be reported with a code from the 46270-46285 range.

A **fissure** is a cleft or a groove, normal or otherwise, as illustrated in Fig. 18–22. An anal fissure is a painful ulcer usually located at the margin of the anus. Code 46200 reports a fissurectomy, which is the excision of the fissure. Sphincterotomy is a surgical incision of a sphincter and if it is performed in conjunction with a fissurectomy, it is bundled into 46200 and not reported separately.

A more complex type of anal repair procedure is the closure of an anal fistula with rectal advancement flap. This procedure is reported with 46288 and often third-party payers bundle many other procedures into the closure procedure. So read the payer guidelines carefully before submitting.

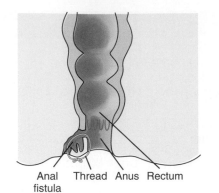

Anal   Thread Anus Rectum
fistula

FIGURE 18–21   Suture threaded through the fistula.

FIGURE 18–22   Anal fissure. (From Townsend CM, Beauchamp RD, Evers BM, Mattox KL: *Sabiston Textbook of Surgery: The Biological Basis of Modern Surgical Practice,* ed 18, Philadelphia, 2008, Saunders.)

NCCI

When reporting 46288 for a Medicare patient, the NCCI edits indicate the following codes are bundled into 46288: 45900, 45905, 45910, 45915, 46040, 46080, 46200, 46220, 46221, 46230, 46250, 46257, 46258, 46260-46262, 46270, 46275, 46280, 46285, 46600, 46940, and 46942. These component codes cannot be reported to Medicare when performed at the same session as code 46288. The edits are posted on the CMS website at www.cms.hhs.gov/NationalCorrectCodInitEd/.

An anoscope is an instrument that is inserted a short distance into the anal canal (Fig. 18–23). Once inserted, various procedures may be performed, such as dilation, biopsy, removal of a foreign body or lesion, and control of hemorrhage. Procedures that utilize an anoscope are reported with endoscopy codes 46600-46615.

Code 46600 describes a **diagnostic anoscopy** (up to 5 cm [2 in]) with dilation and includes collection of specimens. This code is designated as a "separate procedure," which means it cannot be reported if performed with another related service during the same session.

FIGURE 18–23   Stainless steel anoscope. (From Roberts JR, Hedges JR, Chanmugam AS, Chudnofsky CR, Custalow CB, Dronen SC: *Clinical Procedures in Emergency Medicine,* ed 4, Philadelphia, 2004, Saunders.)

The remaining Endoscopy codes describe procedures for foreign body removal, removal of tumor or polyp by different techniques and control of bleeding.

Destruction of anal lesions can be accomplished by various methods, such as chemical, electrodesiccation, cryosurgery, laser surgery, and surgical excision. Destruction of anal lesions is reported with codes 46900-46942, often based on the type of destruction utilized. For example, 46900 reports chemical destruction, 46910 reports electrodesiccation, and 46916 reports cryosurgery. The method of destruction will be documented in the medical record.

Hemorrhoids are a frequent condition of the anus. Hemorrhoids (piles) arise from an inflammation of the venous plexuses (congregation of vessels) around the anus and may be inside or outside of the anal canal. Hemorrhoids are classified into four degrees depending on severity:

- First degree may bleed but do not protrude outside of the anal canal.
- Second degree protrudes outside of the anal canal occasionally but retracts spontaneously.
- Third degree protrudes outside the anal canal more often and must be manually placed back into the anal canal.
- Fourth degree protrudes outside the anal canal but cannot be manually placed back into the anal canal. Fourth degree hemorrhoid may be strangulated or thrombosed as illustrated in Fig. 18–24.

The surgical treatment is determined by the type of hemorrhoid. For example, 46250 reports an external hemorrhoidectomy, whereas 46260 reports a hemorrhoidectomy of both internal and external hemorrhoids.

Sometimes, as an alternative to surgery, hemorrhoids are treated by injection of a sclerosing (caustic) solution, which causes irritation of the tissue that result in increased healing. The sclerosing solution injection is reported with 46500.

FIGURE 18–24 Large thrombosed external hemorrhoid. (From Roberts JR, Hedges JR, editors: *Clinical Procedures in Emergency Medicine,* ed 4, Philadelphia, 2004, Saunders.)

CODING SHOT

The dentate line is the line where the anal mucosal lining meets the skin (mucocutaneous junction or anal verge). An internal hemorrhoid is one that is 1-1.5 cm above this line. The internal hemorrhoid is the one most often treated by a gastroenterologist. An external hemorrhoid is one that is located below the dentate line.

LIVER

Biopsy of the liver may be performed percutaneously (47000) using imaging guidance that is reported separately. If the biopsy is performed at the time of a more major procedure, the biopsy is reported with add-on code 47001. A liver biopsy may also be performed as a wedge biopsy (47100) that involves removal, through an incision, of a small fan-shaped section of tissue for examination.

A liver **transplant** is a complex procedure that usually involves the surgical expertise of several physicians and a trained surgical team. The transplant procedure involves obtaining the graft to be transplanted (from a cadaver or living donor), backbench work (special preparation of the graft before transplantation), and transplantation into the recipient. Each component of the transplant is reported separately. There are extensive notes preceding the transplant codes 47133-47147 that must be carefully read before assigning codes to these complex procedures.

BILIARY TRACT

The gallbladder is connected to the liver and the small intestine by the biliary tract. The tract can be the site of conditions such as calculus and tumor that may obstruct the flow of bile. An incisional procedure (hepaticotomy or hepaticostomy) with exploration of the tract may be performed to determine the cause of obstruction (47400) and may include removal of calculus or drainage of bile from the tract.

A **choledochotomy** is an incision into the biliary tract, and a cholecystostomy is the formation of a stoma between the abdominal wall and the gallbladder. You locate the codes for these procedures in the Incision category of the Biliary Tract subheading (47400-47490).

An **injection** procedure may be necessary to determine if the biliary tract is obstructed. The assignment of a code is based on if the injection is performed percutaneously (47500) or through an existing catheter (47505). The biliary tract may become obstructed due to disease, such as neoplasm. **Stents** may be placed in the obstructed biliary tract to open the area (47511). The stents may also be changed (47525) or revised/reinserted (47530).

Laparoscopic cholecystectomy involves the placement of ports through the abdominal wall into which the laparoscope and instrumentation are inserted to remove the gallbladder. The codes are located in the Laparoscopy category (47560-47579). The operative report will indicate the method used for the removal of the gallbladder, which determines the assignment of the code. For example, 47562 reports a laparoscopic removal of the gallbladder, and 47600 reports an incisional removal of the gallbladder.

Occasionally, the surgeon will begin the procedure using one technique and due to a difficulty convert the procedure to another technique. For example, a procedure that is begun as a laparoscopic procedure (47563) and is converted to an open procedure during the same operative session (47605). Only the successful approach is reported, which in this case is the open procedure (47605). Reporting both a laparoscopic and an open surgical approach to accomplish the same outcome is duplication of services.

PANCREAS

The pancreas is located behind (posterior to) the stomach and produces enzymes and hormones. The pancreas may become inflamed (pancreatitis) and require the placement of drains to remove the excess fluid. If the drain is placed by means of an incision, report 48000, but if the procedure also included cholecystostomy, gastrostomy, and jejunostomy report the service with 48001.

The pancreas can also be the site of a calculus that may be removed through an incision (48020).

Biopsies of the pancreas may be performed by means of an open (48100) or percutaneous (48102) procedure. Guidance is not included in the percutaneous biopsy code, so guidance is reported separately depending on the type of guidance used. If there was an injection portion to the intraoperative pancreatogram (radiography of pancreas during the procedure), the injection is reported separately with add-on code 48400 (Injection procedure, intraoperative pancreatography).

The pancreas can be totally or partially removed and codes for the pancreatectomies (48140-48160) are divided based on the extent of removal and other procedures that may be performed during the same operative session.

The pancreas may be transplanted (48550-48554) and includes harvesting the pancreas graft from a cadaver, backbench work in preparation for transplantation, and transplantation of the graft into the recipient.

ABDOMEN, PERITONEUM, AND OMENTUM

Laparoscopy code 49320 reports a diagnostic laparoscopic procedure. If the procedure was a surgical procedure, the diagnostic laparoscopy is included in the surgical procedure and not reported separately. For example, if the procedure began as a diagnostic laparoscopy but a lymphocele of the peritoneal cavity was identified and drained. The diagnostic laparoscopy converted to a surgical laparoscopy and would be reported with the surgical laparoscopy code 49323.

Hernia codes are listed according to type of hernia (see Repair 49491-49611 and Laparoscopy 49650-49659). Fig. 18–25 is an illustration of an inguinal hernia that would usually be surgically repaired by a herniorrhaphy.

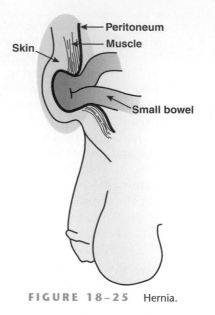

FIGURE 18–25 Hernia.

The defect would be closed with sutures. Other factors in coding hernias are whether the hernia is **strangulated** (the blood supply is cut off) or **incarcerated** (cannot be returned to the abdominal cavity); the repair is an initial or subsequent repair; the hernia is reducible (can be returned to the abdominal cavity); and the age of the patient.

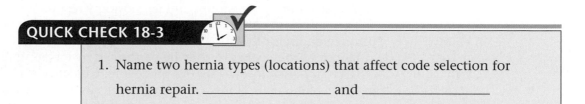

QUICK CHECK 18-3

1. Name two hernia types (locations) that affect code selection for hernia repair. _____ and _____

EXERCISE 18-5 *Anus, Liver, Biliary Tract, Pancreas, Abdomen, Peritoneum, and Omentum*

Using the CPT manual, code the following:

1 Exploratory laparotomy with a cholecystectomy

   CPT Code: _____

2 Cholecystotomy with exploration and removal of calculus

   CPT Code: _____

3 Repair of recurrent reducible incisional hernia, with implantation of a mesh graft, abdominal approach

   CPT Codes: _____, _____

4 Repair of an initial incarcerated inguinal hernia in a 5½ -year-old

   CPT Code: _____

5 Total pancreatectomy

   CPT Code: _____

6 Sphincterotomy and one quadrant hemorrhoidectomy for an anal fissure is performed. During the procedure an enlarged hemorrhoid/sentinel tag was noted at the 10 o'clock position and a fissure right at the base of this. Anoscope and a Kelly clamp were placed, and a sentinel tag excised. The defect was closed with sutures.

   CPT Code: _____

From the Trenches

"Many student coders believe that as soon as they earn their coding certification they'll be making the 'big bucks.' The certification is proof that you have the basic knowledge needed to code, but experience is still needed. Be patient, build your knowledge base, and the increase in pay will follow."

CYNTHIA

CHAPTER REVIEW

CHAPTER 18, PART I, THEORY

Without the use of reference material, complete the following:

1 The codes in the Digestive System subsection begin with this anatomic part, _____, and end with this anatomic part, _____.

2 In the Digestive System, many of the procedures performed to view the esophagus and stomach are performed with this instrument.

_____

3 What type of endoscopy is always included in a surgical endoscopy and would therefore never be reported separately? _____

4 What is the term that describes a surgical opening into the abdomen? _____

5 When a hernia can be returned to the abdominal cavity, it is said to be _____.

CHAPTER 18, PART II, PRACTICAL

Code the following cases using the CPT and ICD-9-CM:

6 Repair of recurrent, reducible incisional hernia

CPT Code: _____

7 Repair of an incarcerated umbilical hernia for a 4-year-old patient

CPT Code: _____

8 Excision of full thickness lip lesion with Abbe-Estlander flap reconstruction

CPT Code: _____

9 Thoracic approach used in a diverticulectomy of hypopharynx

CPT Code: _____

10 Total open abdominal colectomy with ileostomy

CPT Code: _____

11 Multiple biopsies of the small intestine by means of endoscopy with progression past the second portion of the duodenum

CPT Code: _____

12 Proctosigmoidoscopy using rigid endoscope with collection of multiple specimens by brushing

CPT Code: _____

13 A sigmoidoscopy with endoscopic biopsy is performed on a Medicare patient who has an area of ulceration in the rectosigmoid region. The excision of the tissue specimen causes bleeding that is controlled endoscopically.

CPT Code(s): _____

ICD-9-CM Code(s): _____

(ICD-10-CM Code(s): _____)

14 A Medicare patient presents for an EGD with biopsy and dilation of gastric outlet for obstruction both performed during the same endoscopic session. What would the physician report?

CPT Code(s): _____

ICD-9-CM Code(s): _____

(ICD-10-CM Code(s): _____)

15 During a colonoscopy, a mucosal lesion was removed from the mid right colon with snare electrocautery; a colon polyp in the left colon was removed with snare electrocautery; an excrescence 35 cm from the anal verge was removed with biopsy forceps; additional colon polyps were removed by snare electrocautery at 30 and 25 cm from the anal verge; and a hyperplastic lesion was removed with piecemeal polypectomy using hot biopsy forceps.

CPT Code(s): _____

16 This Medicare patient undergoes an EGD with biopsies and dilation of an esophageal stricture. The EGD was placed into the esophagus where stricture and esophagitis was noted. This area was biopsied. The scope was taken to the second portion of the duodenum and slowly withdrawn to the stomach where further biopsies were taken. The scope was withdrawn to the esophagus where a 20-mm balloon was inserted and the esophageal stricture was dilated. The scope and dilator was then withdrawn.

CPT Code(s): _____

QUICK CHECK ANSWERS

QUICK CHECK 18-1
cross

QUICK CHECK 18-2
extent

QUICK CHECK 18-3
Any two of the following: inguinal, lumbar, incisional (ventral), epigastric, umbilical, spigelian, diaphragmatic (hiatal).

Hernia repairs using an abdominal approach are located in the Abdomen, Peritoneum, and Omentum subsection, Repair subheading (49491-49611). Laparoscopic hernia repairs are in the Laparoscopy subheading (49650-49659).

"If someone expresses an interest in becoming a medical coder, I'd advise them to take a position in a physician's office or billing area first, so that they can get a feel for the field. Any experience in the field helps."

Ellen Dooley, BA, CPC-A
Compliance Analyst
University of Missouri Health Care
Columbia, Missouri

Urinary and Male Genital Systems

Chapter Topics

Urinary System

Male Genital System

Chapter Review

Quick Check Answers

Learning Objectives

After completing this chapter you should be able to

1 Understand the format and codes of the Urinary System subsection.

2 Review the subheadings and categories of the Urinary System subsection.

3 Report services with Urinary System codes.

4 Understand the format and codes of the Male Genital System subsection.

5 Review the subheadings and categories of the Male Genital System subsection.

6 Report services with Male Genital System codes.

Make sure to check
evolve
learning system
**for the latest
content updates**

URINARY SYSTEM

The Urinary System subsection (50010-53899) of the CPT manual is arranged anatomically by the subheadings of kidney, ureter, bladder, and urethra (Fig. 19–1), with category codes arranged by procedure (i.e., incision, excision, introduction, repair). A wide range of terminology is used in the subsection. The Glossary at the back of this book includes many of the terms that you will encounter in the CPT manual. Always be certain you know the meaning of all the words in the code description before you assign a code.

Kidney

The first subheading in the Urinary subsection is Kidney (50010-50593).

Incision. The Incision codes (50010-50135) are assigned to report exploration, nephrostomy, drainage, nephrolithotomy, and pyelotomy services.

Renal exploration is a procedure performed if the cause of a patient's condition is unknown. For example, surgical exploration of an injured kidney when the patient is clinically unstable and appears to be having renal blood loss. Access for the exploration procedure is from the side (flank). Note that a parenthetical statement preceding 50010 indicates "For retroperitoneal exploration, abscess, tumor, or cyst, see 49010, 49060, 49203-49205," which are Digestive System codes. Code 49010 reports an exploration of the retroperitoneum. The term **retroperitoneal** refers to that area located behind (retro to) the peritoneum (lines the abdominal walls and covers most of the organs) that is located in the abdominal cavity. The retroperitoneal space may be accessed by means of an abdominal incision. When coding an exploration of the retroperitoneal space, be careful to determine the exact anatomical location(s) explored to report the correct services because there are many organ systems located in the abdominal cavity. For example, the kidney is located in the retroperitoneal space. If only the kidney was explored, report the service with the Urinary System code 50010; if the retroperitoneal area was explored, report the service with the Digestive System code 49010, exploration of retroperitoneal area.

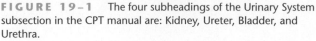

FIGURE 19–1 The four subheadings of the Urinary System subsection in the CPT manual are: Kidney, Ureter, Bladder, and Urethra.

If a procedure begins as an exploratory procedure but becomes a definitive or corrective procedure, such as repair of a lacerated kidney, only the definitive procedure is reported. The exploration is considered a diagnostic procedure that is bundled into the definitive procedure when both are performed during the same operative session.

Open drainage of a perirenal or renal abscess (50020) reports the drainage of a **kidney abscess** or the surrounding kidney tissue. If the drainage was of a retroperitoneal abscess, the service would be reported with the Digestive System code 49060 that reports an open drainage of a retroperitoneal abscess. Again, the exact location of the abscess is the critical factor when assigning the abscess drainage code. The renal abscess can also be accessed percutaneously, in which case the service would be reported with 50021. When performing a percutaneous access to the kidney, fluoroscopy, ultrasound, or computer tomography may be used for guidance of the needle placement and is reported separately with 75989.

CODING SHOT Code 50021 has the symbol next to it to indicate that conscious (moderate) sedation is included with the procedure and not reported separately.

A **nephrostomy** is a procedure used to decompress the renal system by means of the insertion of a catheter into the kidney while leaving the other end of the catheter outside the body to temporarily drain the kidney. The renal collecting system may be obstructed by a calculus or a defect of the renal pelvis or ureter. Code 50040 reports incisional placement of a drainage tube that involves incision into the renal pelvis (pyelotomy). The physician then inserts a catheter into the kidney with the other end carried to the skin surface and sutured in place on the flank.

A **nephrotomy** is exploration of the inside of the kidney. During this exploration (50045), no definitive procedure is performed. If a definitive procedure is performed the exploration is bundled into the definitive procedure. For example, if the surgeon began a procedure as an exploration to determine the cause of urinary obstruction and identified a renal calculus (kidney stone) and removed the calculus, the procedure no longer would be an exploration. The procedure would be reported with 50060, kidney stone removal (nephrolithotomy). The surgeon may also perform a renal endoscopy at the same time as the nephrotomy (such as, to place stents or perform some other type of repair procedure) and the endoscopy is reported separately with a code from range 50570-50580 (Endoscopy, kidney).

Nephrolithotomy procedures include removal of calculus (50060), secondary surgical operation for calculus (50065), procedures complicated by congenital kidney abnormality (50070), and removal of a staghorn calculus (50075). The staghorn calculus (Fig. 19–2) is shaped like a deer antler and can become large and create extensive obstruction. If the calculus involves the renal pelvis and at least two calyces, it is classified as a staghorn calculi. These types of stones account for about 30% of stones reported and are usually associated with urinary infections. With a staghorn, a nephrolithotomy may be performed after extracorporeal shock wave lithotripsy (ESWL), which fragments the stones (52352).

ESWL used to be performed with a machine in which the patient was submersed in a fluid. Newer machines do not require submersion, rather the patient is placed on an x-ray table, and a water-filled cushion is placed under the patient's back (Fig. 19–3). The procedure is performed under general

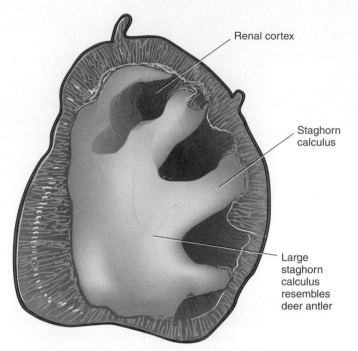

FIGURE 19–2 Large staghorn calculus inside the kidney filling the pelvis and calyceal system.

FIGURE 19–3 Extracorporeal shock wave lithotripsy (ESWL).

anesthesia in an operating room with a built-in ESWL machine. The shock waves are targeted to the stones by means of x-ray and pulverize the stones with repeated shocks. Usually, the particles subsequently pass through the urinary tract.

Percutaneous nephrolithotomy (nephrolithotripsy) is a more invasive method of treating kidney stones and usually is performed with ultrasound. An incision is made over the kidney, a probe is inserted, and shock waves pulverize the stone. Electrohydraulic or mechanical lithotripsy may be used instead of shock waves, but the use of shock waves is the most common method. A tiny basket may also be attached to a probe that is passed into the kidney and the stones removed. Because the stone fragments of a staghorn are so large, they may not pass through the urinary system spontaneously, and an open or percutaneous procedure may need to be performed to remove the fragments. The lithotripsy is reported separately (50590 lithotripsy or 52353 cystourethroscope with lithotripsy).

QUICK CHECK 19-1

1. When lithotripsy is performed to fragment kidney stones, the particles always pass out of the body through the urinary system. True or False?

Percutaneous **nephrostolithotomy** (PCNL) or a **pyelostolithotomy** is a procedure to remove kidney stones. In this procedure, entry is through the patient's back. The procedure is reported based on the size of the stone removed (50080, to 2 cm; 50081, >2 cm). Internal lithotripsy is included in 50080 and 50081 and is not reported separately. External lithotripsy is not included in the codes and can be reported in addition to the 50080 and 50081; but remember to attach modifier -51 to the lesser procedure. The procedure is performed with fluoroscopic guidance that is reported separately with 76000 for the radiologist or 76001 for the radiologist that assists a nonradiological physician.

Excision. There are Excision codes in the Kidney subheading for biopsy, nephrectomy (removal of the kidney), and removal of a cyst. The biopsy codes (50200, 50205) are based on the approach, either percutaneous (through the skin) or by surgical exposure of the kidney.

A **nephrectomy** is the removal of a kidney, either partial or radical (total). A radical nephrectomy includes removal of the fascia and surrounding fatty tissue, regional lymph nodes, and the adrenal gland. The nephrectomy codes (50220-50240) are based on the complexity and extent of the procedure. Nephrectomies can also be performed by means of a laparoscope (50543, 50545-50548), based on whether the procedure was partial, radical, or donor, and whether the procedure included a partial or total ureterectomy.

Ablation is the cutting away or erosion of tissue. Code 50250 reports ablation of a kidney lesion by means of cryosurgery (use of subfreezing temperatures) and is usually performed with ultrasonic guidance. If used, the ultrasonic guidance is not reported separately because it is included in the code description. The surgeon accesses the kidney through an incision and inserts a cryosurgical probe into the lesion. The cryosurgical machine is turned on, and subfreezing temperature is delivered to the lesion (Fig. 19–4). The area is brought back to above freezing, and the treatment is applied again. At times, more than two cycles are applied to ensure the lesion is ablated. This procedure can also be performed percutaneously (50593) or by use of a laparoscope (50542).

Renal Transplantation. Allotransplantation is the transfer of tissue or an organ between two people who are not related (genetically different). Autotransplantation is transfer of tissue from one part of a person's body to another part of that person's body, also known as autograft or autotransplant. A surgeon may perform a renal autotransplant to reposition

FIGURE 19–4   Liquid nitrogen spray. (From White GM, Cox NH: *Diseases of the Skin: A Color Atlas and Text,* ed 2, Edinburgh, 2006, Mosby.)

the kidney, which may be necessary when the kidney has been severely damaged from trauma or disease. A renal autotransplantation is reported with 50380. Backbench work is the work involved in preparation for the transplant surgery and includes:

- Open organ **retrieval** from a deceased (50300) or living (50320) donor; laparoscopic organ retrieval from a living (50547) donor.

- Standard **preparation** based on deceased (50323) or living (50325) donor. As a part of this preparation the surgeon may perform additional surgery on the organ, such as venous, arterial, or ureteral anastomosis (50327-50329).

- **Transplant** service reported with 50360 (without nephrectomy) or 50365 (with nephrectomy) with modifier -50 added for a bilateral procedure.

If backbench procedures were performed, those services would be reported in addition to the transplantation service with modifier -51 added to indicate multiple procedures.

CODING SHOT   If the recipient requires a nephrectomy, the procedure is reported separately with 50340 and with modifier -50 for a bilateral procedure.

Introduction.   Introduction category codes in the Kidney subheading are for aspiration, catheters, injections for radiography, guides, and tube changes. There are also extensive notes within the category.

Codes in the range 50382-50389 are percutaneous, transurethral, or externally accessible procedures that report removal and/or replacement of renal stents and tubes. These stents are not renal artery stents but are ureteral stents that are placed through the renal pelvis. The codes only report a unilateral procedure, so if a bilateral procedure was performed, add modifier -50.

Imaging guidance is used for the codes in this range and is included in the code description, so do not report the guidance separately. If imaging guidance was not used for removal and/or replacement of externally accessible stents, you would report the removal with an E/M code.

QUICK CHECK 19-2

1. An Evaluation and Management (E/M) code is used to report removal of an _____ accessible stent when imaging guidance is not used.

Approximately half of the population over age 50 has renal cysts that are asymptomatic (no symptoms) and are often only discovered as an incidental finding on ultrasound or computed tomography. When these cysts are symptomatic, percutaneous aspiration or injection may be performed. The procedure is performed by use of local anesthetic and on an outpatient basis. A sclerosing agent (such as alcohol) may be injected into the cyst. The code description for 50390 indicates "aspiration and/or injection," which means if both an aspiration and injection are performed during the same operative session, 50390 is reported only one time. Image guidance is not included in the code description, so any guidance used is reported separately.

Repair. Repair category codes (50400-50540) include plastic surgery (pyeloplasty), suturing (nephrorrhaphy), and closure of fistula.

Pyeloplasty is a surgical procedure for an obstruction of the ureteropelvic junction (UPJ), which connects the renal pelvis to the ureter (Fig. 19–5). Usually, this is a congenital condition, but it may also be an acquired condition. If an obstruction occurs the urine will not drain, which results in dilatation of the collecting system and enlargement of the renal pelvis (hydronephrosis). The goal of a pyeloplasty is to remove the obstruction and repair the renal pelvis (Fig. 19–6). As a part of the repair, a nephropexy (surgical fixation of mobile kidney), nephrostomy (a passageway from the kidney to exterior of the body), pyelostomy (a passageway between the renal pelvis and the exterior of the body), and ureteral splinting are included in the codes for a **simple** pyeloplasty (50400). A **complicated** pyeloplasty (50405) includes all of the procedures in the simple pyeloplasty, as indicated by the placement of the semicolon in 50400. (Note that the semicolon is after the term splinting, which means that all the terms that precede the semicolon are included in the code description for the indented code 50405.) In addition to all the procedures in the simple pyeloplasty,

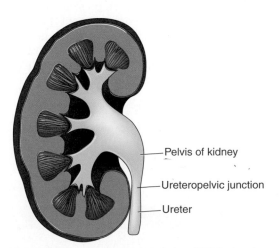

Pelvis of kidney

Ureteropelvic junction

Ureter

FIGURE 19–5 Ureteropelvic junction (UPJ) is the place at which the ureter joins the kidney.

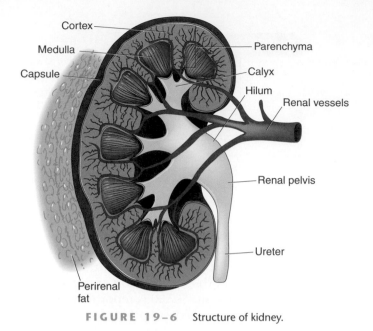

FIGURE 19-6 Structure of kidney.

the complicated pyeloplasty is more difficult, because the procedure may include repair of a congenital kidney abnormality (which can be an extensive procedure), further plastic repair of the pelvis of the kidney, repair of a solitary kidney (patient only has one kidney), or a calycoplasty. A calycoplasty is repair of the calyx (the cup-shaped structure) of the kidney.

Closures of nephrocutaneous, pyelocutaneous, or nephrovisceral fistulas (abnormal openings) are reported with codes from the 50520-50526 range. Code 50520 reports the closure of a fistula between the renal pelvis and the exterior of the body or of the kidney and the exterior. Codes 50525 and 50526 report closure of a fistula between the kidney and another organ, such as the kidney and the bladder. The approach to close the fistula may be abdominal (50525) or thoracic (50526).

TOOLBOX

John, a 43-year-old male patient, presents to his family physician, Dr. Marsh, with complaints of dull groin pain, an ache on the lower left side of his back, and a decrease in urinary output. A pyelogram was ordered and the final diagnosis was hydronephrosis. Antibiotics were prescribed and John is to return for a follow-up in 30 days.

QUESTIONS

1. For this diagnosis, would you expect the renal pelvis, renal column, or renal papilla to be enlarged?_____

2. When you reference "Pyelogram" in the CPT index, what is the "See" direction?

_____

_____

ANSWERS 1. Renal pelvis 2. See Urography, Intravenous; Urography, Retrograde

Laparoscopy. The Laparoscopy codes (50541-50549) report ablation of renal cysts (50541) or lesions (50542). Open cryosurgical ablation of renal tumors is reported with 50250, and percutaneous ablation is reported with 50593.

Laparoscopic nephrectomies and pyeloplasty are also reported with codes from the Laparoscopy category and are based on the extent of the procedure.

Endoscopy. Endoscopy codes (50551-50580) are frequently reported for kidney procedures, because these types of procedures are less invasive than the open procedures and are often performed in an outpatient setting. Renal endoscopies may be performed by means of an established connection between the kidney and the exterior of the body. The codes in the Endoscopy category are divided into those procedures performed through an established nephrostomy or pyelostomy and those that are not. For example, 50555 reports a renal endoscopy through an established nephrostomy/pyelostomy and 50574 reports the same endoscopic biopsy but not through a nephrostomy/pyelostomy. The codes are further divided based on the reason for the procedure: ureteral catheterization, biopsy, fulguration, or foreign body/calculus removal.

The code descriptions in the Endoscopy category code descriptions state "exclusive of radiologic service," which means that the radiologic services are reported in addition to the endoscopic procedures. If, for example, a biopsy (50555) is performed with ultrasound, you would report the biopsy procedure in addition to the ultrasound.

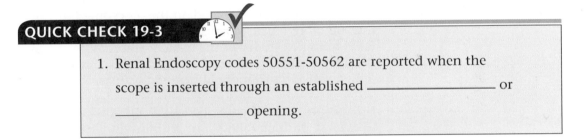

QUICK CHECK 19-3

1. Renal Endoscopy codes 50551-50562 are reported when the scope is inserted through an established _____ or _____ opening.

Kidney Index Locations. You will locate the kidney codes in the CPT manual index under "Kidney"; they are subtermed primarily by category (e.g., insertion, excision, or repair). Another method of locating kidney codes in the CPT manual index is to reference the medical term for the procedure (e.g., nephrostomy or nephrotomy). Again, there are other index location methods; these are just a couple to help you get started locating the codes.

The following kidney codes or code ranges are unilateral and require modifier -50 if the procedure was performed bilaterally:

50020-50290	Incision and Excision Categories
50390-50405	Introduction and Repair Categories
50541-50548	Laparoscopy
50551-50580	Endoscopy
50590	Lithotripsy

The third-party payer may require the use of -RT and/or -LT rather than modifier -50.

EXERCISE 19-1 *Kidney*

Using the CPT manual, code the following:

1 Repeat nephrolithotomy

CPT Code: _____

2 The patient presents for a nephrostomy tube exchange. The patient was placed prone on the angiographic table and has preexisting left nephrostomy tube. The patient did not receive conscious sedation. The back was prepped and draped in the usual sterile fashion. A guidewire was advanced through the nephrostomy tube. The tube was exchanged, and the tube was secured to the skin with suture.

CPT Code: _____

3 The patient presents with right renal calculus with stent for a right ESWL, cystoscopy, and stent removal. The patient was placed on the lithotripsy table and administered a general anesthetic. The stone was targeted, shock head engaged. Total of 2400 shocks at maximum kV of 24 were administered to the stone. Good fragmentation was noted. The patient was then prepped and draped in the supine position. The urethra was anesthetized with 2% Xylocaine jelly. The patient was cystoscoped with the flexible instrument; stent was visualized, grasped, and removed intact.

CPT Codes: _____, _____

Ureter The next subheading (50600-50980) in the Urinary System subsection is Ureter. The codes are based on the procedure (i.e., incision, excision, introduction, repair, laparoscopy, or endoscopy). The ureter is the tube that leads from the kidney to the bladder and may be the site of an assortment of conditions, such as obstruction by calculus, cysts, or lesions in addition to reflux, congenital abnormalities, and fistulas.

Incision. The Incision codes (50600-50630) report open procedures to explore or drain (50600), insert indwelling stent (50605), and removal of calculus (ureterolithotomy) based on the location of the calculus as upper third, middle third, or lower third of the ureter (50610-50630). The incisional procedures also have laparoscopic, endoscopic, and/or transvesical counterparts. For example, to report a laparoscopic ureterolithotomy of the upper third of the ureter report 50945 and for an incisional ureterolithotomy report 50610. It is very important to check the documentation for the method utilized for the procedure to ensure selection of the correct code.

QUICK CHECK 19-4

1. Laparoscopic ureterolithotomy is reported with code

_____, regardless of which portion of the ureter is involved.

Excision. The codes in the Excision category (50650, 50660) report ureterectomy either with bladder cuff or a total excision. The **bladder cuff** is the tissue that connects the ureter to the bladder, and the excision of the bladder cuff is only reported if it is the only procedure performed during the surgical session. A total ureterectomy may be performed by means of an abdominal, vaginal, or perineal approach or a combination of the three approaches. Code 50660 includes all three approaches or a combination of approaches. This means that if two or three approaches were utilized, you still only report 50660 one time.

Introduction.   The Introduction codes (50684-50690) include injection procedures, manometric studies (see paragraph below), and change of tubes and/or stents. Code 50684 reports an **injection** procedure performed through an indwelling catheter to determine the status of the renal collecting system. The physician injects a contrast agent through the catheter and an x-ray is taken. The radiological supervision and interpretation is reported separately with 74425.

Manometric studies (50686) are tests to measure kidney and ureter flow and pressure. The study is conducted by means of a machine (manometer) through an access site (ureterostomy or catheter). A tube carrying sterile fluid is inserted through the access site and into the kidney or bladder and the area is flooded. The pressures and flow are then measured and recorded.

Repair.   Repair procedures (50700-50940) includes ureteroplasty (plastic repair of the ureter), ureterolysis (freeing of fibrous tissue), ureteropyelostomy (connection of upper ureter to renal pelvis), ureterocalicostomy (connection of upper ureter to renal calyx), and ureteroureterostomy (bypass of obstructed ureter), in addition to numerous other procedures to repair the ureter.

CAUTION *Watch the Repair codes for use of modifier -50! Unless stated the procedure is unilateral and requires modifier -50 for bilateral procedures.*

Laparoscopy.   Laparoscopic ureter codes 50947 and 50948 report the placement of a ureteral stent, which may be performed in conjunction with or without cystoscopic placement. The stent is placed because of an obstruction of the ureterovesical junction (UVJ). The surgeon laparoscopically repositions the ureter on the bladder and then by means of the cystoscope places the ureteral stent.

Endoscopy.   The Endoscopy codes (50951-50980) report procedures that are performed through an established stoma (ureterostomy, 50951-50961) or through an incision into the ureter (ureterotomy, 50970-50980). The procedures conducted through a ureterostomy are similar to the types of procedures conducted through a nephrostomy (e.g., 50551-50562, biopsy, catheterization, irrigation, and instillation). Excellent medical terminology skills are essential for working within this subheading, because the words can be intimidating. Keep your medical dictionary close by to look up any words you are not absolutely sure about. You can also refer to the Glossary at the back of the book. The time you spend now increasing the depth and breadth of your medical terminology is an excellent investment and will greatly increase your coding accuracy.

The endoscopy procedures are for irrigation, instillation, catheterization, biopsy, fulguration, and foreign body or calculus removal. The procedures often utilize radiological services, but these services are reported separately. Note that the stand-alone code descriptions in the category (50951, 50970) indicate that the service is "exclusive of radiologic service," meaning that you report those services in addition to the procedure. This also means that all indented codes that follow 50951 and 56970 do not include radiologic services.

When a ureterocystography is performed, the physician injects a radioactive contrast material through a catheter inserted into the bladder via the urethra or through a previously established stoma. The injection procedure is reported in addition to the primary procedure. For example, if the procedure was an endoscopic biopsy of the right ureter through an established stoma, you would report 50955-RT and the injection procedure would be reported with 50684-RT. In addition to the primary and injection procedures, you also report the radiological supervision and interpretation with a Radiology code. For example, 74425 that reports retrograde urography. Retrograde urography is performed by injecting contrast directly into the lower end of the system and the contrast flows backwards through the system allowing for visualization of the tract.

NCCI

According to CMS, 50955 and 50684 cannot be reported together as CMS bundles these codes. Only if the 50684 is a uniquely distinct procedure could you report it with 50955. You must add modifier -59 to the 50684 code. Refer to Fig. 19–7 for an example of the codes that are bundled into 50955. This figure illustrates that 50684 is bundled into 50955. In the far right column, the number 1 indicates that the code can be reported separately with modifier -59 (distinct procedure) added and the 0 indicates that the code cannot be reported with -59 and is always bundled with the primary code.

Code	Bundled	Modifier-59
50955	C8950	1
50955	C8952	1
50955	G0345	1
50955	G0347	1
50955	G0351	1
50955	G0353	1
50955	G0354	1
50955	J2001	1
50955	00910	0
50955	36000	1
50955	36410	1
50955	37202	1
50955	50684	1
50955	50715	1
50955	50951	1
50955	51701	1
50955	51702	1
50955	51703	1
50955	62318	1
50955	62319	1
50955	64415	1
50955	64416	1
50955	64417	1
50955	64450	1
50955	69990	0
50955	90760	1
50955	90765	1
50955	90772	1
50955	90774	1
50955	90775	1
50955	90780	1
50955	96360	1
50955	96365	1
50955	96372	1
50955	96374	1
50955	96375	1

FIGURE 19–7 Codes bundled into 50955.

The following ureter codes or code ranges are unilateral and require modifier -50 if the procedure was performed bilaterally:

50605-50630	Incision
50740-50760	Repair
50780-50840	Repair
50860-50940	Repair
50945-50980	Laparoscopy/Endoscopy

The third-party payer may require the use of -RT and/or -LT rather than modifier -50.

EXERCISE 19-2   *Ureter*

Using the CPT manual, code the following:

1 Ureterolithotomy of the lower one third of the left ureter .

CPT Code: _____

2 Bilateral ureteroneocystostomy

CPT Code: _____

3 Ureteral endoscopic biopsy through an established ureterostomy with injection of contrast

CPT Codes: _____, _____, _____

RT/LT not documented

Bladder   The Bladder subheading (51020-52700) contains codes not only for the usual services, such as incision and excision, but also for some unique services such as urodynamics and procedures performed on the prostate. Review the anatomy of the bladder in Fig. 19–8.

Incision.   Cystotomy (51020-51045) is often performed to fulgurate (use of electric current), insert radioactive material, or cryosurgically to destroy a lesion. In addition, the procedure is used for drainage, placement of catheter/stent, or a cystolithotomy (removal of calculus).

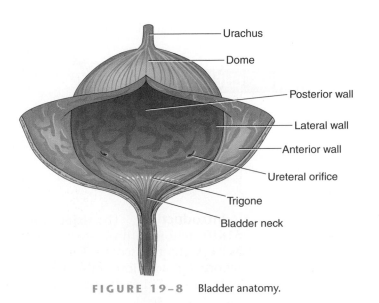

Urachus
Dome
Posterior wall
Lateral wall
Anterior wall
Ureteral orifice
Trigone
Bladder neck

FIGURE 19–8   Bladder anatomy.

A cystolithotomy reported with 51050 is one in which an incision is made in the skin and into the bladder. The physician removes the calculus through the incision, but does not excise the bladder neck. A transvesical ureterolithotomy described in 51060 is a similar procedure to 51050, but the calculus is removed through an incision in the bladder and the ureter. Ureter calculus is removed through an incision in 51065, but the calculus is first fragmented by ultrasound or electrohydraulic means. Electrohydraulic fragmentation is the use of a probe containing two electrodes that are applied, one on each side, of the calculus. Electrical current is then directed through the electrodes, which fragments the calculus.

Removal. **Aspiration** of urine from the bladder may be accomplished by means of needle, trocar (a sharply pointed surgical instrument), or intracatheter (plastic tube with a needle on the end). A suprapubic (above the pubic bone) catheter may also be inserted during the aspiration service (51102). Aspirations are often performed by means of imaging guidance, which is reported separately. If imaging guidance is used, report the guidance separately with 76942, 77002, or 77012.

Excision.   A **urachal cyst** is between the umbilicus and bladder dome and is often diagnosed in young children when the cyst becomes infected. Because of the proximity to the abdominal cavity and potential to rupture, a urachal cyst is a condition that warrants prompt medical attention. A urachal sinus is a congenital abnormality in which prenatal tissue remains, causes drainage to the umbilicus, and results in infection. The excision of a urachal cyst or sinus is reported with 51500 and may or may not include umbilical hernia repair.

Cystotomies and cystectomies (51520-51596) are performed for a variety of reasons, such as excision of a portion of or all of the bladder, repair of a ureterocele, or to replant a ureter into the bladder. The codes are divided based on the extent of the procedure. If the procedure is performed transurethrally, such as a bladder resection, codes from the Transurethral Surgery category (52204-52318) would be reported.

Pelvic exenteration (51597) is also known as total pelvic exenteration (TPE) and is the removal of the pelvic organs and adjacent structures due to malignancy. If TPE is performed due to gynecologic malignancy, report the service with the Female Genital system code 58240. A hysterectomy may be performed with 51597, but the initial and primary reason the procedure is being performed is for other than a gynecological malignancy.

QUICK CHECK 19-5

1. Pelvic exenteration is reported with 51597, unless the diagnosis is a gynecologic malignancy, then code _____ should be reported.

Introduction.   The **injection** procedures reported with codes 51600-51610 are for urethrocystography (x-ray of lower urinary tract, also known as a cystourethroscopy). The radiological supervision and interpretation are reported in addition to the injection procedure. Note that the parenthetical statements after each of the injection codes direct the coder to the correct radiology code(s).

Insertion of bladder catheters may be non-indwelling (51701) or temporary indwelling (51702, 51703). The non-indwelling catheter is the type that is inserted into the urethra and manipulated into the bladder to drain residual urine. The temporary indwelling procedure can be a simple catheterization (such as with a Foley) or a complicated catheterization due to an anatomical anomaly.

Catheter fracturing may occur, for example, when a patient pulls the catheter out while balloon is still inflated. This is a rare complication and does not describe the insertion but rather why it was necessary to reinsert another catheter.

Instillation is a procedure that is performed for bladder cancer. An anticarcinogenic agent is introduced into the bladder by means of a catheter. For example, immunotherapy is the instillation of a nonactive tuberculosis agent into the bladder. The agent is retained in the bladder for a period of time (such as 1 hour) with the patient in a lying position. The agent is then drained and the treatment is concluded. A series of these instillations is performed in a course of treatment. Code 51720 reports the instillation as well as the retention time and drainage.

Urodynamics.
Urodynamics pertains to the motion and flow of urine. Urinary tract flow can be obstructed by renal calculi, narrowing (stricture) of the ureter, cysts, and so forth. The procedures in the Urodynamics subheading (51725-51798) are to be conducted by or under the direct supervision of a physician, and all the instruments, equipment, supplies, and technical assistance necessary to conduct the procedure are bundled into the codes. If the physician performs only the professional service (e.g., interpretation of the results), modifier -26 (professional component) is reported with the code to indicate that the technical portion of the service (performance of test or tests) was provided elsewhere. For example, if a physician provides only the interpretation (-26) of a complex urethral pressure profile (UPP) (51727), report only the professional component of the service as 51727-26.

Repair and Laparoscopy.
Repair procedures (51800-51980) include procedures such as cystoplasty (bladder repair), cystourethroplasty (bladder and urethra), vesicourethropexy/urethropexy (repair for urinary incontinence), and closure of fistulas.

Stress incontinence may be surgically repaired by a colposuspension procedure in which a urethral sling is placed to support and elevate the UVJ (ureterovesical junction, where ureter joins with bladder). There are several types of these sling procedures, such as the Marshall-Marchetti-Krantz (MMK), Burch, paravaginal repair, anterior vesicourethropexy, or urethropexy. These procedures are reported with 51840 for a simple procedure and 51841 for a complicated repair, which would include a secondary repair of the bladder. The urethral suspension and sling operation are also performed by means of laparoscopy (51990, 51992). A sling operation for stress incontinence is also reported with 57288 when vaginal and abdominal incisions are used. A Pereyra procedure (57289) is also known as a needle bladder neck suspension in which sutures are used to support and anchor the bladder. The codes (57287-57289) are in the Female Genital System subsection, Vagina subheading because the procedure includes repair of the vagina. There are also codes in the Urethra subsection (53431-53442) that refer to the creation, removal, or revision of a sling operation for male urinary incontinence and plastic repair of the bladder for incontinence.

Endoscopy. There are codes (52000-52010) for bundled endoscopy procedures (i.e., cystoscopy, urethroscopy, and cystourethroscopy). The codes contain the primary procedure of a cystourethroscopy (endoscopic procedure to view the bladder and urethra) and minor related procedures performed at the same time. For example, if a cystourethroscopy is performed for the biopsy of the ureter with radiography, bundled into the code for the procedure (52007) are the catheterization, endoscopic procedure, and biopsy(ies). To unbundle the code and report the individual components of the procedure separately would not be correct. If the secondary procedure(s) required significant additional time or effort that is documented in the medical record, the procedure can be identified using modifier -22 (increased procedure). There are combination codes that include many components of a procedure bundled into one code. For example, 52005 reports a cystourethroscopy with ureteral catheterization, with/without irrigation, instillation, or ureteropyelography with the one code. Be careful to read each description in this category before assigning a code to be certain you have identified each component included in the code before you assign additional codes. For example, you cannot report a cystourethroscopy (52005) with a catheterization (51701) because a catheterization is included in the code description for 52005. Many third-party payers, such as CMS, have lists of codes (edits) that cannot be reported with other codes. For example, 52000 (cystourethroscopy) cannot be reported with 51701 (catheterization), even though catheterization is not stated in the code description. You need to know not only the limitations set by the notes and codes in the CPT manual but also the limitations set by the third-party payer.

CODING SHOT For a complete list of the CMS Correct Coding Initiative (CCI) edits, check out www.cms.hhs.gov/NationalCorrectCodInitEd/.

A cystourethroscopy is a diagnostic procedure to assess lower urinary tract symptoms (LUTS), such as incontinence or benign prostate hypertrophy (BPH). The procedure is reported only if it is performed as the only procedure during the operative session, because it is designated a separate procedure.

CODING SHOT Usually, third-party payers will not reimburse for more than two cystourethroscopic procedures per episode of illness unless bladder or urethral malignancies are being treated.

QUICK CHECK 19-6

1. To locate endoscopy codes in the CPT index, use the main terms _____, _____, or cystourethroscopy.

Transurethral Surgery. Transurethral Surgery codes (52204-52355) are for the urethra/bladder (52204-52318) and ureter/pelvis (52320-52355).

Code 52204 reports a cystourethroscopy with biopsy and 52000 is also a cystourethroscopy. The difference is that 52000 is a diagnostic procedure only. No additional procedure was performed when reporting 52000. When reporting 52204, a biopsy was performed, so the procedure was not only diagnostic but also a surgical procedure. The procedure may have begun as a diagnostic procedure, but it progressed to a biopsy on identification of a lesion. The diagnostic procedure is then bundled into the surgical procedure and not reported separately.

CODING SHOT

Many third-party payers will bundle 52204 (cystourethroscopy) into many major procedures. For example, Medicare bundles the cystourethroscopy into the transurethral resection of a bladder tumor (52234-52240).

A **transurethral resection of a bladder tumor** (TURBT) is a procedure in which a bladder tumor is removed by fulguration (electric current) or excision. Note that the code descriptions 52234-52240 contain multiple methods of removal of the bladder tumor, that is, "with fulguration (including cryosurgery or laser surgery) and/or resection." If any, or a combination of, these methods has been used to eradicate the tumor, you can assign a code based on the **size** of the bladder tumor. The code description indicates the size as minor (>0.5 cm), small (0.5-2.0 cm), medium (2.0-5.0 cm), and large (>5 cm). Code 52224 is a cystourethroscopy with fulguration or treatment of a minor (<0.5 cm) lesion(s). The lesion(s) are treated with cryosurgery or a laser. This procedure may or may not include a biopsy prior to eradication.

Many of the code descriptions require the coder to be familiar with the anatomy of the bladder and surrounding structures. For example, 52214 (cystourethroscopy) with fulguration (including cryosurgery or laser surgery) of trigone, bladder neck, prostatic fossa, urethra, or periurethral glands. Refer to Fig. 19–8 for bladder anatomy and location of the trigone and bladder neck. To code correctly the coder also needs to know the anatomy surrounding the bladder, such as the prostatic fossa, which is the depression or cavity (prostatic bed) in which the prostate is located.

The codes in the Ureter and Pelvis subsection (52320-52355) all include insertion and removal of temporary stents during the procedure, even though the code descriptions may not all state that fact. You know this only when you read the notes preceding code 52320. That does not mean that insertion and/or removal of temporary stents cannot be reported with other procedures, such as ESWL (50590), only that temporary stents are not reported separately with the codes in the 52320-52355 range. Make a note in your CPT manual next to this range of codes stating "includes insertion/removal of temporary stents" as a reminder of this important point or highlight the paragraph in the notes preceding code 52320 ("The insertion and removal of a temporary uretral catheter...."). Insertion of indwelling stents is reported separately with 52332-51 in addition to the primary procedure. Code 52332 reports **insertion** of unilateral stents, so modifiers to indicate bilateral procedures were performed would also be needed; for example, 52332-51-50. To report **removal** of indwelling stents, use 52310 (simple removal) or 52315 (complicated removal) with modifier -58 (staged or related procedure or service by same physician during the postoperative period). It is a good idea to place a bracket next to codes 52310 and 52315 and write "-58" as a reminder of how to report these codes, because the direction for the use of this modifier is located in notes before code 52320.

Vesical Neck and Prostate. The Vesical Neck and Prostate codes 52400-52700 contain codes to report cystourethroscopy and transurethral procedures. Many of these codes are reviewed in the Male Genital System information because many of these procedures are of the prostate with access through the urethra, such as 52450, transurethral incision of the prostate.

When the procedure is a transurethral **resection** of the bladder neck, report 52500. If a transurethral **incision** of the bladder neck is performed, report 52276 (Bladder, Urethrotomy).

The following bladder code ranges are unilateral and require modifier -50 if the procedure was performed bilaterally:

52005-52010 Endoscopy/Cystoscopy, Urethroscopy and Cystourethroscopy

52320-52355 Ureter and Pelvis

The third-party payer may require the use of -RT and/or -LT rather than modifier -50.

EXERCISE 19-3 *Bladder*

Using the CPT manual, code the following:

1 Needle aspiration of bladder

CPT Code: _____

2 Endoscopy for establishment of a right Gibbons ureteral stent

CPT Code: _____

3 Cystoscopy, left retrograde pyelogram using contrast, under fluoroscopic control, insertion of left ureteral stent

CPT Codes: _____, _____

4 The patient has been diagnosed with incontinence and presents for an urethropexy. The patient was brought to the operating room and placed on the operating table in the supine position, prepped, and draped. A small horizontal incision is made in the abdomen just above the symphysis pubis. The bladder was then suspended by placing sutures bilaterally at the mid-portion of the urethra 1 cm lateral and at the bladder neck 2 cm lateral. The sutures were then suspended to the Cooper's ligament bilaterally. The urethra was then elevated to the horizontal position.

CPT Code: _____

5 The 33-year-old patient has postoperative diagnosis of left ureteral calculus and presents for a cystoscopy, bilateral retrograde pyelograms, left ureteroscopy, and stone extraction. The patient was cystoscoped using a 21-French instrument. There was no evidence of urethral or bladder abnormality. Bilateral retrograde pyelograms were performed that indicated normal collecting system of the right-hand side. There was only a minimal suggestion of a filling defect in the distal ureter on the left. A guidewire was advanced up the ureter under fluoroscopic control and then a rigid short ureteroscope followed this. A stone was visualized and was entrapped in a basket and withdrawn under visual guidance.

CPT Codes: _____, _____

Urethra The subheading Urethra contains codes (53000-53899) for the usual procedures of incision, excision, and repair. For endoscopic procedures of the urethra, refer to codes 52000-52700, which contain cystoscopy, urethroscopy, and cystourethroscopy procedures.

If the physician performs the injection procedure for radiology studies for examination of the urethra, report 51600-51610 based on the type of study being performed. The radiological supervision and interpretation is reported separately with 74430 (cystography), 74450 (retrograde urethrocystography), or 74455 (voiding urethrocystography).

Incision. A meatotomy is surgical incision of the meatus, which is the opening of the urethra to the outside of the body (urethral meatus). This procedure is often bundled into other more major procedures. Codes 53020 (except infant) and 53025 (infant) report a meatotomy if it is performed as a separate procedure. Because 53025 is specifically for infants, do not append modifier -63 (Procedure performed on infants less than 4 kg).

The **Skene's glands** are also known as the paraurethral or the lesser vestibular glands and are located on on either side of the urethra. These glands drain into the urethra near the meatus (urethral opening). When infected, the gland will become enlarged and tender and may require drainage or excision. **Drainage** of an abscess or cyst of the Skene's glands is reported with 53060. **Excision** of the Skene's glands is reported with code 53270.

Excision. The Excision category of codes (53200-53275) includes services such as biopsy, urethrectomy, lesion excision, fulguration, and marsupialization (creating a pouch).

When the urethra is totally surgically removed (urethrectomy), the service is reported with 53210 for a female and 53215 for a male. A urethrectomy involves removal of the urethra and creation of an opening from the bladder to the skin that is then used to drain urine. The procedure would include removal of any tumors of the urethra. If the urethra was not removed and only the tumor was removed, report with 53220.

The bulbourethral gland is also known as the Cowper's gland and is a pair of glands about the size of a pea located beneath the prostate. These glands produce some of the fluid for semen and drain directly into the urethra. Excision of the bulbourethral gland is reported with 53250.

Repair. A urethroplasty may be completed in one stage or two stages (53400-53431). The choice of codes to report a urethroplasty is based on the number of stages and type of repair. Codes 53420 (first stage) and 53425 (second stage) report the two stages of an urethroplasty, and 53415 reports a one-stage urethroplasty.

A tandem cuff or dual cuff is an artifical urinary sphincter (AUS) that is placed due to atrophy, disease, or defect of the urinary sphincter and reported with 53444. An artificial sphincter is inflatable and includes a pump, reservoir, and cuff, is inserted through a subpubic incision, and is illustrated in Fig. 19–9. The small switch in the scrotum can be manipulated to activate the pump and control urinary continence. Codes 53446-53448 report the removal and/or replacement of AUS system, and 53449 reports repair of a previously placed system.

Urethromeatoplasty is repair of the meatus and the urethra (53450, 53460) and is performed to open and/or reconstruct the urethra.

Manipulation. The Manipulation category codes (53600-53665) are a bit different from those you have encountered previously. Manipulation

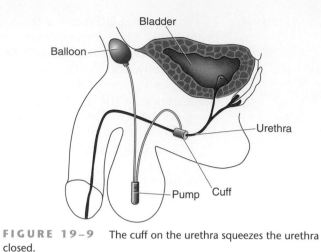

FIGURE 19–9 The cuff on the urethra squeezes the urethra closed.

is performed on the urethra (e.g., dilation or catheterization). Dilation stretches or dilates a passage that has narrowed. The Dilation codes are based on initial or subsequent dilation of a male or female patient.

EXERCISE 19-4 *Urethra*

Using the CPT manual, code the following:

1 Closure of a urethrostomy in a 54-year-old man

  CPT Code: _____

2 Second stage, surgical reconstruction of the urethra, with urinary diversion

  CPT Code: _____

MALE GENITAL SYSTEM

Format

The Male Genital System subsection (54000-55899) of the CPT manual is divided into anatomic subheadings (penis, testis, epididymis, tunica vaginalis, scrotum, vas deferens, spermatic cord, seminal vesicles, and prostate) (Fig. 19–10). The category codes are divided according to procedure. The greatest number of category codes are under the subheading Penis because there are many repair codes in this subheading. The other subheadings are primarily for incision and excision, with only a few repair codes for the remaining subheadings.

Penis

Incisions. Under the Incision category (54000-54015) of the subheading Penis, there is an incision and drainage code (54015). Recall that under the Integumentary System section there are incision and drainage codes. The code from the Penis subheading is for a deep incision, not just an abscess of the skin. For the deep abscess described in 54015, the area is anesthetized, the abscess is opened and cleaned, and often a drain is placed to maintain adequate drainage.

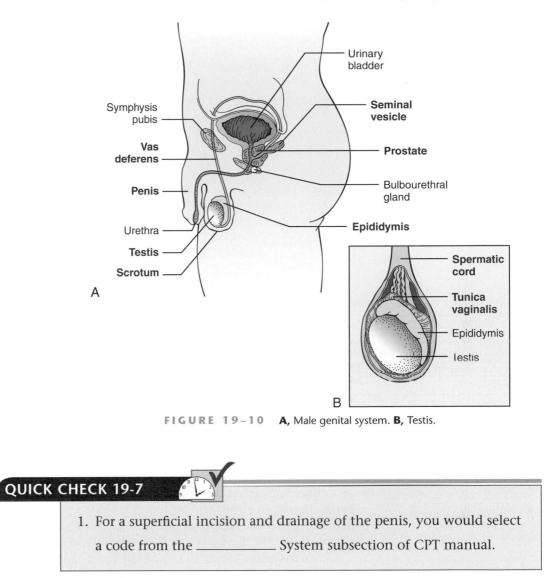

Urinary
bladder

Symphysis
pubis

**Seminal
vesicle**

**Vas
deferens**

Prostate

Penis

Bulbourethral
gland

Urethra

Epididymis

Testis

Scrotum

A

**Spermatic
cord**

**Tunica
vaginalis**

Epididymis

Testis

B

FIGURE 19–10   **A,** Male genital system. **B,** Testis.

QUICK CHECK 19-7

1. For a superficial incision and drainage of the penis, you would select a code from the _____ System subsection of CPT manual.

Destruction. Under the Destruction category (54050-54065) of the subheading Penis there are also destruction codes for lesions of the penis. These lesion destruction codes are divided on the basis of whether the destruction is simple or extensive. Simple destruction is further divided according to the method of destruction (e.g., chemical, cryosurgery, laser). The code for extensive lesion destruction can be reported no matter which method was employed to accomplish the extensive destruction.

Excision. Excision codes (54100-54164) include codes to report biopsy of the penis (54100, 54105). Note that 54100 has a designation of "separate procedure," which means that the code is reported when the biopsy was the only procedure performed during the operative session. To accomplish the biopsy, the physician removes a portion of a lesion by excision of a small section of the lesion (scalpel or scissors) or by a punch biopsy. A punch biopsy is commonly used with skin lesions and is performed with an instrument that is pencil-shaped (Fig. 19–11) that removes a round disk of tissue. The opening left by the punch may require simple closure (suture) depending on the size of the skin defect created by the biopsy. A more complex biopsy (54105) of the penis involves the deeper layers of the penis and may require layered closure, which is reported separately.

FIGURE 19–11 A punch biopsy is used for deeper lesions and the area may require closure.

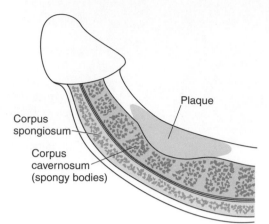

Plaque

Corpus spongiosum

Corpus cavernosum (spongy bodies)

FIGURE 19–12 Curvature of penis due to Peyronie disease.

Peyronie disease is a curvature of the penis that results from plaque formation on the cavernous sheaths of the penis as illustrated in Fig. 19–12. The plaque develops on the lower and upper side of the penis where the erectile tissue is located. Inflammation results and leads to the formation of scar tissue. Over time, this fibrous plaque bends the penis. In severe cases, the penis arches during erection, causing pain. Surgical correction of the curvature involves removal of the penile plaque (54110-54112). Grafting of the defect may be necessary, depending on the extent of the removal. Code 54110 reports the excision of penile plaque when no grafting is required and 54111/54112 report excision when grafting is required.

Penile amputation can occur as a result of trauma or as a surgical procedure for penile cancer. If the procedure is the removal of only the penis (partial or complete), report the service with 54120 or 54125. If the procedure includes removal of the inguinofemoral lymph nodes, report the service based on the extent of the removal (54130, 54135).

Circumcision codes 54150-54161 are divided based on whether the circumcision was accomplished by means of a clamp/other device or surgical excision and whether the procedure was performed on a neonate or non-neonate. A clamp is a device that is used to restrain the foreskin of the penis while the skin is trimmed. Report newborn circumcisions that utilize a clamp or other device with 54150. Surgical excision of the foreskin is a procedure in which a clamp or other device is not used, and the surgeon directly excises the skin from the penis. Once the skin has been removed, the incision is closed with sutures. Report the surgical excision without the use of a clamp or other device with 54160 (neonate) or 54161 (except neonate).

QUICK CHECK 19-8

1. Circumcision code 54160 is assigned for infants aged _____ days or less.

Introduction. Introduction codes (54200-54250) report various injection procedures, irrigations, plethysmography, and other tests. An example would be an injection procedure for Peyronie disease in which steroids are injected into the fibrous tissue of the penis to decrease pain, deformity, and fibrous tissue size. There are two ways the fibrous tissue can be injected: the first way is to inject steroids directly into the area of the lump formed by the fibrous tissue (54200), and the second way is to expose the fibrous tissue through an incision and then inject steroids into the fibrous tissue (54205).

Priapism is a state of prolonged erection that can last from hours to days because of the inability of the blood to flow from the penis, which returns the penis to a flaccid state. The condition may be caused by medications used to treat impotence, such as sildenafil citrate (Viagra) or medical conditions, such as leukemia, multiple myeloma, or tumor infiltrate. If medical intervention is necessary, the surgeon introduces a large needle into the corpus cavernosum and aspirates blood, which is what is keeping the penis erect. The corpus cavernosum is then irrigated with a saline solution. The entire procedure is reported with 54220.

Repair. Repair category (54300-54440) codes are for various repairs made to the penis. The code descriptions often state the condition for which the procedure is being performed. For example, 54304 is plastic repair for correction of chordee or a first-stage hypospadias (defined in next paragraph) repair, and 54380 is plastic repair for epispadias. Many other codes also indicate the stage of the procedure.

Many of the Repair codes refer to repair of chordee and hypospadias. **Chordee** is a condition in which the penis has a ventral (downward) curve and is a congenital deformity. **Hypospadias** is a congenital abnormality in which the urethral meatus (opening) is abnormally placed, usually along the ventral aspect (underside) of the shaft. Degrees of hypospadias are classified according to location: anterior, middle, or posterior. Hypospadias may lead to chordee. The farther from the glans penis the opening is, the greater the chordee. Read the code descriptions for Repair codes carefully as many of the descriptions have only slight differences.

Codes in the range 54400-54417 report insertion, repair, or removal of various types of penile prostheses. The codes are divided based on the type of service and often on the circumstances of the service. Erectile dysfunction (impotence) is a condition in which the penis does not become erect. Impotence may be caused by a variety of conditions, such as obesity, chronic illness, or as a result of medication. One surgical solution to impotence is insertion of a **penile implant**. There are various types of penile implants, but mainly there are two broad categories: non-inflatable (malleable or flexible, 54400) and inflatable (54401). These implants are inserted deep within the penile tissue. If the implant is subsequently removed, the removal procedure is reported with 54406 (inflatable) or 54115 (non-inflatable).

On occasion, removal and replacement are accomplished during the same operative session. Removal of a previously placed prosthesis with insertion of a new prosthesis during the same operative session is reported with 54410, 54411 (inflatable), or 54416/54417 (non-inflatable).

QUICK CHECK 19-9

1. When coding for penile prostheses the code selection is determined by the type of implant, which may be _____ or _____, and the type of service insertion, repair, removal, and/or replacement.

EXERCISE 19-5 *Penis*

Using the CPT and ICD-9-CM manuals, code the following:

1 Extensive electrodesiccation of a condyloma on the penis

CPT Code: _____

ICD-9-CM Code: _____ (ICD-10-CM Code: _____)

2 Patient presents for removal of a previously implanted semi-rigid penile implant

CPT Code: _____

Testis

Excision. The Excision category (54500-54535) codes report services such as biopsy, excision, orchiectomy, and exploration of the testis. Biopsies may be percutaneous (54500) or incisional (54505). If an incisional biopsy of the testis is performed bilaterally, report modifier -50 with 54505.

Extraparenchymal is defined as unrelated to the essential elements of an organ. Removal of an extraparenchymal lesion of the testis is reported with 54512. An incision is made on the scrotum, and the testicle is pulled out through the incision where the tunica vaginalis is opened and the lesion is removed. The testicle is returned to the scrotum and the area is sutured closed.

An **orchiectomy** is the removal of a testis. CPT codes 54520-54535 report orchiectomies based on if the procedure was simple/radical, unilateral/bilateral, with/without testicular prosthesis insertion, and the approach used to gain access to the site. Watch for codes that specify unilateral or bilateral. For example, a simple orchiectomy with or without testicular prosthesis insertion (54520) reports a unilateral procedure. When the procedure is bilateral, modifier -50 must be added to correctly report the procedure. However, a radical orchiectomy as reported with 54530 reports the removal of both testes and does not require modifier -50.

Exploration, Repair, and Laparoscopy. Undescended testis (cryptorchidism) is a congenital condition in which the testis(es) did not descend into the scrotal sac. The condition may be unilateral or bilateral. The testis(es) may remain in the abdominal, inguinal, or prescrotal areas or may move back and forth between areas. Often, undescended testis is associated with a hernia, and if this was the case, during the hernia repair procedure, the undescended testis is brought down into the scrotum and anchored with sutures (orchiopexy). An exploration may be necessary to locate the undescended testis(es) and the choice of codes (54550, 54560) is determined based on the approach used (inguinal/scrotal or abdominal) to gain access to the area. The exploration codes report a unilateral procedure, so if a bilateral procedure was performed, add modifier -50. During an exploration, when no more definitive procedure is performed, it is only reported as an exploration. If the testis was located during the exploration and the surgeon moved the testis into the scrotal sac, the procedure is no longer an exploration, but a corrective procedure (orchiopexy). An orchiopexy is reported with codes from the Repair category or the Laparoscopy category, depending on the technique used. An orchiopexy in which the operative site is opened to the surgeon's view is reported with 54640 or 54650 depending on whether the approach was inguinal or abdominal. If the orchiopexy is performed laparoscopically, report the procedure with 54692.

QUICK CHECK 19-10

1. If during an exploratory procedure the testis is located and moved to the scrotal sac, the procedure becomes this corrective procedure:

_____.

The following testes code ranges are unilateral and require modifier -50 if the procedure was performed bilaterally:

54500-54560   Excision

54640-54680   Repair

54690-54692   Laparoscopy

The third-party payer may require the use of -RT and/or -LT rather than modifier -50.

EXERCISE 19-6 *Testis*

Using the CPT manual, code the following:

1 Simple bilateral orchiectomy with insertion of prosthesis using scrotal approach

CPT Code: _____

2 The diagnosis is azoospermia and the procedure bilateral testicular biopsies. The patient was given a general mask anesthetic, prepped and draped in supine position. Bilateral testicular cord blocks were performed. Beginning on the right side, a scrotal incision was made. The tunica vaginalis was identified, opened, and a stay stitch placed in the testis. A small incision was made, tubules delivered, resected, and sent for permanent section. The testis, vaginalis, and skin were closed with 3-0 chromic. The procedure was repeated in identical fashion on the contralateral side.

CPT Code: _____

Epididymis
The **epididymis** is a narrow, coiled tube that connects the efferent ducts at the back of each testicle to the vas deferens. The epididymis is divided into the caput (head), corpus (body), and cauda (tail). The epididymis can become infected, inflamed, or obstructed. When an abscess or hematoma forms in the epididymis, the surgeon may incise and drain the area (54700). At times, the testis, scrotal space, and epididymis are the site of abscess or hematoma. When any or all of these areas are incised and drained, the service is reported with 54700. For example, if the surgeon incised and drained the scrotal space, the service is reported with 54700. Or, if the surgeon incised and drained the testis, scrotal space, and epididymis, the service is reported with 54700. The one code reports incision and drainage of each or all of the areas.

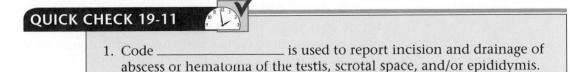

QUICK CHECK 19-11

1. Code _____ is used to report incision and drainage of abscess or hematoma of the testis, scrotal space, and/or epididymis.

Excision. The Excision category (54800-54861) of the Epididymis codes reports biopsy, exploration (with/without biopsy), lesion or spermatocele excision, and unilateral or bilateral removal. A spermatocele is a cyst that contains sperm, and during the excision of the cyst the epididymis may or may not be removed depending on the damage to the area caused by the presence of the cyst. Code 54840 reports the excision of a spermatocele with or without an epididymectomy.

Repair. Repair to the epididymis is an **epididymovasostomy**, also known as vasectomy reversal. During epididymovasostomy, the epididymis is connected to the vas deferens. The surgical procedure is reported with 54900 or 54901 depending if the procedure was unilateral or bilateral. An operating microscope is often used during this procedure and reported separately with 69990.

The following epididymis code range is unilateral and requires modifier -50 if the procedure was performed bilaterally:

54700-54840   Epididymis (Incision)

The third-party payer may require the use of -RT and/or -LT rather than modifier -50.

Tunica Vaginalis

Incision and Excision. The **tunica vaginalis** is a serous sheath of the testis, which can be the site of hydrocele (fluid collection). The physician may aspirate the fluid or inject a substance such as a sclerosing agent (55000) to help prevent further accumulation of fluid. Another method of management of a hydrocele is excision (unilateral, 55040 or bilateral, 55041), which may be accompanied by a hernia repair that is reported separately (49495-49501).

Repair. A Bottle type repair (55060) is a surgical procedure performed to remedy a hydrocele of the tunica vaginalis. An incision is made in the inguinal or scrotal area, and the hydrocele is drained and repositioned. A catheter may be left in place to ensure continued drainage of the area and to prevent further fluid accumulation.

Scrotum

Incision. The scrotum is the sac that contains the testes. If a lesion of the skin of the scrotum is removed, assign codes from the Integumentary System to report the service. However, if the abscess is in the scrotal wall and requires drainage report the procedure with 55100 (Drainage of scrotal wall abscess). If the abscess is of the epididymis, testis, and/or scrotal space, report the service with 54700 because the code reports procedures to any of the three areas.

Repair. Scrotoplasty (also known as oscheoplasty) is repair of a congenital abnormality or traumatic defect of the scrotum. Skin flaps may be utilized during a simple repair (55175) and in the more complex repair (55180) rotational pedicle grafts and/or free skin grafts may be used. Simple skin flaps are included in the scrotoplasty and not reported separately, but the more complex grafts are reported in addition to the scrotoplasty.

Vas Deferens

Incision. The vas deferens is the tube that carries sperm from the testes to the urethra. A vasotomy (55200) is cutting into the vas deferens. Usually the procedure is performed to obtain a semen sample or to determine if there is obstruction. Code 55200 includes cannulization of the vas deferens. The code describes a unilateral or bilateral procedure, so there is no need to report modifier -50 with this code.

Excision. A vasectomy (55250) is a procedure in which a section of the vas deferens is removed for purposes of sterilization. A small incision is made on the scrotum, and the vas deferens is identified and brought out through the incision. A section of the cord is removed, and the vas deferens is returned to its natural position. The procedure includes a unilateral or bilateral procedure and postoperative semen examination(s). The semen is examined at intervals after sterilization to ensure the procedure was a success.

Introduction. A vasotomy (55300) may also be performed for a vasogram, vesiculogram, or epididymogram in which colored dye is traced through the vas deferens to visualize any obstruction. The radiological supervision/interpretation is reported separately with 74440. When a vastomy is combined with a testis biopsy, report 54505-51.

Repair. A vasovasostomy or vasovasorrhaphy is a procedure to remove obstruction from the vas deferens. Injection of dye is used during the procedure to identify the area of blockage. Once the area is identified, it is removed, and the ends of the vas deferens are anastomosed (reconnected end to end). Semen sampling may be conducted to ensure the removal of the blockage. Code 55400 reports a unilateral procedure; modifier -50 should be added to indicate a bilateral procedure. An operating microscope is often used during the procedure and is reported separately with 69990.

EXERCISE 19-7 *Epididymis, Tunica Vaginalis, and Vas Deferens*

Using the CPT and ICD-9-CM manuals, code the following:

1 Epididymis exploration without biopsy due to pain in epididymis

CPT Code: _____

ICD-9-CM Code: _____ (ICD-10-CM Code: _____)

2 Aspiration of fluid sac on the testicular covering

CPT Code: _____

3 Reversal of previously completed vasectomy, bilateral, using an operating microscope

CPT Code: _____

Spermatic Cord

Excision and Laparoscopy. The spermatic cord is a collection of structures that suspends the testes in the scrotum as illustrated in Fig. 19–13. The spermatic cord may be the site of formation of a hydrocele, lesion, or varicocele. Unilateral excision of a spermatic cord hydrocele is reported with 55500 with modifier -50 added to report a bilateral procedure. A **varicocele** is a mass of enlarged vessels that occurs when the valves that control blood flow in and out of the vessel become defective, and the blood is not able to circulate out of the vessel. The trapped blood causes the vessel to swell. Excision of a varicocele by means of a scrotal approach is reported with 55530, and an abdominal approach with 55535. A hernia repair may be performed during the same operative session, and with other procedures in this subsection have been reported separately. However, the single code 55540 reports both the varicocele excision and a hernia repair. If the

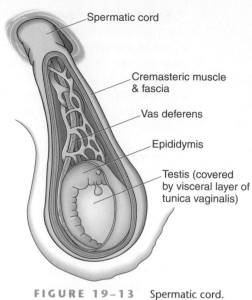

FIGURE 19–13 Spermatic cord.

varicocele is repaired using surgical laparoscopy, report the procedure with 55550.

The following spermatic cord code range is unilateral and requires modifier -50 if the procedure was performed bilaterally:

55500-55550   Spermatic cord (Excision and Laparoscopy categories)

The third-party payer may require the use of -RT and/or -LT rather than modifier -50.

Seminal Vesicles

The seminal vesicles are a pair of glands located posterior to (behind) the bladder. The glands provide the majority of the fluid that becomes semen and empties into the urethra. Seminal vesicles codes are located in the 55600-55680 range.

Incision. A vesiculotomy is surgical cutting into the seminal vesicles. The approach can be by an incision into the lower abdomen or the perineum (between the anus and scrotum). Frequently, the procedure is performed to relieve pressure due to inflammation. There are two codes to report a vesiculotomy based on the extent of the dissection required to accomplish the procedure. If the procedure required **simple** dissection, report 55600, and if **complicated** dissection was required, report 55605. The codes are unilateral, so a bilateral procedure requires modifier -50.

QUICK CHECK 19-12

1. A vesiculotomy may be performed by incision either in the lower _____ area or the _____ (between the anus and scrotum).

Excision.   A vesiculectomy is the removal of one of the seminal vesicles. The procedure is performed to remove a tumor, calculus (stone), or other obstruction. The approach may be through the lower abdomen or perineum, but the choice of codes is the same (55650) because the code description indicates "vesiculectomy, any approach." The code reports a unilateral procedure, so modifier -50 is required for a bilateral procedure.

The **Mullerian ducts** develop prenatally in females, and the Wolffian ducts degenerate. In males it is the opposite, the Wolffian ducts develop, and the Mullerian ducts degenerate. The Mullerian system develops into oviduct, uterus, and upper vagina. The Wolffian ducts develop into epididymis, vas deferens, and seminal vesicles. In some males a remnant of the Mullerian duct remains and a cyst may form at that site. The cyst may be excised using a lower abdominal or perineal approach and reported with 55680.

Prostate

The most common conditions involving the prostate are inflammation (prostatitis), benign enlargement (BPH, benign prostatic hypertrophy), and cancer. Prostate cancer is the most common type of cancer in men.

Benign Prostatic Hyperplasia and Prostatectomy.   The symptoms of BPH are urinary frequency, nocturia, urgency, decreased force of urine stream, and the feeling that the bladder has not completely emptied. These symptoms are a result of the excess prostate tissue pressing against the urethra and bladder. Treatment for BPH is based on the degree of prostate enlargement and severity of symptoms. Minimally invasive treatments include balloon dilation, prostatic stents, and thermal-based therapies. If these treatments are not successful, surgical intervention may be necessary, such as coagulation, transurethral resection, laser vaporization, or open surgical procedure.

BPH treatment and prostatectomies procedures are reported with codes from both the Urinary System and/or the Male Genital System.

Prostatic **stents** (52282 [permanent], 53855 [temporary]) are flexible metal mesh tubes designed to be inserted into the urethra at the level of the prostate and expanded after placement. The stent keeps the urethra open. Over time, the urothelial tissue grows over the stent and the stent becomes incorporated into the urethral wall.

Transurethral microwave heat treatment (**TUMT,** 53850) is the use of microwaves that are sent through a catheter and introduced into the urethra to coagulate excess prostate tissue and allow the urethra to be less constricted.

Transurethral needle ablation (**TUNA,** 53852) is a procedure that utilizes radiofrequency to create heat that is applied to the prostate to destroy excess prostate tissue. During this procedure the urethra is punctured to allow the needles to be placed directly into the prostate. The needles are insulated, so the urethra is not damaged when pierced.

For some patients these less radical treatments are not effective or advisable. For example, for patients with renal insufficiency, recurrent gross hematuria, or bladder stones because of BPH, a surgical procedure is the recommended treatment option. Surgical therapies include transurethral prostate incision, electrovaporization, and laser ablation/coagulation. Let's take a closer look at each of these surgical options:

Transurethral resection of the prostate (**TURP,** 52601, 52630) is the gold-standard of surgical procedures for removal of tumor or prostatic tissue. A special type of cystoscope is inserted through the urethra. The scope has lights, valves for controlling irrigation fluids, and an electrical loop to remove obstructions and cauterize blood vessels.

Transurethral incision of the prostate (**TUIP,** 52450) is used when the prostate is only slightly enlarged. Two incisions are made in the prostate to relieve the pressure on the urethra without removing tissue.

When a laser is used to accomplish the prostatectomy, the choice of codes is first based on whether the procedure was a coagulation (52647) or vaporization (52648). Code 52648 includes with or without transurethral resection of the prostate.

LASER *COAGULATION* (52647)

- Transurethral ultrasound-guided laser induced prostatectomy (**TULIP,** non-contact) is a procedure in which a laser is used to coagulate prostate tissue. There is no direct visualization of the prostate using this method, and the penetration is not as deep as with other more commonly performed methods.

- Visual laser of the prostate (**VLAP,** non-contact) is under the direct vision of the surgeon, but the laser fiber does not come in direct contact with the prostate. This method coagulates the tissue rather than vaporizing it. Once coagulated, the tissue dies and is sloughed off, which relieves the pressure.

- Interstitial laser coagulation of prostate (**ILCP,** contact) uses several laser fibers that are placed directly into the prostate to coagulate the tissue. There is no direct visualization with the ILCP.

QUICK CHECK 19-13

1. Code 52647, laser coagulation of the prostate, may be accomplished by one of three techniques: TULIP (non-contact, no direct

   visualization), _____ (non-contact, direct visualization), or

   _____ (contact, no direct visualization).

LASER *VAPORIZATION* (52648)

- Transurethral vaporization of the prostate (**TUVP** or **TVP,** contact) uses electrical current to vaporize tissue of the prostate by means of a ball that is rolled over the tissue. The ball contains a current that vaporizes the tissue. This procedure is a modification of a TURP.

LASER VAPORIZATION WITH/WITHOUT RESECTION (52648)

- Holmium laser enucleation of the prostate (**HoLEP,** contact), also known as transurethral holmium laser resection **(THLR),** is a procedure used to resect prostate tissue by means of a holmium laser fiber. There is less intraoperative bleeding with this procedure than with a TURP.

There are many different techniques used to remove the prostate (prostatectomy). Codes in the Excision category (55801-55865) represent open surgical procedures. Determination of the correct code to report a prostatectomy (removal of the prostate) is based first on the **approach** (perineal, suprapubic, or retropubic).

- Perineal approach is through the space between the rectum and the base of the scrotum and is used to gain access to a prostate that is located closer to the perineal area.

- Suprapubic approach is through the lower abdominal region, and it is used to gain access to the front (anterior) surface of the bladder. The access to the prostate is gained by an opening in the bladder neck.
- Retropubic approach is also through the lower abdominal region and is used to gain access to the front (anterior) of the prostate.

Once the correct approach has been identified, the **extent** of the procedure will determine code selection. The term subtotal used in many of the code descriptions means anything less than the total removal of the prostate, and the term radical means total removal of the prostate.

QUICK CHECK 19-14

There are different approaches to an open prostatectomy. Match the approach with the definition.

1. Perineal _____

2. Suprapubic _____

3. Retropubic _____

a. Through the lower abdominal region to gain access to the anterior prostate
b. Through the space between the rectum and the base of the scrotum
c. Through the lower abdominal region to gain access to the anterior surface of the bladder, opening the bladder neck to access the prostate

---

Codes 55812-55815 and 55842-55845 include code selection based on the lymph node biopsy/removal performed. If lymph node biopsy (single or multiple) and limited removal of pelvic lymph node(s) was performed, report 55812 (perineal approach) or 55842 (retropubic approach). If lymph nodes were removed bilaterally and include the external iliac, hypogastric and obturator nodes, report 55815 (perineal approach) or 55845 (retropubic approach).

A laparoscopic retropubic prostatectomy (**LRP,** 55866) is a minimally invasive procedure that may be utilized instead of an open procedure. Robotic assisted prostatectomy **(RAP)** is a new instrumentation used with LRP and is designed to assist in the performance of some surgical tasks. Several small incisions are made through which robotic instrumentation is inserted. The surgeon operates the instrumentation from a console. The use of RAP necessitates an assistant during surgery. Surgeons who use a RAP system are extensively trained by the manufacturer of the system before using the system during surgery. The new robotic systems enhance the precision with which the procedure can be performed.

CHECK THIS OUT ☞ One such robotic system is the da Vinci® prostatectomy system and a video about the procedure can be viewed at www.davinciprostatectomy.com/video.html.

Now that you have reviewed BPH treatment and prostatectomies, let's review the remaining codes in the Prostate category.

Biopsy. Biopsy of the prostate may be performed with a needle, punch, or by incision. Report a prostate biopsy with 55700 (needle, punch), 55705 (incisional), or 55706 (transperineal, stereotactic). Do not report these codes during the same procedure. For example, if, during the same operative session, a needle or punch biopsy of the prostate (55700) is undertaken, and it is followed by an incisional biopsy (55705) either to supplement or to obtain adequate tissue, the appropriate CPT code to report is 55705, not both codes. Do not confuse a prostate biopsy with a fine needle aspiration (FNA). During an FNA, fluid is withdrawn for analysis and is reported with 10021 or 10022.

QUICK CHECK 19-15

1. Biopsy of the prostate may be accomplished by one of three

    methods: incision, _____, or _____.

A **prostatotomy** is an incision into the prostate. Codes 55720 and 55725 describe prostatotomies performed to drain an abscess. The surgeon inserts a needle into the prostate via the perineum or through the rectum. Reporting of the procedure is based on if the procedure was simple or complicated. A complicated prostatotomy would document excess bleeding or other factors that increase time and effort necessary to complete the service.

Brachytherapy. Brachytherapy (55860-55865) is a type of radiation treatment for prostate cancer and utilizes high dose rate (HDR, temporary method) or low dose (permanent seeds) and may be used in combination with biopsy/removal of lymph nodes (Fig. 19–14). The placement of the brachytherapy element(s) can be accomplished by transperineal placement (through the area between scrotum and anus) or with open exposure of the prostate. The transperineal placement involves the fastening of a template to the perineal area. The template contains a pattern of holes that indicate where the catheters or needles are to be placed to correctly access the area around the prostate. Approximately 100 permanent seeds are placed for the low-dose method.

For the high dose method of temporary delivery, small catheters are placed into the prostate, and a series of radiation treatments are delivered. For example, a patient would present to an outpatient department of the hospital where a template would be fastened to the perineal area. The

FIGURE 19–14 Brachytherapy for prostate cancer. (Modified from Wein AJ, editor: Campbell-Walsh Urology, ed 9, Philadelphia, 2007, Saunders.)

catheters would be inserted through the holes in the template into the prostate. The treatment plan is established by the physician, and the computer that is attached to the catheters is set to deliver the prescribed dose of radiation. If the prescribed dose cannot be administered in one session, the catheters remain in place, and the patient remains in the hospital overnight. The next day, the patient would receive another radiation treatment. The catheters would be removed, and the patient would be discharged from the hospital. An advantage of the HDR is that the physician can regulate the radiation dosage more precisely than with the low-dose method.

The transperineal placement is reported with 55875 and includes the use of a cystoscope if applicable. The placement of the radioelements is reported separately with 77776-77787. If ultrasound guidance is used during the placement, the guidance is reported separately with 76965, ultrasonic guidance for interstitial radioelement application.

Another approach for placement of radioactive substances is the open approach in which the prostate is viewed by the surgeon. The exposure procedure is reported with 55860, and the application of the radioelements is reported with 77776-77778, based on the number of sources placed: simple (1-4), intermediate (5-10), complex (>10). During the same operative session in which the radioelements are placed, the surgeon may biopsy lymph nodes and/or may perform a lymphadenectomy (55862). If a bilateral pelvic lymphadenectomy is performed and includes the external iliac, hypogastric, and obturator nodes, the procedure is reported with 55865.

Transrectal ultrasound (**TRU,** 76872, 76873) is guidance that is often used when reporting biopsy, evaluation and staging for prostate cancer, delivery of brachytherapy, evaluation or aspiration of prostate abscess, evaluation of infertility, diagnosis of prostate abnormalities, and monitoring of treatment response.

EXERCISE 19-8 *Spermatic Cord and Prostate*

Using the CPT and ICD-9-CM manuals, code the following:

1 A 75-year-old male patient presents with a PSA of 8.1. He has a 100-gram prostate, and 1 out of 10 cores were positive for adenocarcinoma. The patient was placed in the supine position and a number 20 French Foley catheter was inserted into the bladder. A lower abdominal midline incision was made and the retropubic space was entered. Bilateral pelvic lymphadenectomy was performed in the usual manner and included the external iliac, obturator, and hypogastric nodes. Lymph nodes were small and were sent for permanent section to pathology. The prostate was extremely large. The prostate was mobilized using blunt dissection technique. The area was closed in the usual manner. Pathology report later indicated primary malignant neoplasm of the prostate.

   CPT Code: _____

   ICD-9-CM Code: _____ (ICD-10-CM Code: _____)

2 The 68-year-old male patient presents with BPH. Two 18-gauge needles were affixed to the catheter, and by means of a rigid cystoscope, the needles were transurethrally inserted into the prostate. Radiofrequency waves were set at 490 kHz and 99°C was obtained. Ablation of the area was completed and the cystoscope withdrawn.

   CPT Code: _____

CHAPTER REVIEW

CHAPTER 19, PART I, THEORY

Without the use of reference material, complete the following:

1 The greatest number of category codes in the Male Genital System fall under the

_____ subheading because of the numerous repairs made to this anatomic area.

2 In what section of the CPT manual would you find a code for a superficial abscess of the skin of

the penis? _____

3 What is the term that pertains to the motion

and flow of urine? _____

4 What is the modifier that indicates that only the professional portion of the service was

performed? _____

5 The Urinary System subsection is arranged

_____ by the subheadings.

6 The _____ area is located behind the abdominal cavity and during surgical procedures is often accessed by an abdominal incision.

7 A(n) _____ is a procedure that is used to decompress the renal system by means of inserting a catheter into the kidney while leaving the other end of the catheter outside the body to temporarily drain the kidney.

8 A(n) _____ calculus involves at least two calyces and the renal pelvis and accounts for about 30% of the stones reported.

9 You report the removal of an accessible stent of kidney when imaging guidance is not indicated

using a(n) _____ code.

10 If an obstruction occurs, the urine will not drain and may result in dilatation of the collecting system and enlargement of the renal

pelvis, also known as _____.

11 A transvesical ureterolithotomy is one that is performed through the bladder for the removal

of _____.

12 A urethroplasty may be one state or two stages and the choice of codes is based on the number of stages, type of repair, and for some codes the

_____ of the patient.

CHAPTER 19, PART II, PRACTICAL

Code the following cases with CPT and ICD-9-CM codes:

13 Incision and drainage of deep penis abscess

CPT Code: _____

ICD-9-CM Code: _____

(ICD-10-CM Code: _____)

14 Extensive destruction of penile herpetic vesicle lesions using cryosurgery

CPT Code: _____

ICD-9-CM Code: _____

(ICD-10-CM Code: _____)

15 Biopsy of kidney with percutaneous incision by trocar for a patient with a diagnosis of microalbuminuria

CPT Code: _____

ICD-9-CM Code: _____

(ICD-10-CM Code: _____)

16 Physician providing the technical and professional component of a cystography with contrast and four views for a patient with hematuria. Also report the radiology supervision and interpretation.

CPT Codes: _____,

_____

ICD-9-CM Code: _____

(ICD-10-CM Code: _____)

17 A one-stage distal hypospadias repair with circumcision and a V-flap for meatal advancement

CPT Code: _____

ICD-9-CM Code: _____

(ICD-10-CM Code: _____)

18 Needle biopsy with ultrasound guidance of the prostate of a 87-year-old male with an elevated PSA. The pathology results of the biopsy negative for malignancy.

CPT Codes: _____,

_____

ICD-9-CM Code: _____

(ICD-10-CM Code: _____)

19 Dilation of a urethral stricture of male due to syphilis

CPT Code: _____

ICD-9-CM Codes: _____,

_____

(ICD-10-CM Codes: _____,

_____)

20 Injection procedure for Peyronie disease

CPT Code: _____

ICD-9-CM Code: _____

(ICD-10-CM Code: _____)

QUICK CHECK ANSWERS

QUICK CHECK 19-1
1. False, they may not pass spontaneously

QUICK CHECK 19-2
1. externally

QUICK CHECK 19-3
1. nephrostomy, pyelostomy

QUICK CHECK 19-4
1. 50945

QUICK CHECK 19-5
1. 58240

QUICK CHECK 19-6
1. cystoscopy, urethroscopy

QUICK CHECK 19-7
1. Integumentary

QUICK CHECK 19-8
1. 28

QUICK CHECK 19-9
1. non-inflatable, inflatable

QUICK CHECK 19-10
1. orchiopexy

QUICK CHECK 19-11
1. 54700

QUICK CHECK 19-12
1. abdomen, perineum

QUICK CHECK 19-13
1. VLAP, ILCP

QUICK CHECK 19-14
1. b
2. c
3. a

QUICK CHECK 19-15
1. needle, punch

"My motto for my billing and coding students is, 'Persist until you succeed.'"

Patricia Sommerfeld, CPC
Senior Client Manager
HealthMed Inc.
Adjunct Instructor
Mercy College of Health Sciences
Des Moines, Iowa

Reproductive, Intersex Surgery, Female Genital System, and Maternity Care and Delivery

Chapter Topics

Reproductive System Procedures

Intersex Surgery

Female Genital System

Maternity Care and Delivery

Chapter Review

Quick Check Answers

Learning Objectives

After completing this chapter you should be able to

1 Describe reproductive services.
2 Report reproductive services.
3 Report intersex surgery services.
4 Understand the format of the Female Genital System subsection.
5 Identify elements of component coding with Female Genital System codes.
6 Define the critical terms in maternity and delivery services.
7 Define services in the global maternity and delivery package.
8 Understand the format of the Maternity Care and Delivery subsection services.
9 Demonstrate the ability to code the Female Genital and Maternity Care and Delivery subsection.

Make sure to check evolve learning system **for the latest content updates**

REPRODUCTIVE SYSTEM PROCEDURES

The Reproductive System Procedures subsection (55920) is located after the Male Genital System subsection and consists of only one code. Code 55920 reports the placement of needles or catheters into the pelvic organs and/or genitalia for the subsequent interstitial radioelement application (brachytherapy). This procedure is performed with the patient anesthetized. The surgeon examines the diseased areas to determine the area(s) that require treatment. A template device is inserted into the vagina and positioned over the areas to receive the radioelement insertions. The number and depth of the needles or catheters varies depending on the area to be treated, but typically 32 flexiguide catheters are inserted.

This code is not used to report radioelement application for the prostate, which is reported with 55875. Insertion of a vaginal ovoid brachytherapy system is a common type used to treat cervical cancer and is reported with 57155. A Heyman capsule indicated in the parenthetical statement following 55920 directs the coder to 58346 when reporting Heyman capsule insertion. A Heyman capsule was a method of manual loading that was used in the early days of brachytherapy. The physician would manually insert the capsule into the treatment area, which necessitated the physician being in contact with the radioactive source. The newer methods of brachytherapy are safer as the radioelements are inserted via catheters thus reducing the exposure of health care providers.

INTERSEX SURGERY

The Intersex Surgery subsection (55970, 55980) is located before the Female Genital Surgery subsection and contains only two codes: one for a surgical procedure to change the sex organs of a male into those of a female and one to change the sex organs of a female into those of a male. These specialized procedures include a series of procedures that take place over an extended period of time. The procedures are performed by physicians who have special skills and training.

The procedure for changing male genitalia into female genitalia involves removing the penis but preserving the nerves and vessels intact. These tissues are used to form a clitoris and a vagina. The urethral opening is shifted to be in the position of that of a female.

The surgical procedure for changing the female genitalia into male genitalia involves a series of procedures that use the genitalia and surrounding skin to form a penis and testicle structures into which prostheses are inserted.

QUICK CHECK 20-1

1. How many codes are there in the Intersex Surgery subsection?

_____

FEMALE GENITAL SYSTEM

Format

The Female Genital System subsection (56405-58999) is divided according to anatomic site, from the vulva up to the ovaries (Fig. 20–1). The anatomic sites are then divided on the basis of category of procedure (i.e., incision, excision, destruction). Codes for in vitro fertilization are located at the end of the subsection.

FIGURE 20–1 **A,** Female genital system. **B,** Anterior view, female genital system. **C,** External female genital system. **D,** Parts of vulva.

The subsection has a wide variety of codes for minor procedures that are performed in a physician's office as well as for major procedures that are performed in a hospital setting. It is important to read the descriptions of the codes as well as the notes to avoid unbundling in this subsection. For example, if a total abdominal hysterectomy was performed as well as a bilateral oophorectomy (removal of ovaries), only 58150 would be reported because in the code description is the statement "with or without removal of ovary(s)." Bundled into the code are both the abdominal hysterectomy and a bilateral oophorectomy.

There are many screening (well woman) services provided, such as screening mammography, pap tests, and pelvic examination, in addition to colorectal cancer screening and bone mass measurements. In this text, these services are reviewed in the chapter that refers to the codes that would be submitted for the services. For example, mammography is in Chapter 23, Radiology.

Vulva, Perineum, and Introitus

There is a repeated note in the Vulva, Perineum, and Introitus subheading (56405-56821) indicating procedures performed on the Skene's glands are not reported using codes in the Female Genital System subsection but instead are coded using Surgery section, Urinary System subsection codes. That is because Skene's glands, also known as **para-urethral ducts,** are a group of small mucous glands located near the lower end of the urethra and are part of the urinary system. Procedures involving Skene's glands are, therefore, reported using Urinary System codes (53060 or 53270).

Incision.   The vulva includes the following parts: mons pubis, labia majora, labia minora, bulb of vestibule, vaginal orifice or vestibule of the vagina, and the greater (Bartholin's gland) and lesser vestibule glands (see Fig. 20–1, *C* and *D*). When the code description indicates the incision and drainage of an abscess of the vulva, the code reports an abscess of any of those anatomic areas. For example, if a medical record indicates "an incision and drainage of an abscess of Bartholin's gland," you must know that Bartholin's gland is considered a part of the vulva, so the code will be located in that subheading.

Destruction.   Destruction of lesions of the vulva, perineum, or introitus can be accomplished using a variety of methods—laser surgery, cryosurgery, electrosurgery, or chemical destruction. Destruction codes are divided on the basis of whether the destruction is simple or extensive, although the code description does not define simple or extensive. Complexity is based on the physician's judgment of complexity, and the complexity will be stated in the medical record.

> ✋ **CAUTION** *Destruction is not excision. Destruction is obliteration or eradication. Excision is removal. With destruction no tissue is removed, as the tissue is destroyed. There is no pathology report after a lesion has been destroyed because there is nothing for the pathologist to analyze.*

Excision.   The first two codes (56605 and 56606) in the Excision category are for biopsies in which the physician takes a tissue sample by removing a piece of tissue with a scalpel or punch. The area to be biopsied is anesthetized with local anesthetic before the biopsy is performed. The physician may suture the area or use clips for closure. The local anesthesia and closure are included in the package of an excision code, so be careful not to unbundle and report these separately. The codes are also divided on the number of lesions, one and each additional lesion. When using the additional lesions code, be certain to specify the number of lesions biopsied by listing the number of units on the CMS-1500 form in Block 24-G.

> **CODING SHOT** ✏️ If the excision is of a lesion of the skin of the genitalia, report the service with 11420-11426 (Excision of benign lesion) or 11620-11626 (Excision of malignant lesion).

Vulvectomy is the surgical removal of a portion of the vulva. Usually a vulvectomy is performed to treat a malignant or premalignant lesion. The following definitions apply to the vulvectomy codes (56620-56640) and describe the extent and size of the vulvar area removed during the procedure.

EXTENT

Simple	skin and superficial subcutaneous tissue
Radical	skin and deep subcutaneous tissue

SIZE

Partial	less than 80%
Complete	greater than 80%

The vulvectomy codes are divided on the basis of these definitions of extent and size. The extent and size are stated in combination. For example, simple partial vulvectomy describes a superficial subcutaneous tissue **(extent)** removal of 78% **(size)** of the vulvar area. Bundled into the codes is usual closure, but if plastic repair is required, you would report the repair in addition to the procedure. The operative report will indicate the extent of the procedure and the closure.

CODING SHOT

There are two labia: labia minora and labia majora (Fig. 20–2). A partial vulvectomy (less than 80%) pertains to leaving at least 20% of the vulvar area.

The more radical procedures involving the vulva are usually performed because of a demonstrated malignancy, and more extensive removal takes place. This radical removal can include the removal of deep lymph nodes, saphenous veins, ligaments, or large amounts of tissue from the lower abdomen or even from the thigh. The procedure may also be performed bilaterally, so don't forget to add modifier -50 when reporting a bilateral procedure.

CODING SHOT

Most payers do not make a reimbursement adjustment for bilateral procedures. For example, Medicare does not make an adjustment. You must review each payer's guidelines to determine how to submit this code.

Repair.   The procedure codes in the Repair category (56800-56810) describe plastic repair of the vulva, perineum, or introitus. Plastic repair of the **introitus** is surgical repair of the opening of the vagina. The extent and nature of the procedure are determined by the defect being repaired and varies greatly from patient to patient.

Clitoroplasty is surgical reduction of a clitoris (Fig. 20–3) that has become enlarged due to an adrenal gland imbalance.

Perineoplasty is plastic repair of the perineum, usually to provide additional support to the perineal area.

FIGURE 20–2   Labia majora and labia minora. (Modified from Townsend CM, Beauchamp RD, Evers BM, Mattox KL: *Sabiston Textbook of Surgery: The Biological Basis of Modern Surgical Practice*, ed 18, Philadelphia, 2008, Saunders.)

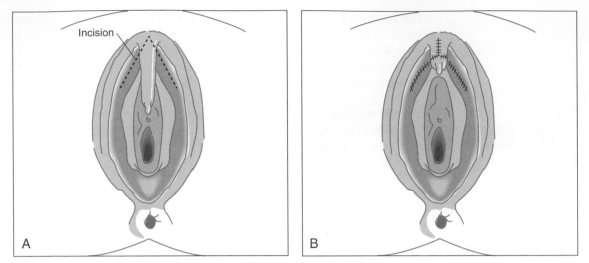

FIGURE 20–3 Reduction clitoroplasty. (From Sanfilippo JS, Muram D, Dewhurst J, Lee PA: *Pediatric and Adolescent Gynecology,* ed 2, Philadelphia, 2001, Saunders.)

Vagina   The Vagina subheading includes the code range 57000-57425. **Colpotomy** (57000-57010) is cutting into the vagina to gain access to the pelvic cavity. The procedure is performed to explore the pelvic cavity or to drain a pelvic abscess. **Colpocentesis** (57020) is the insertion of a long needle (puncture) attached to a syringe through the back wall of the vagina to gain access to the peritoneal cul-de-sac—the area between the uterus and the rectum—to drain fluid. If the colpocentesis is a part of a more major procedure, you do not report it separately, as it is considered to be bundled into the more major procedure. Note that 57020 has "(separate procedure)" after it to designate colpocentesis as a minor procedure that is reported only if it is the only procedure performed of the area.

Destruction.   As with the destruction codes for the vulva, the destruction codes (57061, 57065) for the Vagina subsection are divided on the basis of whether the destruction was simple or extensive, in the judgment of the physician. Any method of destruction is acceptable for assignment of these codes.

Excision.   The Excision category of the Vagina subsection contains codes (57100-57135) for reporting the services of biopsy, vaginectomy (removal of part or all of the vagina), colpocleisis (closure of the vaginal canal), and cyst/lesion removal. The vaginectomy codes are divided according to the extent of the procedure—**partial** or **total**—and the extent to which tissue and adjacent structure(s) are removed.

From the Trenches

"Be willing to learn everything there is to know. Medical terminology and anatomy/ physiology are a must for the successful coder."

PATRICIA

Introduction.   The Introduction category (57150-57180) contains codes for vaginal irrigation. Also included is the insertion of a tandem and/or vaginal ovoid for brachytherapy. The tandem and/or vaginal ovoid are internal implants that contain a radioactive substance and are often used in the treatment of cervical cancer as illustrated in Fig. 20–4. A tandem is a small, hollow metal tube that is inserted through the vagina into the uterus (intrauterine tandem). Vaginal ovoids are small metal cylinders that are placed into the vagina and positioned against the cervix (intravaginal ovoid). The implants then deliver a concentrated dose of radiation to the site of the tumor.

Other codes in the Introduction category report the insertion of a support device (pessary, Fig. 20–5), diaphragm, or cervical cap (to prevent pregnancy); and packing of the vagina (for vaginal hemorrhage). Pessaries are used for vaginal prolapse. The pessary and diaphragm/cervical cap are not included in these Introduction codes. The supply of these devices would be reported using code 99070, supplies, or a HCPCS code (e.g., A4561).

FIGURE 20–4   Tandem and ovoid. (From DiSaia PJ, Creasman WT: *Clinical Gynecologic Oncology,* ed 7, St. Louis, 2007, Mosby.)

FIGURE 20–5   Vaginal pessary (Arabin type). (Modified from Gabbe SG, Niebyl JR, Simpson JL: *Obstetrics: Normal and Problem Pregnancies,* ed 5, Philadelphia, 2007, Churchill Livingstone.)

Repair.   The Repair category (57200-57335) is rather extensive, as the possible forms of repair of the vagina are many. A note in parentheses, "(nonobstetrical)," sometimes follows the code description in the Female Genital System subsection because if the procedure was performed as a part of an obstetric procedure, you would use a code from the Maternity Care and Delivery subsection.

A surgeon performs a **colporrhaphy** to strengthen an area on the wall of the vagina that is weak by pulling together the weakened vaginal area with sutures. Excess tissue can also be removed to tighten the area. The reinforcement might be performed for several reasons, but it is commonly done to prevent the bladder from protruding into the weakened vaginal wall (cystocele) or the rectum from protruding into the vagina (rectocele).

In this Repair category, the codes are often divided on the basis of the approach used. For example, an abdominal approach (open, 57270) to the repair of an enterocele (herniation of intestines through intact vaginal mucosa) has a different code than a vaginal approach (57268) to the same repair; and an anterior colporrhaphy (vaginal repair) (57240) differs from a posterior colporrhaphy (57250). Pay particular attention to the **approach** used. You will find the approach documented in the operative report.

One method of vaginal repair that is not in the Repair category is the laparoscopic repair. Codes for repair of the vagina using a colposcope (microscope) are located in the Vagina subheading, Endoscopy category. The colposcope enables the physician to directly view changes in the vagina and cervix.

> **CAUTION** *Coders need to pay close attention to the **method** as well as to the **approach**. For example, a surgeon might perform an open procedure as opposed to a laparoscopic procedure.*

Notes throughout the Repair category will frequently direct you to the correct code or code range in the Urinary System subsection. Often, the only difference between surgical procedures reported with Female Genital System codes and those reported with the Urinary System codes is the **approach**. For example, Female Genital System code 57330 describes the closure of a vesicovaginal fistula (abnormal channel between bladder and vagina) using a vaginal approach, whereas Urinary System code 51900 describes the same procedure using an abdominal approach. The approach would be documented in the operative report.

Manipulation.   **Manipulation** of the vagina includes dilation (stretching), pelvic examination, and removal of foreign material. What these three different procedures have in common is that they are all performed under **general anesthesia** because a patient cannot tolerate the procedure while awake. If a local anesthetic or no anesthetic was used, which is the usual case, you would not use a Manipulation code (57400-57415); instead, the service would be included in the Evaluation and Management (E/M) service. For example, if a physician removed an impacted tampon from the vagina and used no anesthetic during the procedure, only the office visit at which the removal took place would be reported.

Endoscopy.   As discussed earlier in this chapter, the endoscopic procedure codes (57420-57426) in the Endoscopy category of the Vagina subheading are for colposcopic procedures. The colposcopic procedures are often bundled into other, more major procedures. Fig. 20–6 illustrates an endocervical polyp protruding through the external os (mouth of the cervix)

FIGURE 20–6 Endocervical polyp protruding through the mouth of the cervix as seen through a colposcope. (From Baggish MS: *Colposcopy of the Cervix, Vagina, and Vulva: A Comprehensive Textbook,* Philadelphia, 2003, Mosby.)

as seen by the physician using a colposcope. Only when a colposcopic procedure is performed as the only procedure or is unrelated to another procedure(s) being performed is the colposcopy reported.

If a biopsy of the vagina or cervix is performed with colposcopy, the code to report the service is 57421. The codes specifies "biopsy(s)," so whether one or multiple biopsies were taken, 57421 represents the total service.

Cervix Uteri The Cervix Uteri subheading contains codes (57452-57800) for endoscopy, excision, repair, and manipulation.

Endoscopy. Similar to the vaginal endoscopic codes, the colposcopy codes report procedures of the cervix uteri (57452-57461). A loop electrode excision procedure is referred to as LEEP, LETZ, or cervical loop diathermy and is an office procedure that uses heated wire (Fig. 20–7) to remove cervical tissue. The device is attached to an electric generator that heats the wire. The procedure has a lower risk level and is less expensive than other methods. A LEEP would usually be performed after an abnormal Pap smear result or an abnormal examination. The cervix is moistened, and the loop is positioned over the cervix and drawn across the area. The resulting slice is examined by a pathologist. The device is also used to cauterize the area at the end of the procedure by means of a different attachment.

Excision. The codes in the Excision category often specify "(separate procedure)" because many times, the procedures are bundled into a more

FIGURE 20–7 The loop used in the electrosurgical excision procedure.

major procedure. For example, the excision procedure of a biopsy is often incidental to a more major surgical procedure, such as a hysterectomy, and the biopsy would not be reported separately.

Codes for **conization** of the cervix are divided on the basis of the method used to obtain the tissue (Fig. 20–8). In conization, a cone of tissue is removed from the cervix for a biopsy or treatment of a lesion by means of excision of the lesion. Although a laser is a frequently used method of conization, LEEP technology is also widely used. The code for a LEEP procedure with **cervical biopsy** in the Cervix Uteri subheading, Endoscopy category, is 57460, and the code for a LEEP procedure with **cervical conization** is 57461. The difference between the codes is that the cervical biopsy procedure only removes a sample with return in the future if the lesion is to be completely removed. The conization procedure removes a cone-shaped tissue of the cervix after application of iodine to highlight the abnormal tissue. Also, the cervical biopsy is performed with the use of a colposcope (endoscopy), and the conization is performed using a speculum (Fig. 20–9) (an instrument inserted into a cavity to stretch the opening). Be certain, when coding

FIGURE 20–8   Conization.

FIGURE 20–9   Graves specula. (From Katz VL, Lentz GM, Lobo RA, Gershenson DM: *Comprehensive Gynecology,* ed 5, Philadelphia, 2007, Mosby.)

cervical biopsy and conization, that the information in the medical record provides sufficient detail to allow you to distinguish between a biopsy and a conization. If the record is not complete enough to make the determination, obtain the information from the physician before assigning a code.

Repair. Nonobstetric **cerclage** (repair of the cervix) involves extensive suturing of the cervix to decrease the size of the opening into the vagina (reported with 57700). **Trachelorrhaphy** is a complex cervical repair (57720) in which plastic methods are used to repair a laceration of the cervix. Both Repair codes use a vaginal approach.

Manipulation. Dilation of the cervix is coded separately only if it is the only procedure performed (57800). Dilation of the cervix, like dilation of the vagina, is usually bundled into a more major procedure.

Corpus Uteri

The corpus uteri (58100-58579) is the anatomic area above the isthmus and below the opening for the fallopian tubes. The subheading contains the categories of excision, introduction, repair, and laparoscopy/hysteroscopy procedures. Many of the procedures in the category are very complex, and some of them have several variations. Let's review some of the highlights of corpus uteri coding.

Excision. Endometrial **sampling** is a biopsy of the mucous lining of the uterus. The physician inserts a curet (spoon-shaped instrument) into the endocervical canal to extract tissue samples for pathologic examination. If the sampling is the only procedure performed, it is reported (58100, 58110), but if it is performed as part of a more major procedure involving the cervix, it is considered incidental to the more major procedure and is bundled into the surgical package.

Dilation and curettage (D&C; 58120) can be a diagnostic or therapeutic procedure performed when an endometrial biopsy has failed or was inconclusive or to determine the cause of abnormal bleeding or locate a neoplasm. Clamps are used to manipulate the cervix, a curet is inserted into the uterus, and fragments are removed from the endometrium. The tissue is sent to pathology for analysis. D&C in the Corpus Uteri subheading is for nonobstetric patients only. If a D&C is performed because of postpartum hemorrhage, a code from the subsection Maternity Care and Delivery would be assigned to report the service (59160).

CODING SHOT

Many third-party payers will not reimburse for a dilation and curettage if it is performed with any other pelvic surgery because it is thought to be integral to or a part of the procedure. The CPT manual does not list a D&C as a "(separate procedure)"; therefore, you need to be familiar with the specific reimbursement policies of the payer.

Hysterectomy codes (58150-58294) represent the majority of the codes in the Corpus Uteri subheading. A **hysterectomy** is the removal of the uterus, but in the CPT manual there are many variations of this procedure. The division of the hysterectomy codes is based first on the **approach** (abdominal or vaginal), then on the secondary procedures **(extent)** that were performed (removal of tubes, biopsy, bladder, etc.). You have to read the code descriptions carefully to determine what is bundled into each code.

Because so many procedures are bundled into some of the codes, you also have to be careful not to unbundle and code for items already covered in the main procedure. For example, a total abdominal hysterectomy can include the removal of the ovaries and/or the fallopian tubes; therefore, billing separately for the removal of the ovaries or tubes would be unbundling.

Within the Excision category there are codes for abdominal approaches for hysterectomies. An **abdominal approach** is one in which the surgeon opens the abdomen to view by means of an incision. Review the codes in the range 58150-58240 and underline "abdominal" in each of the codes as a reminder of the approach used in these codes. The other type of surgical approach for hysterectomies listed in the Excision category is the vaginal approach. Using the **vaginal approach,** the surgeon makes an incision in the vagina around the cervix and removes the uterus and/or ovaries/fallopian tubes (salpingo-oophorectomy) through the incision. The cuff of the vagina is then closed with sutures. Review the codes in the range 58260-58294 and underline "vaginal" as a reminder of the approach used in these codes.

QUICK CHECK 20-2

1. What is the difference between codes 58260 and 58290?

_____

2. Locate the myomectomy codes 58140, 58145, 58545, and 58546 in the CPT manual. Review the codes and identify the determining factors when selecting a code.

   a. approach, location, number
   b. approach, number, weight
   c. location, weight, pathological outcome
   d. weight, number, age of patient

Introduction.   It is in the Introduction category (58300-58356) that you will locate the codes for some very common procedures such as the insertion and removal of an **intrauterine device** (IUD) as illustrated in Fig. 20–10 for birth control and for some not-so-common procedures such

FIGURE 20–10   Intrauterine device (IUD). (From Chabner DE: *The Language of Medicine,* ed 8, St. Louis, 2007, Saunders.)

as artificial insemination. There are also several codes that have radiology components—your component coding skills will again be used.

Because intrauterine device (IUD) insertion is reported using Introduction category code 58300, you might think IUD removal would be in a removal category, but it is in the Introduction category (58301).

CODING SHOT The cost of the IUD is not included in the code for the insertion of the IUD. You report the cost of the device separately, using 99070 or a HCPCS code (J7300).

Don't confuse the insertion of an IUD with the placement of an implantable contraceptive such as Norplant, as described in the Integumentary subsection.

The specialized fertility procedure of **artificial insemination** and the preparation of the sperm for insemination are reported with Introduction category codes. During the insemination procedure, sperm is injected into the cervix and often a cervical cap is inserted to keep the sperm in the cervical area. **In vitro fertilization** is a different procedure in which an egg from the female is withdrawn and fertilized with sperm in a laboratory for 2 to 3 days with subsequent implantation into the uterus. There is an In Vitro Fertilization subheading containing codes 58970-58976 to report these services, located at the end of the Female Genital System subsection.

Catheterization and introduction (58340) of saline or contrast material through the cervix and uterus and into the fallopian tubes (hysterosalpingography) is performed by a physician to identify blockage or abnormalities of the fallopian tubes. Ultrasound can also be used for the same procedure (hysterosonography). You need to remember your component coding and report the radiology or ultrasound portion of the procedure with a code from the Radiology section. A note following 58340 in the CPT manual directs you to the correct component code. For the radiographic supervision and interpretation, the component code is 74740; for the ultrasound (sonohysterography), the code is 76831.

A **hysterosalpingraphy** is a diagnostic procedure to test the patency (unblocked) of the fallopian tubes. Saline or contrast material is injected into a tube (58340). A catheter may be introduced (58345) and passed through the fallopian tube using x-ray to show where the catheter encounters an obstruction or a narrowing of the tube. A code from the Radiology section, Gynecological and Obstetrical subsection, would report the radiology portion of the service (74742). **Chromotubation** (58350) is a surgical procedure to open an obstructed or narrowed tube.

Laparoscopy/Hysteroscopy. An increasing number of procedures are being performed by using an endoscope instead of opening the area to complete view. With an endoscopic procedure, usually two or three small incisions are made through which lights, cameras, and instruments may be passed. The surgeon first inserts an instrument into the vagina to grasp the cervix. Another scope is inserted into the abdomen and the uterus and/or ovaries/fallopian tubes may be excised. An incision is made in the vagina and the surgically excised material is removed through the vaginal incision. The vagina is then repaired by means of sutures. Review the codes in the range 58541-58579 and underline "Laparoscopy" or "Hysteroscopy" as a reminder of the approach used in these codes. It is very important to read the full code description to identify the approach. Because endoscopic procedures are less invasive, patients are more accepting of the procedures, and recovery times and risks are reduced. Fig. 20–11 illustrates a laparoscopy procedure and Fig. 20–12 illustrates a laparoscopy/hysteroscopy procedure.

The first rule of a laparoscopy or hysteroscopy is that all surgical procedures include a **diagnostic** procedure. You never unbundle a surgical laparoscopic procedure by also reporting a diagnostic procedure. If a procedure started out as a diagnostic laparoscopic procedure and ended up being a surgical laparoscopic procedure, you report only for the surgical laparoscopy.

> ✋ **CAUTION** *If the laparoscopy is of the peritoneum, you assign a code (49320) from the laparoscopy category of the Digestive System, Abdomen, Peritoneum, and Omentum subheading.*

The codes in the Laparoscopy/Hysteroscopy category are divided on the basis of approach—laparoscopy or hysteroscopy—and further divided by other procedures that might have been performed.

Oviduct/Ovary

The Oviduct/Ovary subheading (58600-58770) is divided into incision, laparoscopy, excision, and repair. Fallopian tube procedures are located in this subheading.

Incision. The Incision category is where you will locate the codes for tubal ligation, which is a permanent, highly effective method of birth control. The codes are divided according to the type of ligation performed and the circumstances at the time of the ligation. The types of ligation are as follows: **tying** off the tube with suture material (ligation), **removing** a portion of the tube (transection), and **blocking** the tube with a device, such as a clip, ring, or band (occlusion). The circumstance under which the procedure is performed affects the choice of codes. For example, a procedure can be performed either on one side (unilateral) or on both sides (bilateral). The procedure can be performed at different times, such as during the same hospitalization period as the period of delivery, during the postpartum period, or during another surgical procedure and these circumstances affect code assignment.

FIGURE 20–11 Laparoscopy.

FIGURE 20–12 Hysteroscopy/laparoscopy.

CODING SHOT Do not use a bilateral procedure modifier (-50) with codes in the Incision category because the code descriptions indicate "tube(s)" or "unilateral or bilateral." Also, do not code tubal ligations performed by means of a laparoscopic procedure using the Incision category codes. There are codes for laparoscopic tubal ligation procedures in the Laparoscopy category of subheading Oviduct/Ovary (58660-58679).

A ligation can be performed by an abdominal or a vaginal approach. If a ligation or transection of the fallopian tube(s) is performed during the same operative procedure as a cesarean delivery or other intra-abdominal surgery, you report the ligation/transection using 58611. Code 58611 only reports the tubal ligation as a component of the more major surgical procedure and is listed in addition to the primary code.

Often at the time of an abdominal tubal ligation, lysis (loosening) of adhesions will be performed. Lysis is not bundled into the ligation code. You report the lysis of adhesions separately, using a Repair category code such as 58660, if allowed by the third-party payer.

CODING SHOT 58740, lysis of adhesions, is performed for restoration of fertility, not for lysis of adhesions at the time of tubal ligation (such as 58660).

Laparoscopy. The procedures described in the Oviduct/Ovary subheading, Laparoscopy category (58660-58679) are surgical laparoscopy and always include a diagnostic laparoscopy. If only a diagnostic laparoscopy was performed, you report 49320 from the Digestive System subsection, Abdomen, Peritoneum, and Omentum category, because the scope is being passed into the abdomen for examination only. Once a definitive procedure such as a tubal ligation has begun, the examination/diagnostic laparoscopic procedure is bundled into the surgical procedure. For example, if a diagnostic laparoscopy was performed and did not lead to a definitive procedure, the diagnostic laparoscopic code 49320 from the Digestive System subsection would be reported to describe the procedure of examining the abdomen using an endoscope. But if a diagnostic laparoscopy was performed and did lead to a fulguration of the oviducts, code 58670 from the Female Genital System subsection would be assigned. The terminal (end or final) procedure dictates the code choice.

The laparoscopy codes are divided on the basis of the procedure performed, for example, lysis of adhesions, oophorectomy, and lesion excision.

Excision. The Excision category codes report salpingectomy (removal of uterine tube) or salpingo-oophorectomy (removal of uterine tube and ovary) and describe unilateral or bilateral procedures that are either complete or partial. An unbundling issue presents itself with the assignment of these codes. If either a salpingectomy or salpingo-oophorectomy is performed with a more major procedure such as a hysterectomy, each is considered bundled into the more major procedure and not reported separately.

Repair. Within the Repair category are codes for lysis of adhesions and various repairs to the fallopian tubes. All of the repairs are performed for the purpose of restoring fertility. Often the repairs are made through small incisions above the pubic hairline, but they can also be performed through a laparoscope, so note the approach used for repairs to the fallopian tubes.

Lysis of adhesions performed on the fallopian tubes (**salpingolysis**) or the ovaries (**ovariolysis**) uses a small incision to insert instrumentation to complete the repairs. Lysis is a procedure that is often performed at the time of another, more major procedure and is usually bundled into the more major procedure. If the lysis takes an extensive amount of time, you can report the service separately with supportive documentation indicating the additional time and effort required to perform the lysis. Another option is the report modifier -22 to indicate that the procedure required more time than normal. The time to complete the lysis portion of the procedure must be clearly documented in the operative report.

From the Trenches

"Teamwork with other coders gives you support with the 'problem' codes. It is extremely important with the physicians because services must be presented accurately and correctly to the insurance companies."

PATRICIA

Ovary   The subheading Ovary (58800-58960) contains the two categories Incision and Excision. The Incision codes report ovarian incision and drainage. The Excision codes report ovarian biopsy, cystectomy, and oophorectomy procedures.

QUICK CHECK 20-3

1. Review code range 58950-58956. Which codes include the statement "total abdominal hysterectomy"? _____

In Vitro Fertilization   In vitro fertilization means to fertilize an egg outside the body. The codes in the In Vitro Fertilization category describe several methods that are used in modern fertility practice. Third-party payers often do not pay for the fertility treatments. You will have to be certain that you know the policy of the payer regarding fertility treatments.

Code 58970, aspiration of the ova, is often performed with ultrasonic guidance and when it is, assign 76948 (Radiology section, Ultrasonic Guidance Procedures) to report the service.

EXERCISE 20-1 *Female Genital System*

Using the CPT manual, code the following:

1 Simple destruction of one lesion of the vaginal vestibule

     CPT Code: _____

2 Biopsy of three lesions of the vulva

     CPT Codes: _____, _____ × _____

3 Closure of rectovaginal fistula, abdominal approach

     CPT Code: _____

4 Cone biopsy (laser) of cervix with dilation and curettage

     CPT Code: _____

5 Unilateral, laparoscopic, ovarian cystectomy

     CPT Code: _____

Using the vulvectomy notes in the CPT manual, match each of the following procedures with its correct definition:

PROCEDURE		THE REMOVAL OF:
6 simple	_____	a. greater than 80% of the vulvar area
7 radical	_____	b. skin and deep subcutaneous tissues
8 partial	_____	c. skin and superficial subcutaneous tissues
9 complete	_____	d. less than 80% of the vulvar area

MATERNITY CARE AND DELIVERY

Format

The Maternity Care and Delivery subsection (59000-59899) is divided according to type of procedure. As a general rule, the subsection progresses from antepartum procedures through delivery procedures. The guidelines are very detailed as to the services included in antepartum and delivery care, not only to facilitate coding but also to help guard against unbundling. Notes at the beginning of this subsection describe, in depth, the services listed in obstetric care. Be certain to read these notes.

Abortion codes, whether for spontaneous abortion, missed abortion, or induction of abortion, are at the end of the subsection. Abortion codes indicate treatment of a spontaneous abortion or missed abortion, including additional division on the basis of **trimester** and induction of abortion by **method**. You must be aware of the gestational age of the fetus to determine the correct code.

Treatment for ectopic pregnancies is based on the site of the pregnancy, the extent of the surgery, and whether the approach was by means of laparoscopy or laparotomy (incision through abdominal wall).

Maternity and Delivery

The gestation of a fetus takes approximately 266 days; but when the estimated date of delivery **(EDD)** is calculated, 280 days are often used, counting the time from the last menstrual period **(LMP).** The gestation is divided into three time periods, called trimesters. The trimesters are as follows:

- First   LMP to week 12
- Second   Weeks 13-27
- Third   Weeks 28-EDD

When a maternity case is uncomplicated, the service codes normally include the antepartum care, delivery, and postpartum care in the global package. **Antepartum care** is considered to include both the initial and subsequent history and physical examinations, blood pressures, patient's weight, routine urinalysis, fetal heart tones, and monthly visits to 28 weeks of gestation, biweekly visits from gestation weeks 29 through 36, and weekly visits from week 37 to delivery when these services are provided by the same physician. If the patient is seen by the same physician for a service other than those identified as part of antepartum care, you would report that service separately. For example, if a patient in week 32 came to the office with a chief complaint of cold symptoms, an E/M service code would be reported for the service and the diagnosis code would further indicate that the service was provided due to a cold not pregnancy.

Admission to the hospital is bundled into the **delivery** codes and includes the admitting history and examination, management of an uncomplicated labor, and delivery that is either vaginal or by cesarean section (including any episiotomy, illustrated in Fig. 20–13, and use of forceps, as illustrated in Fig. 20–14). Included in **postpartum care** are the hospital visits and/or office visits for 6 weeks after a delivery. If the postpartum care is complicated or if services provided to the patient during the postpartum period are not generally part of the postpartum care, you would report those additional services separately.

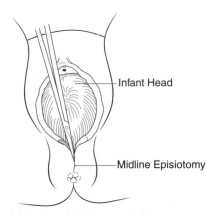

FIGURE 20–13 Midline (median) episiotomy. (From Roberts JR, Hedges JR, eds: *Clinical Procedures in Emergency Medicine,* ed 4, Philadelphia, 2004, Saunders.)

FIGURE 20–14 Use of forceps. (From *Dorland's Illustrated Medical Dictionary,* ed 31, Philadelphia, 2007, Saunders.)

Routine Obstetric Care

There are four codes that describe the global routine obstetric care that includes the antepartum care, delivery, and postpartum care, based on the type of delivery:

- 59400   Vaginal delivery
- 59510   Cesarean delivery
- 59610   Vaginal delivery after a previous cesarean delivery
- 59618   Cesarean delivery following attempted vaginal delivery after previous cesarean delivery

Two abbreviations commonly found on the delivery record are VBAC (vaginal birth after cesarean) and VBACS (vaginal birth after cesarean section), which assist in assigning the correct code.

CODING SHOT

Bundled into the vaginal delivery codes are an episiotomy (cutting of the perineum) and/or the use of forceps during delivery and, therefore, neither is reported separately.

If the physician provided only a portion of the global routine obstetric care, the service is reported with codes that describe that portion of the service as delivery only or postpartum care only, based on the delivery method. For example, if a physician provided only the delivery portion of the service, you would report the service with:

- 59409   Vaginal delivery only
- 59514   Cesarean delivery only
- 59612   Vaginal delivery only, after previous cesarean delivery
- 59620   Cesarean delivery only, following attempted vaginal delivery after previous cesarean delivery

If the global obstetric care is provided and twins are delivered, the same codes are reported but, depending on the third-party payer, modifier -22 (Increased Procedural Services) or -51 (Multiple Procedures) is added. Usually, if both twins are delivered vaginally, report 59400 for Twin A and 59409-51 for Twin B. If one is delivered vaginally and one is delivered cesarean, report 59510 for Twin B and 59409-51 for Twin A. If both are delivered via cesarean, report only 59510 (because only one cesarean was performed).

Delivery Method	Code for TWIN A	Code for TWIN B
Both twins delivered vaginal	59400	59409-51
One twin delivered vaginal Other twin delivered cesarian	59409-51	59510
Both twins delivered cesarian	59510	

Some payers, such as Medicaid in Illinois and Texas, require 59409 (vaginal delivery) or 59410 (cesarean delivery) to be reported since they do not recognize the global obstetric care codes. Each prenatal visit and the delivery is billed separately. Just another reminder that knowledge of the payers' rules will ensure prompt and proper payments.

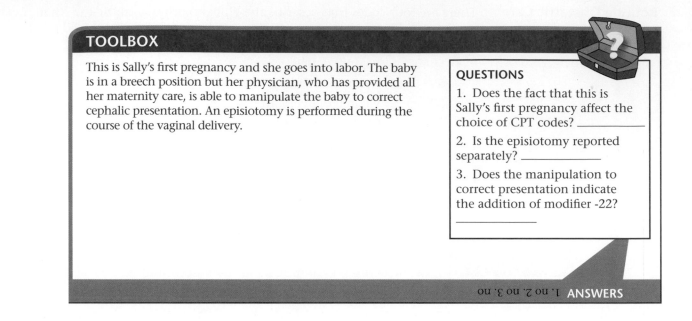

TOOLBOX

This is Sally's first pregnancy and she goes into labor. The baby is in a breech position but her physician, who has provided all her maternity care, is able to manipulate the baby to correct cephalic presentation. An episiotomy is performed during the course of the vaginal delivery.

QUESTIONS

1. Does the fact that this is Sally's first pregnancy affect the choice of CPT codes? _____

2. Is the episiotomy reported separately? _____

3. Does the manipulation to correct presentation indicate the addition of modifier -22? _____

ANSWERS 1. no 2. no 3. no

Antepartum Services

Amniocentesis (59000, 59001) is a procedure in which the physician inserts a needle into the pregnant uterus to withdraw amniotic fluid and is only performed after the first 14 weeks of pregnancy. In this procedure, ultrasound is used to guide the needle, and the supervision and interpretation (S&I) service is reported using 76946 from the Radiology section, Ultrasonic Guidance Procedures subsection.

CODING SHOT

Radiological procedures require a separate medical document before you can submit for reimbursement. Modifier -26 may be required depending on where the service was performed and who owned the radiology equipment.

Several of the antepartum services require component coding in order to fully report the services provided. Attention to the code descriptions and parenthetic statements is necessary to ensure that all services are reported.

Cordocentesis (59012) is a procedure in which fetal blood is drawn. This procedure is performed under ultrasonic guidance to assess the status of the fetus. Cordocentesis is not included in normal antepartum care and should be reported separately. The ultrasonic guidance (76941) would also be reported separately.

Excision. Abdominal **hysterotomy** (59100) may be performed to remove a hydatidiform mole (cystlike structure) (Fig. 20–15) or an embryo. If a tubal ligation is performed at the same time as a hysterotomy, be certain to report 58611 to indicate the ligation.

An **ectopic pregnancy** is one in which the fertilized ovum has become implanted outside of the uterus, as illustrated in Fig. 20–16. The surgical treatment for this condition can use either an abdominal or a vaginal approach (59120-59150); most often, the abdominal approach is used. If the area has not ruptured, the pregnancy is removed. If a rupture has occurred, a more extensive procedure is required. You have to identify the location of

FIGURE 20–15 Hydatidiform. (From Damajnov I, Linder J: *Pathology: A Color Atlas,* St. Louis, 1999, Mosby.)

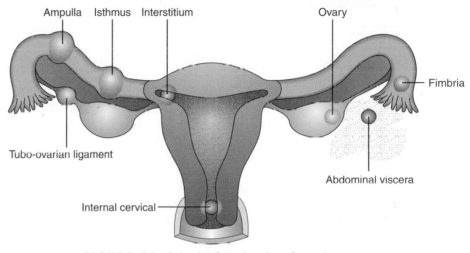

FIGURE 20–16 Implantation sites of ectopic pregnancy.

the ectopic pregnancy, the extent of the necessary repair, and the approach to the repair—vaginal, abdominal, or laparoscopic—to correctly code the procedure.

Postpartum curettage is performed within the first 6 weeks after delivery to remove remaining pieces of the placenta or clotted blood. Code 59160 is only for use with postpartum curettage. If the curettage is nonobstetric, report 58120.

Introduction. A cervical dilator (such as laminaria, which is a compound on a stick that swells from surrounding moisture) may be inserted prior to a procedure in which the cervix is to be dilated; it prepares the cervix for an abortive procedure or a delivery. The dilator initiates uterine contractions, which in turn cause cervical dilatation. Induction can be elective—at the convenience of the patient or the physician—or required, based on a medical risk factor to the mother or fetus. Physicians use a scoring system to measure the stage of cervical ripening, as illustrated in Fig. 20–17.

Score	Dilation (cm)	Effacement (%)	Station	Consistency	Cervical Position
0	Closed	0-30	−3	Firm	Posterior
1	1-2	40-50	−2	Medium	Midposition
2	3-4	60-70	−1, 0	Soft	Anterior
3	>4	>70	+1, +2	—	—

FIGURE 20–17   The Bishop Scoring System of cervical ripening.

To induce cervical ripening (softening and dilation), a preparation such as Prepidil gel is introduced intracervically using a catheter. The cervical ripening takes place in the delivery ward.

CODING SHOT   You can report 59200 (cervical ripening) with an induced abortion (59840 or 59841), but not with an abortion induced by means of vaginal suppositories (59855-59857). Also, do not report an induction procedure using a code that describes a manual dilation as a part of the procedure, such as D&C.

Many third-party payers will not pay separately for an induction procedure, as it is considered to be part of the package for obstetric care. You will have to check with your payers to determine their policies regarding the induction procedure.

Repair.   The obstetric repairs can be to the vulva, vagina, cervix, or uterus. All of these repairs are also located in the Female Genital subsection, but here in the Maternity Care and Delivery subsection, the codes are reported only for repairs made during pregnancy. Repairs made during delivery or after pregnancy are reported using the postpartum codes 59400-59622.

CODING SHOT   Vaginal repairs can be reported separately only by a physician other than the attending physician. When the attending physician performs a procedure such as an episiotomy, it is considered part of the package for obstetric care. Each third-party payer determines what is included in the obstetric package.

Abortion Services.   The abortion codes (59812-59857) include services for treatment for several types of procedures. A **spontaneous** abortion (miscarriage) is one that happens naturally. If the uterus is completely emptied during the miscarriage and the physician manages the postmiscarriage, the services are reported with E/M codes. Sometimes the abortion is **incomplete** and requires intervention to remove the remaining fetal material (59812). A **missed** abortion is one in which the fetus has died naturally sometime during the first half of the pregnancy but remains in the uterus. The physician removes the fetal material from the uterus and reports the service based on the trimester in which the service was provided (59820-59821). A **septic** abortion is similar to a missed abortion but has the added complication of infection. The physician removes the fetal material from the uterus and vigorously treats the infection (59830).

From the Trenches

"Certification means that the coder has been exposed to a lot more knowledge about coding than simply what is used in a particular workplace. It also means more money for the coder."

PATRICIA

The induced abortions are those in which the death of the fetus is brought about by medical intervention (59840-59857). One of three methods is used: dilation with either curettage (scraping) or evacuation (removal by means of suction), intra-amniotic injections, or vaginal suppositories. The selection of the code depends on which of the three methods was used to accomplish the abortion. Dilation and curettage is a procedure in which the cervix is dilated and the fetal material is scraped out by means of a curet. When the dilation and evacuation method is used, the cervix is dilated and the contents are suctioned out by means of a vacuum aspirator. The intra-amniotic injections are of urea or saline, which induces an abortion. Vaginal suppositories (such as prostaglandin) can be inserted into the uterus, with or without cervical dilation, to induce an abortion. A hysterotomy (cutting into the uterus, 59857) may be performed if the medical intervention by injection or vaginal suppositories fails.

EXERCISE 20-2   *Maternity Care and Delivery*

Using the CPT manual, code the following:

1 Laparoscopic salpingectomy for tubal ectopic pregnancy

　　CPT Code: _____

2 Version or breech presentation, successfully converted to cephalic presentation, with normal spontaneous delivery

　　CPT Codes: _____, _____

3 Thirty-year-old woman, 20 weeks' gestation, with cervical cerclage by vaginal approach

　　CPT Code: _____

CHAPTER REVIEW

CHAPTER 20, PART I, THEORY

Without the use of reference material, complete the following:

1 The Female Genital System subsection is divided

by _____ site from the vulva to the ovaries.

2 Skene's glands procedures are reported using

codes from which subsection? _____

3 The vulva includes the following:

mons _____,

labia _____,

labia _____,

bulb of _____,
vaginal orifice or vestibule, greater and

_____

glands.

4 Who is responsible for determining the complexity of destruction of lesions of the

vulva? _____

5 Destruction of a lesion is also known as excision.

True   False

6 Would you expect a pathology report to be available for a lesion that was removed by destruction?

Yes   No

7 The term that describes the removal of a portion

of the vulva is a(n) _____.

8 The removal of the vulvar area is reported

with which two measures? _____ and

_____

9 Vulvar area tissue removal that involves the skin and superficial subcutaneous tissues is

termed _____.

10 Vulvar area tissue removal that involves the skin and deep subcutaneous tissues is termed

_____.

11 A(n) _____ vulvectomy involves less

than 80% of the vulva and a(n) _____
vulvectomy involves more than 80% of the vulva.

CHAPTER 20, PART II, PRACTICAL

Using the CPT and ICD-9-CM manuals, code the following:

12 Sue Lind, age 29, has a Pap test. The pathology report comes back positive for malignancy. Her physician recommends and performs a diagnostic colposcopy. Evidence of further primary malignancy of the uterus is seen and the physician does a laparoscopically assisted vaginal hysterectomy 20 days later of a 236-gram uterus. Report only the hysterectomy and diagnosis code that indicates the medical necessity of the procedure.

CPT Code: _____

ICD-9-CM Code: _____

(ICD-10-CM Code: _____)

13 Laparoscopy with fulguration of obstructed oviducts

CPT Code: _____

ICD-9-CM Code: _____

(ICD-10-CM Code: _____)

14 Oocyte retrieval for in vitro fertilization from a donor by means of a follicle puncture with radiologic assistance

CPT Code: _____

ICD-9-CM Code: _____

(ICD-10-CM Code: _____)

15 The attending physician, who has provided Sally Fisher's obstetric care, performed a cesarean delivery, due to breech presentation, and ligation of the fallopian tubes (sterilization at the request of the patient) and routinely followed up with Sally in the postpartum period. The newborn was an 8 lb 2 oz male.

CPT Codes: _____ (Cesarean delivery, routine care); _____ (Cesarean delivery, tubal ligation)

ICD-9-CM Codes: _____ (Cesarean delivery); _____ (Newborn gestation); _____ (Outcome of delivery); _____ (Sterilization)

(ICD-10-CM Codes: _____, _____, _____, _____)

16 Colpopexy for displaced uterus using an abdominal approach

CPT Code: _____

ICD-9-CM Code: _____

(ICD-10-CM Code: _____)

17 Biopsy of three lesions of the vulva. Pathology report later indicated primary squamous cell carcinoma.

❀ CPT Code(s): _____

❀ ICD-9-CM Code(s): _____

(❀ICD-10-CM Code(s): _____)

18 Fitting and supply of a diaphragm with instructions for use

❀ CPT Code(s): _____

19 Extensive biopsy of mucosa of vagina, requiring closure

CPT Code: _____

20 Using instrumentation, the cervical canal was dilated and examination was completed.

CPT Code: _____

21 Simple incision and drainage of an abscess of the vulva

CPT Code: _____

22 Colpocentesis

CPT Code: _____

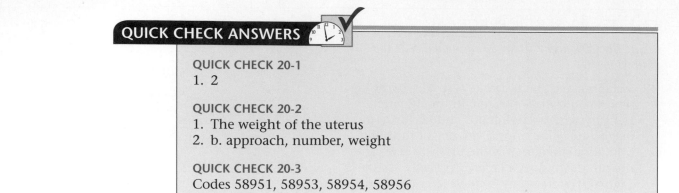

QUICK CHECK ANSWERS

QUICK CHECK 20-1
1. 2

QUICK CHECK 20-2
1. The weight of the uterus
2. b. approach, number, weight

QUICK CHECK 20-3
Codes 58951, 58953, 58954, 58956

"The benefit to working in medical coding is job security, because the field is constantly expanding."

Christine A. Patterson
Coder and Biller
Reinhart Family Healthcare
Monticello, Arkansas

Endocrine and Nervous Systems

Chapter Topics

Endocrine System

Nervous System

Chapter Review

Quick Check Answers

Learning Objectives

After completing this chapter you should be able to

1 Review the Endocrine System subsection format.

2 Understand the Endocrine System subheadings.

3 Demonstrate the ability to code Endocrine System services.

4 Review the Nervous System subsection format.

5 Understand the Nervous System subheadings.

6 Demonstrate the ability to code Nervous System services.

Make sure to check
evolve
learning system
for the latest
content updates

ENDOCRINE SYSTEM

Format

There are nine glands in the endocrine system (Fig. 21–1), but only **four** are included in the Endocrine subsection (60000-60699) of the CPT manual. The four glands in the Endocrine subsection are:

- Thyroid (60000-60300)
- Parathyroid (60500-60512)
- Thymus (60520-60522)
- Adrenal (60540-60545, 60650)

The pituitary and pineal gland codes are in the Nervous System subsection of the CPT manual, the pancreas codes are in the Digestive System subsection, and the ovaries and testes codes are in the respective Female or Male Genital System subsections.

Coding Highlights

The Endocrine System subsection (60000-60699) includes two subheadings of:

- Thyroid Gland
- Parathyroid, Thymus, Adrenal Glands, Pancreas, and Carotid Body (see Fig. 21–2)

The **thyroid** gland is composed of a right and left lobe on either side of the trachea, just below a large piece of cartilage (thyroid cartilage). Two of the hormones secreted by the thyroid gland are T3 (triiodothyronine) and T4 (thyroxine). The thyroid gland normally produces 80% T4 and 20% T3.

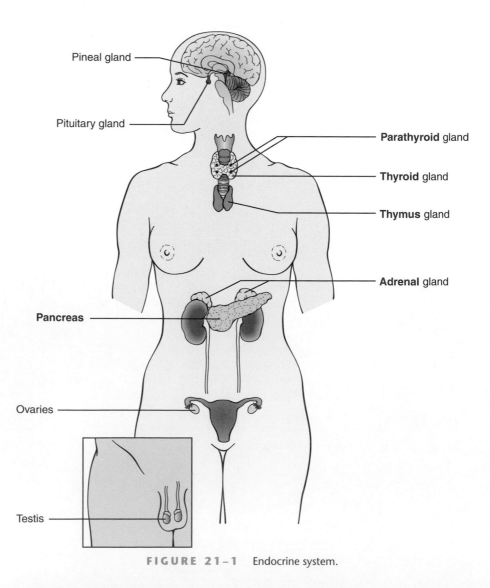

FIGURE 21–1 Endocrine system.

These hormones are necessary to maintain the normal level of metabolism in the cells of the body. Thyroid Function Tests (TFTs) assess the levels of hormones produced by the thyroid gland. Within the Thyroid Gland subheading in the CPT manual (60000-60300) there are the categories of Incision, Excision, and Removal.

Parathyroid glands are four small oval bodies located on the dorsal aspect (back) of the thyroid gland. These glands secrete parathyroid hormone (PTH). That mobilizes calcium from bones into the bloodstream, which is necessary for the proper functioning of body tissues, especially muscles. Within the Parathyroid, Thymus, Adrenal Glands, Pancreas, and Carotid Body subsection (60500-60699) there are categories Excision, Laparoscopy, and Other Procedures.

Adrenal glands (suprarenal) are two small glands situated one on top of each kidney. There are two parts to each gland, the cortex (outer portion) and the medulla (inner portion). The cortex secretes the hormones corticosteroids, and the medulla secretes the hormones catecholamines.

Thymus gland is located behind the breast bone, in front of the heart, and is involved in maturation (development) of the immune system. Thymectomy is removal of the thymus and is usually performed by cutting through the breast bone, similar to heart surgery.

The **pancreas** is an organ that is located behind the stomach and the head of the organ is attached to the duodenum (first section of the small intestine). Although the organ is listed in the heading (Parathyroid, Thymus, Adrenal Glands, Pancreas, and Carotid Body), the codes for procedures involving the pancreas are located in the Digestive System subsection (48000-48999).

The **carotid body** is tissue rich in capillaries that acts as receptors located near the bifurcation (splitting into two) of the carotid arteries as illustrated in Fig. 21–2. The receptors monitor arterial oxygen content and pressure.

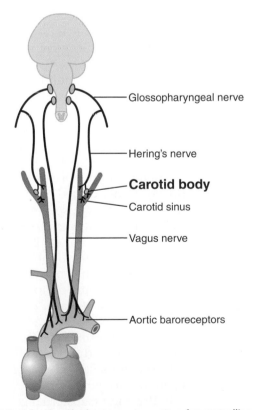

FIGURE 21-2 The baroreceptor system for controlling arterial pressure. (Modified from Guyton AC, Hall JE: *Textbook of Medical Physiology,* ed 11, Philadelphia, 2006, Saunders.)

Tumors that develop in the carotid body may be excised and the service reported with 60600 or 60605.

All **endocrine** glands are ductless, which means they secrete hormones directly into the bloodstream rather than through ducts leading to the exterior of the body. Exocrine glands send their chemical substances into ducts and then out of the body. Examples of **exocrine** glands are sweat, mammary, mucous, salivary, and lacrimal (tear ducts).

From the Trenches

"I think coders automatically network because no one person can know it all. We just help each other as best we can. Teamwork is the difference between a clean, accurate claim for optimum value or a denial."

CHRISTINE

Thyroid Gland Incision and Excision.   A thyroidectomy is the removal of all or part of the thyroid gland. The thyroid gland consists of two lobes, one on each side of the throat, connected by a narrow band of thyroid tissue (isthmus). The term thyroidectomy can apply to a total removal of the gland (total thyroidectomy), removal of one or part of one of the lobes (lobectomy), or the isthmus (isthmusectomy).

A thyroidectomy is performed to assist in treatment of various thyroid diseases, such as thyroid nodules, hyperthyroidism (overactive thyroid gland), cancer of the thyroid gland, or enlargement of the thyroid (goiter) that may cause breathing or swallowing difficulties.

The amount of thyroid tissue removed is determined prior to the surgical procedure. The surgeon works closely with an endocrinologist (a physician specializing in gland tissue disorders) to determine the thyroid gland function and the amount of tissue to remove. Usually thyroid function tests (blood tests) and thyroid scanning are performed before the procedure. For cases in which thyroid cancer is suspected, a biopsy may also be performed.

A partial thyroid lobectomy is reported with 60210 or 60212 and is not performed often. For this to be the technique of choice, the lesion must be located in the upper or lower portion of only one lobe.

Total thyroid lobectomy (60220 or 60225) is typically the least complex operation performed on the thyroid gland. It is performed for solitary nodules that are suspected to be cancerous or those that are indeterminate following biopsy, such as follicular adenomas, solitary nodules, or goiters that are isolated to one lobe (not common). The procedure may or may not include an isthmusectomy (removal of the part that connects the two thyroid lobes) because the code description states "with or without isthmusectomy." An isthmusectomy removes more thyroid tissue than a simple lobectomy and is performed when a larger margin of tissue is needed to assure that all suspect tissue has been removed. Subtotal thyroidectomy (60210, 60212, 60252, 60254) is performed to excise all questionable tissue on the side of the gland as well as the isthmus and the majority of the opposite lobe. This operation is typical for small, non-aggressive thyroid neoplasms. It is also a common operation for goiters that result in problems in the neck or those that extend into the chest (substernal goiters).

Total thyroidectomy (60240, 60252) removes all of the thyroid gland and is often the procedure of choice for thyroid neoplasms that are larger and/or aggressive. Many surgeons prefer the complete removal of thyroid tissue in those patients with thyroid neoplasms regardless of the type of neoplasm.

The technique for a thyroidectomy utilizes a standard neck incision typically measuring about 4-5 inches in length. Many surgeons perform this procedure through an incision as small as 3 inches. The incision is made in the lower part of the central neck and typically involves the removal of that part of the thyroid that contains the suspect tissue. The surgeon must be careful of the laryngeal nerves that are very close to the back side of the thyroid and are responsible for movement of the vocal cords. Damage to a nerve will cause hoarseness of the voice, which although it is usually temporary, may be permanent, although this is an uncommon complication (about 1% to 2%).

A cyst may form on the thyroid and a surgeon may aspirate and/or inject the cyst. The service is reported with 60300. As with other aspiration/injection codes, if the surgeon provides an aspiration and injection, both procedures are reported with one unit of the code (60300), not two units (60300 × 2).

Parathyroid Excision. Parathyroidectomy is an incision made above the collar bone that is approximately 4 inches in length. The four parathyroid glands are located by the surgeon and removed, a drain is inserted at either end of the incision and sutures or surgical clips are applied.

EXERCISE 21-1 *Endocrine System*

Using the CPT manual, code the following. You do not need to assign -RT or -LT to the codes for this exercise.

1 Excision of an adenoma from posterior aspect of the thyroid gland

    Code: _____

2 Surgical removal of a thyroglossal duct cyst

    Code: _____

3 Thymectomy using the transthoracic approach, with radical mediastinal dissection

    Code: _____

4 Removal of tumor affixed to the carotid body

    Code: _____

5 Partial unilateral thyroidlobectomy, with isthmusectomy

    Code: _____

6 Surgical laparoscopy, with partial adrenalectomy, with biopsy, transabdominal approach

    Code: _____

7 Parathyroidectomy, with mediastinal exploration, and sternal split, with parathyroid autotransplantation

    Codes: _____ , _____

8 Re-exploration of parathyroids, with partial thymectomy, transcervical approach

    Code: _____

9 Excision of carotid body tumor with excision of the carotid artery

    Code: _____

NERVOUS SYSTEM

Structure and Function of the Nervous System

Central Nervous and Peripheral Nervous System. The central nervous system includes the brain and spinal cord. The peripheral nervous system contains 12 pairs of cranial nerves and 31 pairs of spinal nerves as illustrated in Fig. 21–3. The peripheral nervous system is divided into the somatic nervous system, autonomic nervous system, and the enteric nervous system. The somatic nervous system coordinates body movements and receives external stimuli and is under conscious control. The autonomic nervous system is divided into the sympathetic (responds to stress), parasympathetic (constricts pupils, slows heartbeat, dilates blood vessels, stimulates digestion), and enteric divisions (manages digestion) and is not under conscious control.

Brain

- Cerebrum—largest part of the brain.
- Cerebral hemispheres—paired halves of the cerebrum. Each hemisphere is subdivided into four major lobes named for the cranial (skull) bones they overlie:

    Frontal

Central Nervous System

• Brain
• Spinal cord

Peripheral Nervous System

• Cranial nerves (12)
• Spinal nerves
  cervical (8)
  thoraic (12)
  lumbar (5)
  sacral (5)
  coccyx (1)

FIGURE 21–3 The central nervous system consists of the brain and spinal cord. The peripheral nervous system consists of nerves that lie outside the skull and spinal cord. (From Stoy WA, Platt TE, Lejeune DA: *Mosby's EMT-Basic Textbook,* ed 2, St. Louis, 2007, Mosby.)

Parietal

Occipital

Temporal

- Cerebellum—posterior part of the brain that coordinates the voluntary muscle movements and maintains balance.
- Cerebral cortex—outer region of the cerebrum (gray matter).
- Fissure—groove in the surface of the cerebral cortex.
- Medulla oblongata—part of the brain located just above the spinal cord and controls breathing, heartbeat, and blood vessel size.
- Ventricles—reservoirs in the interior of the brain filled with cerebrospinal fluid.

The following structures connect the cerebrum with the spinal cord:

- Cerebellum
- Pons (part of brain stem)
- Medulla oblongata (part of brain stem)

These terms are important as they relate to correct code assignment.

Spinal Cord.   The spinal cord is a column of nerve tissue extending from the medulla oblongata to the second lumbar vertebra. Located at the end of the spinal cord is the cauda equina (a group of nerve fibers found below the second lumbar vertebra of the spinal column). The cauda equina carries all the nerves that affect the lower part and limbs of the body and serves as the pathway for impulses going to and from the brain.

Meninges.   The meninges consists of three layers of connective membranes that surround the brain and spinal cord. The outermost membrane of the meninges is the dura mater, which is a thick, tough membrane that contains channels by which blood enters the brain tissue. The subdural space is located below the dural membrane and contains multiple blood vessels. The second layer around the brain and spinal cord is the arachnoid membrane. The third layer of the meninges and the one closest to the brain and spinal cord is the pia mater.

Neurological diseases of this area are classified as:

- Congenital
- Degenerative, movement, and seizure
- Infectious
- Neoplastic
- Traumatic
- Vascular

Code Assignment   The Nervous System subsection (61000-64999) codes report procedures performed on the brain, spinal cord, nerves, and all associated parts. The subheadings are divided according to anatomic site—whether it is a part of the brain or spinal column or a type of nerve. The subheadings are further divided by **type** of procedure. The codes report services on both the central nervous system and the peripheral nervous system.

To assign the correct code, the coder must first know the **purpose** of the procedure, because many of the code descriptions indicate the condition responsible for the procedure. For example, abscess, cyst, hematoma, foreign body, tumor, seizure, aneurysm, vascular malformation, rhinorrhea, hydrocephalus, spondylolisthesis, herniated disc, meningocele, nerve pain, spasm, neuroma, neurofibroma, in addition to the technique used for the procedure. Many of the procedures require radiological supervision and interpretation. Next, the coder must know the **location** of the procedure within the skull, meninges, or brain.

Skull, Meninges, and Brain

Punctures, Twists, or Burr Holes.   The first two categories of codes are Injection, Drainage, or Aspiration (61000-61070) and Twist Drill, Burr Hole(s), or Trephine (61105-61253) that deal with conditions that may require holes or openings be made into the brain to relieve pressure, insertion of monitoring devices, placement of tubing, injection of contrast material, or to drain a hemorrhage. A **ventricular** puncture (61020-61026) requires a puncture through the top portion of the skull, while a **cisternal** puncture (61050, 61055) is an approach at the base of the skull. To accomplish many of these procedures, twist or burr holes are made through the skull, which leaves the skull intact except for the small openings (holes).

Craniectomy/Craniotomy.   Codes in the category Craniectomy or Craniotomy (61304-61576) describe procedures that deal with incision into the skull with possible removal of a portion of the skull to open the operative site to the surgeon. Assignment of these codes is based on the site and condition (e.g., evacuation of hematoma, supratentorial, subdural, 61312).

As in other subsections, many procedures are bundled into one craniectomy/craniotomy code. Only by careful attention to code description can you prevent unbundling surgical procedures and incorrectly report bundled components separately. Carefully review the descriptions of these codes before assigning a code.

When craniectomies are performed, it is not uncommon that additional grafting is required to repair the surgical defect caused by opening the skull. These grafting procedures are reported separately, in addition to the major surgical procedure.

Surgery of Skull Base.   The **skull base** is the area at the base of the cranium where the lobes of the brain rest. When lesions are located within the skull base, it often takes the skill of several surgeons working together to perform surgery dealing with these conditions. The procedures located in the category Surgery of Skull Base (61580-61619) are very involved, taking many hours to complete. The procedures are divided on the approach procedure, the definitive procedure, and the reconstruction/repair procedure.

The **approach procedure** (61580-61598) is the method used to obtain exposure of the lesion (e.g., anterior cranial fossa, middle cranial fossa, posterior cranial fossa). The approach procedure is the anatomical location. The **definitive procedure** (61600-61616) is what was done to the lesion (e.g., biopsy, excision, repair, resection). If one physician did both the approach and the definitive procedures, both would be reported. For example, a neoplasm is excised at the base of the anterior cranial fossa, extradural using a craniofacial approach to the anterior skull base. This would be reported with 61600 for the procedure (definitive procedure, extradural excision of a neoplasm) and 61580 for the approach (approach procedure, craniofacial). Because two procedures (approach and definitive) were performed by the same surgeon, both codes would be reported for the physician—61600 and 61580. The most resource intensive procedure would be listed first without a modifier (definitive), and the lesser procedure (approach) would be listed second with modifier -51 appended.

Code 61613 describes the obliteration (total destruction) of a carotid aneurysm, arteriovenous malformation, or carotid fistula and does not include the approach. Codes 61615 and 61616 report services at the base of posterior cranial fossa and describe the resection or excision of extradural (outside the dura) or intradural (inside the dura) vascular or infectious lesions with or without graft. The approach for the resection is reported separately.

Codes in the Repair and/or Reconstruction of Surgical Defects of the Skull Base (61618, 61619) are performed to rebuild the area used for entry into the skull. This type of repair is the last step of reconstruction and is reported separately, only if the service was documented in the medical record as extensive.

At any point, one or more surgeons may be performing distinctly different portions of these complex procedures. When one surgeon performs the approach procedure, another surgeon performs the definitive procedure, and another surgeon performs the reconstruction/repair procedure, each surgeon's services would be reported with the code for the specific procedure he or she individually performed. Again, if one surgeon performs more than one procedure (e.g., the approach procedure, the definitive procedure, and the reconstruction/repair procedure), each procedure is reported separately, adding modifier -51 to the secondary procedures. For example, one surgeon performs the approach procedure (61580), definitive procedure (61600), and reconstruction/repair (61619). The services are reported as 61600 (the most resource intense), 61619-51, and 61580-51.

Aneurysm, Arteriovenous Malformation, or Vascular Disease.

Aneurysms may develop within the brain and require surgical repair. A arteriovenous malformation is a condition in which the arteries and veins are not in the correct anatomic position. Codes to indicate the definitive procedure or repair of these conditions are located in the category Surgery for Aneurysm, Arteriovenous Malformation, or Vascular Disease (61680-61711). These codes are divided on the basis of the **approach** and **method** of procedure.

CODING SHOT
An electroencephalograph (EEG) is used to monitor currents emanating from the brain and is usually utilized any time a procedure on the brain is performed. Report the EEG service separately with 95950.

Cerebrospinal Fluid (CSF) Shunts.

A **shunt** can be considered a draining device that enables fluids to flow from one area to another. A shunt is necessary when the body is not able to perform the drainage function on its own. In the case of cerebrospinal fluid shunts (62180-62258), the fluid is produced in the ventricles of the brain but does not drain properly and may continue to accumulate in the brain, building pressure and causing brain damage. Drains or shunts are placed from the area of collection to a drainage area to keep the fluid level within a normal range. For instance, code 62223 describes the creation of a shunt from the ventricle to the peritoneal space (ventriculoperitoneal), as illustrated in Fig. 21–4. This means that the shunt originates in the ventricle of the brain and terminates in the peritoneum. Codes in the CSF Shunt category describe all the various types of shunting procedures, including placement of shunting devices and subsequent repair, replacement, and removal. Shunt systems may also be placed to drain obstructed CSF from the spine.

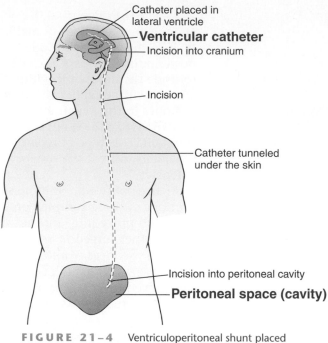

Catheter placed in
lateral ventricle

Ventricular catheter

Incision into cranium

Incision

Catheter tunneled
under the skin

Incision into peritoneal cavity

Peritoneal space (cavity)

FIGURE 21–4 Ventriculoperitoneal shunt placed for chronic hydrocephalus.

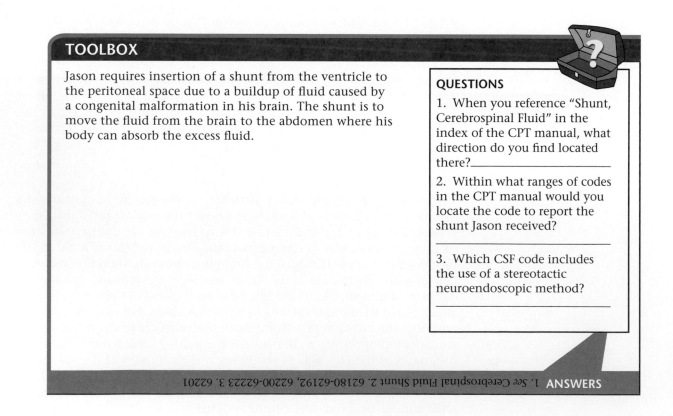

TOOLBOX

Jason requires insertion of a shunt from the ventricle to the peritoneal space due to a buildup of fluid caused by a congenital malformation in his brain. The shunt is to move the fluid from the brain to the abdomen where his body can absorb the excess fluid.

QUESTIONS

1. When you reference "Shunt, Cerebrospinal Fluid" in the index of the CPT manual, what direction do you find located there?_____

2. Within what ranges of codes in the CPT manual would you locate the code to report the shunt Jason received?

_____

3. Which CSF code includes the use of a stereotactic neuroendoscopic method?

_____

ANSWERS 1. *See* Cerebrospinal Fluid Shunt 2. 62180-62192, 62200-62223 3. 62201

Spine and Spinal Cord

The subheading Spine and Spinal Cord (62263-63746) includes codes for injections, laminectomies, excisions, repairs, and shunting. You should be familiar with the terminology for parts of the spinal column (Fig. 21–5). A medical dictionary will help you become familiar with the other parts of the vertebral column, including the lamina, foramina, vertebral bodies, discs, facets, and nerve roots. The basic distinction among the codes in these ranges is the **condition** (such as a herniated intervertebral disc versus a neoplastic lesion of the spinal cord) as well as the **approach** (e.g., anterior, posterior, costovertebral).

The complexity of the procedure is determined by the condition and approach. For example, a patient with a herniated disc at L5-S1 would require less time in surgery for the removal of the disc and decompression of the nerve root than would a patient with a neoplastic growth intertwined in the same area, because removal of a piece of disc would not be as involved as separating a lesion from multiple components of the spinal column. The approaches differ in the amount of expertise and time required. A posterior approach means a surgical opening was formed from the back. An anterior approach means a surgical opening was formed from the front.

When reporting spinal procedures, you must determine the condition, the approach, whether the procedure was unilateral or bilateral, and whether multiple procedures were performed.

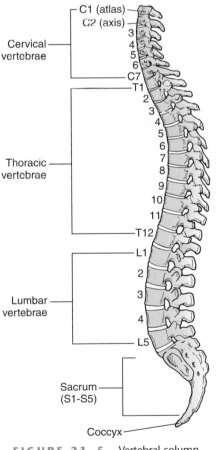

FIGURE 21–5 Vertebral column.

QUICK CHECK 21-1

1. This term describes the approach is from the front _____ and

   this term describes and approach that is from the back _____.

Often when a laminectomy (removal of a lamina) (Fig. 21–6) is performed, an arthrodesis (surgical fusion of joints) is also performed. In some cases spinal instrumentation procedures (the use of rods, wires, and screws to create fusions) are also performed. When multiple procedures are performed, you must review the operative report and confirm all procedures are reported.

A **lumbar puncture** (62270), or spinal tap, obtains cerebrospinal fluid by insertion of a needle into the subarachnoid space in the lumbar region, as illustrated in Fig. 21–7. The fluid is analyzed to diagnose various conditions. For example, if the fluid is pinkish in color and contains erythrocytes, there may be a hemorrhage. A yellowish, cloudy fluid with numerous white blood cells (WBCs) may indicate an infection.

Notes throughout the Spine and Spinal Cord subsection refer you to other code ranges for commonly performed additional procedures (e.g., arthrodesis codes are in the Musculoskeletal subsection). Remember to use the modifier -51 for multiple procedures if more than one procedure is performed during the operative session.

CODING SHOT A sensory evoked study, which monitors the central nervous system, is usually performed with spinal surgery and reported separately with 95925.

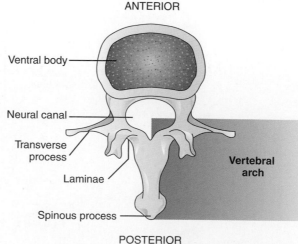

ANTERIOR

Ventral body

Neural canal

Transverse process

Laminae

Vertebral arch

Spinous process

POSTERIOR

FIGURE 21-6 Vertebra viewed from above.

Lumbar
subarachnoid
space

FIGURE 21–7 Lumbar puncture, or spinal tap, in which the cerebrospinal fluid is obtained by inserting a needle into the subarachnoid space. The patient lies laterally with knees drawn up to increase the spaces between the vertebrae.

Destruction by a **neurolytic agent** includes chemical denervation (alcohol or glycerol by injection), radiofrequency (passes a current through an electrode carefully positioned using fluoroscopy), or cryogenic surgery (inserting a probe into tissue, with fluoroscopy guidance, and freezing a region of tissue). Codes 62280-62282 describe neurolytic substances that are injected/infused at specific anatomic sites (e.g., subarachnoid and epidural). Code 62280 reports a subarachnoid injection/infusion of a neurolytic substance. Codes 62281 and 62282 report epidural injection/infusion of a neurolytic substance based on the location as into the cervical or thoracic region (62281) or the lumbar, sacral region (62282).

CODING SHOT Codes 62280-62282 include the injection of contrast material; therefore, the injection of contrast during fluoroscopic guidance and localization is bundled into the codes and is not reported separately.

Codes 62318 and 62319 include the setup and start of the infusion of the therapeutic substance(s). When providing the daily maintenance of the epidural or subarachnoid catheter drug administration, report the service separately with 01996.

Codes in the 62310-62319 range report injection services based on the route of administration (not type of substance administered). These codes exclude injection of a neurolytic substance that are usually reported with codes 62280-62282.

CODING SHOT The injection of contrast material during fluoroscopic guidance and localization are also bundled into the 62310-62319 and not separately reported.

Extracranial Nerves, Peripheral Nerves, and Autonomic Nervous System. Nerves are our sensing devices, and they carry stimuli to and from all parts of the body. Some common procedures performed on nerves include injection, destruction, decompression, and suture/repair and are reported with codes from the Extracranial Nerves, Peripheral Nerves, and Autonomic Nervous System subheading (64400-64999).

The space around the nerves can be injected with anesthetic agents to cause a temporary loss of feeling (64400-64530). The code is assigned according to the type of nerve being injected. Nerves may also be injected to cause destruction of the nerve and permanent loss of feeling in a specific area of the body (64600-64640, 64680-64681). Persons with debilitating pain may undergo this type of procedure and the diagnoses codes must support the medical necessity of the procedure. For example, reporting of 64612 (destruction by neurolytic agent; muscles innervated [supplied] by facial nerve) is supported by diagnosis codes such as 333.81 (blepharospasm) [ICD-10-CM: G24.5], 333.82 (oral mandibular dystonia) [ICD-10-CM: G24.4], or 351.8 (hemifacial spasm nerve) [ICD-10-CM: G51.3].

When reporting Introduction/Injection of Anesthetic Agent (Nerve Block), Diagnostic or Therapeutic codes in the 64400-64907 range, the coder must know the nerves, nerve groupings, and the interaction of the nerve with the body system(s). It is also important to identify the substance injected and the specific nerve the substances was injected into. Let's take a closer look at the origin of these nerves and the interaction each has with the body system(s):

- Trigeminal nerve (5th cranial) emerges from the lateral surface of the pons. The trigeminal nerve is a sensory nerve that supplies the face, teeth, mouth and nasal cavity, and a motor nerve that supplies the muscles of mastication (chewing).

- Facial nerve (7th cranial) consists of the large motor root (supplies the muscles of facial expression) and a smaller root (nervus intermedius).

- Greater occipital nerve is a spinal nerve originating from the cervical spinal nerve C2. It supplies stimuli to the scalp, over the ears, and the parotid gland.

- Vagus nerve (10th cranial) has its origin in the lateral side of medulla oblongata and supplies sensory fibers to the ear, tongue, pharynx, and larynx and motor fibers to the pharynx, larynx, and esophagus.

- Phrenic nerve affects the pleura, pericardium, diaphragm, peritoneum, and sympathetic plexuses. A plexus is a collection (aggregate) of nerves and ganglia.

- Cervical plexus (posterior) is a plexus in the posterior cervical region that is formed by the dorsal rami of the first three or four cervical spinal nerves.

- Axillary nerve originates from the brachial plexus at the axilla (armpit) level and is responsible for sensory information from the shoulder joint and the inferior region of the deltoid muscle.

- Suprascapular nerve has its origin in the brachial plexus at the C5-C6 level that descends through suprascapular and spinoglenoid notches and supplies acromioclavicular and shoulder joints, and supraspinatus muscles.

- Pudendal originates in the sacral plexus at the S2-S4, and sometimes C5 and T1. Divides into the perineal nerve and the dorsal nerve of the penis (clitoris) distributed to the muscles, skin, and erectile tissue of perineum.

Injection of anesthetic into these nerves may be performed to block the pain sensation and provide relief from various pain, such as neck, lower back, myofascial pain syndrome, or cancer pain. There are many types of blocks, such as:

- Brachial plexus block for upper extremity pain.
- Celiac plexus (sympathetic nerve) block for pain in the abdomen.
- Ilioinguinal block for pain from the pelvis area (groin, inguinal, or femoral).
- Intercostal nerve block is for any of the 12 sets of nerves that travel between the spine and the rib cage.
- Sympathetic blocks the nerves that are located along both sides of the spine and supplies the limbs and the abdomen.
- Stellate ganglion block is performed for relief of sympathetic pain of the head or neck. The stellate ganglion is a group of nerves located on each side of the neck and help control blood vessels, sweat glands, and indirectly the temperature of the face, arms and hands.
- Paravertebral nerve block is performed for pain in the cervical, thoracic, or lumbar regions.
- Somatic or sympathetic nerve injection is a rhizotomy. The agent injected may be chemical, thermal electrical, or radiofrequency.

CODING SHOT

Blocks are considered unilateral; modifier -50 should be used for bilateral procedures. When more than one level is involved, use the appropriate add-on code.

Blocks may also be performed when confirming a diagnosis. For example, a lumbar-sacral paravertebral facet joint block (64490-64495) is one method utilized to document or confirm pain of the back. The patient with this condition usually has localized back pain aggravated by motion of the spine. During the procedure, a needle is placed in the facet joint or facet joint nerve under fluoroscopic guidance and a local anesthetic agent is injected. After control of the pain has been obtained, the patient is asked to perform activities that usually aggravate the pain. If the patient has decreased pain or absence of pain, the facet joint is identified as the source of the pain and appropriate treatment may be prescribed.

QUICK CHECK 21-2

List the code ranges for:

1. Nerves injected to cause temporary loss of feeling is reported with

   this range of codes: _____

2. Nerves injected to cause permanent loss of feeling is reported with

   this range of codes: _____

Neuroplasty is the decompression (freeing) of intact nerves (e.g., from scar tissue). If nerves receive excessive pressure from a source, such as scar tissue or displacement of intervertebral disc material, pain may occur. Movement or freeing of nerves is reported with codes from the Neuroplasty (Exploration, Neurolysis, or Nerve Decompression) category (64702-64727). Perhaps the most commonly known neuroplasty procedure is a carpal tunnel release, reported with 64721, during which the median nerve and flexor tendons of the wrist are surgically released (Fig. 21–8).

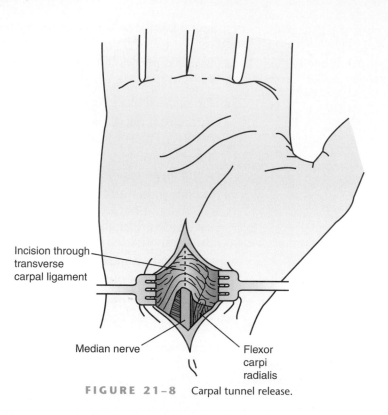

Incision through transverse carpal ligament

Median nerve

Flexor carpi radialis

FIGURE 21–8   Carpal tunnel release.

Nerves can also be removed or they can be repaired (sutured). The codes in the Neurorrhaphy (64831-64876) and the Neurorrhaphy with Nerve Graft (64885-64911) categories describe nerve repairs on the basis of the specific nerve being repaired. This category also includes codes that describe grafting on the basis of the size of the graft.

EXERCISE 21-2 *Nervous System*

Using the CPT manual, code the following:

1 Drainage of a nontraumatic subdural hematoma using burr holes

  CPT Code: _____

  ICD-9-CM Code: _____ (ICD-10-CM Code: _____)

2 Drainage of traumatic subdural hematoma with craniectomy, supratentorial

  CPT Code: _____

  ICD-9-CM Code: _____ (ICD-10-CM Code: _____)

3 Resection of primary, malignant neoplasm, midline skull base, extradural, using infratemporal preauricular approach to middle cranial fossa

  CPT Codes: _____, _____, _____

  ICD-9-CM Code: _____ (ICD-10-CM Code: _____)

4 Removal of complete cerebrospinal fluid shunt system, with replacement due to congenital hydrocephalus

  CPT Code: _____

  ICD-9-CM Code: _____ (ICD-10-CM Code: _____)

CHAPTER REVIEW

CHAPTER 21, PART I, THEORY

Complete the following:

1 How many endocrine glands are included in the Endocrine subsection of the CPT manual?

_____

2 The pituitary and pineal gland procedure codes are in what subsection of the Surgery section?

_____

3 The codes for pancreatic procedures are located in what subsection of the Surgery section?

_____

4 Both subtotal and partial mean something less than _____.

5 Twist or _____ holes are made through the skull to accomplish procedures of the brain.

6 The _____ procedure is the method used to obtain exposure to a lesion of the skull base, and the _____ procedure is what is done to the lesion.

7 CSF means _____.

8 The most commonly known neuroplasty procedure is a(n) _____ _____ release.

9 This term describes the location of the bifurcation of the carotid artery in the neck:

_____ _____

10 Would you report separately the additional grafting required to repair the surgical defect caused by a craniectomy?

Yes   No

CHAPTER 21, PART II, PRACTICAL

Code the following cases:

11 Total thyroidectomy

Code: _____

12 Surgical laparoscopy with partial adrenalectomy using a transabdominal approach

Code: _____

13 Parathyroidectomy with mediastinal exploration

Code: _____

14 Stereotactic creation of a thalamus lesion with multiple staging

Code: _____

15 Torkildsen type operation with CSF shunt insertion

Code: _____

16 Implantation of a tunneled epidural catheter for long-term administration of medication

Code: _____

17 Partial resection of a single segment of a vertebral (cervical) body using an anterior approach with decompression of the spinal cord and nerve roots

Code: _____

18 Therapeutic injection of the greater occipital nerve with an anesthetic agent

Code: _____

19 Complete transaction of the facial nerve

Code: _____

20 Nerve graft of a single strand of nerve, 5 cm in length, to the foot, procedure included procurement of graft

Code: _____

QUICK CHECK ANSWERS

QUICK CHECK 21-1
1. anterior, posterior

QUICK CHECK 21-2
1. 64400-64530
2. 64600-64681

"Most will struggle with terminology, but asking questions will save and often benefit your career. Take my word for it, the best thing you can do is keep asking questions until you understand."

Thomas Mobley, CPC, CPC-H, CEDC, CIRCC, CPC-I

Healthcare Coding Consultants, LLC

Gilbert, Arizona

Eye, Ocular Adnexa, Auditory, and Operating Microscope

Chapter Topics

Eye and Ocular Adnexa

Auditory System

Operating Microscope

Chapter Review

Quick Check Answers

Learning Objectives

After completing this chapter you should be able to

1   Review the Eye and Ocular Adnexa subsection.

2   Understand the Eye and Ocular Adnexa subheadings.

3   Demonstrate the ability to code Eye and Ocular Adnexa services.

4   Review the Auditory System subsection format.

5   Understand Auditory System subheadings.

6   Demonstrate the ability to code Auditory System services.

7   Review reporting use of an operating microscope.

8   Demonstrate the ability to report the use of an operating microscope.

Make sure to check **evolve** learning system **for the latest content updates**

EYE AND OCULAR ADNEXA

Format

The Eye and Ocular Adnexa subsection (65091-68899) includes the subheadings Eyeball, Anterior Segment, Posterior Segment, Ocular Adnexa, and Conjunctiva. There are the typical incision, excision, repair, and destruction categories, but also some that are unique. For example, the subheading Eyeball includes categories for both Removal of Eye (65091-65114) and Removal of Foreign Bodies (65205-65265), although you would expect to find all removal codes in a removal category.

From the Trenches

"The keys to long-term success are flexibility and a lust for knowledge. This field is ever evolving and growing, for to remain relevant you must embrace that change."

TOM

CODING SHOT

Remember to use modifier -50 (bilateral procedure) when the procedure is performed on both eyes. Modifiers -RT and -LT may be assigned for bilateral procedures of anatomic sites that are in pairs; i.e., eyes, breasts, legs, arms, etc.

In this section are codes that include previous surgery to the eye. For example, in the subheading Ocular Adnexa, 67331 is reported for patients who have undergone previous eye surgery or injury. Also, the category Prophylaxis (preventive treatment) (67141, 67145), under the subheading Posterior Segment, has notes regarding the assignment of these codes. The Prophylaxis codes include all the sessions in a treatment period. The Destruction codes in this subcategory include "one or more sessions." Read the code descriptions carefully so you know which elements are included in the code because what is or is not included in the code descriptions varies greatly.

As in all sections of the CPT manual, there are directional notes throughout that will help you think about what defines a particular code. For example, code 67850 is for the "Destruction of lesion of lid margin (up to 1 cm)." This description includes a note in parentheses: "(For Mohs' micrographic surgery, see 17311-17315)." This helpful note gives you the category of codes to refer to if the lesion destruction was performed using Mohs' micrographic surgery.

Refer to Figs. 22–1 through 22–4 as you prepare to code services to the eye and ocular adnexa.

Eyeball

Removal of Eye. The Removal of Eye category contains codes to report **evisceration**, which is removal of the contents of the globe while leaving the extraocular muscles and sclera intact (65091, 65093); **enucleation**, which is removal of the eye while leaving the orbital structures intact, (65101-65105); and **exenteration**, which is removal of the eye, adnexa, and part of the bony orbit (65110-65114). The codes in the Removal of Eye category are divided based on which of these procedures was performed, if an implant was inserted, and in the case of the exenteration, if the bony orbit was removed or a muscle or myocutaneous flap was performed.

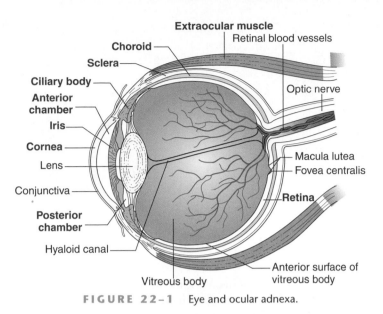

FIGURE 22–1 Eye and ocular adnexa.

FIGURE 22–2 Lacrimal apparatus.

FIGURE 22–3 Eyelid.

Tarsus superior

Tarsus inferior

Lacrimal sac

FIGURE 22–4 Two tarsi.

These codes do not report skin grafting to the orbit. When the operative report indicates skin grafting, report the service separately with codes from the Integumentary System (15120/15121 or 15260/15261). If the eyelid was repaired deeper than skin level, refer to the reconstruction codes 67930/67935 (partial or full thickness repair).

QUICK CHECK 22-1

Match the term with the correct description:

1. Evisceration _____

2. Enucleation _____

3. Exenteration _____

a. Removal of the eye, adnexa, bony structure
b. Removal of the contents of eyeball, structure intact
c. Removal of eyeball only, other structures intact

Secondary Implant(s) Procedures. Implants may be placed inside the muscular cone (ocular implant or fake eye) or outside the muscular cone (orbital implant) as illustrated in Fig. 22–5. The ocular implant is the artificial eye, and the orbital implant replaces the orbit that was occupied by the eyeball before removal. With some implants, the muscles are attached to the implant to enable the artificial eye to move and thus appear more natural. The codes in the 65125-65155 range report a subsequent implantation of ocular implants based on the type of service provided with the implant, such as grafting or attachment of muscles to implant. Removal of an ocular implant is reported with 65175. An orbital implant is a cosmetic device that covers the outer portion of the eye and is also known as a scleral shell prosthesis. Orbital implant insertion is reported with 67550 and removal with 67560.

Removal of Foreign Body. Note the extensive list of parenthetical notes preceding 65205. Take time now to read these notes as they list important concepts that you need to know. The removal codes are for foreign bodies that are located in the external eye or the intraocular eye. A

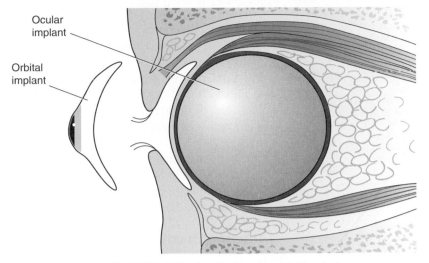

Ocular implant

Orbital implant

FIGURE 22–5 Ocular and orbital implants.

slit lamp is a low-powered microscope with a high-intensity light source that focuses the light as a long narrow beam (slit) and is used to examine eyes (Fig. 22–6). Note that the only difference between 65220 and 65222 is whether a slit lamp is or is not utilized.

Repair of Laceration. The repair codes are assigned to report laceration repair based on where the laceration is located (conjunctiva, cornea, and/or sclera). Code 65286 reports the application of tissue glue for a perforation of the eyeball.

Anterior Segment   The anterior segment includes the cornea, anterior chamber, anterior sclera, iris, ciliary body, and lens.

Slit lamp

Path of light rays

Ophthalmologist

Head rest

Microscope

Chin rest

Mirror

Control lever

FIGURE 22–6   A slit lamp is a microscope with a light attached. The name is derived from the adjustable light beam.

Cornea. The cornea is the transparent part of the eye. The cornea may be the site of a superficial lesion that is completely removed and reported with 65400. If only a portion of the corneal lesion was removed for pathology analysis, report the service as a biopsy with 65410.

A **keratoplasty** is repair of the cornea. Codes 65710-65756 report keratoplasty based on the type of procedure performed and include grafts and preparation of donor material. A penetrating keratoplasty (65730-65755) is the removal of the full thickness of the cornea and replacement with donor cornea. A lamellar keratoplasty (65710) is a procedure in which only a thin layer of the cornea is removed and replaced with donor cornea. **Aphakia** is absence of the lens of the eye, and **pseudophakia** is the presence of an artificial lens after cataract surgery. These terms are in many of the keratoplasty code descriptions.

Anterior Chamber. The anterior chamber of the eye is a fluid-filled (aqueous humor) space, located behind the cornea and in front of the iris. The categories of Incision (65800-65880), Removal (65900-65930), and Introduction (66020-66030) are for procedures performed on the anterior chamber of the eye.

Paracentesis is the removal of fluid. When a physician performs paracentesis of the anterior chamber of the eye, a needle is inserted into the anterior chamber and fluid is withdrawn. The fluid may be withdrawn for diagnostic purposes (65800) or for therapeutic purposes (65805-65815). If an injection procedure is also performed, report 66020 or 66030.

Goniotomy (65820) is a surgical procedure that utilizes an instrument called a goniolens. This procedure may be performed for congenital glaucoma, a condition in which the optic nerve at the back of the eye may be damaged and cause a loss of vision, especially peripheral vision. A note following code 65820 directs the coder not to use modifier -63 (procedure performed on infants less than 4 kg) with the code.

Codes for severing adhesions or scar tissue from the anterior chamber of the eye are based on the location of the adhesion or scar tissue (65860-65880). **Posterior synechiae** are adhesions of the iris to the lens of the eye, and **anterior synechiae** are adhesions of the iris to the cornea. Severing of the adhesions is performed using either laser or incisional technique.

QUICK CHECK 22-2

Match the term with the definition:

1. pseudophakia _____
2. goniotomy _____
3. keratoplasty _____
4. paracentesis _____

a. removal of fluid
b. presence of artificial lens
c. surgical procedure
d. repair of cornea

Anterior Sclera. The sclera is the white, fibrous outer layer of the eyeball and the anterior sclera is the front part of the eye. The anterior sclera may be the site of lesions that are excised (66130) by incision of the conjunctiva to gain access to the lesion. Depending on the size of the lesion, the area of the sclera may not require sutures.

Sometimes, the flow of the aqueous humor is not absorbed or too much fluid is produced and a surgeon may perform a fistulization (creation of a passage) of the sclera to increase the flow. The fistulization can be created by means of removal of a portion of the sclera and iris (e.g., 66150), thermocauterization (e.g., hot probe, 66155), or punch or scissor removal (e.g., 66160). A trabeculotomy ab externo or trabeculectomy ab externo (e.g., 65850, 66170, 66172) is a surgical procedure in which the trabecular meshwork (iris-scleral junction, drains aqueous humor) is reshaped or punctured. This procedure may be performed as a treatment for glaucoma or trauma.

Iris, Ciliary Body.   The ciliary body is located behind the iris (colored part of the eye) and produces aqueous humor. The smooth muscle of the ciliary body attaches to the lens. An iridectomy is usually performed for removal of a lesion (66600) or as a treatment for glaucoma (66625, 66630) by creation of an opening to drain aqueous humor. If the iridotomy is performed by means of laser, report the procedure with 66761 and if it is performed by means of photocoagulation, report the procedure with 66762.

Lens.   A common procedure performed on the lens of the eye is cataract removal. Cataract removal and lens replacements (66830-66990) utilize one of three different approaches:

- Extracapsular cataract extraction (66984) (ECCE) is partial removal and is the most common method. It removes the hard nucleus in one piece and the soft cortex in multiple pieces. The posterior lens capsule is left in place.
- Intracapsular cataract extraction (66983) (ICCE) is total removal that removes the cataract in one piece.
- Phacoemulsification dissolves the hard nucleus by ultrasound then removes the soft cortex in multiple pieces.

Extraocular Muscles.   Under the subheading of Ocular Adnexa are codes for strabismus surgery, which corrects muscle misalignment. The codes are divided based on repair of vertical (67314, 67316) or horizontal (67311, 67312) muscle and are reported by the number of muscles repaired. Vertical muscles move the eye up and down, while the horizontal muscles move the eye side to side.

Orbit.   Under the subheading Orbit are codes for orbitotomy and fine needle aspiration. The orbitotomy codes are divided based on the approach and if a bone flap was or was not placed. Orbitotomy that is performed without a bone flap and with either a frontal or transconjunctival approach (illustrated in Fig. 22–7) are reported with codes 67400-67414. Orbitotomy performed with a bone flap and with a lateral approach are reported with

FIGURE 22–7   Transconjunctival approach. (From Rothrock JC: *Alexander's Care of the Patient in Surgery,* ed 13, St. Louis, 2007, Mosby.)

codes 67420-67450. The codes for a transcranial orbitotomy are located in the Nervous System subsection (61330-61334). Within the Orbit subheading there is also a code (67415) for fine needle aspiration of the orbital contents and it is usually performed as a biopsy method for an orbital mass.

Eyelids. The Eyelid subheading includes procedures performed by incision, excision, destruction, and tarsorrhaphy (suturing the eyelid partial together). There are also codes to report eyelid repair and reconstruction. Eyelid repairs include ectropion (outward sagging/turning, 67914-67917) as illustrated in Fig. 22–8 and entropion (inward turning, 67921-67924) illustrated in Fig. 22–9.

HCPCS modifiers are added to the procedure code to indicate the specific eyelid:

- E1   upper left eyelid
- E2   lower left eyelid
- E3   upper right eyelid
- E4   lower right eyelid

Conjunctiva. The Conjunctiva subheading includes Incision and Drainage (68020, 68040), Excision/Destruction (68100-68135), Injection

FIGURE 22–8 Ectropion is an outward sagging of the eyelid. (**A** from Frazier MS, Drzymkowski JW: *Essentials of Human Diseases and Conditions,* ed 4, St. Louis, 2009, Saunders. **B** from Ignatavicius DD, Workman ML: *Medical-Surgical Nursing: Critical Thinking for Collaborative Care,* ed 5, St. Louis, 2006, Saunders.)

FIGURE 22–9 Entropion is an inward turning of the eyelid. (Note that the patient in **B** has undergone corneal transplantation.) (**A** from Frazier MS, Drzymkowski JW: *Essentials of Human Diseases and Conditions,* ed 4, St. Louis, 2009, Saunders. **B** from Seidel HM, Ball JW, Dains JE, Benedict GW: *Mosby's Guide to Physical Examination,* ed 6, St. Louis, 2006, Mosby Elsevier.)

(68200), Conjunctivoplasty (68320-68340), and the Lacrimal System (68400-68850). Conjunctivoplasty (68326-68328) involves reconstruction of the cul-de-sac with a conjunctival graft or rearrangement. Lacrimal system (see Fig. 22–2) procedures include incision, excision, repair, and probing. The most common procedure performed is nasolacrimal duct probing generally due to an obstruction and reported with 68810 or 68811.

EXERCISE 22-1 *Eye and Ocular Adnexa*

Using the CPT manual, code the following:

1 Emboli removal from anterior segment of the left eye

　　Code: _____

2 New patient strabismus surgery involving the superior oblique muscle of the right eye

　　Code: _____

3 Xenon arc used in three sessions to prevent retinal detachment of left eye

　　Code: _____

4 Corneal incision for revision of earlier procedure that resulted in astigmatism of right eye

　　Code: _____

5 Removal of left eye, with implant, muscles attached to implant

　　Code: _____

AUDITORY SYSTEM

Format

The Auditory System subsection (69000-69979) is divided into the subheadings External Ear, Middle Ear, Inner Ear, and Temporal Bone/Middle Fossa Approach. The first three subheadings represent the anatomic divisions of the auditory system: external, middle, and inner ear (Fig. 22–10). The categories listed under each subheading include introduction, incision, excision, removal, repair, and other procedures, depending on the particular subheading. The subheading Temporal Bone/Middle Fossa Approach (69950-69970) contains codes that describe various surgical procedures in which the surgeon makes an incision in front of the ear. Through this incision, the surgeon performs a craniotomy and exposes the brain. The surgeon then repairs the nerve, removes a tumor, or otherwise treats the area.

OPERATING MICROSCOPE

The code for reporting the use of an operating microscope, 69990, is in a subsection of a single code following the Auditory System subsection. This code is an add-on code and is never reported alone; rather, it is reported with the procedure in which the operating microscope was used. Code 69990 is assigned with codes from any subsection within the Surgery section. Read the extensive notes preceding the code to better understand when this code should or should not be reported.

EXERCISE 22-2 · *Auditory System*

Using the CPT manual, code the following:

1 Left labyrinthotomy with cryosurgery with multiple perfusions, transcanal

　　Code: _____

2 Bilateral insertion of pressure equalization tubes, using general anesthesia

　　Codes: _____, _____

3 Transcranial approach with sectioning of the left vestibular nerve

　　Code: _____

4 Reconstruction of the right auditory canal, due to injury

　　Code: _____

5 Establishment of an opening in the inner wall of the right inner ear, semicircular canal

　　Code: _____

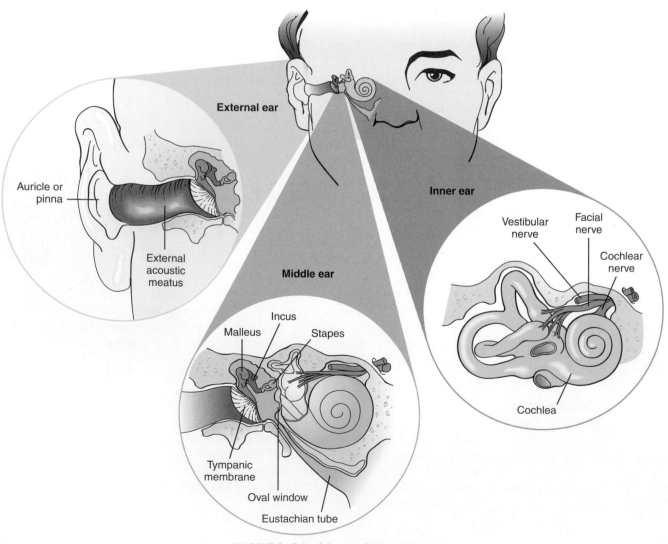

FIGURE 22–10　Auditory system.

External Ear

Incision. The external ear may be the site of an abscess or hematoma and the incision and drainage may be simple (69000) or complicated (69005). If the abscess drained is within the auditory canal, report the service with 69020. Be careful when reporting 69020 as it can be bundled into a major procedure and not reported separately.

Excision. Codes for the external ear include biopsy by location of external ear (69100) or external auditory canal (69105), excision of the external ear, either partially or complete (69110, 69120). If the external ear was reconstructed after the excision, report the repair with split thickness autograft codes (15120, 15121) from the Integumentary System based on the square centimeters used in the repair.

Exostosis is a bony growth and when present in the external auditory canal it is termed "surfer's ear," because it is associated with chronic cold water exposure. An incision is made behind the ear to gain access to the canal, and the bony growth is excised (69140).

Removal of Foreign Body. With the shape of the ear, it is easy to see how foreign bodies and cerumen (earwax) can become lodged in the external ear. When a foreign body is removed from the ear, the code reported is based on whether general anesthesia was or was not used (69200, 69205). Removal of impacted cerumen (69210) is reported whether the procedure was unilateral or bilateral.

Repair. An **otoplasty** is a procedure performed for a protruding ear that may or may not include a decrease in the size of the ear. This procedure is usually performed with the use of conscious sedation, which is included in 69300. When an otoplasty is performed bilaterally, modifier -50 is added to code.

Reconstruction of the external auditory canal (canalplasty/canaloplasty) may be performed for conditions such as stenosis due to injury or infection (69310) or for a congenital defect (69320). Canaloplasty is bundled into some middle ear repair codes, such as 69631-69646 and not reported separately.

Middle Ear

Myringotomy and Tympanostomy. The eustachian tube connects the middle ear to the back of the throat and allows for drainage of fluid. When a eustachian tube dysfunctions, fluid collects in the middle ear. The tube can also become inflamed from allergies or infection. Eustachian tube dysfunction is a fairly common condition in children, because the tube does not always mature to the level of normal function and therefore does not function properly. The fluid or inflammation prevents air from entering the middle ear, resulting in a pressure increase in the middle ear. Surgical intervention is an inflation of the eustachian tube with access through the nose (transnasal, 69400, 69401). **Myringotomy** is the incision into the tympanic membrane (69420, 69421) and reinflation of the eustachian tube. **Tympanostomy** is the insertion of a small plastic or metal tube (PE [pressure equalization] tube) that allows the fluid to drain (69433, 69436). The tubes may later be removed, fall out naturally, or sometimes be left in place. Surgical removal of a ventilation tube is reported with 69424, which is a procedure that requires general anesthesia. Ventilation tube removal is bundled into many major procedures, in which case the removal is not reported separately.

CODING SHOT Code 67424 is unilateral, so if the tubes were removed bilaterally, add modifier -50.

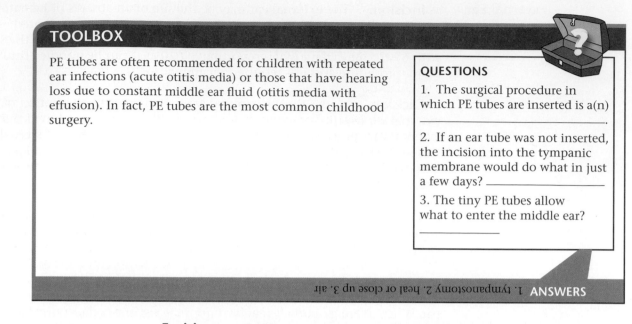

TOOLBOX

PE tubes are often recommended for children with repeated ear infections (acute otitis media) or those that have hearing loss due to constant middle ear fluid (otitis media with effusion). In fact, PE tubes are the most common childhood surgery.

QUESTIONS

1. The surgical procedure in which PE tubes are inserted is a(n) _____.

2. If an ear tube was not inserted, the incision into the tympanic membrane would do what in just a few days? _____

3. The tiny PE tubes allow what to enter the middle ear? _____

ANSWERS 1. tympanostomy 2. heal or close up 3. air

Excision.   Middle ear excision procedures include antrotomy (simple mastoidectomy, 69501), mastoidectomy (complete, modified radical, or radical, 69502-69511), polyp removal (69540), and tumor removal (69550-69554).

Also included in the Excision category is a petrous apicectomy. The petrous apex (Fig. 22–11) of the temporal bone may be the site of infection (petrous apicitis) that can lead to more complicated infection, such as brain abscess or meningitis. Sometimes, to remove the infected bone, a mastoidectomy is performed and is included in the petrous apicectomy code 69530.

Repair.   Middle ear repair procedures include revision mastoidectomies based on the extent of the procedure. For example, a simple mastoidectomy is performed on a patient with cholesteatoma of the middle ear. A **cholesteatoma** is a benign growth of skin in an abnormal location, in this case in the middle ear. The growth may reoccur and the surgeon may perform a complete mastoidectomy (69601). If the disease has progressed to the point where the tympanic membrane is damaged and requires repair, the procedure is reported with 69604.

The two major divisions in the tympanoplasty codes are with or without removal of the mastoid bone (mastoidectomy). When no mastoidectomy

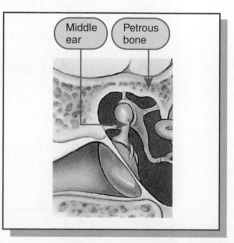

FIGURE 22–11   The bony structure is the petrous bone. (Modified from Christensen BL, Kockrow ED: *Adult Health Nursing,* ed 5, St. Louis, 2006, Mosby.)

is performed, choose the code from the 69631-69633 range, based on the extent of the procedure. When a mastoidectomy is performed, report the service with codes from the 69641-69646 range, based on the extent of the procedure. The **ossicular chain** is the bones of the ear that include the malleus (hammer), incus (anvil), and stapes (stirrup). The chain may be eroded and repaired as a part of a tympanoplasty (69632 or 69642). The repair may be so extensive that it may require the use of prosthesis, such as a partial ossicular replacement prosthesis (PORP, incus and malleus are absent or damaged) or total ossicular replacement prosthesis (TORP, incus and arch of the stapes are damaged, or the malleus, incus and arch of the stapes are absent). PORP and TORP are reported with 69633 or 69637 depending upon other repairs performed during the tympanoplasty.

Inner Ear

Incision and/or Destruction.   A **labyrinth** is a cavelike structure, located in the inner ear. The labyrinth is dominated by two fluid-filled spaces that contain endolymph and perilymph. These spaces contain the nerve tissue responsible for hearing and balance. When the pressure within the space is altered, vertigo, ringing in the ears, and hearing loss may occur. A **labyrinthotomy** is a procedure in which the labyrinth is surgically incised, and various procedures performed to return the labyrinth to functional condition. Codes 69801 and 69802 are reported for a labyrinthotomy based on whether a mastoidectomy was performed.

Excision.   A **labyrinthectomy** is a procedure in which the incus and stapes are removed. If a transcanal approach is used, report 69905. If a postauricular incision (behind the ear) is used as the approach, report 69910.

Introduction.   A **cochlear device implant** (Fig. 22–12) is a computerized device that restores partial hearing in those who are profoundly hearing impaired. A receiver on the outside of the skin behind the ear picks up sound waves. The receiver is placed over the transmitter, which is surgically implanted under the skin behind the ear. A sound

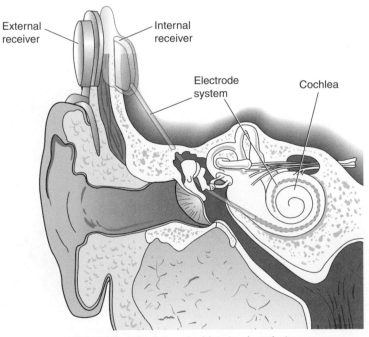

FIGURE 22-12   Cochlear implant device.

processor is connected to an electrode implanted between the processor and the cochlea and it receives a signal from the transmitter and transfers the signal to the cochlear nerve. The implantation of the cochlear device is reported with 69930.

Temporal Bone, Middle Fossa Approach.   The middle fossa approach is used by surgeons to excise acoustic neuromas, to decompress the facial nerve (proximal temporal), and repair nerves in the vestibular labyrinth. The codes in the Temporal Bone, Middle Fossa Approach subheading report removal of the vestibular nerve (69950), relief of pressure (decompression) of the facial nerve and/or repair (69955), decompression of the internal auditory canal (69960), and removal of tumors of the temporal bone (69970).

Operating Microscope.   An operating microscope (Fig. 22–13) is used in microsurgical procedures and is reported separately with add-on code 69990, unless the code indicates the inclusion of use of an operating microscope. This does not include magnifying loupes (Fig. 22–14) that are used to enlarge the area being viewed.

FIGURE 22–13   The operating microscope allows for visualization of minute structures, such as nerve fibers and blood vessels. (From Microsurgery Instruments Inc.: The Economic Operating Microscope (website): www.microsurgeryusa.com/EOM. htm. Accessed June 1, 2006.)

FIGURE 22–14   Magnifying loupes are produced in a range of powers. (From Mopec: Magnifying Loupe (website): www.mopec.com/product/523/binocular_magnifying_loupe/. Accessed July 7, 2009.)

QUICK CHECK 22-3

1. Use of the operating microscope is used only with procedures on the ear.
   True or False?

EXERCISE 22-3 *Ear and Operating Microscope*

Complete the following:

1 This is a bony growth that is also known as surfer's ear. _____

2 For a protruding ear, the surgeon may perform this procedure. _____

3 This is a benign growth of the skin in an abnormal location, such as the middle ear. _____

4 The code to report the use of an operating microscope in addition to the procedure is _____.

CHAPTER REVIEW

CHAPTER 22, PART I, THEORY

Complete the following:

Match the terms for the ossicular chain:

1 hammer _____   a. incus

2 anvil _____   b. stapes

3 stirrup _____   c. malleus

4 This is a benign growth of skin in an abnormal location.

   a. cholesteatoma
   b. glucogonomas
   c. TSH-oma
   d. schwannoma

5 This is the removal of the eye, adnexa, and part of the bony orbit.

   a. evisceration
   b. enucleation
   c. exenteration
   d. none of the above

6 This is a low-powered microscope with a high-intensity light source that focuses the light as a long narrow beam and is used to examine the eyes.

   a. goniolens
   b. otoscope
   c. ophthalmoscope
   d. slit lamp

7 This is a cosmetic implant that covers the outer portion of the eye and is also known as a scleral shell prosthesis.

   a. ocular
   b. orbital
   c. conjunctival
   d. intraocular

8 This is a bony growth that is also known as surfer's ear because it is associated with chronic cold water exposure.

   a. vestibular
   b. mastoiditis
   c. exostosis
   d. labyrinthitis

9 During this procedure, small plastic or metal tubes are inserted through the tympanic membrane to allow for the drainage of fluid. Later the tubes may be removed, fall out naturally, or are left in place.

   a. myringotomy
   b. antrotomy
   c. tympanostomy
   d. mastoidectomy

10 This is a cavelike structure that is dominated by two fluid-filled spaces.

   a. labyrinth
   b. auricle
   c. external acoustic meatus
   d. malleus

CHAPTER 22, PART II, PRACTICAL

Code the following cases:

11 Excision of corneal lesion of right eye

Code: _____

12 Iridectomy with corneal section for removal of lesion from left eye

Code: _____

13 Left lamellar keratoplasty with replacement of a thin layer of the cornea with donor cornea

Code(s): _____

14 Corneal biopsy of the right eye

Code(s): _____

15 Diagnostic paracentesis of aqueous the anterior chamber of the left eye

Code: _____

16 A one stage, right eye ECCE with insertion of intraocular lens prosthesis using a manual technique

Code: _____

17 A one stage ICCE of the left eye with insertion of intraocular lens prosthesis

Code: _____

18 Iridotomy for removal of a primary lesion by means of corneal section, right

Code: _____

19 A male patient, age 69, with type II diabetes and progressive diabetic retinopathy resulting in retinal hemorrhage. The physician provides three sessions of photocoagulation to his right eye over the course of 2 weeks

CPT Code: _____

ICD-9-CM Codes: _____,

_____

20 Repair of a detached right retina by means of an encircling procedure and including scleral dissection, implant, cryotherapy, and drainage of subretinal fluid

CPT Code: _____

ICD-9-CM Code: _____

QUICK CHECK ANSWERS

QUICK CHECK 22-1
1. b
2. c
3. a

QUICK CHECK 22-2
1. b
2. c
3. d
4. a

QUICK CHECK 22-3
1. False

"Try not to stay in just one specialty. Become educated and learn other specialties so you can grow in all types of coding."

Patricia Champion, CPC

Licensed PMCC Instructor, Educator/Trainer

AAPC National Advisory Board

Nashville, Tennessee

Radiology

Chapter Topics

Format

Radiology Terminology

Terms

Planes

Guidelines

Diagnostic Radiology

Breast, Mammography

Diagnostic Ultrasound

Radiation Oncology

Nuclear Medicine

Chapter Review

Quick Check Answers

Learning Objectives

After completing this chapter you should be able to

1 Demonstrate an understanding of Radiology terminology.

2 Analyze the elements of component coding in reporting radiology services.

3 Identify elements of the global procedure.

4 State the appropriate coding of contrast material.

5 Explain the format of the Radiology section.

6 Demonstrate the ability to code Radiology services and procedures.

Make sure to check
evolve
learning system
for the latest
content updates

FORMAT   **Radiology** is the branch of medicine that uses radiant energy to diagnose and treat patients. The term originally referred to the use of x-rays to produce radiographs but is now commonly applied to all types of medical imaging. A physician who specializes in radiology is a **radiologist.** Radiologists can provide services to patients independent of or in conjunction with another physician of a different specialty. The Radiology section of the CPT manual is divided into subsections:

- Diagnostic Radiology (Diagnostic Imaging)
- Diagnostic Ultrasound
- Radiologic Guidance
- Breast, Mammography
- Bone/Joint Studies
- Radiation Oncology
- Nuclear Medicine

RADIOLOGY TERMINOLOGY   The suffix -*graphy* means "making of a film" using a variety of methods. **Radiography** is a broad term used to indicate any number of methods used by radiologists to do diagnostic testing. The following exercise will familiarize you with some of the numerous radiographic procedures in the CPT manual.

EXERCISE 23-1   *Radiology Terminology*

The following words end in "-graphy," meaning "making of a film." For example, in angiocardiography, "angio" means vessels and "cardio" means heart, so angiocardiography is the making of a film of the heart and vessels. What do the other "-graphy" words mean?

angiocardiography _____ heart and vessels _____

1 aortography _____
2 arthrography _____
3 cholangiopancreatography _____
4 cholangiography _____
5 cystography _____
6 dacryocystography _____
7 duodenography _____
8 echocardiography _____
9 encephalography _____
10 epididymography _____
11 hepatography _____
12 hysterosalpingography _____
13 laryngography _____
14 lymphangiography _____
15 myelography _____
16 pyelography _____

Continued

17 sialography _____

18 sinography _____

19 splenography _____

20 urography _____

21 venography _____

22 vesiculography _____

TERMS

Here are just a few more radiographic terms for your review:

1. **Fluoroscopy** is an x-ray procedure that allows the visualization of internal organs in motion. It uses real-time video images. After x-rays pass through the patient, instead of using film, the images are captured by a device called an image intensifier and converted into light. The light is then captured by a camera and displayed on a video monitor. Fluoroscopy allows the study of the function of the organ (physiology) as well as the structure of the organ (anatomy).

2. **Magnetic resonance imaging (MRI)** is a radiology technique that uses magnetism, radio waves, and a computer to produce images of body structures. The MRI scanner is a tube surrounded by a giant circular magnet. The patient is placed on a moveable bed that is inserted into the magnet. The magnet creates a strong magnetic field that aligns the protons of hydrogen atoms, which are then exposed to a beam of radio waves. This spins the various protons of the body and produces a faint signal that is detected by the receiver portion of the MRI scanner. The received information is processed by a computer, and an image is then produced.

3. **Tomography** is the process of producing a tomogram, a two-dimensional image of a slice or section, through a three-dimensional object. Tomography achieves this result by simply moving an x-ray source in one direction as the x-ray film is moved in the opposite direction. The tomogram is the picture, tomograph is the apparatus, and tomography is the process.

4. **Biometry** is the application of a statistical method to a biologic fact. For example, the application of this science in radiology has resulted in analysis of data, for example, of the effectiveness of radiation used in the treatment of brain tumors—science applied to biology.

PLANES

Terminology referring to planes of the body and the positioning of the body is often used in the Radiology section. A **position** is how the patient is placed during the x-ray examination (such as lying down or standing up), and a **projection** is the path of the x-ray beam. An example of a projection is anteroposterior, which denotes that the x-ray beam enters the patient's body at the front (anterior) and exits from the back (posterior). An example of a position is **prone,** which means the patient is lying on his or her anterior (front), but the entrance and exit of the x-ray beam are not specified. Familiarity with this terminology will aid you as you review the Radiology section and begin to choose the correct codes for physician services. Fig. 23–1 illustrates the major planes and the surfaces of the body that can be accessed by positioning the body.

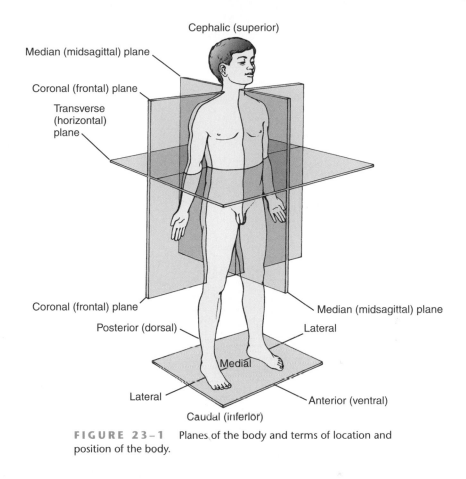

Cephalic (superior)

Median (midsagittal) plane

Coronal (frontal) plane

Transverse (horizontal) plane

Coronal (frontal) plane

Median (midsagittal) plane

Posterior (dorsal)

Lateral

Medial

Lateral

Anterior (ventral)

Caudal (inferior)

FIGURE 23–1 Planes of the body and terms of location and position of the body.

From the Trenches

"We have a very strong camaraderie. Through networking, when coders have problems with their notes or some questions they may have in coding, they can always call someone they have networked with to get an answer."

PATRICIA

Fig. 23–2 shows proximal and distal body references. **Proximal** and **distal** are directional body references that mean closest to (proximal) or farthest from (distal) the trunk of the body. These terms are relative, meaning they are used to describe the position of the part as compared with another part. Therefore, the term "proximal" describes a part as being closer to the body trunk than another part, and the term "distal" describes a part as being farther away from the body than another part. The knee would be described as being proximal to the ankle, and it would also be described as being distal to the thigh or hip. Fig. 23–3 illustrates the **anteroposterior (AP)** (front to back) position, in which the patient has his or her front (anterior) closest to the x-ray machine, and the x-ray travels through the patient from the front to the back. In Fig. 23–4, the **posteroanterior (PA)** position, the patient has his or her back (posterior) located closest to the machine, and the beam travels through the patient from back to front.

Lateral positions are side positions. When the patient's right side is closest to the film, it is called *right lateral*. When the patient's left side is

FIGURE 23-2 Proximal and distal.

FIGURE 23-3 Anteroposterior (AP) projection.

FIGURE 23-4 Posteroanterior (PA) projection.

closest to the film, it is called *left lateral.* For example, Fig. 23–5 shows a left lateral position, and Fig. 23–6 shows a right lateral position. The use of these various positions allows the physician to view the body from a variety of angles. Fig. 23–7 shows posteroanterior and lateral positions used to view a patient's lung with emphysema.

Dorsal (more commonly refers to the "back" but may be stated to mean "supine") means lying on the back; **ventral** (more commonly refers to the "anterior" but may be stated as "prone") means lying on the stomach; and **lateral** means lying on the side.

Decubitus positions are recumbent (lying) positions; the x-ray beam is placed horizontally. Ventral decubitus (prone) is the act of lying on the stomach (Fig. 23–8, *A*), and dorsal decubitus (supine) is the act of lying on the back (Fig. 23–8, *B*). The term "decubitus," generally shortened to "decub," has a special meaning in radiology. The simple act of lying on one's

FIGURE 23-5   Left lateral projection.

FIGURE 23-6   Right lateral projection.

FIGURE 23-7   Posteroanterior and lateral radiographs of the thorax in a patient with emphysema. (From Goldman L, Ausiello D, eds: *Cecil Medicine*, ed 23, Philadelphia, 2008, Saunders.)

back would be referred to as lying supine, but if a horizontal x-ray beam is used, the position becomes decubitus. The type of decubitus is determined by the body surface the patient is lying on.

Recumbent means lying down. Thus, right lateral recumbent means the patient is lying on the right side (Fig. 23–8, *C*), and left lateral recumbent means the patient is lying on the left side (Fig. 23–8, *D*). In the ventral decubitus position, the patient is positioned prone and the x-ray beam comes into the patient from the right side and exits on the left (Fig. 23–8, *E*).

In the left lateral decubitus position, the patient is lying on the left side with the beam coming from the front and passing through to the back (anteroposterior) (Fig. 23–8, *F*).

When the patient is positioned on his or her back (dorsal decubitus) and the x-ray beam comes into the left side of the patient, the positioning is dorsal decubitus, but the view obtained is a right lateral (because the right side is closest to the film) (Fig. 23–8, *G*).

Oblique views refer to those obtained while the body is rotated so it is not in a full anteroposterior or posteroanterior position but somewhat diagonal. Oblique views are termed according to the body surface on which the patient is lying. The left anterior oblique *(LAO)* position is depicted in

FIGURE 23-8 Radiographic positions. **A,** Prone (ventral decubitus). **B,** Supine (dorsal decubitus). **C,** Right lateral recumbent. **D,** Left lateral recumbent. **E,** Ventral decubitus. **F,** Left lateral decubitus. **G,** Dorsal decubitus. **H,** Left anterior oblique (LAO). **I,** Right anterior oblique (RAO). **J,** Left posterior oblique (LPO). **K,** Right posterior oblique (RPO).

Fig. 23–8, *H* with the patient's left side rotated forward toward the table. The patient is lying on the left anterior aspect of his or her body. The right anterior oblique (RAO) position has the patient on his or her right side rotated forward toward the table, as in Fig. 23–8, *I*.

Two more oblique views are left posterior oblique and right posterior oblique. In the left posterior oblique (LPO) view, the patient is rotated so that the left posterior aspect of his or her body is against the table, as in Fig. 23–8, *J*. The right posterior oblique (RPO) view has the patient with the right side rotated back, as in Fig. 23–8, *K*.

The last two terms that describe projections are tangential and axial. **Tangential** is the position that allows the beam to skim the body part, which produces a profile of the structure of the body (Fig. 23–9, *A*). Fig. 23–9, *B* illustrates the **axial** projection, which is any projection that allows the beam to pass through the body part lengthwise.

EXERCISE 23-2 *Planes*

Fill in the blanks with the correct words:

1 What is the word that indicates how the patient is placed during the x-ray examination?

   _____

2 What is the term that indicates the path the x-ray beam travels?

   _____

What do the following abbreviations mean?

3 AP _____

4 PA _____

5 RAO _____

6 LPO _____

7 What term indicates that a patient is lying supine, or on his or her back? _____

8 What term indicates that a patient is lying prone, or on his or her stomach? _____

9 What term indicates that a patient is lying on his or her right side? _____

10 What is the term that indicates when a patient is on his or her back and the x-ray beam comes into the right side of the patient? _____

A Tangential projection   B Axial projection

FIGURE 23–9 Radiographic projections. **A,** Tangential projection. **B,** Axial projection.

GUIDELINES

As with all Guidelines, the Radiology Guidelines should be read carefully before radiologic procedures or services are reported. The Guidelines contain the unique instructions used within the section and the indications for multiple procedures, separate procedures, unlisted radiology procedure codes, and applicable modifiers.

Guidelines that are used more commonly in this section than in others are those explaining the professional, technical, and global components of a procedure. These components are as follows:

1. **Professional:** describes the services of the physician, including the supervision of the taking of the x-ray film and the interpretation with report of the x-ray films.

2. **Technical:** describes the services of the technologist, as well as the use of the equipment, film, and other supplies.

3. **Global:** describes the combination of the professional and technical components (1 and 2).

For example, if a patient undergoes a radiology procedure in a clinic that owns its own equipment, employs its own technologist(s), and also employs the radiologist who supervises, interprets, and reports on the radiologic results, the global procedure is reported. But if the radiologist is reading and interpreting films that were taken at another facility, only the professional component would be reported for physician services.

CODING SHOT

Third-party payment is generally 40% for the professional component, 60% for the technical component, and 100% for the global service.

When only the professional component of the service is provided, modifier -26 is placed after the CPT code. Modifier -26 alerts the third-party payer to the fact that only the professional component was provided. If, for example, an independent radiology facility takes a complete chest x-ray (71030) and sends the x-rays to an independent radiologist who reads the x-rays and writes a report of the findings in the x-rays, the coding for the independent radiologist would be the professional component only:

71030-26   Complete chest x-ray, four views

There is no CPT modifier to indicate the technical component of radiologic services. The modifier most commonly used is the HCPCS Level II modifier -TC, which reports the technical component. When submitting claims for radiologic services in which only the technical component was provided, use a code followed by -TC. For example, if you were the coder for the independent radiology facility that took the chest x-ray (71030) but sent it elsewhere to be interpreted, you would report the technical component only:

71030-TC   Complete chest x-ray, four views

CODING SHOT

TC (Technical Component) and -26 (Professional Component) are terms used by third-party payers. When contacting a payer regarding payment of a service, first determine if there is a separate allowance for the -TC and -26.

Supervision and Interpretation

The other coding practice most commonly used in the Radiology section is called **component** or **combination coding,** which means that a code from the Radiology section as well as a code from one of the other sections must be reported to fully describe the procedure. For example, interventional radiologists may inject contrast material; place stents, catheters, or guidewires; or perform any number of procedures found throughout the CPT manual. Many times, before radiology procedures can be performed, a contrast material must be injected into the patient to make certain organs or vessels stand out more clearly on the radiographic image. When this contrast material is injected into the patient by the radiologist, a CPT code from the Surgery section must be used to indicate the injection procedure and a code is reported for the contrast substance, such as A4643.

CODING SHOT

Codes in the Radiology section describe only the radiology procedures, not the injections or placement of other material necessary to perform the procedure.

Suppose, for example, a voiding urethrocystography with contrast medium enhancement is performed. In this procedure, a physician injects a radioactive material into the bladder. An x-ray of the bladder (cystography) is then obtained; the x-rays show filling, voiding, and post-voiding. The injection portion of the procedure is reported with a surgery code (51600: Injection procedure for cystography or voiding urethrocystography); the cystography is reported with a radiology code (74455: Urethrocystography, voiding, radiologic supervision and interpretation).

As a new coder, you will need to pay special attention to the information in parentheses below the codes in the Radiology section. This parenthetic material gives you information about other components of procedures and other codes to consider. Previous editions of the CPT manual had combination codes that were used when the physician did both components of some procedures. Using the combination code replaced the use of one code from surgery and one code from radiology; but many of these combination codes have been deleted to allow the physicians to more specifically indicate the services provided. There are many parenthetic phrases throughout the Radiology section and you will want to refer to them when coding component procedures.

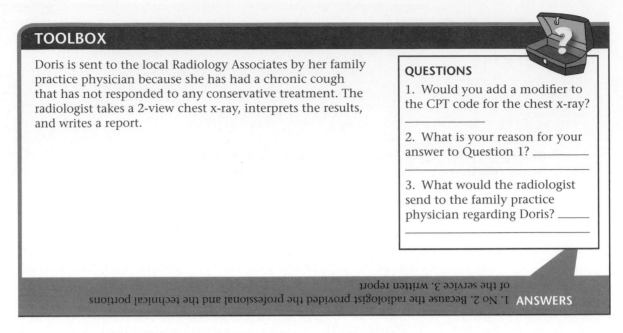

TOOLBOX

Doris is sent to the local Radiology Associates by her family practice physician because she has had a chronic cough that has not responded to any conservative treatment. The radiologist takes a 2-view chest x-ray, interprets the results, and writes a report.

QUESTIONS

1. Would you add a modifier to the CPT code for the chest x-ray? _____

2. What is your reason for your answer to Question 1? _____

3. What would the radiologist send to the family practice physician regarding Doris? _____

ANSWERS 1. No 2. Because the radiologist provided the professional and the technical portions of the service 3. written report

Odds and Ends

Many of the code descriptions state "radiologic supervision and interpretation" and alert you to component coding, letting you know that -26 or -TC may be appropriate. Always read the parenthetic information that follows these component codes.

Some codes are divided based on the extent of the radiologic examination, such as procedures that specify "with KUB" (kidney, ureter, and bladder). You must read the radiologist's report or the details in the medical record to understand the extent of the procedure.

NCCI

The Comprehensive Coding Initiative (CCI) bundles some x-rays into a main x-ray procedure. For example, code 74241 (radiologic examination, gastrointestinal tract, upper; with or without delayed films, with KUB). According to the CCI edits, all the following codes are bundled into 74241:

- 74000 – x-ray of the abdomen, single anteroposterior
- 74010 – x-ray of abdomen, anteroposterior and additional oblique and cone views
- 74210 – x-ray exam, pharynx and/or cervical esophagus
- 74220 – x-ray exam of the esophagus
- 74240 – x-ray exam, gastrointestinal tract, upper, with or without delayed films, without KUB
- 74245 – radiologic examination, gastrointestinal tract, upper; with small intestine, includes multiple serial films
- 74249 – radiologic examination, gastrointestinal tract, upper, air contrast, with specific high-density barium, effervescent agent, with or without glucagon; with small intestine follow through

Some of these codes may be reported if a modifier (ex, -59) is added to indicate the service was separate and distinct from the main service reported with 74241.

Codes are also often divided on the basis of whether contrast material was or was not used. The phrase "with contrast" in the CPT manual means contrast that was administered intravascularly, intra-articularly, or intrathecally (into the subarachnoid space). If the procedure indicates that contrast was administered orally or rectally, the service is reported as "without contrast."

CODING SHOT

Report the supply of contrast material with Medicine section code 99070, supplies, or a HCPCS code. The injection of the contrast material is included in the "with contrast" radiology procedure code, unless guidelines state that a surgical code should also be listed to report the injection procedure. Avoid reporting 99070 if there is a more definite HCPCS code available.

There are new guidelines issued by CMS that were originally titled Medically Unbelievable Edits (MUEs). CMS changed the name to Medically Unlikely Edits. This information is included in a software system that allows Medicare to reduce the number of claims that contain medically improbable information, such as a hysterectomy on a male patient. There are approximately 3000 edits in the software, and 60 of those directly relate to radiology service. One type of edit is the maximum number of units that can be reported. If the MUE indicated that the maximum number of units for a particular radiology service was two for a particular service and you submitted three units, the claim would be automatically edited (kicked out). Unlike some edits, you cannot override the MUEs by addending a modifier. Denied claims must be appealed with supporting documentation that indicates the service was medically necessary, was administered in a separate session, or was a repeat procedure by the same physician.

Radiographic procedures are located in the CPT manual index under the main term "X-ray," with subterms for the anatomic part (e.g., hand, spine).

EXERCISE 23-3 *Guidelines*

Fill in the blanks using the Radiology Guidelines of your CPT manual:

1 What procedure is one that is "performed independently of, and is not immediately related to, other services"? _____

2 What is the name of the Medicare edit software?

_____

3 Using your CPT manual, list at least four of the subsections of the Radiology section.

_____

_____

_____

_____

DIAGNOSTIC RADIOLOGY

The most standard radiographic procedures are contained in the Diagnostic Radiology subsection (70010-76499) of the Radiology section. This subsection describes diagnostic imaging, including plain x-ray films, the use of computed axial tomography (CAT or CT) scanning, magnetic resonance imaging (MRI), magnetic resonance angiography (MRA), and angiography. CT scanning uses an x-ray beam that rotates around the patient, as illustrated in Fig. 23–10. Fig. 23–11 shows the detail that can be obtained with MRI and CT scans. Special computer software is used with CT scanners to produce three-dimensional images that enable the study of internal structures. Tomography, CT scanning, and MRI may include the use of injectable dyes (radiographic contrast) to aid in imaging, and the codes are divided on the basis of whether or not contrast was used. For example, under the subheading Spine and Pelvis (72010-72295), the codes for CAT, MRI, and MRA are divided as follows:

72192 Computerized tomography, pelvis; without contrast material

72195 Magnetic resonance (e.g., proton) imaging, pelvis; without contrast material(s)

72198 Magnetic resonance angiography, pelvis, with or without contrast material(s)

Note one of these codes is for CAT, one code for the MRI, and one code for the MRA. The codes are divided by CAT, MRI, and MRA throughout the Diagnostic Radiology subsection. So you must read carefully to ensure that you report the correct type of imaging. Fig. 23–12 is an example of a magnetic resonance image of the brain.

FIGURE 23–10 **A,** Computed tomography scanner. **B,** Principles of computed tomographic (CT) scanning. The x-ray tube produces a fan-shaped beam that passes through a section (slice) of the patient. This fan-shaped beam is received by a circular array of detectors at the opposite side. These detectors receive x-rays along the path through the patient's body. The detector and x-ray source rotate around the axis, producing exposures at 1-degree intervals of rotation. (**A** from Drake RL, Vogl W, Mitchell AWM: *Gray's Anatomy for Students,* Philadelphia, 2005, Elsevier Inc. **B** from Stimac GK: *Introduction to Diagnostic Imaging,* Philadelphia, 1992, WB Saunders.)

FIGURE 23–11 Axial MRI frame. *Arrows* highlight the descending aorta. (From Bragg DG, Rubin P, Hricak H: *Oncologic Imaging,* ed 2, Philadelphia, 2002, Saunders.)

From the Trenches

What are the benefits to working in medical coding?
"Feeling that you have not just helped doctors improve their bottom line, but you also have helped patients not to have to worry about their bills."
PATRICIA

FIGURE 23–12 Magnetic resonance imaging (MRI) scan slice in the axial, coronal, and sagittal planes from a patient with subcortical aphasia. The lesion is an infarction involving the anterior caudate, putamen, and anterior limb of the left internal capsule. (Modified from Bradley WG, Daroff RB, Fenichel GM, Jankovic J: *Neurology in Clinical Practice,* ed 5, Philadelphia, 2008, Butterworth-Heinemann.)

In **angiography,** dyes are injected into the vessels to add contrast that facilitates the visualization of vessels' lumen size and condition. The lumen is the cavity or channel within the vessel. Angiography is performed to view blood vessels after injecting them with a radio-opaque dye that outlines the vessels on x-ray. Angiography is used to identify abnormalities inside the vessels. Fig. 23–13 shows an angiogram of the aortic arch and brachiocephalic vessels. The radiologist studies the vessels using angiography to detect conditions such as malformations, strokes, or myocardial infarctions.

There are some combination codes in the angiography codes; so you must carefully read the complete procedure descriptor and parenthetical information to assure correct coding.

Codes in the Diagnostic Radiology subsection are divided according to anatomic site, from the head down. Some of the codes indicate a specific number of views, such as a minimum of three views or a single view. You should pay special attention to the description in each code and understand clearly how many views are specified in the code.

CODING SHOT

If fewer than the total number of views specified in the code are taken, modifier -52 would be used to indicate to the third-party payer that less of the procedure was performed than is described by the code, unless a code already exists for the smaller number of views.

BREAST, MAMMOGRAPHY

Mammography (77051-77059) is the use of diagnostic radiology to detect breast tumors or other abnormal breast conditions, such as these codes used to report mammography services:

77055   Mammography; unilateral

77056   bilateral

77057   Screening mammography, bilateral (2-view film study of each breast)

Codes 77055 and 77056 report mammography performed to detect a suspected tumor. For example, a patient who upon examination has demonstrated an abnormality in a breast would appropriately have the service reported with 77055. If, however, a patient has presented for the

FIGURE 23–13 Angiography of the aortic arch and brachiocephalic vessels. (From Stimac GK: *Introduction to Diagnostic Imaging,* Philadelphia, WB Saunders, 1992, p 447.)

usual screening mammography, report the service with 77057. Note that the description for the usual screening mammography indicates "bilateral," because screening mammography is performed on both breasts.

When new codes are published, their submission requires special attention. Under radiology guidelines, if a service is rarely provided, unusual, variable, or new, when submitting for reimbursement of the service a special report may be necessary. The report would include the complexity of symptoms, final diagnosis, pertinent physical findings, diagnostic/therapeutic procedures, concurrent problems, and follow-up care.

EXERCISE 23-4 *Diagnostic Radiology and Breast Mammography*

Code the radiology portion of the procedures unless otherwise directed:

1 What is the code for a diagnostic mammography, bilateral?

   CPT Code: _____

2 What is the code for an unlisted diagnostic radiologic procedure?

   CPT Code: _____

3 What is the code for the supervision and interpretation of an aortography, thoracic, by serialography?

   CPT Code: _____

DIAGNOSTIC ULTRASOUND

Another subsection in Radiology is Diagnostic Ultrasound (76506-76999). **Diagnostic ultrasound** is the use of high-frequency sound waves to image anatomic structures and to detect the cause of illness and disease. It is used by the physician in the diagnostic process. Ultrasound moves at different speeds through tissue, depending on the density of the tissue. Forms and outlines of organs can be identified by ultrasound as the sound waves move through or bounce back (echo) from the tissues.

QUICK CHECK 23-1

1. According to the information in Diagnostic Ultrasound, Pelvis codes 76805 and _____ include determination of the number of fetuses.

There are many uses for ultrasound in medicine, such as showing a gallstone (Fig. 23–14) and showing first trimester twins (Fig. 23–15). You may think that these ultrasound procedures do not produce a picture clear enough to be of use to the physician in the diagnostic process, but a professional trained in the interpretation of ultrasound images is able to read them clearly.

Codes for ultrasound procedures are found in three locations:

■ Radiology section, Diagnostic Ultrasound subsection, 76506-76999, is usually divided on the basis of the anatomic location of the procedure (chest, pelvis)

FIGURE 23–14 Ultrasound showing a gallstone. (From Goldman L, Ausiello D, editors: *Cecil Medicine,* ed 23, Philadelphia, 2008, Saunders.)

FIGURE 23–15 Twins on first trimester ultrasound scan. (From James DK, Steer PJ, Weiner CP, Gonik B: *High Risk Pregnancy: Management Options,* ed 3, Philadelphia, 2006, Saunders.)

- Medicine section, Non-Invasive Vascular Diagnostic Studies subsection, 93875-93990, divided on the basis of the anatomic location of the procedure (cerebrovascular, extremity)
- Medicine section, Echocardiography (ultrasound of the heart and great arteries), 93303-93352

An **interventional radiologist** is a physician who is skilled in both the surgical procedure and the radiology portion of an interventional radiologic service. The interventional radiologist is a board-certified physician who specializes in minimally invasive treatments performed using image guidance. These procedures have less risk, pain, and recovery time compared with open surgery. For example, an interventional radiologist who performed a liver biopsy using CT guidance to locate the lesion would report the services with a surgery code (47000) and a radiology code (77012-26). The interventional radiologist provided the surgical portion of the service, reported with a surgery code, and provided the professional portion of the CT guidance service, reported with a code from the Radiology section with modifier -26.

Most of the services in the Diagnostic Ultrasound subsection are located in the index of the CPT manual under the main term "Ultrasound." These terms are subdivided anatomically and by procedure (e.g., guidance or drainage).

EXERCISE 23-5 *Diagnostic Ultrasound*

In the CPT manual, Diagnostic Ultrasound is usually divided into subheadings.
Locate and list the subheadings:

1 _____

2 _____

3 _____

4 _____

5 _____

6 _____

7 _____

8 _____

9 _____

The ultrasound sound waves are sent through body tissues with a device called a **transducer.** The transducer is placed directly on the skin to which a gel has been applied. The sound waves that are sent by the transducer through the body are then reflected by internal structures that return an echo to the transducer. The echoes are then transmitted electronically to the viewing monitor. The echo images are recorded on film or video tape. The technical term for ultrasound testing and recording is sonography. Ultrasound testing is painless and involves no radiation and produces no harmful side effects.

Ultrasound examinations can be utilized in various areas of the body for a multitude of purposes. These purposes can include examination of the chest, abdomen, and blood vessels (such as to detect blood clots in veins). Ultrasound can obtain detailed images of the size and function of the heart and detect abnormalities of the valves (such as mitral valve prolapse and aortic stenosis) and endocarditis (infection of the heart). Ultrasound is commonly used to guide fluid withdrawal (aspiration) from the chest, lung, or heart. Other uses of ultrasound include gallstone detection and viewing of the ureter, liver, spleen, pancreas, and aorta within the abdomen. Ultrasound can detect fluid, cysts, tumors, or abscesses in the abdomen or liver, aortic aneurysms, evaluate the structure of the thyroid gland in the neck, arteriosclerosis in the legs, and evaluation of the size, gender, movement, and position of the growing baby during pregnancy.

Modes and Scans

There are four different types of ultrasound listed in the CPT manual: A-mode, M-mode, B-scan, and real-time scan.

A-mode: one-dimensional display reflecting the time it takes the sound wave to reach a structure and reflect back. This process maps the outline of the structure. "A" is for amplitude of sound return (echo).

M-mode: one-dimensional display of the movement of structures. "M" stands for motion.

B-scan: two-dimensional display of the movement of tissues and organs. "B" stands for brightness. The sound waves bounce off tissue or organs and are projected onto a black and white television screen. The strong signals display as black and the weaker signals display as lighter shades of gray. B-scan is also called gray-scale ultrasound.

Real-time scan: two-dimensional display of both the structure and the motion of tissues and organs that indicates the size, shape, and movement of the tissue or organ.

Codes are often divided on the basis of the scan or mode that was used and the medical record will indicate the scan or mode used.

Several codes within the subsection include the use of Doppler ultrasound. **Doppler ultrasound** is the use of sound that can be transmitted only through solids or liquids and is a specific version of ultrasonography, or ultrasound. Doppler ultrasound is named for an Austrian physicist, Johann Doppler, who discovered a relationship between sound and light waves—a relationship upon which ultrasound technology was built. Doppler ultrasound is used to measure moving objects and as such is ideal for measuring bloodflow. Codes often state "with or without Doppler." Doppler ultrasound can be standard black and white or color. Color Doppler translates the standard black and white into colored images. Just imagine how much easier it is to see a leak in a vessel when the vessel is yellow and the blood is red. The code descriptions will specifically state "color-flow Doppler."

There is some component coding necessary, but it occurs mostly under the subheading of Ultrasonic Guidance Procedures (76930-76999). The parenthetic information will refer you to the surgical procedure code. For example, 76945 is for the radiologic supervision and interpretation of ultrasonic guidance for chorionic villus sampling, which is an aspiration of cells for analysis to determine any cell abnormalities. The physician guides the insertion of a needle to withdraw the sample. If the physician performed both the radiologic portion of the procedure and the surgical procedure, you would report 59015 from the Surgery section and 76945 from the Radiology section. The radiology service reported with 76945 is not bundled into the surgical service (59015) and would be separately reimbursed. Modifier -26 would be reported with 76945, unless the radiologist owned the equipment.

EXERCISE 23-6 *Modes and Scans*

Assign codes using the CPT and ICD-9-CM manuals for the following:

1 An ultrasound of the spinal canal

   CPT Code: _____

2 An ultrasound of the chest and mediastinum, real time

   CPT Code: _____

3 A complete abdominal ultrasound in real time with image documentation

   CPT Code: _____

4 A uterine ultrasound in real time with image documentation of a 32-week pregnant female with twins

   CPT Code: _____

   ICD-9-CM Code: _____ (ICD-10-CM Code: _____)

5 A fetal profile, biophysical, with nonstress testing in a mother with Type 1 Diabetes mellitus

   CPT Code: _____

   ICD-9-CM Codes: _____, _____ (ICD-10-CM Code: _____)

[handwritten margin note: answer wrong / Quest. Changed]

RADIATION ONCOLOGY

The Radiation Oncology subsection (77261-77799) of the Radiology section reports both professional and technical treatments utilizing radiation to destroy tumors and special attention must be given to reporting the components. The subsection is divided on the basis of treatment. Read all of the definitions carefully to make certain you know what is bundled into the code. Many third-party payers have developed strict guidelines determining the number of times some procedures are allowed within each treatment course. You should work closely with third-party payers to understand their preferred reporting.

From the Trenches

"There are so many opportunities and not enough skilled coders to fill the positions for physician's offices, clinics, hospitals, as health care consultants, and also in colleges to teach coding at a college level."

PATRICIA

The codes within this subheading include codes for the initial consultation through management of the patient during the course of treatment. When the initial consultation occurs, the code for the service would be an E/M code. For example, the patient might be an inpatient when the therapeutic radiologist first sees the patient for evaluation of treatment options and before a decision for treatment is made. You would report this consultation service with an Inpatient Consultation code from the E/M section.

Clinical Treatment Planning

Clinical Treatment Planning (77261-77263) reflects professional services by the physician. It includes interpretation of special testing, tumor localization, treatment volume determination, treatment time/dosage determination, choice of treatment modality (method), determination of number and size of treatment ports, selection of appropriate treatment devices, and any other procedures necessary to adequately develop a course of treatment. A treatment plan is established for all patients requiring radiation therapy.

There are three types of clinical treatment plans: simple, intermediate, and complex.

Simple planning requires that there be a single treatment area that is encompassed by a single port or by simple parallel opposed ports with simple or no blocking.

Intermediate planning requires that there be three or more converging ports, two separate treatment areas, multiple blocks, or special time/ dose constraints.

Complex planning requires that there be highly complex blocking, custom shielding blocks, tangential ports, special wedges or compensators, three or more separate treatment areas, rotational or special beam consideration, or a combination of therapeutic modalities.

Simulation

Simulation (77280-77299) is the service of determining treatment areas and the placement of the ports for radiation treatment, but does not include the administration of the radiation. A simulation can be performed on a simulator designated for use only in simulations in a radiation therapy treatment unit, or on a diagnostic x-ray machine. Codes are divided into four levels of service:

Simple simulation of a single treatment area, with either a single port or parallel opposed ports and simple or no blocking

Intermediate simulation of three or more converging ports, with two separate treatment areas and multiple blocks

Complex simulation of tangential ports, with three or more treatment areas, rotation or arc therapy, complex blocking, custom shielding blocks, brachytherapy source verification, hyperthermia probe verification, and any use of contrast material

Three-dimensional (3D) computer-generated reconstruction of tumor volume and surrounding critical normal tissue structures based on direct CT scan and/or MRI data in preparation for non-coplanar or coplanar therapy. This is a simulation that utilizes documented three-dimensional beam's-eye view volume dose displays of multiple or moving beams. Documentation of three-dimensional volume reconstruction and dose distribution is required.

After the initial simulation and treatment plans have been established for a patient, if any change is made in the field of treatment, a new simulation billing is required. When coding for a treatment period, you will have codes for planning, simulation, the isodose plan, devices, treatment management (the number of treatments determines the number of times billed), and the radiation delivery.

The codes in Clinical Treatment Planning are located in the index of the CPT manual under the main term "Radiology Therapy." Codes can also be located under the main term of the specific service, such as "field set-up."

EXERCISE 23-7   *Clinical Treatment Planning*

Using the CPT manual, code the following:

1 Complex therapeutic radiology simulation-aided field setting

    CPT Code: _____

2 Therapeutic radiology treatment planning; simple

    CPT Code: _____

Medical Radiation Physics, Dosimetry, Treatment Devices, and Special Services

Medical Radiation Physics, Dosimetry, Treatment Devices, and Special Services (77300-77370, 77399) reports the decision making of the physician as to the type of treatment (modality), dose, and development of treatment devices. It is common to have several dosimetry or device changes during a treatment course. **Dosimetry** is the calculation of the radiation dose and placement.

Codes in this subheading are divided mostly on the basis of the level of treatment (simple, intermediate, complex). The codes are located in the index of the CPT manual under the main term "Radiation Therapy" and the subterm of the specific service, such as dose plan or treatment.

EXERCISE 23-8 *Medical Radiation, Physics, Dosimetry, Treatment Devices, and Special Services*

Using the CPT and ICD-9-CM manuals, code the following:

1 Design and construction of a bite block, intermediate

CPT Code: _____

2 Calculation of an isodose for brachytherapy, single plane, two sources, simple

CPT Code: _____

3 Teletherapy, isodose plan, to one area, simple, for cancer of the prostate, primary malignant

CPT Code: _____

ICD-9-CM Code: _____ (ICD-10-CM Code: _____)

Radiation Treatment Delivery

Stereotactic Radiation Treatment Delivery (77371-77373) and Radiation Treatment Delivery (77401-77423) reflect **technical components** only. These codes report the actual delivery of the radiation. Radiation treatment is delivered in units called megaelectron volts (MeV). A megaelectron volt is a unit of energy. The radiation energy **delivered** by the machine is measured in megaelectron volts; the energy that is **deposited** in the patient's tissue is measured in Gray (one Gray = 100 rads; 1 centigray [cGy] = 1 rad). A rad is a radiation-absorbed dose. The therapy dose in a cancer treatment would typically be in the thousands of rads.

To report Radiation Treatment Delivery services, you need to know the amount of radiation delivered (6-10 MeV, 11-19 MeV) and the number of the following:

- **Areas** treated (single, two, three or more)
- **Ports** involved (single, three or more, tangential)
- **Blocks** used (none, multiple, custom)

EXERCISE 23-9 *Radiation Treatment Delivery*

Using the CPT and ICD-9-CM manuals, code the following:

The patient receives radiation treatment delivery:

1 To a single area at 4 MeV

CPT Code: _____

2 With superficial voltage only

CPT Code: _____

3 To four separate areas with a rotational beam at 4 MeV

CPT Code: _____

4 For two separate areas, using three or more ports with multiple blocks at 5 MeV

CPT Code: _____

5 For three or more separate areas using custom blocks, wedges, rotation beams, up to 5 MeV for bone metastasis of the thoracic and lumbar spine (unknown primary)

CPT Code: _____

ICD-9-CM Codes: _____, _____

(ICD-10-CM Codes: _____, _____)

Radiation Treatment Management

Radiation Treatment Management codes (77427-77499) report the **professional component** of radiation treatment management. The codes report weekly management of radiation therapy. The notes under the heading Radiation Treatment Management state that clinical management is based on five fractions or treatment sessions regardless of the time interval separating the delivery of treatment. This means that these codes may be reported if the patient receives a treatment at least five times within a week (7-day); it also means that if the patient receives five treatments at any time during this week (i.e., skipping a day or two between treatments), these codes may still be reported.

If the patient receives five treatments and then receives an additional one or two fractions, you do not report the additional fractions. Only if three or more fractions beyond the original five are delivered would you report 77427 to indicate the additional treatment management.

Bundled into the Radiation Treatment Management codes are the following physician services:

- Review of port films
- Review of dosimetry, dose delivery, and treatment parameters
- Review of patient treatment setup
- Examination of the patient for medical evaluation and management (e.g., assessment of the patient's response to treatment, coordination of care and treatment, review of imaging and/or lab test results)

CODING SHOT Services related to and covered under Radiation Treatment Management are based on the third-party payer.

The following can be reported in addition to the 77427 (treatment management) because none of the following are bundled into the treatment management:

- 77417 Port films can be reported, two per week per treatment course
- 77300 Basic plan calculation at the onset of treatment
- 77263 Complex planning reported at the beginning of treatment
- E/M code: Usually on the first day of treatment as either an office visit or a consultation service

CODING SHOT The 77427 is reported once per each unit of five fractions or treatment sessions. All five sessions/treatments must be completed to report code 77427. The continuing medical physics consultation code 77336 is reported by the physicist once per every fifth fraction. This is a facility/technical service code and is not reported by the radiation oncologist.

It would be inappropriate to report these items individually. For example, the physician sees the patient in the office to evaluate the patient's response to treatment. You might think you should use an E/M code to report the office visit, but that would be incorrect because the management codes already include the office visit service.

Proton Beam Treatment Delivery

The delivery of radiation treatment (77520-77525) using a proton beam utilizes particles that are positively charged with electricity. The use of the proton beam is an alternative delivery method for radiation in which proton (electromagnetic) radiation would be used. The codes in the subheading are divided according to whether the delivery was simple, intermediate, or complex.

Hyperthermia

Hyperthermia (77600-77615) is an increase in body temperature and is used as an adjunct to radiation therapy or chemotherapy for the treatment of cancer. The heat source can be ultrasound, microwave, or another means of increasing the temperature in an area. When the temperature of an area is increased, metabolism increases, which boosts the ability of the body to eradicate the cancer cells. The location of the heat source can be external (to a depth of greater or less than 4 cm), interstitial (within the tissues), or intracavitary (inside the body). External treatment would be the application to the skin of a heat source. Interstitial treatment is the insertion of a probe that delivers heat directly to the treatment area. Codes 77600-77615 report external or interstitial treatment delivery.

Intracavitary hyperthermia treatment delivery requires the insertion of a heat-producing probe into a body orifice, such as the rectum or vagina. Code 77620 reports intracavitary treatment and is the only code listed under the heading Clinical Intracavitary Hyperthermia.

QUICK CHECK 23-2

1. Hyperthermia is used as an independent treatment modality.
   True or False?

EXERCISE 23-10 *Clinical Treatment Management*

Using the CPT manual, code the following management services:

1 Five radiation treatments

   CPT Code: _____

2 Unlisted procedure code for therapeutic radiation clinical treatment management (Submission of this unlisted procedure code would necessitate a special report and assumes that no Category III code exists for the procedure.)

   CPT Code: _____

Clinical Brachytherapy

Clinical **brachytherapy** (77750-77799) is the placement of radioactive material directly into or surrounding the site of the tumor as discussed earlier in this text. Placement may be intracavitary or interstitial, and material may be placed permanently or temporarily.

The terms "source" and "ribbon" are used in the Clinical Brachytherapy codes. A **source** is a container holding a radioactive element that can be inserted directly into the body where it delivers the radiation dose over time. Sources come in various forms, such as seeds or capsules, and are placed in a cavity (intracavitary) or permanently placed within the tissue (interstitial). Fig. 23–16 illustrates the results of a single permanent seed implanted into

FIGURE 23–16   **A,** MR image scan of 80-year-old man with large petroclival meningioma previously treated with radiosurgery 6 years earlier. **B,** Results 3 months after placement of single permanent I-125 seed. **C,** Results 9 months after placement of single seed. (From Crownover RL, ed: *Hematology/Oncology Clinics of North America,* Vol 13, Number 3, June 1999, p 645.)

the cranial posterior fossa of a patient with a meningioma. A ribbon is another source and ribbons are seeds embedded on a tape. The ribbon is cut to the desired length to control the amount of radiation the patient receives. Ribbons are inserted temporarily into the tissue.

Codes are divided on the basis of the number of sources or ribbons used in an application:

- Simple   1-4
- Intermediate   5-10
- Complex   11 or more

The Clinical Brachytherapy codes include the physician's work related to the patient's admission to the hospital as well as the daily hospital visits.

EXERCISE 23-11   *Clinical Brachytherapy*

Using the CPT and ICD-9-CM manuals, code the following:

1 A simple application of a radioactive source, intracavitary

   CPT Code: _____

2 A simple application of a radioactive source, interstitial

   CPT Code: _____

3 Surface application of a radiation source for ovarian cancer, primary

   CPT Code: _____

   ICD-9-CM Code: _____ (ICD-10-CM Code: _____)

NUCLEAR MEDICINE   Nuclear medicine (78000-79999) reports placement of radionuclides within the body and the monitoring of emissions from the radioactive elements. Nuclear medicine is used not only for diagnostic studies but also for therapeutic treatment, such as treatment of thyroid conditions.

Stress tests are an example of nuclear medicine techniques. Radioactive material may be used during stress tests to monitor coronary artery bloodflow.

Radioactive material (called a tracer) adheres to red blood cells (such as thallium or technetium sestamibi [Cardiolite]). The radioactive materials on the red blood cells allow an image of the heart to be seen and indicate areas where blood is flowing. The radioactive materials are injected 1 minute before the end of a stress test and then again 24 hours later for a comparison study. If the bloodflow is decreased or absent, the image will show a blank area. If the coronary arteries are clear and allow blood to flow to the heart muscle, the image will show blood dispersement to all areas. If the arteries are partially blocked, the flow may be decreased but would be adequate during rest. During exercise, however, the necessary amount of oxygenated blood may not be adequate to keep the heart functioning properly, and that is when chest pain may occur. During a stress test, if radionuclide dispersement is absent during exercise (showing inadequate blood supply to the area during peak demand) but is present during resting periods (showing adequate flow at rest), this is called **reversible ischemia,** meaning that heart muscle death has not occurred. With intervention, arteries may be opened or bypassed to increase the supply of blood to the muscle before heart muscle death does occur. If the radionuclide is absent during rest and exercise, the ischemia is considered **irreversible,** meaning that heart muscle death has already occurred. A stress test is one of the many uses of nuclear medicine for diagnostic purposes. As you code, you will become familiar with these various diagnostic tests and how they are reported.

CODING SHOT None of the codes in the subsection includes the radio-pharmaceutical(s) used for diagnosis or therapy services. When radiopharmaceutical(s) are supplied for diagnostic purposes, report 79005 (oral), 79101 (intravenous), 79440 (intra-articular) or 79445 (intra-arterial) or use the specific Level II HCPCS code. The oral and intravenous administration codes include the administration service. For intra-arterial, intra-cavity, and intra-articular administration also report the appropriate injection/procedure codes in addition to the imaging guidance and radiological supervision/interpretation when appropriate.

Two other subheadings within the Nuclear Medicine subsection are Diagnostic (78000-78999) and Therapeutic (79005-79999). The subheading Diagnostic is further divided into category codes based on system, such as the endocrine system and the cardiovascular system.

EXERCISE 23-12 *Nuclear Medicine*

Which subheading in the Nuclear Medicine subsection would you reference to locate codes for the following?

1 Liver _____

2 Thyroid _____

3 Spleen _____

4 Bone _____

5 Brain _____

CHAPTER REVIEW

CHAPTER 23, PART I, THEORY

Without the use of the CPT manual, complete the following:

1 What is a branch of medicine that uses radiant energy to diagnose and treat patients?

_____

2 The CPT manual divides the Radiology section into subsections of Radiologic Guidance, Breast Mammography, Bone/Joint Studies, Diagnostic

Radiology, _____,

_____,

and Nuclear Medicine.

3 What type of procedure is "performed independently of, and is not immediately related to, other services"?

_____

4 One Gray equals how many rads? _____

5 The modifier used to indicate the Professional

Component is _____.

6 The two words that mean supervising the taking of the x-rays and reading/reporting the results of

the films are _____ and _____.

7 The name for the use of high-frequency sound waves in an imaging process that is used to diagnose patient illness is

_____.

8 The Radiation Oncology section of the CPT manual is divided into subsections based on

the _____ of service provided to the patient.

9 The scientific study of energy is

_____.

10 The scientific calculation of the radiation emitted from various radioactive sources is

_____

11 Radiation treatment delivery codes are based on the treatment area involved and further divided based on levels of what?

_____.

12 MeV stands for

_____.

13 Radiation Treatment Management is reported

in units of _____ fractions.

14 Nuclear Medicine uses these to image organs for diagnosis and treatment:

_____

Identify the planes of the body on the figure on the next page:

15 _____

16 _____

17 _____

CHAPTER 23, PART II, PRACTICAL

The coding exercise that follows uses codes from a variety of CPT sections.

Using the CPT and ICD-9-CM manuals, code the following:

18 An established patient is seen in the physician's office with the chief complaint of a persistent cough. Otherwise, the patient claims to be in good health. The physician collects a history, including the chief complaint and the history of the present illness. The physical examination performed focuses on the respiratory tract. The decision making is straightforward because the physician wants to evaluate the patient for a possible case of bronchitis.

CPT Code: _____

The patient is sent to the clinic's radiology department for a two-view chest x-ray study, frontal and lateral.

CPT Code: _____

The radiologist sends the x-ray results to the physician, who reviews them and decides to order a consultation with a pulmonologist from another clinic. The patient sees the other clinic's pulmonologist, who performs a comprehensive history and a comprehensive examination with moderate complexity.

CPT Code: _____

A bronchoscopy with transbronchial lung biopsy is performed.

CPT Code: _____

Then there is radiologic supervision and interpretation of a unilateral bronchography.

CPT Code: _____

19 A new patient is seen in the office for unilateral ear pain. In the expanded problem focused history and the physical examination, the physician focuses his attention on the head, ears, nose, and throat. The physician's provisional diagnoses include otalgia and

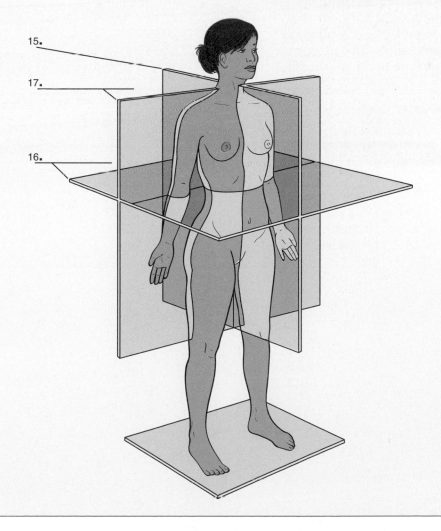

15.

17.

16.

possible ear infections. The decision making is straightforward for the physician.

CPT Code: _____

The patient is sent to the clinic's radiologist for an x-ray of the ear.

CPT Code: _____

The patient is then sent to the clinic's ear specialist, who inserts a ventilation tube (tympanostomy) using local anesthesia.

CPT Code: _____

ICD-9-CM Code: _____

(ICD-10-CM Code: _____)

20 A new patient is seen in the office for a variety of complaints, but in particular a swelling and heaviness of his right leg. The physician documents the patient's complaints, collects a comprehensive history of the present illness, performs a comprehensive review of systems, and inquires about the patient's past, family, and social history. A complete multisystem physical examination is performed. The physician's working diagnosis is edema of the lower extremity, cause to be determined. Given the nature of the problem, the physician

considers the decision making process to be highly complex.

CPT Code: _____

ICD-9-CM Code: _____

(ICD-10-CM Code: _____)

21A The patient is sent to radiology for a unilateral lymphangiography of one extremity due to swelling of the arm. The patient has a history of breast cancer.

CPT Code: _____

ICD-9-CM Codes: _____,

_____

(ICD-10-CM Codes: _____,

_____)

21B Another physician performs the injection procedure for the lymphangiography.

CPT Code: _____

ICD-9-CM Codes: _____,

_____

(ICD-10-CM Codes: _____,

_____)

QUICK CHECK ANSWERS

QUICK CHECK 23-1
1. 76810

QUICK CHECK 23-2
1. False

"Coding is a diverse field, so there are a lot of opportunities in many areas . . . . Find an area of interest and become an expert in it; make yourself valuable."

Keith Russell, CPC, CPC-H
Senior Compliance Analyst
Baylor College of Medicine
Houston, Texas

Pathology/Laboratory

Chapter Topics

Format

Organ or Disease Oriented Panels

Drug Testing

Therapeutic Drug Assays

Evocative/Suppression Testing

Consultations (Clinical Pathology)

Urinalysis and Chemistry

Hematology and Coagulation

Immunology

Transfusion Medicine

Microbiology

Anatomic Pathology

Cytopathology and Cytogenic Studies

Surgical Pathology

Other Procedures

Chapter Review

Quick Check Answers

Learning Objectives

After completing this chapter you should be able to

1 Explain the format of the Pathology and Laboratory section.

2 Understand the information in the Pathology and Laboratory Guidelines.

3 Demonstrate an understanding of Pathology and Laboratory terminology.

4 Differentiate amongst the Organ or Disease Oriented Panels codes.

5 Recognize Drug Testing codes.

6 Identify Therapeutic Drug Assays codes.

7 Classify Evocative/Suppression Testing codes.

8 Explain Consultations (Clinical Pathology) codes.

9 Interpret Urinalysis and Chemistry codes.

10 Evaluate Hematology and Coagulation codes.

11 Describe Immunology codes.

12 Discriminate amongst Transfusion Medicine codes.

13 Interpret Microbiology codes.

14 Evaluate Anatomic Pathology codes.

15 Summarize Cytopathology and Cytogenic Studies codes.

16 Explain Surgical Pathology codes.

17 Choose Other Procedures codes.

18 Demonstrate the ability to code Pathology and Laboratory services.

Make sure to check
evolve
learning system
for the latest content updates

FORMAT

The Pathology and Laboratory section of the CPT manual is formatted according to type of test performed—automated multichannel, panels, assays, and so forth. To familiarize yourself with the content of the Pathology and Laboratory section, review the subsections in the CPT manual. This will help you get a broad overview of the contents of this important section as you prepare to learn the specifics.

Laboratories have built-in **indicators** that allow additional tests to be performed without a written order from the physician. These standards are set by the medical facility and imply that when a certain test is positive, it is assumed that the physician would want further information on the condition and specific additional tests are to be performed. For example, if a routine urinalysis is performed, a culture is performed if the test is positive for bacteria. If a culture is performed to identify the organism, a sensitivity test is performed if the bacteria are of a certain type or count, as predetermined by the medical facility to warrant the additional laboratory studies. You will code only after the tests are performed, because an order for a laboratory test does not ensure that the test will be performed. This standard ensures that all laboratory tests performed are reported. Remember that what the physician ordered may not be all the laboratory work performed, depending on the facility's policy concerning indicators.

The services in the Pathology and Laboratory section include the laboratory **tests** only. The **collection** of the specimen is reported separately from the analysis of the test. For example, if a technician in a clinic laboratory withdraws blood by means of a venipuncture from the arm, and the blood sample was then analyzed in the laboratory, you would report 36415 for the venipuncture as shown in Fig. 24–1 in addition to a code to report the test performed on the blood in the laboratory.

Most Pathology and Laboratory subsections contain notes. Whenever notes are available, be sure to read them before assigning codes from the subsection because specific information pertinent to the codes is contained in these notes.

ORGAN OR DISEASE ORIENTED PANELS

The codes in the Organ or Disease Oriented Panels subsection (80047-80076) are grouped according to the usual laboratory work ordered by a physician for the diagnosis of or screening for various diseases or conditions. Groups of tests may be performed together using automated equipment, depending on the situation or disease. For example, during the first obstetric visit, a mother is commonly asked to have baseline laboratory tests performed to ensure that appropriate antepartum care is provided. CPT code 80055 describes an obstetric panel that would typically be performed during the first obstetric visit.

FIGURE 24–1   Venipuncture. (From Young AP, Proctor DB: *Kinn's The Medical Assistant,* ed 10, St. Louis, 2007, Saunders.)

To assign a panel code, each test listed in the panel description must be performed. Additional tests are reported separately. The development of panels saves the facility from having to report each test separately, and it is often more economical for the patient. You cannot assign modifier -52 (reduced service) with a panel. For example, if all of the tests in the obstetric panel were done except the syphilis test, you could not report 80055 (Obstetrical Panel) with modifier -52. You would instead list each of the tests separately.

CODING SHOT

Be careful when coding multiple panels on the same day for the same patient. Sometimes several panels include some of the same tests. For example, a hepatitis B surface antigen test is included in both the obstetric panel and the acute hepatitis panel. It would be inappropriate to report the same test twice.

The laboratory and pathology reports in the patient medical record will describe the method by which the test was performed. There are many different methods of performing the same test. For example, a urinalysis can be automated or nonautomated and can include or exclude a microscopy. It is necessary to know these details if you are to assign the correct urinalysis code. If the details you need are not in the medical record, ask the laboratory staff or physician for further clarification.

EXERCISE 24-1 *Organ or Disease Oriental Panels*

Complete the following:

1 Hepatic function panel code in a patient with hepatitis B serum virus, chronic

   CPT Code: _____

   ICD-9-CM Code: _____ (ICD-10-CM Code: _____)

2 How many laboratory tests must be included in a hepatic function panel? _____

3 Does an obstetric panel include a rubella antibody test? _____

4 Is blood typing ABO included in an obstetric panel? _____

DRUG TESTING   Laboratory drug testing (80100-80103) is performed to identify the presence or absence of a drug. Testing that determines the presence or absence of a drug is **qualitative** (the drug is either present or not present in the specimen).

From the Trenches

Why should a coder consider getting certified?
"Certification indicates a level of competence and many employers now require applicants to be certified. Plus, salary surveys have shown that certified coders command higher salaries than non-certified coders."

KEITH

When the presence of a drug is detected in the qualitative test, a confirmation test is usually performed by using a second testing method. Code 80102 is used to report a confirmation test. Codes from the Therapeutic Drug Assay and Chemistry subsections are used to further identify the exact amount of the drug that is present **(quantitative).** For example, a patient who has been on a medication for a long time might need to undergo testing to determine whether the drug level is at the correct therapeutic level. The CPT manual lists the drugs most commonly tested for, although the use of the codes is not limited to the drugs listed.

Modifier -51 is not assigned to pathology or laboratory codes; instead, each test is listed separately. For example, if a confirmation test was conducted for both alcohol and cocaine, report 80102 twice and append modifier -91, repeat clinical diagnostic laboratory test, to the second code.

QUICK CHECK 24-1

1. What is the repeat clinical laboratory test modifier? _____

TOOLBOX

Jason has been sent to the clinic to have a drug test, as are all employees of the company for which he works. The company requests all employees be screened for barbiturates and antidepressants.

QUESTIONS

1. Your clinic uses a chromatograph to determine two drug classes (80100). How would you report the service chromatographic determination of two drugs? _____

2. If your clinic did not use a chromatography, but rather did a test for each of the two tests, how would you report the tests? _____

ANSWERS 1. 80100, chromatographic determination 2. 80101 × 2, other than chromatograph

---

THERAPEUTIC DRUG ASSAYS

Drug assays (80150-80299) test for a specific drug and for the amount of that drug. Many types of drugs are listed in this subsection. If the drug is not listed, it is possible that quantitative analysis may be listed under the methodology (e.g., immunoassay, radioassay).

Therapeutic drug assays are performed to help the physician monitor the level of medication in the patient's system or to monitor the patient's compliance. For example, levels may be measured to make certain the patient is getting the correct level of antibiotics. Blood specimens for drug monitoring are usually taken during the drug's highest therapeutic concentration (peak level) and at the drug's lowest therapeutic concentration (trough or residual level). Peak and trough levels should be within the therapeutic range directed by the physician.

The drugs are listed by their generic names, not their brand names. For example, 80152 describes the generic drug amitriptyline, also sold under the brand names of Elavil and Endep. A *Physician's Desk Reference* that lists pharmaceuticals by the generic and brand name will be helpful as you code drug testing and assays.

One location of Drug Testing codes in the index of the CPT manual is under the main term "Drug," subtermed by the reason for the tests—analysis or confirmation. Therapeutic Drug Assay subsection codes can be found under the main term "Drug Assay" and subterms of the material examined, for example, amikacin, digoxin.

EXERCISE 24-2 *Therapeutic Drug Testing and Drug Assays*

Assign the correct CPT and ICD-9-CM codes for the following drug tests:

1 Confirmation of cocaine (qualitative)

 CPT Code: _____

2 Identify the amount of digoxin in the blood (quantitative)

 CPT Code: _____

3 Quantitative examination of blood for amikacin in a patient with fever and immune neutropenia

 CPT Code: _____

 ICD-9-CM Code: _____ (ICD-10-CM Code: _____)

4 Examination of blood, quantitative for lithium in a patient with manic depression syndrome

 CPT Code: _____

 ICD-9-CM Code: _____ (ICD-10-CM Code: _____)

EVOCATIVE/ SUPPRESSION TESTING

Evocative/Suppression (80400-80440) testing is performed to measure the effect of evocative or suppressive agents on chemical constituents. For example, 80400 is reported when a patient undergoes testing to determine whether adrenocorticotropic hormone (ACTH) is being produced in the body. The patient may have adrenal gland insufficiency. Note that following each of the code descriptions is a statement of the services that must have been provided for the code to be reported. For example, the requirement to report 80400 ACTH stimulation panel is "Cortisol (82533 × 2)" or two cortisol tests were performed. Code 80400 bundles two units of 82533 into one code. Before you can assign 80400, however, you must read the code description for 82533 to ensure that the code reports the correct test.

> ✋ **CAUTION** *Remember that the codes from the Pathology and Laboratory section are only for the tests performed and do not reflect the complete service provided to the patient.*

To code the components of Evocative/Suppression Testing consider the following:

- If the physician **supplied** the agent, report the supply using 99070 from the Medicine section or a HCPCS code.
- If the physician **administered** the agent, report the infusion or injection with codes 96365-96379 from the Medicine section.
- If the test involved **prolonged attendance** by the physician, report the service with the appropriate E/M code.

CONSULTATIONS (CLINICAL PATHOLOGY)

A clinical pathologist, upon request from a primary care physician, will perform a consultation to render additional medical interpretation of test results. For example, a primary care physician reviews lab test results and requests a clinical pathologist to review, interpret, and prepare a written report on the findings, which represents a clinical pathology consultation.

There are two codes under the subsection Consultations (80500, 80502). These consultations are based on whether the consultation was limited or comprehensive. A **limited consultation** is one that was done without the pathologist's review of the medical record of the patient, and a **comprehensive consultation** is one in which the medical record was reviewed as a part of the consultative services. When either of these consultation codes is submitted to a third-party payer, the submission is accompanied by a written report.

These are not the only consultation codes in the Pathology and Laboratory section of the CPT manual. There are also consultation codes toward the end of the section in the Surgical Pathology subsection (88321-88334) that report the services of a pathologist who reviews and gives an opinion or advice concerning pathology slides, specimens, material, or records that were prepared elsewhere or for pathology consultation during surgery. Pathology consultations during surgery are provided to examine tissue removed from a patient during a surgical procedure. If the pathologist did not use a microscope to examine the tissue, report 88329. If a microscope was used to examine the tissue, report 88331 or 88332, depending on the number of specimens that were examined.

A **specimen** is a sample of tissue from a suspect area; a **block** is a frozen piece of a specimen; and a **section** is a slice of a frozen block. A pathologist prepares a specimen by cutting it into blocks and taking sections from the blocks. The preparation of a frozen section is illustrated in Fig. 24–2. The number of sections taken depends on the judgment of the pathologist as to the number of areas of the specimen that need to be examined. The frozen section is placed (mounted) on a slide or held by other means that allow the pathologist to view the tissue under a microscope.

CODING SHOT 🖊 Each specimen may be reported separately, but each slide from that specimen may not.

FIGURE 24–2 Frozen section preparation. (Courtesy National Institute of Environmental Health Sciences—National Institutes of Health.)

When one block is sectioned and examined, the service of examining that first section is reported using 88331. The second and subsequent sections of the same block are included in the reporting of 88331. If another block from another area (a second block) was sectioned, the first section would be reported using 88331, and subsequent sections from the second block using 88332. You cannot use 88332 without first reporting 88331. Although 88332 is not marked as an add-on code (one that is used only with another code), its function is that of an add-on code because it is for subsequent sections that were examined.

NCCI

The edits bundle **88329** (pathology consultation during surgery) with **88331** (first tissue block) and **88332** (each additional tissue block). By issuing this guideline, CMS includes the frozen sections in the consultation bundle, which would usually be reported separately.

URINALYSIS AND CHEMISTRY

Many types of tests are located under the Urinalysis and Chemistry subsections (81000-84999). Urinalysis codes are for **nonspecific** tests performed on urine. Chemistry codes are for **specific** tests performed on material from any source (e.g., urine, blood, breath, feces, sputum) (Fig. 24–3). For example, a urinalysis using a dipstick (81000-81003) would report the presence and quantity of the following constituents: bilirubin, glucose,

FIGURE 24–3 Urinalysis with chemical reagent strips. (From Young AP, Proctor DB: *Kinn's The Medical Assistant,* ed 10, St. Louis, 2007, Saunders.)

hemoglobin, ketones, leukocytes, nitrite, pH, protein, specific gravity, and urobilinogen. Any number of these constituents may be analyzed and reported using a code from the Urinalysis subsection (81000-81099). However, if the physician ordered an analysis of the urine specifically to determine the presence of urobilinogen (reduced bilirubin) and the exact amount of urobilinogen present (quantitative analysis), you would choose a code (84580) from the Chemistry subsection. The main things to remember when coding from these two subsections are:

1. Identify specific tests
2. Determine if the test was automated (by machine) or nonautomated (manual)
3. Number of tests performed
4. Identify combination codes for similar types of tests
5. Whether the results are qualitative or quantitative
6. Method of testing

EXERCISE 24-3 *Urinalysis and Chemistry*

Code the following:

1 An automated urinalysis without microscopy

    CPT Code: _____

2 Urinalysis, microscopic only

    CPT Code: _____

3 Albumin, serum

    CPT Code: _____

4 Total bilirubin

    CPT Code: _____

5 Gases, blood pH only, in a patient with respiratory failure

    CPT Code: _____

    ICD-9-CM Code: _____ (ICD-10-CM Code: _____)

6 Sodium, urine, in a patient with congestive heart failure

    CPT Code: _____

    ICD-9-CM Code: _____ (ICD-10-CM Code: _____)

7 Uric acid, blood in a patient with acute gouty arthritis

    CPT Code: _____

    ICD-9-CM Code: _____ (ICD-10-CM Code: _____)

HEMATOLOGY AND COAGULATION The Hematology and Coagulation subsection contains codes (85002-85999) based on the various blood-drawing methods and tests. The method used to perform the test is often what determines code assignment. A blood count is used to measure the kind and number of cells in the blood, such as red and white blood cells. It is a commonly used test to detect various abnormalities in the blood. Blood counts can be manual or automated (Fig. 24–4), with many variations of the tests. For example, codes in the range 85004-85049 are blood count codes divided by method (manual or automated) and type of count, such as white blood count (WBC, 85004-85009) or a complete blood count (CBC, 85025, 85027). To accurately code a blood count, the method and the type of the count must be documented.

There are codes within the Hematology and Coagulation subsection for bone marrow smear and smear interpretations (85060, 85097). When a physician procures the bone marrow by means of aspiration, the service is reported with codes from the Surgery section (38204-38242); but that is only part of the service. The other part of the service is the pathology analysis of the aspirated specimen. As the coder in a clinic setting, you may be reporting only the surgical services or only the pathology/laboratory services or a combination of both. When reporting the surgical services always review the pathology report as a part of the code assignment and when reporting the pathology services, always review the operative report.

There are many blood coagulation tests located in the Hematology and Coagulation subsection. The codes are divided based on the particular factor being tested. Great care must be taken to ensure that the correct coagulation factor has been reported based on the information in the medical record. Coagulation factor tests analyze the level of certain proteins in the blood that enable the blood to congeal properly. Low levels of a factor may result in excessive bleeding and high levels may lead to clot formation (thrombosis). For example, 85610 reports a test to assess the level of factor II (also known as a prothrombin). This test is often performed when a patient is on a blood thinning medication and the physician wants to determine if the factor is at the optimal level.

Most of the tests in the Hematology and Coagulation subsection can be located in the index of the CPT manual under the name of the test, such as prothrombin time, coagulation time, or hemogram.

FIGURE 24-4 Hematology analyzer. (From Clinical Diagnostic Solutions, Inc.: *M-Series Hematology Analyzer CAP.* (website): http://cdsolinc.com/new_site/index.php?main_page=product_info&cPath=7_44&products_id=97. Accessed July 7, 2009.)

EXERCISE 24-4 *Hematology and Coagulation*

Code the following:

1 Blood count by an automated hemogram (RBC, WBC, Hgb, Hct, and platelet count)

CPT Code: _____

2 Blood count by an automated hemogram and platelet count with complete differential white blood cell count in a patient with anemia due to acute blood loss

CPT Code: _____

ICD-9-CM Code: _____ (ICD-10-CM Code: _____)

3 Automated RBC

CPT Code: _____

4 Interpretation of a bone marrow smear in a patient with acute leukemia, in remission

CPT Code: _____

ICD-9-CM Code: _____ (ICD-10-CM Code: _____)

As you can see, there are many variations of just a blood count test! Read the medical record and code descriptions carefully before assigning the codes.

IMMUNOLOGY Immunology codes (86000-86804) report identification of conditions of the immune system caused by the action of antibodies (e.g., hypersensitivity, allergic reactions, immunity, and alterations of body tissue).

EXERCISE 24-5 *Immunology*

Code the following:

1 ANA (antinuclear antibody) titer

CPT Code: _____

2 ASO (antistreptolysin O) screen

CPT Code: _____

3 Cold agglutinin screen in a patient with acute upper respiratory infections

CPT Code: _____

ICD-9-CM Code: _____ (ICD-10-CM Code: _____)

TRANSFUSION MEDICINE The Transfusion Medicine subsection codes (86850-86999) report tests performed on blood or blood products. Tests include screening of blood (Fig. 24–5) for antibodies, Coombs testing, autologous blood collection and processing, blood typing, compatibility testing, and preparation of and treatments performed on blood and blood products.

Transfusion of blood and blood components is reported with codes from a variety of locations. For example, to report the actual blood transfusion, assign 36430 from the Surgery section of the CPT manual. You must also report the

FIGURE 24–5   Blood transfusion.

substance being transfused, such as whole blood, HCPCS code P9010 per unit or red blood cells, P9021 per unit. The blood bank would provide and report the collection, processing, and storing of the autologous blood with 86890.

EXERCISE 24-6   *Transfusion Medicine*

Code the following:

1 ABO and Rh blood typing

   CPT Codes: _____, _____

2 Irradiation of blood product, 3 units

   CPT Code: _____

MICROBIOLOGY   Microbiology codes (87001-87999) report the study of microorganisms and includes bacteriology (study of bacteria), mycology (study of fungi), parasitology (study of parasites), and virology (study of viruses). For example, Fig. 24–6 illustrates a Petri dish used to culture microbes. Culture codes for the identification of organisms as well as the identification of sensitivities of

FIGURE 24–6   Mold growing in petri dish. (Courtesy United States Environmental Protection Agency.)

the organism to antibiotics (called culture and sensitivity) are located in this subsection. Culture codes must be read carefully because some codes report screening only to detect the presence of an organism; some codes indicate the identification of specific organisms; and others indicate additional sensitivity testing to determine which antibiotic would be best for treatment of the specified bacteria. You report all tests performed on the basis of whether they are quantitative or qualitative and/or a sensitivity study.

QUICK CHECK 24-2

1. According to the Microbiology Guidelines, how do you report multiple procedures rendered on the same day?

_____

EXERCISE 24-7 *Microbiology*

Code the following:

1 HIV-1, quantification

    CPT Code: _____

2 Streptococcus, group A, using an amplified probe method in a patient with headache and fever

    CPT Code: _____

    ICD-9-CM Codes: _____, _____

    (ICD-10-CM Codes: _____, _____)

3 Quantification of *Gardnerella vaginalis,* herpes simplex, and *Candida* species, in a patient with bacterial vaginosis

    CPT Codes: _____, _____, _____

    ICD-9-CM Code: _____ (ICD-10-CM Code: _____)

4 Direct probe method of mycobacterial tuberculosis, herpes simplex virus, and *Chlamydia trachomatis*

    CPT Codes: _____, _____, _____

5 Bacterial culture of urine, quantitative with colony count for urination frequency

    CPT Code(s): _____

    ICD-9-CM Code(s): _____ (ICD-10-CM Code(s): _____)

ANATOMIC PATHOLOGY

Anatomic Pathology codes (88000-88099) report examination of body fluids or tissues in postmortem (after death) examination. Postmortem examination involves the completion of gross microscopic and limited autopsies. Codes are divided according to the extent of the examination. This subsection also contains codes for forensic examination and coroners' calls, which means that some codes report an examination without the central nervous system (88000, 88020), with the brain (88005, 88025), with the brain and the spinal cord (88007, 88027), etc. There are two codes for each extent because one is a gross examination and one is a microscopic examination.

CYTOPATHOLOGY AND CYTOGENIC STUDIES

The Cytopathology subsection codes (88104-88199) report the laboratory work performed to determine whether cellular changes are present. For example, a very common cytopathology procedure is the Papanicolaou smear (Pap smear). Cytopathology may also be performed on fluids that have been aspirated from a site to identify cellular changes. Cytogenetic Studies (88230-88299) include tests performed for genetic and chromosomal studies.

QUICK CHECK 24-3

1. Where are the modifiers for cytogenic studies located? _____

SURGICAL PATHOLOGY

Surgical Pathology codes (88300-88399) describe the evaluation of specimens to determine the pathology of disease processes. When choosing the correct code for pathology, identify the source of the specimen and the reason for the surgical procedure. The Surgical Pathology subsection codes are divided into six levels (Levels I through VI) based on the specimen examined and the level of work required by the pathologist. Pathology testing is performed on all tissue removed from the body. The surgical pathology classification level is determined by the complexity of the pathologic examination.

From the Trenches

"Being certified opens many doors, but it also gives a level of credibility and confidence to your work, which makes a difference when dealing with other professions."

KEITH

Level I pathology code 88300 identifies specimens that normally do not need to be viewed under a microscope for pathologic diagnosis (e.g., a tooth)—those for which the probability of disease or malignancy is minimal.

Level II pathology code 88302 deals with those tissues that are usually considered normal tissue and have been removed not because of the probability of the presence of disease or malignancy, but for some other reason (e.g., a fallopian tube for sterilization, foreskin of a newborn).

Level III pathology code 88304 is assigned for specimens with a low probability of disease or malignancy. For example, a gallbladder may be neoplastic (benign or malignant), but when the gallbladder is removed for cholecystitis (inflammation of the gallbladder), it is usually inflamed from chronic disease and not because of cancerous changes.

Level IV pathology code 88305 designates a higher probability of malignancy or decision making for disease pathology. For example, a uterus is removed because of a diagnosis of prolapse. There is a possibility that the uterus is malignant or that there are other causes of disease pathology.

Level V pathology code 88307 classifies more complex pathology evaluations (e.g., examination of a uterus that was removed for reasons other than prolapse or neoplasm).

Level VI pathology code 88309 includes examination of neoplastic tissue or very involved specimens, such as a total resection of a colon.

For example, 88305 reports examination of tissue from a breast biopsy that does not require microscopic evaluation of the margins or tissue from a breast reduction; 88307 reports examination of tissue from the excision of a breast lesion that does require microscopic evaluation of the margins and a partial/simple mastectomy; and 88309 reports examination of tissue from a mastectomy with regional lymph node. The probability of cancer increases with each code.

CODING SHOT

A specimen is defined as tissue submitted for examination. If two specimens of the same area are received and examined, each specimen is reported. For example, if two separately identified anus tags are received and each is examined, report 88304 × 2. If one anus tag is received and two different areas of the tag are examined, report 88304 only once.

The remaining codes at the end of the subsection classify specialized procedures, utilization of stains, consultations performed, preparations used, and/or instrumentation needed to complete testing.

The surgical pathology codes are located in the index under the main term "Pathology" and subterms "Surgical" and "Gross and Micro Exam."

EXERCISE 24-8 *Surgical Pathology*

Code the following using one of the six surgical pathology codes in the CPT manual:

1 The specimen is a uterus, tubes, and ovaries. The procedure was an abdominal hysterectomy for ovarian cancer.

   CPT Code: _____

2 The specimen is a portion of a lung. The procedure was a left lower lobe segmental resection.

   CPT Code: _____

3 The specimen is the prostate. The procedure was a transurethral resection of the prostate.

   CPT Code: _____

4 What is the surgical pathology code for the following pathology report?

   CPT Code: _____

PATHOLOGY DEPARTMENT

Patient:	Alice C. Fisher	**Date Collected:**	02/09/0X
DOB:	12/06/37	**Date Received:**	02/09/0X
Sex:	F	**Date Examined:**	02/10/0X
Record Number:	5909890	**Access Number:**	P4218
Account:	MP8352	**Surgeon:**	Dr. White

CLINICAL HISTORY: UMBILICAL HERNIA, INFLAMED

TISSUE RECEIVED: UMBILICAL HERNIA

GROSS DESCRIPTION: The specimen is labeled with the patient's name and "umbilical hernia" and consists of yellow-white fibrofatty tissue approximately 3.5 × 2 × 1 cm. Representative sections are processed in two slides.

MICROSCOPIC DIAGNOSIS: Mature adipose tissue with fibrovascular and fibrotendinous tissue with focal reactive fibrous tissue consistent with umbilical hernia.

Alberto Matusa, MD

Alberto Matusa, MD
Head, Pathology Department
Merry Brook Hospital

OTHER PROCEDURES   Other Procedures includes miscellaneous testing on body fluids, the use of special instrumentation, and testing performed on oocytes and sperm.

CHAPTER REVIEW

CHAPTER 24, PART I, THEORY

Without the use of the CPT manual, complete the following:

1 The Pathology and Laboratory section of the CPT manual is formatted according to the type of _____ performed.

2 Laboratories have built-in _____ that allow additional tests to be performed without the written order of the physician.

3 Codes that are grouped according to the usual laboratory work ordered by a physician for diagnosis or screening of various diseases or

    conditions are _____.

4 Can you use a reduced service modifier with pathology or laboratory codes?

  Yes   No

5 Will the medical record contain the method used to perform the test?

  Yes   No

CHAPTER 24, PART II, PRACTICAL

Answer the following:

6 The Hematology and Coagulation subsections contain codes based on the various testing methods and tests. The method used to do the test is often the code determiner. Blood cell counts can be manual or automated, with many variations of the tests. What would the code be for an automated blood count (hemogram) with automated differential WBC count? A manual blood count (hemogram) with manual cell count?

Automated CPT Code: _____

Manual CPT Code: _____

Code the following three cases with the correct pathology code from the CPT:

7 The specimen is tonsils and adenoids. The procedure is a tonsillectomy with adenoidectomy.

☙ CPT Code(s): _____

8 The specimen is an appendix. The procedure is an incidental appendectomy.

☙ CPT Code(s): _____

9 The specimen is a tooth. The procedure is an odontectomy, gross examination only.

☙ CPT Code(s): _____

Code the following:

10 Western Blot of blood, with interpretation and report

☙ CPT Code(s): _____

11 Vitamin K analysis of blood

☙ CPT Code(s): _____

12 Quantitative analysis of urine for alkaloids

☙ CPT Code(s): _____

13 Three specimens of gastric secretions for total gastric acid

☙ CPT Code(s): _____

14 Blood analysis for HGH

☙ CPT Code(s): _____

15 Total insulin

☙ CPT Code(s): _____

16 LDL cholesterol using direct measurements

☙ CPT Code(s): _____

17 Blood count: one manual cell count

☙ CPT Code(s): _____

18 Blood smear interpretation

☙ CPT Code(s): _____

19 PTT of whole blood

☙ CPT Code(s): _____

20 Sedimentation rate, automated for fever and swelling in hand

☙ CPT Code(s): _____

☙ ICD-9-CM Code(s): _____

(☙ ICD-10-CM Code(s): _____)

21 Lee and White coagulation time

☙ CPT Code(s): _____

22 Clotting factor XII (Hageman factor) for excessive bleeding menopausal onset

☙ CPT Code(s): _____

☙ ICD-9-CM Code(s): _____

(☙ ICD-10-CM Code(s): _____)

23 Blood typing for paternity test, ABO, Rh, and MN

☙ CPT Code(s): _____

24 Culture of urine for bacteria with colony count for pain on urination

☙ CPT Code(s): _____

☙ ICD-9-CM Code(s): _____

(☙ ICD-10-CM Code(s): _____)

25 Schlichter test for complaints of leg pain and fever

⊛ CPT Code(s): _____

⊛ ICD-9-CM Code(s): _____

(⊛ ICD-10-CM Code(s): _____)

26 Postmortem examination, gross only, with brain and spinal cord

⊛ CPT Code(s): _____

27 Therapeutic drug assay for digoxin and vancomycin, patient has chronic sinus bradycardia

⊛ CPT Code(s): _____

⊛ ICD-9-CM Code(s): _____

(⊛ ICD-10-CM Code(s): _____)

28 Pathology consultation during surgery

⊛ CPT Code(s): _____

QUICK CHECK ANSWERS

QUICK CHECK 24-1
1. modifier -91

QUICK CHECK 24-2
1. report separate entries

QUICK CHECK 24-3
1. Appendix I

"Teamwork is so important! You have to be able to work with other people, and keep your mind open at all times . . . . Coding can be subjective; there is no one who knows everything."

Stephanie A. Lewis, CPC, ACS-EM, CCP
Compliance Analyst
University of Missouri Health Care
Columbia, Missouri

Medicine

Chapter Topics

Format

Introduction to Immunizations

Psychiatry

Biofeedback

Dialysis

Gastroenterology

Ophthalmology

Special Otorhinolaryngologic Services

Cardiovascular

Pulmonary

Allergy and Clinical Immunology

Endocrinology

Neurology and Neuromuscular Procedures

Central Nervous System Assessments/Tests

Health and Behavior Assessment/Intervention

Chemotherapy Administration

Photodynamic Therapy

Special Dermatological Procedures

Learning Objectives

After completing this chapter, you should be able to

1   Analyze the format of the Medicine section.

2   Report psychiatric services.

3   Identify biofeedback services.

4   List components of dialysis reporting.

5   Demonstrate ability to report gastrointestinal services.

6   Understand ophthalmology and otorhinolaryngologic reporting.

7   Report cardiovascular services.

8   Identify services reported with pulmonary codes.

9   List the important elements of coding allergy and clinical immunology services.

10   Report endocrine services.

11   Define neurology and neuromuscular services.

12   Demonstrate an understanding of central nervous system assessment and intervention.

13   Analyze chemotherapy services.

14   Report special services and dermatologic procedures.

15   Code physical medicine and rehabilitation services.

16   Report active wound management.

17   Define osteopathic and chiropractic services.

18   Understand non-face-to-face services.

19   Code special services, procedures, and reports.

20   Report medical services using Medicine section codes.

Make sure to check
evolve
learning system
for the latest content updates

Physical Medicine and Rehabilitation

Medical Nutrition Therapy

Osteopathic Manipulative Treatment (OMT)

Chiropractic Manipulative Treatment (CMT)

Non-Face-to-Face Nonphysician Services

Special Services, Procedures, and Reports

Other Services and Procedures

Home Health Procedures/ Services

Medication Therapy Management Services

Chapter Review

Quick Check Answers

The Medicine section (90281-99607) reports diagnostic and therapeutic services that are generally **noninvasive** (not entering a body cavity), but there are also **invasive** (entering a body cavity) procedures in the section, such as cardiac catheterization. The section begins with Guidelines applicable to all of the Medicine section codes, such as Multiple Procedures, Add-on Codes, Separate Procedures, Subsection Information, Unlisted Service/Procedure, Special Report, and Materials Supplied by Physician.

The various subsections of Medicine contain many specific notes to be applied with a certain group of codes, so be certain to read all notes that pertain to the group of codes with which you are working.

FORMAT Take a moment now to review the Medicine section in the CPT manual to have an overview of the subsections.

Many specialized types of tests are located in the Medicine section (e.g., biofeedback, audiologic function tests, electrocardiograms). Codes in this section do not usually include the supplies used in the testing, therapy, or diagnostic treatments unless specifically stated in the code description or guidelines. You report supplies, including drugs, separately unless otherwise instructed in the code information. CPT code 99070 is the supplies and materials code used to identify the supplying of drugs, trays, supplies, or materials needed to provide the service or the specific HCPCS supply code, which is usually what the payer will require. For example, Fig. 25–1 illustrates the code for the service of a prescription for corneal contact lenses (also known as contacts, see Fig. 25–2) for both eyes (92310). When the lenses and the prescription services are provided, both the lenses and

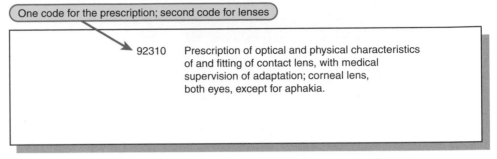

One code for the prescription; second code for lenses

92310   Prescription of optical and physical characteristics of and fitting of contact lens, with medical supervision of adaptation; corneal lens, both eyes, except for aphakia.

FIGURE 25–1   Some codes are for the supply only.

FIGURE 25–2   Contact lenses.

the prescription service are reported. The supply of contact lenses may be reported as part of the service of fitting or reported separately using the appropriate HCPCS Level II supply code (V2500-V2599). Reporting the supply of the lens depends on the third-party payer guidelines.

INTRODUCTION TO IMMUNIZATIONS

There are two types of immunization—active and passive. **Active immunization** is the type given when it is anticipated that the person will be in contact with the disease. Active immunization agents can be toxoids or vaccines. Toxoids are bacteria that have been made nontoxic and when injected, they produce an immune response that builds protection against a disease. Vaccines are viruses that are given in small doses and cause an immune response. **Passive immunization** does not cause an immune response; rather, the injected material contains a high level of antibodies against a disease (e.g., rabies, hepatitis B, tetanus), called immune globulins.

The first three subsections in the Medicine section are:

- Immune Globulins
- Immunization Administration for Vaccines/Toxoids
- Vaccines, Toxoids

Immune Globulins

The immune globulins (90281-90399) are passive immunization agents obtained from pooled human plasma that is immune to a particular disease.

The codes in this subsection identify only the immune globulin **product** and must be reported with the appropriate **administration** code (96365-96368, 96372, 96374, or 96375 as appropriate).

1. Immune globulins are _____ injections.
   a. active
   b. passive
   c. both a and b
   d. neither a nor b

Codes in the Immune Globulins subsection are categorized according to the:

- Type of immune globulin (rabies, hepatitis B, etc.)
- Method of injection (IM, IV, SC, etc.)
- Type of dose (full dose, mini-dose, etc.)

Immunization Administration for Vaccines/Toxoids

The Immunization Administration subsection codes (90465-90474) are reported in conjunction with the Vaccines, Toxoids subsection codes (90476-90749). Immunization reporting requires two codes: one to report the **administration** and one to report the **substance** administered. A variety of administration methods are utilized to deliver the vaccine/toxoid: percutaneous, intradermal, subcutaneous, intramuscular, intranasal, or oral. The administration codes are divided based on the **method** of administration and in some codes, the patient **age**. Report each dose administered—single or combination with the appropriate administration code.

- Codes 90465-90468 report immunization administration for patients under the age of 8 and for which the physician has counseled the patient's family regarding the injection.
- Codes 90465 and 90466 report percutaneous, intradermal, subcutaneous, or intramuscular injection.
- Codes 90467 and 90468 report intranasal or oral routes of administration.

For example, you can report multiple administrations by reporting 90471 for the first administration and then reporting 90472 for each administration after the first.

Example

90471	**Administration** service for tetanus
90703	Tetanus toxoid (substance injected, IM)
90472	**Administration** service for rubella
90706	Rubella virus (substance injected, SC)
90472	**Administration** service for diphtheria (may require -59, based on payer guidelines)
90719	Diphtheria toxoid (substance injected, IM)

Or you can report the first administration with 90471, as you would usually do, and then report 90472 times the number of injections after the first one.

Example—Administration

90471	Administration service for tetanus
90472 × 2	Administration service, rubella and diphtheria

If several vaccines were administered, report the service as:

Example—Multiple Vaccines

90471	Administration service for tetanus and diphtheria
90702	Tetanus and diphtheria toxoids (substances injected, IM)
90472	Administration service for rubella
90706	Rubella virus (substance injected, SC)

NCCI

Medicare reimburses for tetanus injections (90703 [tetanus, age 7>, IM], and 90718 [tetanus/diphtheria, age 7>, IM]) when given for an acute injury to a person who is incompletely immunized. When a tetanus booster is given to a patient in the absence of an injury, the injection (90703) is not covered by Medicare.

Vaccines, Toxoids

The Vaccines, Toxoids subsection codes (90476-90749) report vaccine products for immunizations. The subsection contains many codes for a single disease (e.g., 90703 for tetanus toxoid) as well as codes for a combination of diseases (e.g., 90701 for diphtheria, tetanus, and pertussis [DTP]). In many of the code descriptions, specific ages are identified. For example, 90658, influenza vaccine, specifies age 3 and above, whereas code 90657, influenza vaccine, specifies ages 6 to 35 months. Vaccines have pediatric or adult listed on the label of the vial. You must carefully review the description of the vaccine product to determine which disease is specified in the code you are assigning. When one code is available to describe multiple products given, the combination code must be assigned. If each vaccine were to be listed separately when a combination vaccine was administered, it would be considered unbundling.

NCCI

Medicare does not reimburse for the pediatric dose of a pneumococcal vaccine reported with 90669. When reporting an adult dose of a pneumococcal vaccine (90732) to Medicare, the pneumococcal administration code is **G0009** with a diagnosis code of **V03.82** (prophylactic vaccination, streptococcus pneumoniae). Once Medicare has assigned a HCPCS Level II administration code for a vaccine, the CPT administration code is not accepted.

From the Trenches

"I often tell coders and auditors I work with that they are detectives and should think and act like a detective, never giving up until they have dug up all the information that they can to back up what they are telling a physician or non-physician practitioner."

STEPHANIE

✋ **CAUTION**   *There are often multiple codes available for variations of the product. For example, there are eight codes with combinations of diphtheria. Read all descriptions carefully before assigning a code.*

There are codes with schedules for a vaccine, such as a three-dose or four-dose schedule. For example, 90633 is a two-dose hepatitis A vaccine that is intended to be administered on a two-dose schedule. Each time the vaccine is administered, 90633 is reported along with the date of the injection. The term schedule refers to the number of doses provided and the timing of the administration. The doses and timing must be exactly as specified in the code.

The CPT Guidelines state that modifier -51 (multiple procedures) should not be reported for the vaccines/toxoids when performed with administration procedures. Most payers want you to report the administration codes multiple times or use the "times" symbol (×) to indicate the number of injections given.

If a patient is given a vaccine in the course of an E/M service, the administration and Vaccine/Toxoids codes are assigned in addition to the E/M code. Some third-party payers require a -25 modifier on the E/M code, so be certain to check with your local payer on how to submit the E/M code.

CODING SHOT   If the only service is administration of a vaccine and no other service was provided, do not report an E/M service.

CPT INFLUENZA VACCINE CODES:

CPT	90657	Influenza virus vaccine split, virus when administered to children **6-35 months of age,** for intramuscular use
	90658	Influenza virus vaccine, split virus when administered to individuals **3 years of age and older,** for intramuscular use

REPORT ADMINISTRATION OF INFLUENZA VACCINE:

HCPCS	G0008	Administration of influenza vaccine (Medicare only)
CPT	90471	Intramuscular administration, one vaccine
	90472	Intramuscular administration, each additional vaccine

CPT PNEUMOCOCCAL VACCINE CODE:

	90732	Pneumococcal polysaccharide **vaccine,** 23-valent, 2 years of age and older, for subcutaneous or intramuscular use

REPORT ADMINISTRATION OF PNEUMOCOCCAL VACCINE:

HCPCS	G0009	Administration of pneumococcal vaccine (Medicare only)
CPT	90471	Intramuscular administration, one vaccine
	90472	Intramuscular administration, each additional vaccine

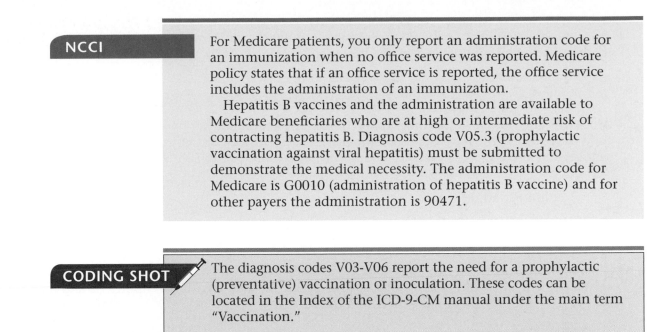

NCCI

For Medicare patients, you only report an administration code for an immunization when no office service was reported. Medicare policy states that if an office service is reported, the office service includes the administration of an immunization.

Hepatitis B vaccines and the administration are available to Medicare beneficiaries who are at high or intermediate risk of contracting hepatitis B. Diagnosis code V05.3 (prophylactic vaccination against viral hepatitis) must be submitted to demonstrate the medical necessity. The administration code for Medicare is G0010 (administration of hepatitis B vaccine) and for other payers the administration is 90471.

CODING SHOT

The diagnosis codes V03-V06 report the need for a prophylactic (preventative) vaccination or inoculation. These codes can be located in the Index of the ICD-9-CM manual under the main term "Vaccination."

EXERCISE 25-1 *Immunizations*

To report an E/M service with a vaccine service, a separate identifiable E/M service must have been provided and documented in the medical record. The following vaccines were administered to a variety of patients. If they have a brief history and examination performed to assess vaccine needs and general health status no E/M service will be reported except if the question indicates there was a "separate service" provided.

1 A parent takes a 9-year-old child to the child's physician for an oral poliomyelitis vaccine. The physician's assistant evaluates the child (established patient) and administers the vaccine orally to the child.

    CPT Codes: _____ (poliovirus vaccine), _____ (administration)

    ICD-9-CM Code: _____ (ICD-10-CM Code: _____)

2 An established patient (10 years old); the only service for the visit is an injection of DTP (diphtheria, tetanus toxoid, pertussis) and oral poliovirus. Services were provided by the nurse, at the direction of the physician.

    CPT Codes: _____ (DT vaccine), _____ (poliovirus vaccine),

    _____ _____ (administrations)

    ICD-9-CM Code: _____ (ICD-10-CM Code: _____)

3 An established patient, a 1-year-old, is brought in for a well-baby checkup (separate service) by the physician, and the following are given: DT and IM injectable poliomyelitis. The physician counseled the parent on the vaccines. A comprehensive preventative medicine evaluation was provided by the physician.

    CPT Codes: _____ (E/M), _____ (vaccine), _____

    (vaccine), _____ _____ (administrations)

    ICD-9-CM Codes: _____ (vaccinations), _____ _____ (routine

    examination) (ICD-10-CM Codes: _____ _____, _____)

Continued

4 A 64-year-old established patient comes in for an influenza virus (not preservative-free) vaccine that is administered intramuscularly by the nurse. The vaccine is the only service provided at that visit.

   CPT Codes: _____ (vaccination), _____ (administration)

   ICD-9-CM Code: _____ (ICD-10-CM Code: _____)

5 A new patient, 30 years old, comes for an office visit to evaluate her hypothyroid status at which time the physician does an expanded problem focused history and physical examination (separate service) and also administers a DTP and *Haemophilus influenzae* B (Hib) vaccine.

   CPT Codes: _____ (E/M), _____ (vaccine), _____ (administration)

   ICD-9-CM Codes: _____, _____, _____

   (ICD-10-CM Code: _____)

6 A parent brings an 18-month-old infant (established patient) for a well-baby examination (separate service) at which the physician administers a vaccine intramuscularly for diphtheria and tetanus toxoid (DT) after counseling the parent on the vaccines.

   CPT Codes: _____ (E/M), _____ (vaccine), _____ (administration)

   ICD-9-CM Codes: _____, _____

   (ICD-10-CM Codes: _____, _____)

7 A 50-year-old established patient presents to the nurse for a flu shot.

   CPT Codes: _____, _____

   ICD-9-CM Code: _____ (ICD-10-CM Code: _____)

PSYCHIATRY The Psychiatry subsection (90801-90899) has a lengthy note under the heading detailing the use of psychiatric codes in conjunction with hospital and clinic E/M services. If psychiatric treatments are rendered on the same day as E/M services, both the E/M service and the psychiatric treatment are reported with one code from the Psychiatry subsection. For example, if a patient is admitted to the hospital with a drug overdose secondary to depression, and the physician spends 25 minutes in supportive psychotherapy with the patient several hours after he was admitted to the hospital, services are reported with 90817 (Individual Medical Psychotherapy) for the psychiatric treatment and medical evaluation/management on the same day. Code 90817 includes the development of orders, the review and interpretation of laboratory work or other diagnostic studies, and the review of therapy reports and other information from the medical record. If the psychiatric treatment is provided on a different day than the E/M service, a code from the E/M section would be reported in addition to the psychiatry code. You will work closely with third-party payers to determine any specific regional instructions for coding psychiatric services.

Partial hospitalization refers to a hospital setting in which the patients are in the hospital during the day and return to their homes in the evenings and on weekends. The facilities may be open only during the day, 5 days a week, although there are also facilities that are open 7 days a week. When a physician admits a patient to a partial hospital facility, the physician is responsible for preparing all of the admission paperwork that is prepared for admission to an acute care hospital. E/M Initial Hospital Care and Subsequent Hospital Care codes (99221-99233) report inpatient stays. The psychiatric services the physician provides to the patient are listed separately unless the E/M service and psychiatric service are provided on the same day. These same-day services are reported with codes from the Psychiatry subsection.

Specific descriptions of services included in each of the codes appear in the Psychiatry subsection. Some codes reflect evaluation or diagnostic services, such as CPT code 90801 (psychiatric diagnostic interview evaluation); some reflect therapeutic procedures, such as 90804 (individual psychotherapy); and still others, located in the Central Nervous System Assessments/Tests, report psychological testing, such as code 96101 (psychological testing, per hour).

A **psychiatrist** is a physician who specializes in psychiatry. A **psychologist** is not a physician but is a qualified specialist in psychiatry. States have varying regulations about how a psychologist reports services provided, and some states require a psychologist to provide and report services only under the supervision of a psychiatrist. Third-party payers may also restrict the types of service a psychologist may report for reimbursement.

Time is the major billing factor in the Psychiatry subsection. Diagnostic and therapeutic time must be documented in the patient's record to provide accurate billing.

Code 90801, comprehensive psychiatric service is described as the elicitation (gathering) of a complete medical (including past, family, social) and psychiatric history, establishment of a tentative diagnosis, and an evaluation of the patient's ability and willingness to work to solve the mental problem. This service includes a complete mental status exam. Information may be obtained from the patient, other physicians and/or family. There may be overlapping of the medical and psychiatric history depending on the problem. An E/M service may be substituted for the initial interview procedure, including consultation codes (99241-99245), provided the required elements of the E/M service are provided. Consultation services require, in addition to the history and examination, a written report of the consultation's opinion or advice. Consultation does not include psychiatric treatment.

Interactive psychiatric diagnostic interview examination using play equipment, physical devices, language interpreter, or other mechanisms of communication is reported with 90802.

Insight-oriented, behavior modifying, and/or supportive psychotherapy is reported with 90804-90809, 90816-90822, or 90853. These services refer to the development of insight or understanding through the use of behavior modification techniques, supportive interactions, discussion of reality, or any combination of these to result in a change in the patient's behavior.

Interactive psychotherapy (90810-90815, 90823-90829, 90857) is typically furnished to children. It involves the use of physical aids and non-verbal communication to overcome the communication barriers between the physician and a patient who has lost, or has not yet developed, the language or communication skills to explain his/her symptoms, response to treatment, or to understand the physician.

Some patients receive psychotherapy only and others receive psychotherapy and medical E/M services. E/M services involve a variety of responsibilities unique to the medical management of psychiatric patients, such as medical diagnostic evaluation, drug management when indicated, physician orders, interpretation of laboratory or other medical diagnostic studies and observations, review of activity therapy reports, the supervision of nursing and ancillary personnel, and scheduling of hospital resources for diagnosis and treatment, and leadership or direction of a treatment team.

To report psychotherapy, the code is chosen on the basis of the **type** of psychotherapy (interactive using nonverbal techniques vs. insight-oriented, behavior modifying, and/or supportive using verbal techniques), the **place** of service (office vs inpatient), the face-to-face time spent with the patient during psychotherapy, and whether E/M services were furnished on the same **date** of service as psychotherapy.

The medical record must indicate the **time** spent in the psychotherapy encounter and the therapeutic maneuvers, such as behavior modification, supportive interactions, and interpretation of unconscious motivation, that were applied to produce the therapeutic change.

The medical record should document the symptoms, the goals of therapy, and the methods of monitoring the outcome. It should also document why the chosen therapy is the appropriate treatment modality either instead of or in addition to another form of psychiatric treatment.

EXERCISE 25-2 *Psychiatry*

Using the CPT manual and ICD-9-CM, code the following:

1 Individual medical psychotherapy in office for 30 minutes. The patient was diagnosed with chronic paranoid psychosis.

   CPT Code: _____

   ICD-9-CM Code: _____ (ICD-10-CM Code: _____)

2 Psychological testing, 2 hours, administered by a physician. The patient presents with moderate undersocialized aggressive outburst conduct disorder.

   CPT Code: _____ × _____

   ICD-9-CM Code: _____ (ICD-10-CM Code: _____)

3 Psychiatric evaluation of tests, medical records, or hospital data to make appropriate diagnosis for a 16-year-old male. Documentation supports an overanxious disorder.

   CPT Code: _____

   ICD-9-CM Code: _____ (ICD-10-CM Code: _____)

4 An initial psychiatric interview examination is provided for a patient that presents in a depressive state with tremors.

   CPT Code: _____

   ICD-9-CM Codes: _____, _____

   (ICD-10-CM Codes: _____, _____)

BIOFEEDBACK   **Biofeedback** is the process of giving a person self-information. The information can be used by patients to gain control over physiologic processes, such as blood pressure, heart rate, or pain. Patients are trained to use biofeedback by a professional and then continue the use of the therapy on their own. Biofeedback training is often incorporated in individual psychophysiologic therapy. When biofeedback is part of the individual psychophysiologic therapy, one code is reported for both the biofeedback training and the individual psychophysiologic therapy (90875).

Biofeedback codes (90901, 90911) are located in the CPT manual index under the main terms "Training" and "Biofeedback."

EXERCISE 25-3   *Biofeedback*

Using the CPT manual and ICD-9-CM, code the following:

1 A 40-year-old woman has been seen by the physician for several individual psychiatric sessions as the patient attempts to give up a two-pack-a-day cigarette **addiction** of 15 years' continuous duration. The patient is experiencing increased **anxiety** and **insomnia**, which is the reason for this visit. As a part of the last 30-minute psychiatric session, the physician teaches the patient to use biofeedback in an attempt to help her alleviate the generalized anxiety and idiopathic insomnia. The patient is instructed to use the biofeedback techniques three times a day until the next session.

   CPT Code: _____

   ICD-9-CM Codes: _____, _____, _____

   (ICD-10-CM Codes: _____, _____, _____)

2 A 52-year-old man is referred to the physician by his primary care physician for biofeedback to help regulate his blood pressure. The patient was diagnosed with hypertensive heart disease. There is no evidence of heart failure. The physician conducts a 60-minute session during which the patient is trained in the use of biofeedback.

   CPT Code: _____

   ICD-9-CM Code: _____ ___ (ICD-10-CM Code: _____)

DIALYSIS   Dialysis is the cleansing of the blood of waste products when it is not possible for the body to perform the cleansing function adequately on its own. Dialysis may be temporary, as in the case of a patient who has acute renal failure from which he or she recovers, or permanent, as in the case of a patient with end-stage renal disease (ESRD) who will not recover without a kidney transplant.

   The Dialysis subsection of the Medicine section (90935-90999) is divided into types of dialysis (see Table 25–1).

Hemodialysis   **Hemodialysis** is the routing of blood and its waste products to the outside of the body where it is filtered. After the blood is cleansed, it is returned to the body. Hemodialysis codes (90935 and 90937) are reported for each day the service is provided. The codes in the hemodialysis category are based on the number of times the physician evaluates the patient during the procedure.

Peritoneal Dialysis   **Peritoneal dialysis** (90945, 90947) involves using the peritoneal cavity as a filter. Dialysis fluid is introduced into the cavity and left there for several hours so cleansing can take place (Fig. 25–3). The dialysis fluid is then drained from the peritoneal cavity. Peritoneal dialysis is reported on the basis of each day the service is provided. Some patients learn how to perform dialysis for themselves. Dialysis teaching codes are located under Other Dialysis Procedures.

End Stage Renal Disease   The subheading (End Stage Renal Disease Services) deals with dialysis of a permanent nature. The 90951-90966 codes reflect all services included in treating a patient with ESRD and are listed according to patient age (e.g., younger than 2 years of age, 2-11 years of age) and number of visits (1, 2-3, 4+) per month. Dialysis services are reported as a monthly fee. For those cases in which a patient may be, for example, visiting the area and will not require a full month of dialysis, daily fees may be reported using codes 90967-90970 in the ESRD category. Few third-party payers allow E/M codes to be reported in addition to dialysis service codes. Most payers consider

TABLE 25–1

TYPES OF DIALYSIS

The codes to report physician services for patients with end-stage renal disease are located in the 90951-90970 range. Codes 90951-90962 report a full month of physician service that includes monitoring the nutritional needs of the patient, assessing the status of the patient, and counseling. The monthly services are reported based on the age of the patient and number of face-to-face visits that occurred during the month.

Age	Visits per Month	Code
≤2	4+	90951
	2-3	90952
	1	90953
2-11	4+	90954
	2-3	90955
	1	90956
12-19	4+	90957
	2-3	90958
	1	90959
20+	4+	90960
	2-3	90961
	1	90962

If the physician provides the same evaluation and management to a patient receiving home dialysis, the monthly service is reported based on the age of the patient.

Age	Code
≤2	90963
2-11	90964
12-19	90965
20+	90966

If the physician provides these same services for less than a total month, the services are also reported based on the age of the patient.

Age	Code
≤2	90967
2-11	90968
12-19	90969
20+	90970

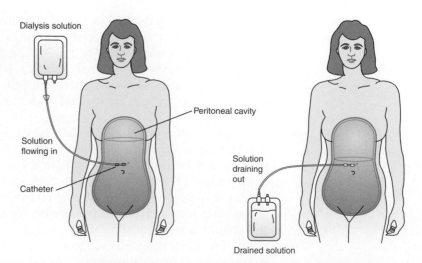

Dialysis solution

Peritoneal cavity

Solution flowing in

Catheter

Solution draining out

Drained solution

FIGURE 25–3   Peritoneal dialysis can be done by the patient. The dialysis solution enters the peritoneal cavity by a catheter. After the solution has been inside the patient for several hours, it is drained out through the catheter.

the dialysis codes to be bundled to include all the treatment necessary for a patient with renal disease, including the E/M services. To report a separate E/M service, the condition would have to be unrelated to the renal condition and modifier -25 must be added to the E/M code. The diagnosis code reported would also indicate that the E/M service was unrelated to the ESRD service.

Dialysis is usually performed in an outpatient setting at a hospital or other outpatient dialysis facility (Fig. 25–4). The physician services are reported based on the **type** of dialysis the patient is receiving, the **complexity** of the service, and the **number** of visits the physician provides to the patient. The reporting of just one code covers all physician visits to the dialysis laboratory during that month. During a physician's visit to the dialysis laboratory, the physician assesses the patient while the patient is receiving dialysis. The monthly services also include nutrition assessment and telephone calls.

Dialysis patients must sometimes be admitted to the hospital and while in the hospital must continue to receive dialysis treatments. When the physician assesses the inpatient while the patient is undergoing dialysis, report 90935 (single visit) or 90937 (multiple visits). Code 90937 may include a significant revision of the dialysis prescription. If a hospitalized patient receiving peritoneal dialysis is assessed by the physician, the physician services are reported with 90945 (single visit) and 90947 (multiple visits). Code 90947 may also include a significant revision of the dialysis prescription. Modifier -26 is not used on these codes, as the code descriptions describe only the physician service to the dialysis patient.

CODING SHOT

If a patient is admitted to the hospital and requires management of his/her dialysis while in the hospital, the physician can report those services, but then cannot report the monthly service for the time period the patient is in the hospital. The monthly services for services provided when the patient was not in the hospital is then reported with 90967-90970, which are per day codes.

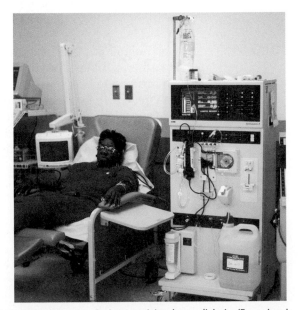

FIGURE 25–4 Patient receiving hemodialysis. (From Lewis SM, Heitkemper MM, Dirksen SR: *Medical-Surgical Nursing: Assessment and Management of Clinical Problems*, ed 6, St. Louis, 2004, Mosby.)

When a patient does not receive a full month of dialysis in the outpatient setting because of a kidney transplant, relocation, or death, report the number of days the patient had dialysis. For example, a 50-year-old patient receives peritoneal dialysis from March 1 through 10. On March 11, the patient receives a kidney transplant. The 10 days of service are reported with 90970 × 10.

"Dialysis" is the main term to be referenced in the CPT manual index.

EXERCISE 25-4 *Dialysis*

Using the CPT manual and ICD-9-CM, code the following dialysis services:

1 A 10-year-old patient with end-stage renal disease has 3 encounters during a full month of hemodialysis treatment

   CPT Code: _____

   ICD-9-CM Code: _____ (ICD-10-CM Code: _____)

2 Hemodialysis for an inpatient with a single physician evaluation for acute renal failure

   CPT Code: _____

   ICD-9-CM Code: _____ (ICD-10-CM Code: _____)

3 Peritoneal dialysis provided for an inpatient with repeated physician evaluations. The patient has acute renal failure with tubular necrosis.

   CPT Code: _____

   ICD-9-CM Code: _____ (ICD-10-CM Code: _____)

Define the following terms or abbreviations:

4 peritoneal _____

5 hemofiltration _____

6 ESRD _____

GASTROENTEROLOGY   The Gastroenterology subsection (91000-91299) contains many types of tests and treatments that are performed on the esophagus, stomach, and intestine. Several intubation codes are listed in the Gastroenterology subsection. You must carefully review the code descriptions to determine which services are bundled into the code. For example, CPT code 91055 includes intubation, collection, and preparation of specimens. Because these three services are bundled into one code, it would be incorrect to code each service individually.

EXERCISE 25-5 *Gastroenterology*

Using the CPT manual and ICD-9-CM, code the following:

1 A 2-hour gastroesophageal reflux test with nasal catheter intraluminal impedance electrode for detection of reflux. The patient was diagnosed with gastroesophageal reflux.

   CPT Code: _____

   ICD-9-CM Code: _____ (ICD-10-CM Code: _____)

2 Gastric intubation and aspiration for treatment of ingested poison

   CPT Code: _____

3 Gastric intubation with washings and slide preparation for cytology. The patient has persistent abdominal pain and loss of appetite.

   CPT Code: _____

   ICD-9-CM Codes: _____, _____

   (ICD-10-CM Codes: _____, _____)

Define the following terms:

4 motility study _____

5 manometric studies _____

OPHTHALMOLOGY

The notes located at the beginning of the Ophthalmology subsection (92002-92499) describe the services included in the various types of ophthalmologic services. Ophthalmology is a very specialized field and ophthalmologists treat patients for a variety of diseases and injuries. Often the services provided and documented do not adequately fall into an E/M definition. Therefore, the AMA developed specialized codes that deal specifically with ophthalmology services. There are extensive subsection notes that are required reading before you code in the subsection. The notes explain the levels of service and present excellent examples to clarify the assignment of the codes.

The general ophthalmologic services (e.g., routine yearly eye examinations) are located in the subheading General Ophthalmological Services. The codes in this subsection are based on whether the patient is a new or an established patient and on the complexity of service provided. There are two levels of service (intermediate and comprehensive). Of special note are the definitions of new and established patients.

The definitions of the terms "new" and "established" patient are the same as those used in the E/M section. You will recall that those definitions are as follows:

New patient: One who has not received any face-to-face professional service from the physician, or another physician of the same specialty who belongs to the same group practice, within the past 3 years.

Established patient: One who has received face-to-face professional services from the physician, or another physician of the same specialty who belongs to the same group practice, within the past 3 years.

The subheading Special Ophthalmological Services contains **bilateral** codes. Each service in this subheading is performed on both eyes, and the codes do not require a modifier to indicate that two eyes were examined or tested. In fact, should you need to report only one eye from these codes, you add modifier -52 to indicate a reduced service. It is a good idea to make a note next to the codes that are bilateral in the CPT manual and also to make a note of modifier -52, to reduce the service if it was performed for only one eye.

Special Ophthalmological Service codes are those services that are not normally performed in a general eye examination. Services in this group are performed for medically indicated reasons. For example, an ophthalmological examination under general anesthesia with manipulation of the globe of the eye to determine the range of motion (92018). The definitions of the codes are very comprehensive in detailing the services involved with each code.

Other codes that are located in the Ophthalmology subsection under the subheading Spectacle Services report the provision of materials to the patient (e.g., spectacles, contact lenses, or ocular prostheses). The refraction that is performed to determine the lens prescription may be reported separately, depending on the policies set by third-party payers.

The decision to assign an ophthalmology code or an E/M code is determined by the level of E/M service documented. The ophthalmology codes have specific notes prior to code 92002 that serve as a guideline for an intermediate or comprehensive service. Documentation should include the chief complaint, history, and general medical examination. Testing may include the following types of measures:

- External examination, ophthalmoscopy, and biomicroscopy for an acute complicated condition
- Visual acuity (clarity of vision)
- Basic sensorimotor examination (tests sensory and motor coordination)
- Confrontation visual fields (peripheral vision)
- Tonometry (intraocular pressure)
- Evaluation of complete visual system
- May include mydriasis (excess dilation of pupil) for ophthalmoscopy
- Initiation of diagnosis and treatment programs

An **intermediate** ophthalmological service (92002, 92012) describes an evaluation of a new or existing condition complicated with a new diagnosis or management problem not necessarily relating to the primary diagnosis.

A **comprehensive** service (92004, 92014) describes a general evaluation of the complete visual system (Fig. 25–5). The comprehensive services

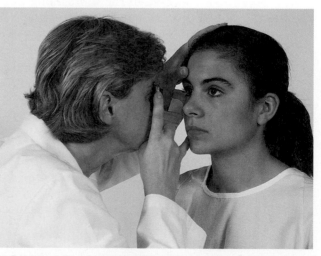

FIGURE 25–5   Examination of the eye. (From Jarvis C: *Physical Examination & Health Assessment,* ed 5, St. Louis, 2008, Saunders.)

constitute a single service that may be performed at different sessions, but is reported only once.

The initiation of diagnostic and treatment program includes the prescription of medication, and arranging for special ophthalmological diagnostic or treatment services, consultations, laboratory procedures and radiological services.

From the Trenches

"Coding is an evolving science; in order to be successful a coder needs to be willing to use every day to the fullest by continuing their education and learning something new and useful."

STEPHANIE

QUICK CHECK 25-2

1. Many of the codes for Contact Lens and Spectacle services are selected based on the diagnosis of aphakia. Define aphakia.

EXERCISE 25-6 *Ophthalmology*

Using the CPT manual and ICD-9-CM, code the following:

1 Established patient, comprehensive ophthalmologic examination

    CPT Code: _____

2 Fitting of contact lens for treatment of a cataract, including the lens

    CPT Code: _____

3 Tonography (indention method) with interpretation and report. The patient presented with preglaucoma.

    CPT Code: _____

    ICD-9-CM Code: _____ (ICD-10-CM Code: _____)

4 New patient, comprehensive ophthalmologic examination. The patient presented with proliferative diabetic retinopathy. The patient has Type I diabetes mellitus under good control.

    CPT Code: _____

    ICD-9-CM Codes: _____ (diabetes with ophthalmic manifestation), _____

    (proliferative retinopathy) (ICD-10-CM Codes: _____, _____)

SPECIAL OTORHINOLARYN-GOLOGIC SERVICES

The services in this subsection (92502-92700) are special tests or studies of the ears, nose, and larynx. Audiology (hearing) testing is also located in the Special Otorhinolaryngologic Services subsection. An audiology test may be performed by a physician or an audiologist trained in this area.

Otorhinolaryngologic diagnostic and treatment services are usually reported using codes from the Surgery section. Special services are reported using the otorhinolaryngologic codes from the Medicine section. For example, a nasopharyngoscopy with endoscopy provided during an office visit would be reported with 92511 (nasopharyngoscopy with endoscopy, the procedure) and a code from the E/M section for the office visit (with -25).

EXERCISE 25-7 *Special Otorhinolaryngologic Services*

Using the CPT manual and ICD-9-CM, code the following:

1 Monaural hearing aid check in ear (monaural: "mon," one and "aural," ear)

CPT Code: _____

2 Screening test, pure tone, air only

CPT Code: _____

3 A nasopharyngoscopy with endoscope due to recent bloody sputum

CPT Code: _____

ICD-9-CM Code: _____ (ICD-10-CM Code: _____)

4 Nasal function study due to inadequate respiratory air flow

CPT Code: _____

ICD-9-CM Code: _____ (ICD-10-CM Code: _____)

 CONGRATULATIONS! Keep up the hard work; you will soon be finished with the entire CPT manual!

CARDIOVASCULAR

The Cardiovascular subsection is discussed in Chapter 16, but there are also some services that are reported with Medicine codes that you have not reviewed yet. Let's take a closer look at these services.

Therapeutic Services

Under this heading you will find invasive and noninvasive cardiovascular service codes (92950-92998), such as cardiopulmonary resuscitation (CPR) and cardioconversions (changing [converting] an abnormal heart rhythm to a normal one). Transluminenal coronary angioplasty (PTCA) codes 92982 and 92984 are also located in here. For PTCA, two catheters are placed; one a central venous catheter inserted through the femoral or brachial artery and a second catheter with a balloon tip is threaded up to the heart. The balloon is inflated in the area of occlusion and the occlusive material is pressed back, thereby widening the vessel.

Cardiography (93000-93278), Implantable and Wearable Cardiac Device Evaluations (93279-93299), and Echocardiography (93303-93352) were reviewed in Chapter 16 of this text.

Cardiac Catheterization

Codes 93501-93533 report cardiac catheterization, which is a diagnostic medical procedure performed on the heart. Cardiac Catheterization codes were also reviewed in Chapter 16 of this text. In this section you report the catheter placement, injection, and guidance services with the following codes:

- Catheter placement 93501-93533
- Injection 93539-93545
- Guidance 93555-93556

The right side of the heart may be accessed by entering the right femoral vein and advancing through the inferior vena cava or entering the basilic vein in the arm and advancing through the superior vena cava. Right heart catheters are used to measure and record right atrial, right ventricular, pulmonary artery, and pulmonary capillary wedge pressures. Right-sided pressure measurements help diagnose congestive heart failure and right-sided valve disease.

The left side of the heart is approached through the arterial system. Access is commonly through the right femoral artery and advancing through the ascending aorta, the aortic valve, and into the left ventricle. A left heart catheterization will help to diagnose coronary artery disease, left ventricular dysfunction, and valve disease.

Fig. 25–6 shows examples of both right and left cardiac catheters.

Noninvasive Vascular Diagnostic Studies

The codes in this subsection (93875-93990) report procedures that are conducted to study veins and arteries other than the heart and great vessels. These studies use the same devices as are used in heart and great-vessel echocardiography, except that the divisions are based on the location of the vein or artery being studied.

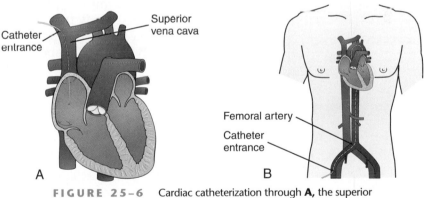

FIGURE 25–6 Cardiac catheterization through **A,** the superior vena cava, or **B,** the femoral artery.

EXERCISE 25-8 *Noninvasive Vascular Diagnostic Studies*

Using the CPT and ICD-9-CM manuals, code the following:

1 A patient is referred for a single-level, bilateral venous occlusion plethysmography of the legs. The patient has complained of intermittent leg claudication.

CPT Code: _____

ICD-9-CM Code: _____ (ICD-10-CM Code: _____)

2 A 34-year-old patient presents with a history of inability to sustain an erection due to organic impotence. The physician uses a duplex scan to conduct a complete study of the arterial and venous flow of the penis.

CPT Code: _____

ICD-9-CM Code: _____ (ICD-10-CM Code: _____)

PULMONARY Codes in the Pulmonary subsection (94002-94799) report therapies, such as nebulizer treatments, incentive spirometry (illustrated in Fig. 25–7), and diagnostic tests, such as pulmonary function tests. A nebulizer (Fig. 25–8) is a device that produces a spray, which is inhaled; it is used to treat patients with, for example, asthma. Pulmonary function tests monitor the function of the pulmonary system and examine the lung capacity of patients with, for example, emphysema. In most cases, several pulmonary function tests are performed together. The data are then compiled, and a diagnosis is made. Several indicators must be present from a variety of tests, and those tests must be performed many times and produce the same result each time for the results to be considered conclusive. In most cases, each type of test is reported separately, unless it is specifically stated otherwise in the code description.

FIGURE 25–7 Incentive spirometry is used to promote alveolar inflation and lung capacity.

FIGURE 25-8 An acute asthmatic patient in hospital, receiving nebulized β_2 agonist (the nebulizer is driven by oxygen). (From Forbes CD, Jackson WF: *Color Atlas and Text of Clinical Medicine,* ed 3, 2003, Mosby.)

CODING SHOT Add -26 to the code when reporting only the physician interpretation of the test if the physician does not own the testing equipment.

EXERCISE 25-9 *Pulmonary*

Using the CPT and ICD-9-CM manuals, code the following:

1 Pulmonary stress test, simple

    CPT Code: _____

2 Vital capacity, total

    CPT Code: _____

3 Bronchodilation responsiveness evaluation with spirometry before and after bronchodilator treatment. The patient has a cough and a 20-year smoking dependence.

    CPT Code: _____

    ICD-9-CM Codes: _____, _____

    (ICD-10-CM Codes: _____, _____)

ALLERGY AND CLINICAL IMMUNOLOGY

Read the notes that appear at the beginning of the Allergy and Clinical Immunology subsection (95004-95199). The subsection is divided into two parts. The **first** is Allergy Testing, which describes allergy testing by various methods (percutaneous, intracutaneous, inhalation) and the type of tests (allergenic extracts, venoms, biologicals, food). The number of tests must always be specified for reporting purposes because for most of these codes, payment is made per test.

Allergy testing consist of the performance, evaluation, and interpretation of allergens placed under the skin. The testings should be based on a complete history and physical examination of the patient and correlated with signs and symptoms related to the presence of possible allergy diagnoses during allergy testing (95004-95075).

The **second** subheading is Allergen Immunotherapy and the codes specify three types of services:

1. Injection only
2. Prescription and injection
3. Provision of antigen only

All the codes in Allergen Immunotherapy have specific notes that you must read to know whether the code is for injection, prescription and injection, or antigen only. For example, code 95115 reports the injection of antigen only and does not include the extract, but code 95120 reports the prescription, extract, and injection. So careful reading of the descriptions is a necessity.

The professional service necessary to provide the immunotherapy is bundled into the code, so an office visit code would not usually be reported. If the physician provided another identifiable service at the time of the immunotherapy, an office visit may be reported. But for the patient who has only the injection, prescription, antigen, or any combination of these three, the codes already contain the professional service.

Allergy Immunotherapy is the repeated administration of allergens to patients for the purpose of providing protection against the allergic symptoms and reactions associated with exposure to these allergens. Immunotherapy (hyposensitization) may extend over a period of months, usually on an increasing dosage scale. This is followed by a build-up of tolerance to the antigen (as evidenced by the higher doses that can be administered) and a decline in the symptoms and medication requirements.

Indications for immunotherapy are determined by diagnostic testing appropriate to the individual needs of each patient and his/her clinical history of allergic diseases.

EXERCISE 25-10 *Allergy and Clinical Immunology*

Using the CPT and ICD-9-CM manuals, code the following:

1 Direct nasal mucous membrane allergy test

   CPT Code: _____

2 Percutaneous test using allergen extracts, immediate type reaction, 10 tests

   CPT Code: _____ × _____

3 Single injection of allergen using extract provided by the patient. Patient has documented allergy to ragweed.

   CPT Code: _____

   ICD-9-CM Code: _____ (ICD-10-CM Code: _____)

4 Physician prepares a 10-dose multi-vial allergenic extract for a patient. At the same encounter, one dose from this vial is administered by one injection to the patient.

   CPT Code: _____, _____

ENDOCRINOLOGY   This subsection contains only codes used to report glucose monitoring (95250, 95251). Continuous glucose monitoring is a procedure in which a probe is inserted subcutaneously and attached to a monitor that is worn by the patient. The monitor records the glucose level for a 72-hour period at which time the probe is removed and the data are downloaded from the monitor. The patient records his or her insulin administration, meals, exercise, and any hypoglycemic events during the monitoring period, in addition to performing the usual finger stick glucose four times a day during the 3-day period. The service includes the initial hookup, calibration of the monitor, patient training, recording, and downloading of data with printout of results.

NEUROLOGY AND NEUROMUSCULAR PROCEDURES

There are codes in the Neurology and Neuromuscular Procedures (95803-96020) subsection for sleep testing, muscle testing (electromyography), range of motion measurements (Fig. 25–9), cerebral seizure monitoring, and a variety of neurologic function tests. The codes in this subsection are usually reported by physicians who specialize in neurology (neurologists). Sleep studies in newborns are performed by pediatric pulmonologists. A neurologist usually is a consultant to a physician who is seeking the advice and input of another physician concerning a patient with suspected neurologic problems.

One of the specialized tests conducted in the neurology specialty area is sleep studies (95805-95811). **Sleep studies** are the monitoring of a patient's sleep for 6 or more hours. The studies include the tracing (technical component) and the physician's review, interpretation, and report (professional component). If a physician performs only the professional component, modifier -26 is reported.

Sleep studies diagnose various sleep disorders and measure a patient's response to therapy. An electroencephalogram (EEG) is a procedure that records changes in brain waves. **Polysomnography** (Fig. 25–10) is the measurement of the brain waves during sleep but with the added feature of

FIGURE 25–9 Range-of-motion measurements. **A,** Palmar flexion. **B,** Dorsiflexion. **C,** Ulnar deviation. **D,** Radial deviation. (From DeLee JC, Drez D: *DeLee & Drez's Orthopaedic Sports Medicine: Principles and Practice,* ed 2, Philadelphia, 2003, Saunders.)

FIGURE 25-10 Example of a patient set up to undergo polysomnography. (From Albert RK, Spiro SG, Jett JR: *Clinical Respiratory Medicine*, ed 2, Philadelphia, 2004, Mosby.)

recording the various stages of sleep (i.e., excited, relaxed, drowsy, asleep, or deep sleep). During each of these stages, the rate and amplitude (height) of the brain waves are measured and compared with normal ranges. Certain neurologic conditions may be identified by the degree to which brain waves vary from normal ranges.

Nerve conduction tests (95900-95905) are usually performed in conjunction with conventional motor nerve conduction studies of the same nerve and may include F-wave studies. F-waves assess motor nerve function along the entire extent of that nerve. An impulse generated at the stimulating electrode travels up the motor nerves to the motor neuron cell bodies in the spinal cord. The impulse then travels down the same motor nerves to the neuromuscular junction, and then to the muscle. Codes 95900, 95903, and 95904 are intended to be reported for each nerve tested, regardless of the number of stimulation sites along the sensory or motor nerve being tested. For a given patient, multiple motor or sensory nerve conduction codes may be assigned if multiple motor or sensory nerves are tested.

A nerve conduction test with F-wave study reported with 95903 bundles the services of a test report without F-wave study (95900). Procedure codes 95900 and 95903 may not be reported for the same nerve on the same day. If, during the same session, one nerve is tested without an F-wave study and a different nerve is tested with an F-wave study, report the test with an F-wave study using a -59 modifier.

Code 95905 reports motor and/or sensory nerve conduction using preconfigured electrodes that have been customized to specific anatomic sites.

H-reflex studies (95934-95936) usually involve assessment of the tibial motor nerve and the gastrocnemius-soleus muscle complex, and are not often performed in conjunction with conventional nerve conduction studies of this nerve-muscle pair. Although additional H-reflex studies of other muscles are occasionally indicated, typically only one or two H-reflex studies are

QUICK CHECK 25-3

1. According to the Sleep Testing Guidelines, polysomnography includes sleep staging with:

   a. EEG, EOG, EMG, ECG

   b. Monitoring snoring, continuous blood pressures, and body positions

   c. ECG, Extended EEG, NCPAP

   d. EEG, EOG, EMG

performed on a patient during a given encounter. Bilateral gastrocnemius-soleus H-reflex abnormalities are often early indications of spinal stenosis, bilateral S1 radiculopathies, and peripheral polyneuropathies.

Parameters are what are being measured during a sleep test. For example, parameters include the measurement of snoring or blood pressure. The number of parameters measured is listed in the code description. The patient's medical record will contain the parameters, or measurements, recorded during the test. To report sleep tests accurately, you must know the parameters and stages of testing. Additionally, many codes include a time component (such as 95803); so it is important to have the duration of the test stated in the medical record.

Electromyographic (EMG) studies use needles and electric current to stimulate nerves and record the results. Assessments of dysphasia, developmental testing, neurobehavior status, and neuropsychological test codes are also located in this subsection.

EXERCISE 25-11 *Neurology and Neuromuscular Procedures*

Using the notes under the Sleep Testing subheading and the code descriptions following the notes, identify the following abbreviations:

1 NCPAP _____

2 EEG _____

3 EMG _____

4 EOG _____

Using the CPT and ICD-9-CM manuals, code the following:

5 Awake and drowsy EEG and photic stimulation in clinic. The patient presents with episodes of sleep apnea.

   CPT Code: _____

   ICD-9-CM Code: _____ (ICD-10-CM Code: _____)

6 Needle electromyography, three extremities and related paraspinal areas. The patient complains of numbness in arms and legs.

   CPT Code: _____

   ICD-9-CM Code: _____ (ICD-10-CM Code: _____)

7 Range-of-motion measurement and report on both legs. The patient is experiencing muscular incoordination.

   CPT Code: _____ × _____

   ICD-9-CM Code: _____ (ICD-10-CM Code: _____)

CENTRAL NERVOUS SYSTEM ASSESSMENTS/TESTS

The Central Nervous System Assessments/Tests codes (96101-96125) identify psychological testing, speech/language (aphasia) assessment, developmental progress assessments, and thinking/reasoning status examination (neurobehavioral). Except for the basic developmental testing, the codes are defined on a per-hour basis. The results of all the tests are to be developed into a report that is included in the patient record.

EXERCISE 25-12 *Central Nervous System Assessments/Tests*

Using the CPT and ICD-9-CM manuals, code the following (code all cases at 60 minutes in length):

1 A mother presented to the office of a psychiatrist with a 10-year-old who had been referred by the child's pediatrician for his nonconformist conduct disturbance. At the psychiatric office visit, the mother expressed great concern about the child's inability to behave as she and the child's father believed appropriate. One week later the psychiatrist conducted several limited developmental tests of this patient. The psychiatrist then discussed the results of the tests with the mother. Code only the developmental testing.

    CPT Code: _____

    ICD-9-CM Code: _____ (ICD-10-CM Code: _____)

2 A young executive is referred for an 80-minute psychologist administered Minnesota Multiphasic Personality Inventory (MMPI) test by his employer. The employer requests the testing for all newly hired executives who will be working with highly sensitive government documents.

    CPT Code: _____

    ICD-9-CM Code: _____ (ICD-10-CM Code: _____)

3 A 14-year-old is seen in the office for a 70-minute assessment of the child's attention span. The child is experiencing increasingly severe episodes of lethargy. The physician conducts a clinical assessment of the child's cognitive function.

    CPT Code: _____

    ICD-9-CM Code: _____ (ICD-10-CM Code: _____)

HEALTH AND BEHAVIOR ASSESSMENT/ INTERVENTION

The codes in this subsection (96150-96155) do not report preventive medicine services, nor do they report psychiatric treatments. Instead, these codes report assessment and/or intervention for behavioral, emotional, social, psychological, or knowledge factors that are affecting the patient's health. Examples of **assessments** are clinical interview, behavior observation, and questionnaires. Examples of **interventions** are individual, group, or family sessions. All services are based on 15-minute increments. These services are not performed by a physician. If these services are performed by a physician they are reported with E/M codes.

Hydration

Codes 96360 and 96361 report hydration services. The physician's work related to these services usually involves oversight of the treatment plan and staff supervision. When the physician provides a significant separately identifiable E/M service, report the service with an appropriate E/M service reporting modifier -25. Modifier -25 must be added to the E/M code or the service will be assumed to be related to the physician's service for the hydration, injection, or infusion service.

Bundled into the hydration services are local anesthesia, placing the intravenous line, accessing an indwelling access line/ catheter/port, flushing at the end of the infusion, and all standard supplies.

Codes 96360 and 96361 report intravenous hydration infusions that include the **prepackaged** fluid and electrolytes. If other than a prepackaged substance is used, that substance would be reported separately. Saline is not reported separately unless given alone for hydration. If the drugs are mixed into the saline, then only the drug is reported and the saline is bundled into the cost of the drug and not reported separately. Included in these hydration codes are the physician supervision and oversight of the staff providing the service. Code 96360 reports 31 minutes to 1 hour of intravenous infusion hydration service and 96361, the add-on code, reports each additional hour. You can only report 96361 if the service is at least 31 minutes over the 1 hour that was reported with 90760. Time under 31 minutes is not reported.

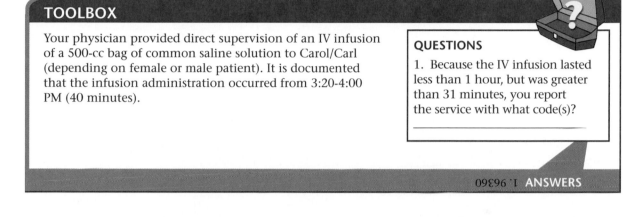

TOOLBOX

Your physician provided direct supervision of an IV infusion of a 500-cc bag of common saline solution to Carol/Carl (depending on female or male patient). It is documented that the infusion administration occurred from 3:20-4:00 PM (40 minutes).

QUESTIONS

1. Because the IV infusion lasted less than 1 hour, but was greater than 31 minutes, you report the service with what code(s)?

ANSWERS 1. 96360

Therapeutic, Prophylactic, and Diagnostic Injections and Infusions

Codes 96365-96379 report the administration of therapeutic, prophylactic, or diagnostic intravenous infusion or injection. Intravenous **infusions** are reported with 96365-96368 and are divided based on the time and type of infusion. The initial infusion is reported with 96365 (up to 1 hour) and each additional hour (over 30 minutes) is reported with 96366. Sometimes one infusion is provided followed by another infusion with a different medication (sequential infusions), in which case the initial infusion is listed first and the **sequential** infusion (96367) is listed second. There are times when more than one infusion is provided at the same time, which is a concurrent infusion. A **concurrent** infusion is when there is one site and two lines infusing at the same time. Report the initial infusion first and then the concurrent infusion (96368).

Subcutaneous infusions are reported with codes 96369-96371. Initial set up and first hour are reported with 96369. Each additional hour is reported with 96370. Additional set up for a new infusion site is reported with 96371.

To report therapeutic, prophylactic, and diagnostic **injections** (96372-96376), the physician must be present. Therapeutic, prophylactic, and diagnostic injections are divided based on the method used for the administration (Fig. 25–11). **Subcutaneous** and **intramuscular** injections are reported with 96372 in addition to a code to report the substance injected. For example, if the injection was a subcutaneous human rabies immune globulin, report 90375 for the substance and 96372 for the administration. The vaccines/toxoids are reported with 90465/90466 or 90471/90472. Code 96372 is not used to report chemotherapy administration (see 96401-96549). Injections for allergen immunotherapy are reported with 95115/95117, not with therapeutic, prophylactic, or diagnostic injection codes. **Intra-arterial** (96373) and **intravenous push** (96374/96375/96376) are reported with therapeutic, prophylactic, and diagnostic injection codes.

CHEMOTHERAPY ADMINISTRATION

Chemotherapy codes 96401-96549 report a variety of chemotherapy services. The Injection and Intravenous Infusion Chemotherapy codes (96401-96417) report subcutaneous/intramuscular, intralesional, and

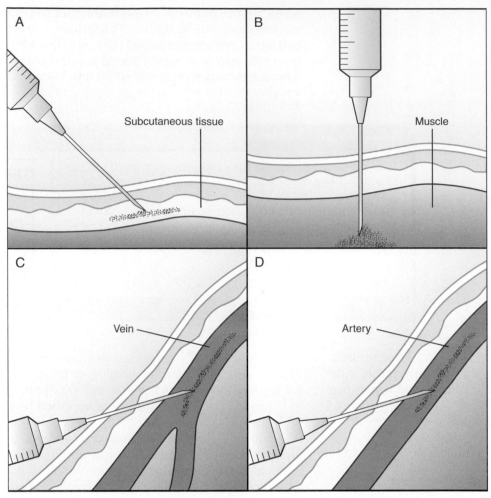

FIGURE 25–11 Injection methods. **A,** Subcutaneous (SC). **B,** Intramuscular (IM). **C,** Intravenous (IV). **D,** Intra-arterial.

intravenous chemotherapy. Intra-Arterial Chemotherapy codes (96420-96425) report various forms of chemotherapy administered via the arteries. Other Injection and Infusion Services codes (96440-96549) report other types of chemotherapy, such as pleural (96440), peritoneal (96445), and central nervous system (96450), in addition to refilling/maintenance of portable or implantable pumps or reservoirs (96521, 96522).

There are two other sets of codes used to report chemotherapy services: Hydration (96360-96361) and Therapeutic, Prophylactic, and Diagnostic Injections and Infusions (96365-96379), which you learned about earlier in this chapter. In addition to these CPT codes, HCPCS "J" codes report the substances injected or infused.

Included (not reported separately) with chemotherapy infusion or injection codes 96401-96549 are the following:

1. Use of local anesthesia
2. IV start
3. Access to indwelling intravenous, subcutaneous catheter or port
4. Flush at the conclusion of infusion
5. Standard tubing, syringes, and supplies
6. Preparation of the chemotherapy agent(s)

If other services are provided, they may be reported separately.

The initial intravenous infusion (the treatment) is reported with 96365 and each additional hour of infusion, up to 8 hours, is reported with 96366. If a sequential (one after another) intravenous therapy is provided, the service is reported with 96367. When a concurrent (at the same time as another) intravenous therapy is provided the service is reported with 96368. A concurrent infusion is one in which multiple infusions are provided through the same intravenous line. A concurrent infusion can be billed only once per patient encounter.

If more than one substance is placed in the **one** bag, it is considered **one** infusate and **one** infusion. You would report **one** administration code and a Level II HCPCS J code for each substance or drug.

Any administration that is 15 minutes or less is considered a push, not an infusion. The administration of an initial or single intravenous push is reported with 96374 and each additional push is reported with 96375. Report only one push per drug. For example, if a patient is given a push of morphine 2 mg at the beginning of a service and morphine 2 mg later in the service, bill one administration code for the two IV pushes of morphine. The appropriate units of the J code (J2270—morphine up to 10 mg × 1) would also be billed for the total dose.

If two drugs are mixed in the same bag and administered for 15 minutes or less, the service is reported with the appropriate push CPT code (initial or subsequent) × 1 unit. The drug(s) or substance would be separately reported with the appropriate J code based on the amount and type.

A patient will often receive hydration and ancillary medications before or after chemotherapy. Only one initial administration code can be reported for each encounter; other services are reported with secondary or subsequent codes.

Example

A patient presents for a chemotherapy session and is given a 40-minute hydration prior to chemotherapy reported with 96361. If the patient receives hydration before and after chemotherapy, calculate the entire time of hydration infusion and code the appropriate number of units for 96361. For example, a patient received 1 hour of hydration before chemotherapy and 40 minutes of hydration after chemotherapy. The total hydration time is 100 minutes. Code 96361 × 2 units.

Modifier -59 should be reported to indicate that hydration was provided prior to or following chemotherapy. Hydration provided at the same time as chemotherapy to facilitate drug delivery is not reported separately. All infusions must have a documented start and stop time.

The patient may also receive medications before and/or after chemotherapy, such as anti-nausea medications. These medications are reported in addition to the chemotherapy because chemotherapy is always the primary service. When the patient receives multiple intravenous infusions of medications and these medications are administered individually, each is reported separately; but if the medications are mixed together and given in one infusion, they are reported as one infusion.

Code 96375 is an add-on code and is only reported with another code, such as 96413, Chemotherapy administration. The charges for the patients in the examples that follow would list the chemotherapy administration first, followed by the other service codes since the chemotherapy is the primary service.

Example

After chemotherapy, a patient received Aloxi (J2469), Benadryl (J1200), and Decadron (J1100) in three separate infusions of less than 15 minutes (pushes). The J codes are reported along with 96375 × 3.

If the medications are all mixed together and administered in one infusion of less than 15 minutes, the J codes are reported along with 96375 × 1.

Example

A patient presents for chemotherapy and receives two pushes, one of Aloxi, 0.25 mg, and one of Benadryl, 50 mg. Chemotherapy with Rituximab, 100 mg, is administered for 3 hours by means of an intravenous infusion. After therapy, the patient is administered Decadron, 1 mg, by intravenous push. The services are reported as follows:

Pre- and post-medications: 96375 × 3 (three total IV pushes); J2469 (Aloxi) × 10 units; J1200 (Benadryl) × 1 unit; and J1100 (Decadron) × 1 unit. NOTE: 1 unit of Aloxi = 25 mcg, therefore, 0.25 mg = 250 mcg = 10 units.

Chemotherapy: 96413 (initial hour); 96415 × 2 (2 additional hours); J9310 × 1 (Rituximab). Chemotherapy is the initial infusion and the hydration and pushes are secondary/subsequent.

If a significant identifiable office visit service was provided, in addition to the chemotherapy administration, report that service with an E/M code adding -25 to indicate the service was separate and significant.

CODING SHOT

Chemotherapy administration codes (96401-96459) include the use of local anesthesia, initiating the intravenous therapy, access to an indwelling port, flush at conclusion, tubing/supplies/syringes, and preparation of the chemotherapy agent(s). These services and are not reported separately.

EXERCISE 25-13 *Chemotherapy Administration*

Using the CPT and ICD-9-CM manuals, code only the chemotherapy administration:

1 Chemotherapy injected into the pleural cavity with thoracentesis. The patient has documented primary cancer of the lungs.

    CPT Code: _____

    ICD-9-CM Code: _____ (ICD-10-CM Code: _____)

2 Refilling and maintenance of a patient's portable pump. The patient has primary adenocarcinoma of the colon.

    CPT Code: _____

    ICD-9-CM Code: _____ (ICD-10-CM Code: _____)

3 Chemotherapy administered subcutaneously with local anesthesia. The patient has melanoma of the chest wall.

    CPT Code: _____

    ICD-9-CM Code: _____ (ICD-10-CM Code: _____)

4 Chemotherapy administered intravenously using the infusion technique for 50 minutes. The patient has breast cancer with metastasis (secondary site) to the bone of the spinal column.

    CPT Code: _____

    ICD-9-CM Codes: _____, _____

    (ICD-10-CM Codes: _____, _____)

5 Chemotherapy injected into the central nervous system using a lumbar puncture. Patient has cancer of the brain, primary.

    CPT Code: _____

    ICD-9-CM Code: _____ (ICD-10-CM Code: _____)

6 An established patient is seen in the office for pernicious anemia. The nurse administers an injection of vitamin B$_{12}$, 900 mcg. Report the substance with a HCPCS Level II code. The service was not significant enough to report a separate E/M code for the office visit.

    CPT Codes: _____ (therapeutic injection), _____ (substance HCPCS code)

PHOTODYNAMIC THERAPY

The photodynamic therapy services (96567-96571) are reported in conjunction with the bronchoscopy or endoscopy services. An agent is injected into the patient that remains in cancerous cells longer than in the normal cells. After the agent has dissipated from the normal cells, the patient is exposed to laser light. The agent absorbs the light and the light produces oxygen, destroying the cancerous cells.

Codes for endoscopic application are divided on the basis of time—the first 30 minutes and each additional 15 minutes. External application is based on each exposure session.

SPECIAL DERMATOLOGICAL PROCEDURES

The dermatology codes (96900-96999) are usually reported by a dermatologist who provides services to a patient in an office on a consultation basis. The dermatology codes for special procedures would typically be reported in addition to an E/M consultation code. For example, if a patient is referred by his family physician to a dermatologist for treatment of acne. The dermatologist conducts a history and examination and treats the patient with ultraviolet light (actinotherapy). The reporting would be an Office or Other Outpatient Consultation code, depending on the level of service provided, and 96900 to report the actinotherapy.

EXERCISE 25-14 *Special Dermatological Procedures*

Using the CPT and ICD-9-CM manuals, code the following:

1 A 16-year-old patient sees a dermatologist in consultation, at which time the physician does a problem focused history and physical examination regarding the patient's acne vulgaris. The physician prescribes and provides a treatment of ultraviolet light therapy.

   CPT Codes: _____, _____

   ICD-9-CM Code: _____ (ICD-10-CM Code: _____)

2 Photochemotherapy is provided for a 34-year-old consultative patient with severe bullous dermatosis. The patient receives 8 hours of treatment. The physician provides a comprehensive history and physical examination with moderately complex medical decision making.

   CPT Codes: _____, _____

   ICD-9-CM Code: _____ (ICD-10-CM Code: _____)

From the Trenches

"Having good working relationships with physicians is the #1 priority. You need to be confident that what you are telling them is correct, and when they realize that you know what you are talking about, they will respect you."

STEPHANIE

PHYSICAL MEDICINE AND REHABILITATION

The codes in the Physical Medicine and Rehabilitation subsection (97001-97799) are reported by a physician or therapist. The subsection includes codes for different modalities of treatments (e.g., traction, whirlpool, electrical stimulation) as well as various types of patient training (e.g., functional activities, gait training, massage). The codes are reported on the basis of time or treatment area, as stated in the description of the code. Codes are divided by supervision or constant attendance. Unit coding (i.e., ×2, ×3) is necessary if the time spent administering the treatment exceeds the time listed in the code.

Example
Reporting for patient's prosthetic training of 60 minutes would be:
97761 × 4   Prosthetic training, each 15 minutes

CODING SHOT An **orthotic** is a support, splint, or brace used to align a body part, such as an elbow brace (L3700-L3766). A **prosthetic** is a replacement, such as a breast prosthesis (L8000-L8039).

All services provided by independent physical therapists and occupational therapists require a written referral from a physician that includes documentation of the disease or injury being treated and the diagnosis.

The services are rendered according to a written treatment plan determined by the provider after an appropriate assessment of the illness or injury. All providers rendering therapy must document the appropriate history, examination, diagnosis, related physician orders, therapy goals and potential for achievement, any contraindications, functional assessment, type of treatment, the body areas to be treated, the date that therapy initiated, and expected frequency and duration of treatments. This documentation must be maintained in the patient's medical record.

Documentation should indicate the prognosis for restoration of function and the medical necessity of the treatment.

Physical therapy test and measurement codes are listed by the type of testing and the time the testing requires. The type of test would be such as functional capacity. Note the use of type and time in the following CPT code.

Example

97750   Physical performance test or measurement (e.g., musculoskeletal, functional capacity, with written report, each 15 minutes)

CODING SHOT   For all codes that are time based, the time must be documented in the patient's medical record.

The codes in Physical Medicine and Rehabilitation are reported for physical medicine and therapy as well as for other rehabilitation, for example, community/work reintegration (97537).

Active Wound Care Management

Nonphysician personnel perform the procedures described in Active Wound Care Management codes (97597-97606). The codes are not reported with or to replace the surgical debridement represented by 11040-11044. If a physician performed the procedures, the services would be reported with 11040-11044.

Wound management codes are based on nonselective or negative pressure procedures. **Nonselective** debridement is that in which healthy tissue is removed along with necrotic tissue. The tissue is gradually loosened with water (hydrotherapy). Loosened tissue may be cut away with sharp instruments. Nonselective debridement is usually done over the course of several visits.

Negative Pressure Wound Therapy (NPWT, 97605, 97606), as illustrated in Figs. 25–12 and 25–13, may include vacuuming the drainage and tissue from the wound area, application of topical medications or ointments, assessment of the wound, and directions to the patient for continued care of the wound. Choice of codes is dependent on the square centimeters treated.

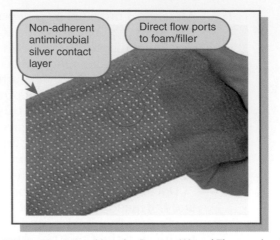

FIGURE 25-12 Negative Pressure Wound Therapy dressing. (Modified from Argentum Medical, LLC: *Silverlon® Negative Pressure Therapy Wound Dressing.* (website): http://www.silverlon.com/ pressure_dressing_vac.html. Accessed June 15, 2009.)

FIGURE 25-13 Negative pressure-assisted wound closure sponge in place on patient's abdomen. (From Townsend CM, Beauchamp RD, Evers BM, Mattox KL: *Sabiston Textbook of Surgery: The Biological Basis of Modern Surgical Practice,* ed 18, Philadelphia, 2008, Saunders.)

EXERCISE 25-15 *Physical Medicine and Rehabilitation*

Using the CPT and ICD-9-CM manuals, code the following:

1 Application of cold packs to one area (modality)

 CPT Code: _____

2 Initial prosthetic training, 30 minutes

 CPT Codes: _____ × _____

3 Physical medicine treatment procedure, gait training, 30 minutes. Patient status is post-acute Cerebrovascular Accident.

 CPT Code: _____

 ICD-9-CM Code: _____ (ICD-10-CM Code: _____)

MEDICAL NUTRITION THERAPY

These codes (97802-97804) are reported by nonphysician personnel for medical nutritional therapy assessment (NTA) or intervention. If a physician provides the service, the service is reported using E/M codes or Preventive Medicine codes.

The codes report face-to-face services with the patient based on time of 15 minutes for initial or re-assessments and 30 minutes for group assessments. The provider would review the patient's medical record, including the history of present illness and past medical history, along with pertinent laboratory data. The nutritional history would be obtained from the patient and an appropriate examination would be conducted. Documentation would indicate the nutritional assessment and prescription recommended to the patient and this information would be communicated to the health care provider.

OSTEOPATHIC MANIPULATIVE TREATMENT (OMT)

Osteopathic manipulative treatment (98925-98929) is a form of manual treatment applied by a physician to eliminate or alleviate somatic (body) dysfunction and related disorders. The codes are listed according to body regions. These body regions are the head; cervical, thoracic, lumbar, sacral, and pelvic regions; lower extremities; upper extremities; rib cage; abdomen and viscera region. Codes are separated on the basis of the number of body regions treated. These codes are usually reported by osteopathic physicians (doctors of osteopathy, DO).

CHIROPRACTIC MANIPULATIVE TREATMENT (CMT)

The Chiropractic Manipulative Treatment subsection (98940-98943) is divided by the number of regions manipulated. For this subsection, the **spine** is divided into five regions (cervical, thoracic, lumbar, sacral, and pelvic), and the **extraspinal** regions are divided into five regions (head, lower extremities, upper extremities, rib cage, and abdomen). Chiropractic manipulation is the manipulation of the spinal column and other structures. Each of the codes in the Chiropractic Manipulative Treatment subsection has a professional assessment bundled into the code. An office visit code is reported only if the patient had a significant separately identifiable service provided; otherwise, the service of the office visit is bundled into the code.

EXERCISE 25-16   *Manipulative Treatment*

Using the CPT manual and ICD-9-CM, code the following therapies:

1 Sally, a 43-year-old woman, presents with the complaint of a seizing pain in the area of her lower left hip. The chiropractor conducts an assessment of the patient and provides a chiropractic alignment to two spinal regions.

　　CPT Code: _____

　　ICD-9-CM Code: _____ (ICD-10-CM Code: _____)

2 Osteopathic lumbar manipulation (OMT), one region. Patient has chronic low back pain.

　　CPT Code: _____

　　ICD-9-CM Code: _____ (ICD-10-CM Code: _____)

NON-FACE-TO-FACE NONPHYSICIAN SERVICES

This subsection is divided into Telephone Services (98966-98968) and On-Line Medical Evaluation (98969) services provided by qualified health care professionals. The notes and the code descriptions for these codes indicate that the telephone or online service cannot originate from a related assessment that was provided within the previous 7 days or result in an appointment within the next 24 hours or the soonest available appointment. The telephone services are reported based on the documented time, and the online service is per incident.

SPECIAL SERVICES, PROCEDURES, AND REPORTS

Special Services, Procedures, and Reports (99000-99091) is a miscellaneous subsection that includes codes for services that are not reported with codes from other sections. The codes report services that are, for example, rendered at unusual hours of the day or on holidays. These codes are considered adjunct codes and are to be reported in addition to the codes for the major service. For example, if a physician goes to the office on a Sunday to meet an established patient and provide urgent, but not emergency, service, the E/M service code for the office visit would be reported in addition to 99050 to indicate the unusual time at which the service was provided.

An often reported code is 99024 for an office visit provided during a global period. Third-party payers do not reimburse for the submission of this code; however, it communicates that the service was provided to the patient during the follow-period of a previous surgical procedure.

You have assigned 99070, supplies, from this subsection before. One of the big advantages of the HCPCS coding system is that you specifically identify the supply reported rather than the more general 99070. For example, you may report 99070 for a body sock for a patient. With the HCPCS coding system, you can specify the body sock with a code L0984. It is best to use HCPCS codes when reporting supplies since most third party payers will request additional information when 99070 is submitted.

The subsection also contains codes for medical testimony, the completion of complicated reports, education services, unusual travel, and supplies. Although this subsection is small, it contains codes that are reported often. Take a few minutes to become familiar with the codes listed within Special Services, Procedures, and Reports and mark the subsection for future use.

The codes for Special Services are located in the CPT manual index under the main term "Special Services."

EXERCISE 25-17 *Special Services, Procedures, and Reports*

Using the CPT manual and ICD-9-CM, code the following:

1 What medicine code is reported in addition to the basic service code when a service is provided after hours on Monday?

   CPT Code: _____

2 Conveyance of a specimen from the physician's office to a laboratory

   CPT Code: _____

3 Supplies provided for an office visit exceeding those usually used

   CPT Code: _____

Qualifying Circumstances for Anesthesia.   Anesthesia is discussed in Chapter 11.

Moderate Sedation.   Sedation reported with 99143-99150 is discussed in Chapter 11.

OTHER SERVICES AND PROCEDURES

A wide variety of codes (99170-99199) is located in this subsection of the Medicine section. For example, you will find codes for anogenital examination with a colposcope of a child in a case of suspected trauma, visual function screenings, pumping poison from the stomach, and therapeutic phlebotomy treatments. Because the codes are so varied, the way in which they are divided is also varied. For example, the code range 99190-99192 is divided on the basis of time, whereas other codes are divided according to the extent of the service.

HOME HEALTH PROCEDURES/ SERVICES

These codes (99500-99602) report nonphysician services provided at the patient's residence. The residence may be an assisted living apartment, custodial care facility, group home, or other nontraditional residence. The codes are divided based on the reason for the service (e.g., injection, hemodialysis).

Home Infusion Procedures Services

The codes 99601 and 99602 represent services of administration of a variety of therapies (e.g., nutrition, chemotherapy, pain management). The services are provided by nonphysician allied health professionals. Codes are divided based on the time spent providing the infusion.

MEDICATION THERAPY MANAGEMENT SERVICES

These codes (99605-99607) are for patient assessments and interventions by a pharmacist, upon request. These codes do not describe the product-specific information that a pharmacist would ordinarily provide to a patient regarding a medication; but rather to assist in the management of treatment-related medication complications or interactions. The codes are reported by the pharmacist based on the patient status (new or established) and the time spent in assessment and intervention.

CHAPTER REVIEW

CHAPTER 25, PART I, THEORY

Without the use of the CPT manual, answer the following questions:

1 There are two types of services in the Medicine section. One is diagnostic and the other is

_____.

2 What do the following abbreviations mean?

  a IV _____

  b IM _____

  c SC _____

3 The routing of blood, including the waste products, outside of the body for cleansing is

_____.

4 The dialysis that involves using a cavity as a filter is known as what kind of dialysis?

_____

5 What is the name of the test that checks the intraocular pressure of the eye?

_____

6 What is the name of the scope that is used to

examine color vision? _____

7 What is the word that means the body of knowledge about the ear, nose, and larynx?

_____

8 In what subsection of the Medicine section would you find CPR, coronary atherectomies,

and heart valvuloplasties? _____

9 What kind of scanning uses ultrasonic technology with a display of both structure and

motion with time? _____

10 What is the name of the ultrasonic documentation that records velocity mapping

and imaging? _____

11 In what Medicine subsection would you find therapies such as nebulizer treatments?

_____

12 Percutaneous, intracutaneous, and inhalation are examples of what from the Allergy

subsection? _____

13 Allergenic extracts, venoms, biologicals, and food are examples of what from the Allergy

subsection? _____

14 If you were looking for the code number to indicate the circumstance in which a physician sees a patient between the hours of 10 PM and 8 AM, in what subsection of the Medicine section would you find that code?

_____

CHAPTER 25, PART II, PRACTICAL

Using the CPT manual and ICD-9-CM, code the following:

15 An 18-month-old established patient receives a DT that is administered intramuscularly by the physician, after the physician counseled the parents on the vaccine.

CPT Codes: _____,

_____

ICD-9-CM Codes: _____,

_____

(ICD-10-CM Codes: _____,

_____)

16 A 30-year-old established patient receives a tetanus toxoid that is administered intramuscularly by the physician's assistant.

CPT Codes: _____,

_____

ICD-9-CM Code: _____

(ICD-10-CM Code: _____)

17 A DTP and an oral poliomyelitis vaccine (live) are administered to a new 10-year-old patient. A problem focused history and examination are performed for an acute URI, and the medical decision making is straightforward (separate identifiable service).

CPT Codes: _____,

_____, _____,

_____, _____

ICD-9-CM Codes: _____,

_____

(ICD-10-CM Codes: _____,

_____)

18 An established, 70-year-old Medicare patient presents to the nurse for a pneumonia and a flu immunization (2 injections).

☣ CPT Code(s): _____

☣ ICD-9-CM Code(s): _____

(☣ ICD-10-CM Code(s): _____)

19 A patient brings his allergy medication into the office, and a single injection service is provided by the nurse. The patient is allergic to primrose.

CPT Code: _____

ICD-9-CM Code: _____

(ICD-10-CM Code: _____)

20 A patient receives the initial 30-minute training for her prosthetic arm. Patient has a congenital absence of forearm.

CPT Code: _____ × _____

ICD-9-CM Code: _____

(ICD-10-CM Code: _____)

21 The patient presents for a bronchospasm evaluation before and after a spirometry that is administered to monitor his lung capacity. The patient has episodes of shortness of breath.

CPT Codes: ___ _____,

_____

ICD-9-CM Code: ___ _____

(ICD-10-CM Code: _____)

22 Nasopharyngoscopy with endoscope. The patient has persistent nosebleeds.

CPT Code: _____

ICD-9-CM Code: _____

(ICD-10-CM Code: _____)

23 A 30-year-old with end-stage renal disease receives a full month of dialysis with eight encounters.

CPT Code: _____

ICD-9-CM Code: _____

(ICD-10-CM Code: _____)

24 Ophthalmology Clinic Progress Note

Today, I saw a new patient who is a 46-year-old white female who was diagnosed with Graves', toxic diffuse goiter, early last year. She had some swelling of the eyes and was originally told she had an allergy; then the same person, after he found out she had Graves', put her on prednisone. It was unknown what the dose was, but the patient showed me her bottles and it is obvious that she was on 20 mg a day, taken at suppertime. She has now come down from this. She was also on prednisone acetate eye drops. The patient denies any history of any problems except that she became quite depressed and her head felt funny on the steroids. The patient had a history of an ulcer problem in the past, which was treated with diet. The patient allegedly had a positive Mantoux test years ago, but her chest x-rays have always been negative.

Today when I saw her, she was 20/80 in the right and 20/40 in the left with her refraction. The lids are markedly swollen, and she has marked inferior ptosis from the sagging lids, the water collection, and the redness. There is marked chemosis of the conjunctivae and thickening of the lids. The patient has full extraocular motility, except she cannot converge. There is marked swelling of the globes on the retropulsion exam. The pressures are 21 and 20 in primary gaze and 30 and 24 in up gaze. The discs are flat. The patient has pseudoexfoliation in the right eye and nuclear sclerotic cataracts in both eyes, right greater than left.

I counseled the patient about the treatment of this and offered her radiation therapy along with the proper dose of steroids of 100 mg a day for a week and then taper down from the 100 mg. I will send her to see Dr. Zapata for consultation radiation therapy, and then I think we would see her weekly as we get this problem under control. I did not feel she needed any topical medication, and she definitely does not need surgery now since there is no proptosis at this time. We will see her again in 1 week. I counseled her about the side effects of the high dose of steroids and how to take them.

Code: _____

ICD-9-CM Codes: _____,

_____, _____,

_____, _____

(ICD-10-CM Codes: _____,

_____, _____,

_____, _____)

QUICK CHECK ANSWERS

QUICK CHECK 25-1
1. b

QUICK CHECK 25-2
1. absence of the lens of the eye

QUICK CHECK 25-3
1. d. EEG, EOG, EMG

A good coder has to be able to work independently and like to solve puzzles, while sometimes a coder will have to figure out which parts of the puzzle are missing and clarify with the physician. Coding is even more rewarding when you know that you can positively impact a facility's bottom line by doing a great job.

Karla R. Lovaasen, RHIA, CCS, CCS-P

Coding and Consulting Services
Abingdon, Maryland

Inpatient Coding

Karla R. Lovaasen, RHIA, CCS, CCS-P
Co-author: ICD-9-CM Coding: Theory and Practice, 2010 Edition
(St. Louis, 2010, Saunders)

Chapter Topics

Differences between Inpatient and Outpatient Coding

Selection of Principal Diagnosis

Reporting Additional Diagnoses

Present on Admission (POA)

Chapter Review

Learning Objectives

After completing this chapter you should be able to

1 Explain the differences between inpatient and outpatient coding.

2 Define principal diagnosis and procedure.

3 Examine the Official Guidelines for Coding and Reporting.

4 Review the Guidelines for Selection of a Principal Diagnosis.

5 Determine when a condition should be reported as an additional diagnosis.

6 Explain the purpose of the present on admission indicators.

Make sure to check
evolve
learning system
for the latest
content updates

DIFFERENCES BETWEEN INPATIENT AND OUTPATIENT CODING

One difference between inpatient and outpatient coding is the use of CPT codes. In the outpatient setting (physician or outpatient hospital/facility), CPT codes are used to report services and procedures that were provided. The CPT codes drive outpatient reimbursement so physician and outpatient coders pay greater attention to the CPT codes that are assigned. Although ICD-9-CM codes are assigned, there has not been as much emphasis on the accuracy and specificity of ICD-9-CM coding in the outpatient setting. Although more emphasis will need to be given to ICD-9-CM coding in the future with the initiatives such as Value-Driven Health Care, physician rankings and profiling, pay for performance and various other projects. Also payer claims electronic editing processes (scrubbers) and edits make correct ICD-9-CM codes an important part of correct coding for reimbursement.

Another difference is in the guidelines that affect both settings. In Chapter 3, The Official Guidelines for Coding and Report for Outpatients were covered. This chapter will review some of the Guidelines and terminology that are specific to inpatient coding. For more in-depth training in ICD-9-CM, chapter-specific guidelines and inpatient reimbursement, the publication *ICD-9-CM Coding: Theory and Practice, 2009 Edition,* by Karla R. Lovaasen and Jennifer Schwerdtfeger (2009, Elsevier Saunders) is recommended.

There are several Uniform Hospital Discharge Data Set (UHDDS) definitions that must be learned and applied when coding inpatient records. In the outpatient setting, the primary diagnosis for the encounter is the first-listed diagnosis. In the inpatient setting, the primary or first-listed diagnosis is termed the principal diagnosis. The **principal diagnosis** is defined as "that condition established after study to be chiefly responsible for occasioning the admission of the patient to the hospital for care." The principal diagnosis is important in determining the Medicare Severity Diagnosis Related Group (MS-DRG) for services and may determine the amount the hospital is reimbursed (depending on the third-party payer).

ICD-9-CM OFFICIAL GUIDELINES FOR CODING AND REPORTING

Introduction (Paragraph 3)

These guidelines are based on the coding and sequencing instructions in Volume I, II and III of ICD-9-CM, but provide additional instruction. Adherence to these guidelines when assigning ICD-9-CM diagnosis and procedure codes is required under the Health Insurance Portability and Accountability Act (HIPAA). The diagnosis codes (Volumes 1-2) have been adopted under HIPAA for all healthcare settings. Volume 3 procedure codes have been adopted for inpatient procedures reported by hospitals.

In the inpatient setting, ICD-9-CM procedure codes (Volume 3) are assigned instead of CPT codes. Procedure codes need to be sequenced properly with the principal procedure as the first-listed procedure. The **principal procedure** is one that is performed for definitive treatment rather than for diagnostic or exploratory purposes, or one necessary for a complication. If two procedures appear to meet this definition, then the one most closely related to the principal diagnosis should be assigned as the principal procedure. A procedure is considered to be significant if it:

- Is surgical in nature
- Carries a procedural risk
- Carries an anesthetic risk
- Requires specialized training to perform

For a procedure to be significant it does not have to be performed in the operating room. Many procedures are performed in the emergency department, at a patient's bedside, treatment room, or in an interventional radiology department. Any procedure that affects reimbursement should be coded and reported. Most facilities will have a policy regarding what procedures should be coded.

SELECTION OF PRINCIPAL DIAGNOSIS

ICD-9-CM OFFICIAL GUIDELINES FOR CODING AND REPORTING

SECTION II. Selection of Principal Diagnosis

The circumstances of inpatient admission always govern the selection of principal diagnosis. The principal diagnosis is defined in the Uniform Hospital Discharge Data Set (UHDDS) as "that condition established after study to be chiefly responsible for occasioning the admission of the patient to the hospital for care."

The UHDDS definitions are used by hospitals to report inpatient data elements in a standardized manner. These data elements and their definitions can be found in the July 31, 1985, Federal Register (Vol. 50, No. 147), pp. 31038-40.

Since that time the application of the UHDDS definitions has been expanded to include all non-outpatient settings (acute care, short term, long term care and psychiatric hospitals; home health agencies; rehab facilities; nursing homes, etc).

In determining principal diagnosis the coding conventions in the ICD-9-CM, Volumes I and II take precedence over these official coding guidelines. *(See Section I. A., Conventions for the ICD-9-CM)*

The importance of consistent, complete documentation in the medical record cannot be overemphasized. Without such documentation the application of all coding guidelines is a difficult, if not impossible, task.

The **principal** diagnosis is sequenced **first** in inpatient coding. In an outpatient setting, it is important to indicate as the primary diagnosis the main reason for the visit, as well as subsequent diagnoses to substantiate adjunct services (such as laboratory and radiology) and to sequence the **primary** diagnosis **first.** The terminology "principal diagnosis" refers only to an acute care setting and is used in conjunction with the MS-DRG payment scheme; "first-listed diagnosis" refers only to outpatient settings. There are specific guidelines that assist with the selection of the principal diagnosis.

Symptoms, Signs, and Ill-Defined Conditions

ICD-9-CM OFFICIAL GUIDELINES FOR CODING AND REPORTING

SECTION II.

A. Codes for symptoms, signs, and ill-defined conditions

Codes for symptoms, signs, and ill-defined conditions from Chapter 16 *(Symptoms, Signs, and Ill-Defined Conditions)* are not to be used as a principal diagnosis when a related definitive diagnosis has been established.

EXERCISE 26-1 *Symptoms, Signs, and Ill-Defined Conditions*

1 A 63-year-old male is admitted with chest pain. Cardiac enzyme levels are elevated and the ECG indicates an acute myocardial infarction. The principal diagnosis is acute myocardial infarction. Chest pain is not coded, because it is a code from Chapter 16 of the ICD-9-CM and a symptom of the definitive diagnosis of acute myocardial infarction.

Let's code this case together.

a For an acute myocardial infarction, infarction is the **manifestation.** "Acute" indicates the **episode** of care and "myocardial" indicates the general **site** of the infarction.

b Locate the term "Infarct, infarction" in the Index.

c Under the term "Infarct, infarction" locate the subterm "myocardium." Note after "myocardium, myocardial" you find "(acute...)" and are directed to code 410.9. You can never stop at the Index. You must always refer to the Tabular, otherwise you will miss important notes, such as "a fifth digit is required."

d Now turn to 410.9 in the Tabular, Volume 1.

e Under "410.9 Unspecified site" you are presented with a notation that a fifth digit is required.

f Go back to the three-digit category code 410 where the fifth digits are listed. The fifth digit 0 is for an unspecified episode of care; the fifth digit 1 is for the initial episode of care; and the fifth digit 2 is for a subsequent episode of care. The myocardial infarction was diagnosed during this visit, so that would be the initial episode of care as defined in the ICD-9-CM. The correct fifth digit is 1.

g The complete, correct code is 410.91.

Now you try one.

2 A patient is admitted to the hospital with severe flank pain and hematuria. A urinalysis is done and it is positive for *Escherichia coli*. The discharge summary states acute pyelonephritis due to *E. coli*.

a What is the principal diagnosis? _____

b Locate the principal diagnosis in the Index. What code does the Index direct you to locate?

   ICD-9-CM Code: _____ (ICD-10-CM Code: _____)

c Locate the code in the Tabular. What is the three-digit category code and the title of the category you were directed to?

   ICD-9-CM Code and title: _____

d Was there a mention of a lesion in the case above? _____

e What is the correct principal code for this case?

   ICD-9-CM Code: _____ (ICD-10-CM Code: _____)

f Why do you think "severe flank pain and hematuria" are noted on this patient's case?

   _____

🛑 **STOP** *Wait, you're not finished with this case yet. Go back to the three-digit category code 590 and look at the entry immediately under "Infections of kidney." A note states, "Use additional code to identify organism, such as Escherichia coli [E. coli] (041.4)." You also code 041.4 to indicate the type of infection present. You have to be very careful to read all notes in the category before coding. If, in the end, you arrived at codes 590.10 (acute pyelonephritis) and 041.4 (Escherichia), you did a fine job.*

Two or More Interrelated Conditions

ICD-9-CM OFFICIAL GUIDELINES FOR CODING AND REPORTING

SECTION II.

B. Two or more interrelated conditions, each potentially meeting the definition for principal diagnosis

When there are two or more interrelated conditions (such as diseases in the same ICD-9-CM chapter or manifestations characteristically associated with a certain disease) potentially meeting the definition of principal diagnosis, either condition may be sequenced first, unless the circumstances of the admission, the therapy provided, the Tabular List, or the Alphabetic Index indicate otherwise.

EXERCISE 26-2 *Two or More Interrelated Conditions*

1 A patient is admitted with chest pain, shortness of breath, and a heart murmur. The patient undergoes a diagnostic cardiac catheterization, which shows two-vessel coronary artery disease (native coronary arteries) and severe mitral (valve) stenosis. It is recommended that bypass surgery with mitral valve replacement be performed as soon as possible.

The patient has two conditions, each of which has the potential to be the principal diagnosis: mitral valve stenosis and coronary artery disease.

   a Locate stenosis in the Index: both "mitral" and "valve" indicate the site of the stenosis the patient has—the condition is stenosis. Under the main term "Stenosis," locate the subterm "mitral." The words in parentheses indicate the kinds of mitral stenosis, such as valve, chronic, or inactive. You are looking for valve, so the correct four-digit subcategory code for the mitral valve stenosis is likely to be 394.0.

   b Locate coronary artery disease by locating the main term "Disease" and the subterms "artery" and "coronary." The entry directs you to "*see* Arteriosclerosis, coronary." Under the main term "Arteriosclerosis" and the subterm "coronary (native artery)" you will be directed to code 414.01. If the Tabular validates codes 394.0 (mitral valve stenosis) and 414.01 (coronary artery disease, native artery), either code could be sequenced first because none of the information indicates one condition warranted more care than the other.

Now you do one.

2 A patient is involved in a car accident and is admitted with an open fracture of the right humerus and an open fracture of the distal femur. Both fractures require open reduction, which means that the fracture will be repaired using an open incision into the fracture site.

   a What are the two diagnoses? _____

Either of these diagnoses may be principal, because both are addressed and plans are made to treat both surgically. They were equally the reason for admission to the hospital.

   b Under what main term in the Index would you locate both diagnoses? _____

   c After the main term "Fracture," what would be the first applicable subterm for the fracture of the

     right humerus? _____

   d What is the word that appears in parentheses after humerus? _____

Continued

Because the patient's case states "open," you know that 812.20 is not the correct code because 812.20 specifies "closed." Go farther down the list of subterms to "Fracture, humerus, open." What is the code for "open"?

     ICD-9-CM Code: _____ (ICD-10-CM Code: _____)

e In the Tabular, does the code you chose in the Index match the description and if it does, why?

_____

You still have to locate the code for the open fracture of distal femur.

f After looking in the Index using the main term "Fracture," what is the subterm you would locate?

_____

g What is the word in parentheses after the first subterm?

_____

h What is the next subterm?

_____

i What does this subterm direct you to do?

_____

j When you take the subterm direction, what is the next subterm that you must use to locate the correct code? _____

Note: If "open" or "closed" fracture is not stated, assume it is a "closed" fracture.

k What is the code that you are directed to look up under "Fracture, femur, lower end, open"?

     ICD-9-CM Code: _____ (ICD-10-CM Code: _____)

l After checking the code in the Tabular, is the code correct? _____

Two or More Diagnoses

If two or more diagnoses are equally responsible for the outpatient visit, either can be sequenced as the principal diagnosis. The same is applicable in the inpatient setting.

> ## ICD-9-CM OFFICIAL GUIDELINES FOR CODING AND REPORTING
>
> **SECTION II.**
> **C. Two or more diagnoses that equally meet the definition for principal diagnosis**
>
> In the unusual instance when two or more diagnoses equally meet the criteria for principal diagnosis as determined by the circumstances of admission, diagnostic workup and/or therapy provided, and the Alphabetic Index, Tabular List, or another coding guidelines does not provide sequencing direction, any one of the diagnoses may be sequenced first.

EXERCISE 26-3   *Two or More Diagnoses*

1 A patient is admitted with weakness, diarrhea of 2 days' duration, diaphoresis, and abdominal pain. The attending physician lists the diagnoses as viral gastroenteritis and dehydration. Intravenous fluids with electrolyte supplements are ordered.

    a Locate "Gastroenteritis" as the main term in the Index and then the subterm "viral." When you do this you will be directed to code 008.8 (unspecified) because the record does not specify the organism type.

    b After you have located code 008.8 in the Tabular and made sure it is the correct code, look for any notes under the three-digit category code to see if there are any fifth digits that need to be assigned.

    c The correct code is 008.8 and there is no fifth digit to assign. Now you need to code the other diagnosis of dehydration. It seems almost too good to be true: There is only one word in the diagnosis. "Dehydration" is the main term. Dehydration appears in the Index, and it points to only one code. Check out the code 276.51 in the Tabular.

    d The Tabular confirms that 276.51 is for dehydration and there is no note regarding any *Excludes* that concern this case. The correct code is 276.51.

    e Remember, when two equally important diagnoses are indicated, it does not matter which code is sequenced first. So, the two codes for this case can be stated as 008.8 and 276.51 *or* 276.51 and 008.8. The order of the codes may not seem too earth-shattering right now, but the order of the codes is significant. One of these diagnoses may be reimbursed at a higher rate than the other; therefore, selection of the principal diagnosis is critically important.

Now you have the opportunity to do the next case.

2 A patient was admitted with heavy menstrual bleeding of 2 days' duration, severe abdominal pain, and anemia due to acute blood loss. The patient was given medication intravenously to control the pain and bleeding. She also received two units of packed cells for the anemia. Investigations were performed to determine a cause of the heavy bleeding.

    a What is the medical term for heavy menstrual/uterine bleeding?

        _____

    b The medical term from the question above is one of the diagnosis that you will need to locate. What code does the Index indicate and the Tabular of the text confirm as a code for the first diagnosis?

        ICD-9-CM Code: _____ (ICD-10-CM Code: _____)

    c What is the second diagnosis? _____

    d Locate the second diagnosis code and confirm your finding in the Tabular. (Hint: The subterms for the second code are "blood loss" and "acute.") What is the code?

        ICD-9-CM Code: _____ (ICD-10-CM Code: _____)

Comparative or Contrasting Conditions

ICD-9-CM OFFICIAL GUIDELINES FOR CODING AND REPORTING

SECTION II.

D. Two or more comparative or contrasting conditions.

In those rare instances when two or more contrasting or comparative diagnoses are documented as "either/or" (or similar terminology), they are coded as if the diagnoses were confirmed and the diagnoses are sequenced according to the circumstances of the admission. If no further determination can be made as to which diagnosis should be principal, either diagnosis may be sequenced first.

EXERCISE 26-4 *Comparative or Contrasting Conditions*

1 A patient is admitted to the hospital with chest pain, nausea, and dyspnea. The patient has a history of a prior myocardial infarction 2 years earlier. The pain is atypical (irregular). An ECG and cardiac enzyme study (creatine phosphokinase) are ordered, as well as an upper gastrointestinal series to rule out esophageal reflux. The admitting diagnosis by the attending physician is unstable angina or esophageal reflux.

   a Angina is located by the main term "Angina" and the subterm "unstable." The correct code is 411.1.

   b The second diagnosis is reflux, esophageal, located in the Index under the main term "Reflux" and the subterm "esophageal." You are directed to code 530.81. After checking this in the Tabular to be sure this is the correct code and has no exclusions or additions, you have the second of the two contrasting conditions, 530.81. Only further evaluation by the physician will finally determine what the principal diagnosis is; but for now, the case has been coded to the greatest specificity possible with the information available in the patient record as 530.81 and 411.1 or 411.1 and 530.81. Either diagnosis may be selected as the principal diagnosis.

Here's a case for you to code.

2 A 75-year-old man is admitted with severe low back pain. He is known to have prostate cancer as well as severe spondylosis. Spine x-ray films and a bone scan are ordered. Differential diagnoses are compression fracture versus bone metastases from prostate cancer. (Note: The physician would have to be consulted to determine whether prostate cancer is "current" prostate cancer or "history of" prostate cancer.)

   a What is the main term for compression fracture?

   _____

   b Using "Fracture" as the main term and "compression" as the subterm, what are you directed to

   do? _____

Before you continue to look up other possible subterms, you need to consider why the patient has severe low back pain. You may need to query the physician or review the record to determine whether or not the compression fracture was due to trauma. The term "idiopathic" means of unknown cause; the term "pathologic" means due to a disease or accompanying a disease. Let us assume that the patient record substantiates a diagnosis of a fracture due to a disease (pathologic). Under Fracture, locate pathologic and then the subterm "vertebrae." You are then forwarded to 733.13, which is the correct code according to the Tabular.

   c The second diagnosis in the differential diagnoses is metastasis from prostate cancer. Locating cancer in the Index, you find: "*see also* Neoplasm, by site, malignant." The potential neoplasm is of the bone. "Neoplasm" is the main term and "bone" is a subterm. Secondary is the type of malignancy because the record states that this patient has prostate cancer (primary) and now has the potential to have bone (secondary) cancer. Under the "Secondary" column, what is the correct code for "Neoplasm, bone" for this patient?

   ICD-9-CM Code: _____ (ICD-10-CM Code: _____)

An additional code would be assigned for the prostate cancer.

⬣ **STOP** *The difference between Guidelines Section II, D (Two or More Comparative or Contrasting Conditions), and Section II, E (Symptom[s] Followed by Contrasting/Comparative Diagnosis) is the way the physician states the final diagnosis. In the Guideline Section II, D, symptoms are documented but the physician states "X versus Y" instead of listing the symptoms. In Guideline Section II, E, the physician states the diagnosis as "symptoms due to X versus Y."*

Symptom(s) Followed by Contrasting/ Comparative Diagnoses

ICD-9-CM OFFICIAL GUIDELINES FOR CODING AND REPORTING

SECTION II.

E. A symptom(s) followed by contrasting/comparative diagnoses

When a symptom(s) is followed by contrasting/comparative diagnoses, the symptom code is sequenced first. All the contrasting/comparative diagnoses should be coded as additional diagnoses.

EXERCISE 26-5 *Symptom(s) Followed by Contrasting/Comparative*

1 The patient presents with knee pain of 3 months' duration, with no known trauma, either bucket-handle tear of medial meniscus or loose body in the knee joint. The final diagnosis is knee pain due to bucket-handle tear of medial meniscus versus loose body in the knee joint.

There will be three codes for this case: one for the **pain** in the knee joint, one for the **tear** in the meniscus, and one for the **loose body** in the knee joint.

   a Using "Pain, joint, knee" for the first condition, what is the correct code?

      ICD-9-CM Code: _____ (ICD-10-CM Code: _____)

   b Using "Tear, meniscus, bucket handle, old," what is the correct second code?

      ICD-9-CM Code: _____ (ICD-10-CM Code: _____)

   c Using "Loose, body, joint, knee," what is the correct third code?

      ICD-9-CM Code: _____ (ICD-10-CM Code: _____)

Original Treatment Plan Not Carried Out

ICD-9-CM OFFICIAL GUIDELINES FOR CODING AND REPORTING

SECTION II.

F. Original treatment plan not carried out

Sequence as the principal diagnosis the condition, which after study occasioned the admission to the hospital, even though treatment may not have been carried out due to unforeseen circumstances.

EXERCISE 26-6 *Original Treatment Plan Not Carried Out*

1 A patient is admitted to the hospital for an elective cholecystectomy. The patient has chronic cholecystitis, and gallstones were visualized on x-ray films. After admission, it is noticed that the patient has a fever, is coughing, and shows some patchy infiltrates on the chest x-ray film. Surgery is canceled because the patient may have pneumonia.

This case will have three codes: the cholecystitis with gallstones (cholelithiasis), pneumonia, and surgery not done.

  a Cholelithiasis with cholecystitis, without mention of obstruction. What is the code?

     ICD-9-CM Code: _____ (ICD-10-CM Code: _____)

  b What is the pneumonia code?

     ICD-9-CM Code: _____ (ICD-10-CM Code: _____)

  c The surgery that was not done is located in the Index under "Surgery, not done because of."

     Why was the surgery not done? _____

  d What is the code for the surgery not done?

     ICD-9-CM Code: _____ (ICD-10-CM Code: _____)

No procedure code is submitted because no procedure was done.

2 A patient is admitted for elective sterilization by tubal ligation. The patient and her husband decide not to go through with the surgery, and the surgery is canceled.

  a How many codes will there be for this case and what are the main terms for each?

     _____

  b What is the V code for the sterilization?

     ICD-9-CM Code: _____ (ICD-10-CM Code: _____)

  c What is the code for the surgery not done?

     ICD-9-CM Code: _____ (ICD-10-CM Code: _____)

Complications

ICD-9-CM OFFICIAL GUIDELINES FOR CODING AND REPORTING

SECTION II.

G. Complications of surgery and other medical care

When the admission is for treatment of a complication resulting from surgery or other medical care, the complication code is sequenced as the principal diagnosis. If the complication is classified to the 996-999 series and the code lacks the necessary specificity in describing the complication, an additional code for the specific complication should be assigned.

EXERCISE 26-7   *Complications of Surgery and Other Medical Care*

1 A patient is admitted to the hospital because of a postoperative ileus. The patient had a colectomy for colon cancer at another facility last week. On admission patient has abdominal pain with distension and nausea and vomiting.

Patient has not had a bowel movement for 3 days. Patient is scheduled to see an oncologist regarding adjunctive treatment for colon cancer.

a Patient was admitted for a complication due to surgery. What is the complication?

_____

b What code is assigned as the principal diagnosis?

ICD-9-CM Code: _____ (ICD-10-CM Code: _____)

c Is there an additional code that should be assigned to indicate the exact nature of the

complication? _____

d What is the additional code?

ICD-9-CM Code: _____ (ICD-10-CM Code: _____)

e Are there any secondary diagnosis codes that should be assigned? _____

If so, what are those codes? _____

2 A patient is admitted because of a malfunction of insulin pump. The patient is a type I diabetic and the pump has not been delivering an adequate dose of insulin.

a What is the principal diagnosis and code for this case? _____

b What is the V code for long-term use of insulin?

ICD-9-CM Code: _____ (ICD-10-CM Code: _____)

c What additional codes should be assigned in this case?

_____

No ICD-9-CM procedure code is submitted because no procedure was done.

Uncertain Diagnosis

ICD-9-CM OFFICIAL GUIDELINES FOR CODING AND REPORTING

SECTION II.

H. Uncertain Diagnosis

If the diagnosis documented at the time of discharge is qualified as "probable", "suspected", "likely", "questionable", "possible", or "still to be ruled out", or other similar terms indicating uncertainty, code the condition as if it existed or was established. The bases for these guidelines are the diagnostic workup, arrangements for further workup or observation, and initial therapeutic approach that correspond most closely with the established diagnosis.

Note: This guideline is applicable only to inpatient admissions to short-term, acute, long-term care and psychiatric hospitals.

The basis for this guideline is that the diagnostic workup and arrangements for further workup, observation, or therapies are the same whether treating the confirmed condition or ruling the condition out.

Because hospitals are reimbursed a set payment (Medicare Severity Diagnosis-Related Groups amount) for each hospitalization for Medicare patients, the facility resources used are averaged across the entire patient stay in the hospital. In an outpatient setting, only confirmed diagnoses may be reported, and rule-out, possible, or probable diagnoses are not reported if there is a chief complaint, sign, or symptom that occasioned the visit. In an outpatient setting, each visit in the process of confirming a diagnosis is reported.

Examples

UNCERTAIN DIAGNOSIS

Hospital Inpatient

Diagnosis: <u>Probable</u> bronchitis (code as bronchitis)

Index: **Bronchitis 490**

Tabular: **490 Bronchitis**

Hospital Inpatient

Diagnosis: <u>Rule out</u> Graves' disease (code as Graves' disease)

Index: **Graves' Disease 242.0**

Tabular: **242.00 Toxic diffuse goiter** (Graves' disease)

Clinic Outpatient

Diagnosis: Chest pain, <u>rule out</u> myocardial infarction (code as chest pain)

Index: **Pain(s), chest 786.50**

Tabular: **786.50 Chest pain, unspecified**

Clinic Outpatient

Diagnosis: Cough and fever, <u>probably</u> pneumonia (code as cough and fever)

Index: **Cough 786.2**

Index: **Fever 780.60**

Tabular: **786.2 Cough**

780.60 Pyrexia of unknown origin (fever)

There are two exceptions to this guideline that are identified in the chapter-specific guidelines. The exceptions are:

- Code 042, AIDS should only be assigned for confirmed cases.
- Code 488.0, Avian influenza should only be assigned for confirmed cases.

EXERCISE 26-8 *Uncertain Diagnoses*

1 Patient was admitted from the nursing home with fever, cough, and shortness of breath. Patient has a history of previous cerebrovascular accident with resultant dysphagia. Patient is being treated for hypertension. The physician documents the discharge diagnosis as probable aspiration pneumonia.

   a What is the principal diagnosis? _____

   b How do you code probable aspiration pneumonia?

   ICD-9-CM Code: _____ (ICD-10-CM Code: _____)

   c Are there any additional diagnosis codes that should be assigned in this case? _____

   ICD-9-CM Codes: _____, _____, _____

   (ICD-10-CM Codes: _____, _____, _____)

2 Patient is admitted with hematuria. Investigations show that the patient likely has a malignant neoplasm of the right kidney. The patient refused any further interventions or workup. The physician's final diagnosis is suspected malignancy right kidney.

   a What is the principal diagnosis? _____

   b How do you code suspected malignancy right kidney?

   ICD-9-CM Code: _____ (ICD-10-CM Code: _____)

   c Are there additional diagnosis codes that should be assigned in this case? _____

   ICD-9-CM Code: _____ (ICD-10-CM Code: _____)

ICD-9-CM OFFICIAL GUIDELINES FOR CODING AND REPORTING

SECTION II.
I. Admission from Observation Unit

   1. Admission Following Medical Observation
   When a patient is admitted to an observation unit for a medical condition, which either worsens or does not improve, and is subsequently admitted as an inpatient of the same hospital for this same medical condition, the principal diagnosis would be the medical condition which led to the hospital admission.

   2. Admission Following Post-Operative Observation
   When a patient is admitted to an observation unit to monitor a condition (or complication) that develops following outpatient surgery, and then is subsequently admitted as an inpatient of the same hospital, hospitals should apply the Uniform Hospital Discharge Data Set (UHDDS) definition of principal diagnosis as "that condition established after study to be chiefly responsible for occasioning the admission of the patient to the hospital for care."

ICD-9-CM OFFICIAL GUIDELINES FOR CODING AND REPORTING

SECTION II.

J. Admission from Outpatient Surgery

When a patient receives surgery in the hospital's outpatient surgery department and is subsequently admitted for continuing inpatient care at the same hospital, the following guidelines should be followed in selecting the principal diagnosis for the inpatient admission:

- If the reason for the inpatient admission is a complication, assign the complication as the principal diagnosis.
- If no complication, or other condition, is documented as the reason for the inpatient admission, assign the reason for the outpatient surgery as the principal diagnosis.
- If the reason for the inpatient admission is another condition unrelated to the surgery, assign the unrelated condition as the principal diagnosis.

EXERCISE 26-9 *Admission from Observation Unit or Outpatient Surgery*

1 Patient is admitted after outpatient percutaneous needle biopsy of the kidney. Patient developed atrial fibrillation in the recovery room and decision was made to admit to ICU. Patient was treated and monitored on telemetry. The atrial fibrillation resolved and the patient's biopsy showed that the patient had lupus nephritis.

a What is the principal diagnosis? _____

b What code is assigned to the principal diagnosis?

   ICD-9-CM Code: _____ (ICD-10-CM Code: _____)

c What secondary diagnosis codes are assigned?

   ICD-9-CM Codes: _____, _____, _____

   (ICD-10-CM Codes: _____, _____, _____)

d Should a procedure code be assigned? _____

   If so, what code is assigned? _____

e What E codes would be assigned?

   ICD-9-CM Code: _____ Complication of other surgical operation

   ICD-9-CM Code: _____ Place of occurrence, facility

   (ICD-10-CM Code: _____ Complication of other surgical operation

   ICD-10-CM Code: _____ Place of occurrence, facility)

REPORTING ADDITIONAL DIAGNOSES

After determining and coding the principal diagnosis and any procedures that were performed, a thorough review of the record is necessary to determine if any additional diagnoses should be coded and reported. These additional diagnoses have the potential to affect reimbursement so it is important to capture these conditions.

ICD-9-CM OFFICIAL GUIDELINES FOR CODING AND REPORTING

SECTION III. Reporting Additional Diagnoses

GENERAL RULES FOR OTHER (ADDITIONAL) DIAGNOSES

For reporting purposes the definition for "other diagnoses" is interpreted as additional conditions that affect patient care in terms of requiring:

> clinical evaluation; or
> therapeutic treatment; or
> diagnostic procedures; or
> extended length of hospital stay; or
> increased nursing care and/or monitoring.

The UHDDS item #11-b defines Other Diagnoses as "all conditions that coexist at the time of admission, that develop subsequently, or that affect the treatment received and/or the length of stay. Diagnoses that relate to an earlier episode which have no bearing on the current hospital stay are to be excluded." UHDDS definitions apply to inpatients in acute care, short-term, long term care and psychiatric hospital setting. The UHDDS definitions are used by acute care short-term hospitals to report inpatient data elements in a standardized manner. These data elements and their definitions can be found in the July 31, 1985, Federal Register (Vol. 50, No. 147), pp. 31038-40.

Since that time the application of the UHDDS definitions has been expanded to include all non-outpatient settings (acute care, short term, long term care and psychiatric hospitals; home health agencies; rehab facilities; nursing homes, etc).

The general rule is that for reporting purposes, the term "other diagnoses" is interpreted to refer to additional conditions that affect patient care in terms of requiring:

- Clinical evaluation; or
- Therapeutic treatment; or
- Diagnostic procedures; or
- Extended length of hospital stay, or
- Increased nursing care and/or monitoring

ICD-9-CM OFFICIAL GUIDELINES FOR CODING AND REPORTING

SECTION III. Reporting Additional Diagnoses (Paragraph 3)

The following guidelines are to be applied in designating "other diagnoses" when neither the Alphabetic Index nor the Tabular List in ICD-9-CM provide direction. The listing of the diagnoses in the patient record is the responsibility of the attending provider.

A. Previous conditions

If the provider has included a diagnosis in the final diagnostic statement, such as the discharge summary or the face sheet, it should ordinarily be coded. Some providers include in the diagnostic statement resolved conditions or diagnoses and status-post procedures from previous admission that have no bearing on the current stay. Such conditions are not to be reported and are coded only if required by hospital policy.

However, history codes (V10-V19) may be used as secondary codes if the historical condition or family history has an impact on current care or influences treatment.

EXERCISE 26-10 *Previous Conditions*

Circle the conditions in the following diagnostic lists that would NOT be coded:

1 Herpes zoster

   History of hysterectomy

   Diabetes

2 Influenza

   Hypertension (currently controlled by medication)

   History of peptic ulcer disease

3 Congestive heart failure

   Remote history of appendectomy

   Previous arthroscopic surgery to left knee

ICD-9-CM OFFICIAL GUIDELINES FOR CODING AND REPORTING

SECTION III.
B. Abnormal findings

Abnormal findings (laboratory, x-ray, pathologic, and other diagnostic results) are not coded and reported unless the provider indicates their clinical significance. If the findings are outside the normal range and the attending provider has ordered other tests to evaluate the condition or prescribed treatment, it is appropriate to ask the provider whether the abnormal finding should be added.

Please note: This differs from the coding practices in the outpatient setting for coding encounters for diagnostic tests that have been interpreted by a provider.

EXERCISE 26-11 *Abnormal Findings*

1 If the physician documents that a patient's potassium level is 2.5 and orders potassium supplements with a repeat potassium lab test, is it acceptable to query the physician about the

   2.5 potassium level? _____

2 On review of the record the coder notices that the patient's sodium level is slightly below normal. There is no documentation of any treatment, evaluation, or monitoring. Is it acceptable to query

   the physician about the abnormal sodium level? _____

The guideline for uncertain diagnoses is repeated in Section III, Reporting Additional Diagnoses. Sometimes a physician will document "rule out" as a final diagnostic statement, but upon review of the record it is apparent that the diagnosis was actually ruled out. A diagnosis that has been ruled out should not be coded as if it exists.

ICD-9-CM OFFICIAL GUIDELINES FOR CODING AND REPORTING

SECTION III.

C. Uncertain Diagnosis

If the diagnosis documented at the time of discharge is qualified as "probable", "suspected", "likely", "questionable", "possible", or "still to be ruled out", or other similar terms indicating uncertainty, code the condition as if it existed or was established. The bases for these guidelines are the diagnostic workup, arrangements for further workup or observation, and initial therapeutic approach that correspond most closely with the established diagnosis.

Note: This guideline is applicable only to inpatient admissions to short-term, acute, long-term care and psychiatric hospitals.

PRESENT ON ADMISSION (POA)

The Deficit Reduction Act (DRA) mandated that all acute-care facilities that are reimbursed under MS-DRGs identify and report diagnoses that were present at the time of a patient's admission. This policy was implemented October 1, 2007, and expected to save lives and healthcare dollars by no longer paying for the treatment of preventable errors, injuries, and infections that can occur in the hospital setting. CMS will not pay for conditions considered preventable, such as pressure ulcers, falls resulting in injury, infections due to genitourinary or central line catheters, or other complications.

The Present on Admission (POA) indicator distinguishes between conditions that develop during a particular hospital stay and those conditions present at the time of admission. Hospitals were allowed a 1-year grace time and after October 1, 2008, a hospital's reimbursement may be affected if certain complications develop after admission to the hospital. Coding staff will have to assign the POA indicators to the ICD-9-CM codes that are assigned. This requirement makes it even more important to have accurate and complete documentation in the health record. In some instances, it may be necessary to query the physician if a condition was present at the time of admission. The Cooperating Parties have developed POA guidelines that are supplemental to the ICD-9-CM Official Guidelines for Coding and Reporting to assist with the application of the POA requirement.

CHAPTER REVIEW

CHAPTER 26, PART I, THEORY

1 Codes can be assigned to diagnoses that are documented as being "probable," "suspected," "likely" in which setting?

   Inpatient   Outpatient

2 In which setting can any confirmed or definitive diagnoses be coded from the interpretation of a diagnostic test result?

   Inpatient   Outpatient

3 In which setting would a CPT code be assigned for a herniorrhaphy?

   Inpatient   Outpatient

4 Which statement about a significant procedure is NOT true?

  a. Requires specialized training
  b. Carries an anesthetic risk
  c. Is surgical in nature
  d. Must be performed in an operating room

5 The physician documents flank pain due to renal stone. The flank pain is the principal diagnosis.

   True   False

6 In the inpatient setting, the physician documents suspected cholelithiasis in the discharge summary. The cholelithiasis is coded as if it exists.

   True   False

7 If the coder doesn't know if a diagnosis is present on admission, a POA indicator is not assigned.

   True   False

8 A patient is admitted with low-grade fever and right upper quadrant pain. The physician documents that the patient's right upper quadrant pain is due to chronic cholecystitis versus peptic ulcer disease. Which diagnoses should be reported?

  a. Chronic cholecystitis
  b. Peptic ulcer disease
  c. Chronic cholecystitis, peptic ulcer disease
  d. Right upper quadrant pain, chronic cholecystitis, peptic ulcer disease

9 Patient is admitted with hyperglycemia due to new-onset diabetes, type II. Patient has had polydipsia, polyuria, and unexplained weight loss. Which diagnoses should be reported?

  a. Hyperglycemia, diabetes, type II
  b. Diabetes, type II
  c. Diabetes, type II, polydipsia, polyuria, weight loss
  d. Hyperglycemia, diabetes, type II, weight loss

10 Patient is admitted with heartburn due to gastroesophageal reflux disease (GERD). Which diagnoses should be reported?

  a. Heartburn
  b. Heartburn and GERD
  c. GERD and heartburn
  d. GERD

CHAPTER 26, PART II, PRACTICAL

Assign and sequence codes to the following inpatient diagnoses.

11 Headache due to malignant neoplasm of the brain

ICD-9-CM Code: _____

(ICD-10-CM Code: _____)

12 Patient was admitted with shortness of breath. Patient was found to have both pneumonia and decompensated congestive heart failure. The pneumonia was treated with IV antibiotics and the congestive heart failure with IV Lasix. Both were present on admission.

ICD-9-CM Codes: _____,

_____

(ICD-10-CM Codes: _____,

_____)

13 Acute cholecystitis versus acute pancreatitis

ICD-9-CM Codes: _____,

_____

(ICD-10-CM Codes: _____,

_____)

14 Epigastric pain due to acute cholecystitis versus acute pancreatitis

ICD-9-CM Codes: _____,

_____, _____

(ICD-10-CM Codes: _____,

_____, _____)

15 Patient was admitted for elective D&C because of post-menopausal bleeding. The surgery was cancelled because the surgeon became ill. The patient's surgery was rescheduled for next week.

ICD-9-CM Codes: _____,

_____

(ICD-10-CM Codes: _____,

_____)

16 Patient was admitted for dehiscence of abdominal incision.

ICD-9-CM Code(s): _____

(ICD-10-CM Code(s): _____)

17 Patient was admitted for medical observation for chest pain. After the patient was determined to have suffered a NSTEMI (Non-ST Elevation Myocardial Infarction), the patient was admitted to acute care.

ICD-9-CM Code(s): _____

(ICD-10-CM Code(s): _____)

18 Patient was admitted for suspected avian influenza. Avian influenza was ruled out and it was determined that the patient's symptoms were due to viral pneumonia.

ICD-9-CM Code(s): _____

(ICD-10-CM Code(s): _____)

19 Patient was admitted to the observation unit for exacerbation of COPD. The patient did not improve and was admitted for continued care and treatment.

ICD-9-CM Code(s): _____

(ICD-10-CM Code(s): _____)

20 Patient was admitted following an outpatient esophagogastroduodenoscopy for dilatation of an esophageal stricture. The patient was unable to void and was admitted because of urinary retention.

ICD-9-CM Code(s): _____

(ICD-10-CM Code(s): _____)

Online Resources

The most current coding guidelines and code system updates are posted to the Evolve website at http://evolve.elsevier.com/Buck/step.

Once registered for your free Evolve resources, go to the *Course Documents* section, then select *Coding Updates, Tips, and Links* to reference the following:

- ICD-9-CM Official Guidelines for Coding and Reporting
- 1995 Guidelines for E/M Services
- 1997 Documentation Guidelines for Evaluation and Management Services

- CPT Updates
- ICD-9-CM Updates
- HCPCS Updates

- Study Tips
- WebLinks

Exercise Answers

CHAPTER 1

Exercise 1-1
1. the government
2. 1965
3. A
4. B

Exercise 1-2
1. October
2. November or December
3. Department of Health and Human Services
4. January 26, 2009
5. Ambulatory Surgical Center
6. Alberta Dwivedi

Exercise 1-3
1. Resource-Based Relative Value Scale
2. *Federal Register*
3. OBRA

Exercise 1-4
1. fraud
2. Office of the Inspector General or OIG
3. gatekeeper
4. Program for All-Inclusive Care of the Elderly

CHAPTER 2

Exercise 2-1
1. morbidity or sickness (also acceptable for morbidity is mortality or death rate)
2. ICD-9
3. Clinical Modification
4. Any four of the following six (or similar wording):
   a. facilitate payment for health services
   b. evaluate patients' use of health care facilities (utilization patterns)
   c. study health care costs
   d. research the quality of health care

           e. predict health care trends

           f. plan for future health care needs

    5. verbal, narrative

Exercise 2-2
1. Endocrine, Nutritional and Metabolic Diseases, and Immunity Disorders (240-279)
2. Disorders of Thyroid Gland (240-246)
3. 240 Simple and unspecified goiter
4. 240.0 Goiter, specified as simple

Exercise 2-3
1. **711.06**
2. no
3. by adding fourth and fifth digits to the codes

Exercise 2-4
1. a. Appendix B
   b. Appendix D
   c. Appendix A
   d. Appendix E
   e. Appendix C
2. Appendix D: Industrial Accidents

Exercise 2-5
1. Normocytic <u>anemia</u>
2. Acute <u>prostatitis</u>
3. Severe protein calorie <u>malnutrition</u>
4. <u>Granuloma</u> lung
5. <u>Pain</u> in neck

Exercise 2-6
1. essential
2. nonessential
3. essential
4. nonessential
5. nonessential

Exercise 2-7
1. no, 205.10 per Excludes note and remember to assign the fifth digit
2. yes
3. no, 754.70 per Excludes note see codes 754.5-754.7
4. yes
5. per Excludes note see category 532

Exercise 2-8
1. No answer required
2. a. **710.0 *[424.91]***
   b. **710.0**
   c. Diffuse disease of connective tissue
   d. all collagen diseases whose effects are not confined mainly to a single system
   e. **424.91**
   f. **710.0**
   g. **710.0, 424.91**

Exercise 2-9
1. *see* Human immunodeficiency virus
2. no cross reference is listed
3. *see also* Pruritus
4. *see also* Adenitis
5. *see* condition

Exercise 2-10
1. **331.11, 294.11**
2. **117.3, 484.6**
3. **440.23, 707.13**
4. **600.01, 788.20**
5. **695.10, 713.3**

Exercise 2-11
1. f
2. b
3. c
4. d
5. a
6. e
7. g

Exercise 2-12
1. f
2. g
3. a
4. h
5. k
6. i
7. e
8. d
9. j
10. b
11. c
12. false
13. true

Exercise 2-13
1. Obstetrical Procedures
2. Miscellaneous Diagnostic and Therapeutic Procedures
3. Procedures and Interventions, Not Elsewhere Classified

Exercise 2-14
1. referring to a vein
2. pertaining to the lungs or pulmonary artery
3. joining together of two openings
4. pertaining to the heart and lungs
5. circulation that occurs outside of the body
6. a surgical procedure that joins the superior vena cava and pulmonary artery
7. manages the heart and lung functions of a patient during a surgical procedure

Exercise 2-15
1. **45.24** (Sigmoidoscopy, flexible)
2. **63.73** (Vasectomy)
3. **76.73** (Reduction, fracture, maxilla)
4. **99.04** (Transfusion, packed cells)
5. **21.03** (Cauterization, nose, for epistaxis (with packing))

CHAPTER 3

Exercise 3-1
1. Urinary tract infection
2. Crohn's disease
3. Sprain knee
4. COPD and CHF (either could be first-listed)
5. Pneumonia

Exercise 3-2
1. **789.00** (Pain, abdominal, unspecified), **787.91** (Diarrhea)
   Either diagnosis could be listed first
2. **556.9** (Colitis, ulcerative, unspecified)
3. **780.79** (Fatigue), **782.4** (Jaundice, unspecified)
   Either diagnosis could be listed first
4. **070.70** (Hepatitis C, unspecified)

Exercise 3-3
1. Admission for elective sterilization
2. Benign prostatic hypertrophy
3. Hematuria

Exercise 3-4
1. Pelvic pain
2. Biliary duct stricture
3. Post-menopausal bleeding

Exercise 3-5
1. Contact, smallpox; **V01.3**
2. Vaccination, prophylactic, smallpox; **V04.1**
3. History, malignant neoplasm, tongue; **V10.01**
4. **V53.31** (Cardiac, device, pacemaker, cardiac, fitting or adjustment)
5. **V25.5** (Insertion, subdermal implantable contraceptive)
6. **V10.46** (History (personal), malignant neoplasm, prostate)
7. **V06.5** (Vaccination, mumps, with measles and rubella [MMR])
8. **V76.12** (Screening, mammogram)
9. **V70.5** (Examination, medical, pre-employment)

Exercise 3-6
1. **V71.4, 913.0**
2. **V71.5** (Rape)

Exercise 3-7
1. Palpitations **785.1**, rheumatoid arthritis **714.0**
2. Memory loss **780.93**, diabetes mellitus, type II **250.00**
3. Urinary tract infection **599.0**, psoriasis **696.1**

Exercise 3-8

1. Pain, knee **719.46,** Stiffness, knee **719.56.** Osteoarthritis is not coded because it has not been confirmed.

2. Pain, wrist **719.43,** numbness **782.0.** Carpal tunnel syndrome is not coded because it has not been confirmed.

3. Amenorrhea **626.0,** galactorrhea **611.6.** Pituitary tumor is not coded because it has not been confirmed.

4. Breast lump **611.72.** Breast cancer is not coded because it has not been confirmed.

Exercise 3-9

1. a, c (asthma, systemic lupus erythematous)

2. e, f, d (diabetes, atherosclerosis, status post op CABG)

3. i, j (contact dermatitis, colostomy)

4. k (eye exam)

5. g, h (acquired absence of uterus, personal history of primary malignancy of cervix uteri)

CHAPTER 4

Exercise 4-1

1. category code, subcategory code, subclassification code

2. category code, subcategory code, subclassification code

Exercise 4-2

1. Abdominal pain, nausea and sometimes vomiting, loss of appetite, low-grade fever, constipation, diarrhea, inability to pass gas, abdominal swelling (any two of these)

2. chest pain

3. False

4. False

5. chest pain, shortness of breath

6. hip pain, contusion of hip

Exercise 4-3

1. **601.1** (Prostatitis, chronic); **041.00** (Infection, streptococcal) [in this order]

2. **466.0** (Bronchitis, with acute or subacute); **041.7** (Infection, *Pseudomonas* NEC) [in this order]

3. **250.71** (Diabetes, with gangrene); **785.4** (Gangrene) [in this order]

4. **599.0** (Infection, urinary [tract] NEC); **041.4** (Infection, *Escherichia coli* NEC) [in this order]

5. **277.39** (Cardiomyopathy, amyloid); **425.7** (Cardiomyopathy, metabolic NEC, amyloid)

Exercise 4-4

1. **482.2** (Pneumonia, due to, *Haemophilus influenzae*)

2. **112.0** (Thrush)

3. **008.45** (Enteritis, *Clostridium difficile*)

4. **003.0** (Gastroenteritis, *salmonella*)

5. **823.82** (Fracture, tibia (closed), with fibula)

Exercise 4-5

1. Residual: scars, face
   Cause: third-degree burns

2. Residual: constrictive pericarditis
   Cause: tuberculosis infection

3. Residual: foreign body, femur
   Cause: gunshot injury, femur
4. Residual: mental retardation
   Cause: poliomyelitis
5. Residual: leg pain
   Cause: fracture, femur

Exercise 4-6
1. Residual: arthritis, ankle, traumatic
   Code: **716.17** (Arthritis, traumatic)
   Cause: fracture, ankle
   Code: **905.4** (Late effect, fracture, extremity, lower)
2. Residual: dysphasia
   Code: There is no code for the residual because there is one combination code that reports both the residual and the cause.
   Cause: cerebrovascular accident
   Code: **438.12** (Late effect, cerebrovascular disease with dysphasia)
3. Residual: deafness, sensorineural
   Code: **389.10** (Deafness, sensorineural)
   Cause: meningitis
   Code: **326** (Late effect, meningitis, unspecified cause)

Exercise 4-7
1. **435.9** (Stroke, in evolution)
2. **291.0** (Impending, delirium tremens)
3. **640.00** (Threatened, miscarriage, unspecified)
4. **644.10** (Labor, threatened unspecified)
5. **411.1** (Impending, coronary, syndrome)

CHAPTER 5

Exercise 5-1
1. **008.8** (Gastroenteritis, viral NEC)
2. **038.43** (Septicemia, *Pseudomonas*); **995.92** (Severe sepsis); **785.52** (Septic, shock)
3. **045.90** (Poliomyelitis, unspecified type)
4. **112.1** (Candidiasis, vagina)

Exercise 5-2
1. i
2. c
3. h
4. g
5. a
6. b
7. e
8. f
9. d

Exercise 5-3
1. **V58.11** (Chemotherapy, encounter for); **183.0** (Neoplasm, ovary, primary)

2. **V58.0** (Admission, radiation management); **198.5** (Neoplasm, bone, secondary); **V10.3** (History, malignant neoplasm, breast)

3. a. metastatic carcinoma of bronchus

   b. primary, unknown

   c. secondary

   d. **197.0** (Neoplasm, lung, main bronchus, secondary); **199.1** (Neoplasm, unknown site or unspecified, primary)

4. a. Two

   b. Uncontrolled nausea and vomiting

   c. Lung cancer

   d. **787.01** (Nausea, with vomiting)

   e. **162.9** (Neoplasm, lung, primary); **E933.1** (Table of Drugs and Chemicals, Antineoplastic Agents, Therapeutic Use)

Exercise 5-4
1. **203.00** (Myeloma, multiple)
2. **233.1** (Neoplasm, cervix)
3. **153.3** (Neoplasm, intestinal, colon, sigmoid, primary); **197.6** (Neoplasm, peritoneum, secondary)
4. **185** (Neoplasm, prostate, primary); **198.5** (Neoplasm, bone, secondary)
5. **198.3** (Neoplasm, brain, secondary); **199.1** (Neoplasm, unknown, primary)
6. **197.0** (Neoplasm, lung, secondary); **V10.3** (History (of), malignant neoplasm (of), breast). Note: This is personal history, not family history, V16.3.

Exercise 5-5
1. **255.41** (Disease, Addison's)
2. **276.51** (Dehydration)
3. **250.30** (Diabetes, coma, hypoglycemic)
4. **242.01** (Goiter, toxic, with mention of thyrotoxic crisis or storm)

Exercise 5-6
1. **281.0** (Anemia, pernicious)
2. **286.6** (Coagulation, intravascular)
3. **286.0** (Hemophilia)
4. **285.1** (Anemia, blood loss, acute)
5. **289.6** (Polycythemia, familial)

Exercise 5-7
1. **331.0** (Alzheimer's, disease or sclerosis); **294.11** (Alzheimer's, dementia, with behavior disturbance) [in this order]
2. **300.4** (Depression, anxiety)
3. **318.2** (Retardation, mental, profound, IQ under 20)
4. **307.1** (Anorexia, nervosa)
5. **291.0** (Delirium, withdrawal, alcoholic, acute); **303.91** (Dependence, alcohol, alcoholic)

Exercise 5-8
1. **320.82** (Meningitis, *Proteus morganii*)
2. **340** (Sclerosis, multiple)
3. **382.9** (Otitis, media, acute)
4. **365.11** (Glaucoma, chronic, open angle)
5. **351.0** (Palsy, Bell's)

Exercise 5-9
1. **428.0** (Failure, heart, congestive)
2. **410.71** (Infarction, subendocardial)
3. **446.0** (Periarteritis); **405.99** (Hypertension, due to, periarteritis nodosa)
4. **434.01** (Infarction, brain, thrombotic)
5. **430** (Hemorrhage, subarachnoid)

Exercise 5-10
1. **464.4** (Croup)
2. **518.81** (Respiratory, failure); **428.0** (Disease, heart, congestive)
3. **491.20** (Disease, lung, obstructive with, bronchitis)
4. **487.1** (Influenza, with, bronchitis)
5. **482.2** (Pneumonia, due to, Hemophilus influenzae)

CHAPTER 6

Exercise 6-1
1. **540.0** (Appendicitis, with perforation, peritonitis or rupture)
2. **532.00** (Ulcer, duodenum, acute, with hemorrhage)
3. **574.00** (Cholelithiasis, with cholecystitis, acute); **574.10** (Cholelithiasis, with cholecystitis, chronic). Note acute before chronic.
4. **558.9** (Gastroenteritis)
5. **530.81** (Reflux, gastroesophageal)

Exercise 6-2
1. **614.9** (Disease, pelvis, inflammatory)
2. **599.70** (Hematuria, unspecified)
3. **590.10** (Pyelonephritis, acute); **590.00** (Pyelonephritis, chronic). Note acute before chronic.
4. **600.00** (Hypertrophy, prostate, benign)
5. **610.1** (Disease, breast, fibrocystic)

Exercise 6-3
1. **631** (Blighted ovum)
2. **634.91** (Abortion, spontaneous)
3. **644.13** (Labor, false)
4. **664.31** (Laceration, perineum, complicating delivery, fourth degree); **V27.0** (Outcome of delivery, single, liveborn)
5. **660.11** (Delivery, complicated by, deformity, fetus, causing obstructed labor); **653.41** (Delivery, complicated, cephalopelvic disproportion); **V27.0** (Outcome of delivery, single, liveborn)

Exercise 6-4
1. **698.9** (Pruritus)
2. **705.1** (Rash, heat)
3. **696.1** (Psoriasis)
4. **707.05** (Ulcer, skin, decubitus buttock); **707.20** (Unspecified stage)
5. **692.6** (Dermatitis, due to, poison ivy)

Exercise 6-5
1. **714.0** (Arthritis, rheumatoid)
2. **723.1** (Pain, neck)
3. **718.31** (Dislocation, shoulder, recurrent)
4. **733.11** (Fracture, pathologic, humerus); **198.5** (Neoplasm, bone, secondary); **V10.3** (History (of), malignant neoplasm, breast)

Exercise 6-6
1. **744.21** (Absence, ear, lobe)
2. **V30.00** (Newborn, single, born in hospital, without mention of cesarean delivery or section); **752.51** (Undescended, testis)
3. **759.83** (Syndrome, fragile X)
4. **754.30** (Dislocation, hip, congenital)

Exercise 6-7
1. **780.91** (Fussy infant)
2. **786.52** (Pain, chest, wall)
3. **793.80** (Abnormal, mammogram)
4. **780.39** (Seizure)
5. **796.2** (Blood, pressure, high, incidental reading, without diagnosis of hypertension)

Exercise 6-8
1. Derailment, railway; **E802.0**
2. Accident, motor vehicle, not involving collision; **E816.0**
3. Collision, off-road vehicle and other object, fixed; **E821.0**
4. Collision, animal being ridden; **E828.2**
5. Collision, watercraft, causing, injury; **E831.1**

Exercise 6-9
1. **980.0** (Alcohol, grain, beverage, Poisoning), **E980.9** (Poisoning, Alcohol, grain, beverage, Undetermined)
2. **989.89** (Antifreeze, Poisoning), E980.9 (Poisoning, antifreeze, Undetermined)
3. **969.4** (Valium, Poisoning), **E853.2** (Poisoning, Valium, Accidental)
4. Due to drugs and medicines

Exercise 6-10
1. **942.33** (Burn, abdomen, third degree); **945.26** (Burn, thigh, second degree); **E924.0** (Burning, hot, liquid); **948.11**—15% with 10% third degree (Burn, extent)
2. **945.36** (Burn, thigh, third degree); **958.3** (Burn, infected); **948.00**—4½% (Burn, extent) (No E code is required for subsequent treatment.)
3. **945.22** (Burn, foot, second degree) (Note that only the highest-level burn is coded when burns are in the same area.); **948.00**—2¼% (Burn, extent); **E897** (Fire, controlled, bonfire)
4. **944.30** (Burn, hand, third degree); **948.00**—2¼% (Burn, extent) (No E code is required for subsequent treatment.)
5. **942.32** (Burn, chest wall, third degree); **943.21** (Burn, forearm, second degree); **944.10** (Burn, hand, first degree); **948.10**—11% (Burn, extent) [in this order] (No E code is required for subsequent treatment.)

Exercise 6-11
1. **996.69** (Complications, breast implants, infection or inflammation)
2. **996.85** (Rejection, transplant, bone marrow)
3. **998.59** (Abscess, postoperative), **682.9** (Abscess, postoperative, stitch, unspecified site)
4. **996.01** (Complications, mechanical, implant, electrode NEC, cardiac)

CHAPTER 7

Exercise 7-1
1. F
2. 1
3. B
4. 0

5. D
6. 0

Exercise 7-2

1. 7
2. L
3. M
4. G
5. N
6. 1
7. R
8. 5
9. T
10. 8

Exercise 7-3

1. transfer
2. excision
3. inspection
4. transplantation
5. insertion
6. removal
7. fragmentation
8. occlusion
9. revision
10. release

Exercise 7-4

1. complete
2. expandable
3. multiaxial
4. standardized in terminology (in any order)
5. 7
6. alphanumeric
7. 34
8. O and I
9. procedure

CHAPTER 8

Exercise 8-1

1. American Medical Association or AMA
2. Current Procedural Terminology
3. services
4. 1966
5. 1983

Exercise 8-2

1. c
2. a
3. g
4. b
5. d

6. e

7. f

8. Appendix B

9. Appendix E

10. Appendix D

Exercise 8-3

1. Surgery

2. Respiratory System

3. Nose

4. Excision

Exercise 8-4

1. A concise statement describing the symptom, problem, condition, diagnosis, or other factor that is the reason for the encounter, usually stated in the patient's words

2. different

3. interpreting physician

4. a physician

5. **99070**

Exercise 8-5

1. those codes that have full description (or similar wording)

2. those codes that include their own description as well as that portion of the stand-alone code description found before the semicolon in a preceding code (or similar wording)

3. alternative anatomic site, alternative procedure, or description of the extent of service (in any order and similar wording)

Exercise 8-6

1. -62

2. **43820-62**

3. -50

4. -78

5. -57

6. -51

7. -66

8. -80

Exercise 8-7

1. **69799, 29999, 43499**

2. **88299, 81099, 84999**

3. **99199**

4. **77799, 78999**

Exercise 8-8

1. **49900**

2. **27303**

3. **27786-27814, 27792**

Exercise 8-9

1. a. Emergency

   b. **99288** (Emergency Department Services, Physician Direction of Advanced Life Support)

2. a. Fracture

   b. **27238** (Fracture, Femur, Intertrochanteric, Closed Treatment)

3. a. Removal

   b. **47480** (Removal, Calculi, Gallbladder)

4. a. Lung

   b. **32141** (Lung, Bullae, Excision)

Exercise 8-10

1. *See* Dialysis
2. *See* Antinuclear Antibodies (ANA)
3. *See* Radius; Ulna; Wrist

Exercise 8-11

1. into the subarachnoid space
2. into a vein
3. into a muscle
4. under the skin
5. through the respiratory system

Exercise 8-12

1. a. Current Procedural Terminology or CPT, Level I
   b. National Codes, Level II
2. K, G, Q, S (in any order)
3. No
4. J codes
5. oral
6. E codes
7. a. -NU
   b. -E2
   c. -AM
8. IM
9. up to 5 mg
10. **J1730**
11. **A4918**

CHAPTER 9

Exercise 9-1

1. **57270-22**
2. **54535-22; 186.9** (Neoplasm, testis, testes, Malignant, Primary); **998.11** (Complications, hemorrhage)
3. -23; **578.0** (Hematemesis); **331.0, 294.11** (Alzheimer's, dementia, with behavioral disturbance). Suspected peptic ulcer is not reported since it has not been confirmed.
4. -24; **294.8** (Dementia)
5. -25
6. -26

Exercise 9-2

1. -32; **V70.3** (Examination, medical, insurance certification)
2. -47
3. -50; **354.0** (Carpal tunnel syndrome)
4. **17274** and **17264-51; 173.4** (Neoplasm, skin, neck, Malignant, Primary); **173.6** (Neoplasm, skin, arm, Malignant, Primary) (Code 17274 is more resource-intensive and listed first without the modifier.)

5. **61250** and **61250-50**; **852.20** (Hematoma, subdural unspecified state of consciousness)
6. **28450** and **28450-51**
7. **27447** and **27447-50** (Arthroplasty, Knee)
8. **-52**
9. **24006** and **24006-50** or **24006-50** or **24006-RT** and **24006-LT**
10. **19305-50** or **19305** and **19305-50** or **19305-RT** and **19305-LT**

Exercise 9-3
1. **-58**; **202.91** (Neoplasm, lymph, gland, primary, any site, NEC)
2. **43124-54**
3. **19306-55**
4. **19306-56**

Exercise 9-4
1. -62
2. -66, **070.54** (Hepatitis, viral type C, chronic); **571.5** (Cirrhosis)
3. -80
4. -81
5. -78
6. -79
7. -77

Exercise 9-5
1. -99
2. -90
3. -91

CHAPTER 10

Exercise 10-1
1. office
2. office visit or other outpatient service
3. new
4. **99201**
5. five
6. five

Exercise 10-2
1. problem focused
2. expanded problem focused
3. detailed
4. comprehensive
5. comprehensive

Exercise 10-3
1. problem focused
2. expanded problem focused
3. detailed
4. comprehensive
5. comprehensive

Exercise 10-4
1. OS
2. BA

3. OS

4. OS

5. OS

6. OS

7. OS

8. BA

9. BA

10. BA

11. OS

12. OS

13. BA

14. OS

15. OS

16. BA

17. OS

18. OS

19. OS

20. OS

Note: Some terms—thorax, lungs, heart, vagina, blood vessels, neurologic—are specifically presented in the text as being a body area or an organ system. For other terms, you have to make the connection; for example, the thorax is examined as a body area but the lungs are examined as an organ system.

21. a. expanded problem focused (CC, brief HPI, problem pertinent ROS, and no PFSH required)

    b. expanded problem focused (the constitutional and one organ system, equals 2 for an expanded problem focused examination)

22.   CC: Cold

      HPI: Quality (dry, hacking)

             Location (nasal)

             Duration (9 days)

             Associated Signs and Symptoms (sleeplessness)

             HPI ELEMENTS (4) = COMPREHENSIVE

      PFSH: Personal

             Family

             PFSH ELEMENTS (2) = COMPREHENSIVE

      ROS: Constitutional (fever, aching)

             Respiratory (coughing)

             ROS ELEMENTS (2) = DETAILED

    a. detailed (Level 3)

       General survey: Minor distress

       Vital signs: Temperature, BP, pulse

       CONSTITUTIONAL (no matter how many elements checked off it only counts as 1) = 1

       BODY AREAS: Head = 1

       ORGAN SYSTEMS: Respiratory (mucous membranes, lungs clear to percussion and auscultation), Otolaryngologic (ears, nose) = 2

b. Expanded Problem Focused
Detailed history
EPF Exam

Exercise 10-5
1. limited (Some chart audit forms classify a new problem with no further follow-up planned as multiple.)
2. limited (The data could be moderate if the patient has brought records that the physician would have to review.)
3. moderate
4. low
5. **99203; 722.73** (Myelopathy, due to or with, intervertebral disc disorder, lumbar, lumbosacral)
   ICD-10-CM: **M51.07** (Myelopathy, due to or with, intervertebral disc disorder, lumbar, lumbosacral)
6. straightforward or low; **381.01** (Otitis, media, serous, acute)
   ICD-10-CM: **H65.00** (Otitis, media, serous, acute, unspecified ear)
7. low (risks are increased for the elderly); **461.9** (Sinusitis, acute)
   ICD-10-CM: **J01.90** (Sinusitis)

Exercise 10-6
1. b or c; **381.00** (Otitis, media, acute, with effusion)
   ICD-10-CM: **H65.191** (Otitis, media, acute, with effusion, right ear)
2. d or e; **491.21** (Disease, lung, obstructive, with, exacerbation NEC)
   ICD-10-CM: **J44.1** (Disease, lung, obstructive, with, exacerbation)
3. e; **786.05** (Short, breath); **425.4** (Cardiomyopathy, congestive)
   ICD-10-CM: **R06.02** (Shortness, breath), **I42.0** (Cardiomyopathy, congestive)
4. c; **842.10** (Sprain, thumb)
   ICD-10-CM: **S6392.xA** (Sprain, thumb, left, initial encounter)
5. a; **401.0** (Hypertension, Malignant)
   ICD-10-CM: **I10** (Hypertension, Malignant)
6. b; **477.0** (Allergy, grass)
   ICD-10-CM: **J30.1** (Allergy, grass)

Exercise 10-7
1. detailed, detailed, low
2. comprehensive, comprehensive, moderate
3. comprehensive, comprehensive, high
4. **99203** (Office and/or Other Outpatient Services, Office Visit, New Patient); **V26.52** (Sterilization, status, vasectomy)
   ICD-10-CM: **Z98.52** (Sterilization, status, vasectomy)
5. **99201** (Office and/or Other Outpatient Services, Office Visit, New Patient); **V58.32** (Suture, removal)
   ICD-10-CM: **Z48.02** (Suture, removal)
6. **99205** (Office and/or Other Outpatient Services, Office Visit, New Patient); **311** (Depression); **780.52** (Sleeplessness); **305.1** (Abuse, tobacco) (Note that some coders may assign 90801, Psychiatric Diagnostic or Evaluation Interview Procedures, subject to the credentials of the provider.)
   ICD-10-CM: **F32.9** (Depression), **G47.00** (Sleeplessness), **F17.200** (Abuse, tobacco)

7. **99203** (Office and/or Other Outpatient Services, Office Visit, New Patient); **844.1** (Sprain, strain; medial collateral, knee)

   ICD-10-CM: **S83.419A** (Sprain, strain; medial collateral, knee, unspecified knee, initial encounter)

8. **99202** (Office and/or Other Outpatient Services, Office Visit, New Patient); **477.0** (Allergy, grass, pollen)

   ICD-10-CM: **J30.1** (Allergy, grass, pollen)

Exercise 10-8

1. yes

2. **99212** (Office and/or Other Outpatient Services, Office Visit, Established Patient) (Note: Some chart audit forms would assign 99213 because of the antibiotic prescription.)

3. **99211** (Office and/or Other Outpatient Services, Office Visit, Established Patient); **717.83** (Sprain, knee, old, cruciate, anterior)

   ICD-10-CM: **S83.519D** (Sprain, knee, cruciate, anterior, unspecified knee, subsequent encounter)

4. **99215** (Office and/or Other Outpatient Services, Office Visit, Established Patient); **780.2** (Fainting)

   ICD-10-CM: **R55** (Fainting)

5. **99213** (Office and/or Other Outpatient Services, Office Visit, Established Patient); **780.79** (Malaise); **995.20** (Effect, adverse, drug/medicinal); **401.9** (Hypertension, Unspecified) (Note: Although the MDM complexity is at the level of code 99214, the history and examination were at the level of code 99213; because two of the three key components must be documented in order to use 99214, you must assign the lower level, 99213.)

   ICD-10-CM: **R53.81** (Malaise), **T46.5X5** (Effect, adverse, drug/medicinal), **I10** (Hypertension, Unspecified)

6. **99212** (Office and/or Other Outpatient Services, Office Visit, Established Patient); **701.9** (Tag, skin)

   ICD-10-CM: **L91.8** (Tag, skin)

7. **99213** (Office and/or Other Outpatient Services, Office Visit, Established Patient); **787.91** (Diarrhea)

   ICD-10-CM: **R19.7** (Diarrhea)

Exercise 10-9

1. **99219** (Hospital Services, Observation, Initial Care); **850.11** (Concussion, with, loss of consciousness, brief)

   ICD-10-CM: **S06.0X1A** (Consciousness, with, loss of consciousness, unspecified duration, initial encounter)

Exercise 10-10

1. **99221** (Hospital Service, Initial Hospital Care)

2. **99223** (Hospital Service, Initial Hospital Care)

3. comprehensive, moderate

4. **99221** (Hospital Service, Inpatient Services, Initial Hospital Care); **595.0** (Cystitis, acute); **590.10** (Pyelitis, acute)

   ICD-10-CM: **N30.00** (Cystitis, acute), **N10** (Pyelitis, acute)

Exercise 10-11

1. 30 minutes or less, more than 30 minutes

2. no

Exercise 10-12

1. **99244** (Consultation, Office and/or Other Outpatient); **733.13** (Fracture, pathologic); **V10.3** (History, personal, malignant neoplasm, breast)

   ICD-10-CM: **M84.68xA** (Fracture, pathological, other site, initial encounter for fracture), **Z85.3** (History, personal, malignant, breast)

2. **99241** (Consultation, Office and/or Other Outpatient); **726.90** (Tendinitis); **726.33** (Bursitis, elbow)

   ICD-10-CM: **M77.9** (Tendinitis), **M70.21** (Bursitis, elbow, right elbow)

3. **99242** (Consultation, Office and/or Other Outpatient); **715.16** (Osteoarthritis)

   ICD-10-CM: **M17.11** (Osteoarthritis, knee, right)

4. **99241** (Consultation, Office and/or Other Outpatient); **455.2** (Hemorrhoids, internal, bleeding)

   ICD-10-CM: **I84.111** (Hemorrhoids, internal, bleeding)

5. **99244** (Consultation, Office and/or Other Outpatient); **786.09** (Dyspnea), **780.79** (Fatigue), **780.4** (Dizziness), **424.0** (Insufficiency, mitral), **V45.01** (Status, cardiac, device, pacemaker)

   ICD-10-CM: **R06.00** (Dyspnea), **R53.83** (Fatigue), **R42** (Dizziness), **I34.0** (Insufficiency, mitral), **Z95.0** (Status, cardiac, device, pacemaker)

6. **99252** (Consultation, Inpatient); **427.31** (Fibrillation, atrial)

   ICD-10-CM: **I48.0** (Fibrillation, atrial)

7. **99255-57** (Consultation, Inpatient) (Modifier -57 indicates the decision to perform surgery.)

8. **99252** (Consultation, Inpatient)

9. **99255** (Consultation, Inpatient); **780.31** (Febrile, convulsion)

   ICD-10-CM: **R56.00** (Febrile, convulsion)

10. **99233** (Hospital Inpatient Services, Subsequent Hospital Care); **410.11** (Infarction, myocardial) (Note that the angina and tachycardia are not reported as both of these are symptoms of myocardial infarction.)

    ICD-10-CM: **I21.09** (Infarction, myocardial)

11. **99233** (Hospital Inpatient Services, Subsequent Hospital Care); **780.39** (Febrile, convulsion)

    ICD-10-CM: **R56.9** (Febrile, convulsion)

12. **99244** (Consultation, Office); **745.2** (Tetralogy of Fallot)

    ICD-10-CM: **Q21.3** (Tetralogy of Fallot)

13. **99242-32** (Consultation, Office) (Modifier -32, insurance company requested)

14. **99244-32** (Consultation, Office) (Modifier -32 indicates a mandatory consultation.)

Exercise 10-13

1. self-limited or minor
2. high
3. moderate
4. low to moderate
5. **99285** (Emergency Department Services); **427.5** (Arrest, cardiac)

   ICD-10-CM: **I46.9** (Arrest, cardiac)

6. **99285** (Emergency Department Services); **518.82** (Distress, respiratory, acute [adult])

   ICD-10-CM: **J80** (Distress, respiratory, acute [adult])

7. **99283** (Emergency Department Services)

8. **99288** (Emergency Department, Physician Direction of Advanced Life Support)

Exercise 10-14
1. **99291** (Critical Care Services)

2. no

3. **99291** and **99292 × 4** (180 minutes of care) (Critical Care Services); **949.2** (Burn, unspecified site, multiple, second degree); **948.50** (Burn, unspecified site, multiple, 50-59 percent)

   ICD-10-CM: **T30.0** (Burn, unspecified site, multiple, second degree), **T31.50** (Burn, unspecified site, multiple, 50-59 percent)

Exercise 10-15
1. moderate

2. **99306** (Nursing Facility Services, Initial Care); **434.91** (Accident, cerebral), **250.00** (Diabetes), **401.9** (Hypertension, unspecified)

   ICD-10-CM: **I63.50** (Accident, cerebral), **E11.9** (Diabetes), **I10** (Hypertension, unspecified)

3. c

4. b

5. a

6. **99308** (Nursing Facility Services, Subsequent Care); **518.89** (Infection, respiratory); **780.09** (Unconscious)

   ICD-10-CM: **J06.9** (Infection, respiratory), **R40.20** (Unconscious)

Exercise 10-16
1. **99347** (Home Services, Established Patient)

Exercise 10-17
1. no

2. no, in addition to another E/M code

3. no, the physician has to spend at least 30 minutes

4. whether the patient is an inpatient or an outpatient

5. no, by time

6. no

Exercise 10-18
1. 30 minutes or more

2. 99366, 99367, 99368

Exercise 10-19
1. age

2. -25

Exercise 10-20
1. Basic Life and/or Disability Evaluation Services

2. Work-Related or Medical Disability Evaluation Services

3. whether the treating physician or a physician other than the treating physician conducted the evaluation

4. **99455** (Insurance Examination); **V70.3** (Examination, medical, insurance certification); **492.8** (Disease, lung, obstructive, with, emphysema NEC)

   ICD-10-CM: **Z02.71** (Examination, medical, insurance disability), **J43.9** (Disease, obstructive, with, emphysema NEC)

Exercise 10-21
1. very low birth weight

2. **99466** (Critical Care Services, Interfacility Transport)

3. **99463** (Newborn Care, Normal)

4. **99476** (Critical Care Services, Pediatric, Subsequent)

5. **99478** (Critical Care Services, Neonatal, Low Birth Weight Infant)

Exercise 10-22

1. **99201** (Office and/or Other Outpatient Services, Office Visits, New Patient); **383.00** (Mastoiditis, acute)

   ICD-10-CM: **H70.009** (Mastoiditis, acute, unspecified ear)

2. **99212** (Office and Other Outpatient Visits, Office Visits, Established Patient); **382.9** (Otitis, media, acute)

   ICD-10-CM: **H66.90** (Otitis, media, acute, unspecified ear)

3. **99211** (Office and/or Other Outpatient Services, Office Visits, Established Patient)

4. **99306** (Nursing Facility Services, Initial Care)

5. **99202** (Office and/or Other Outpatient Services, Office Visits, New Patient); **706.1** (Acne)

   ICD-10-CM: **L70.9** (Acne)

6. **99211** (Office and/or Other Outpatient Services, Office Visits, Established Patient)

7. **99285** (Emergency Department Services); **427.0** (Tachycardia, paroxysmal, nodal)

   ICD-10-CM: **I47.1** (Tachycardia, paroxysmal, nodal)

8. **99291** (Critical Care Services)

9. **99291** (Critical Care Services) and **99292** (Critical Care Services)

10. **99214** (Office and/or Other Outpatient Services, Established Patient)

11. **99254** (Consultation, Inpatient)

CHAPTER 11

Exercise 11-1

1. Radiologic Procedures, Burn Excisions or Debridement, Obstetrics, and Other Procedures

2. absence of pain

3. induction or administration of a drug to obtain partial or complete loss of sensation (or similar wording)

4. general, regional, local, sacral, caudal, lumbar, endotracheal, epidural, and patient controlled

5. moderate or conscious sedation

6. Medicine

Exercise 11-2

1. P2

2. P3

3. 99116

4. actual

5. Stop

6. start

Exercise 11-3

1. -22

2. -23

3. -AD

4. -QS

5. -QX

Exercise 11-4

1. **01999** (Anesthesia, Unlisted Services and Procedures)

2. Anesthesia, Thyroid, **00322**

3. Anesthesia, Cesarean Delivery, **01961**

4. Anesthesia, Prostate, or Anesthesia, Transurethral Procedures, **00914**

5. Anesthesia, Cleft Palate Repair, **00172**

6. Anesthesia, Achilles Tendon Repair, **01472**

7. **$98.50** (B = 3, T = 1, M = 1; total 5; 5 $19.70)

8. a. **$203.85** (B = 5, T = 4, M = 0; total 9; 9 $22.65)

   b. **$182.07** (B = 5, T = 4, M = 0; total 9; 9 $20.23)

9. a. **$199.10** (B = 7, T = 2, M = 1; total 10; 10 $19.91)

   b. **$219.01** (B = 7, T = 3, M = 1; total 11; 11 $19.91)

CHAPTER 12

Exercise 12-1

1. **20999**

2. **69949**

3. **17999**

4. **27899**

5. **64999**

6. **67999**

Exercise 12-2

1. pre-, intra-, and postoperative services, or similar wording

2. no

3. no

Exercise 12-3

1. **10021** (Aspiration, Fine Needle)

2. **10022** (Aspiration, Fine Needle), **76942** (Ultrasound, Guidance)

CHAPTER 13

Exercise 13-1

1. **11056** (Lesion, Skin, Paring/Curettement); **078.19** (Wart, common)

2. **11200** (Lesion, Skin Tags, Removal); **701.9** (Tag, skin)

3. **11311** (Lesion, Skin, Shaving); **709.9** (Lesion, dermal)

Exercise 13-2

1. **13121** (Repair, Wound, Complex); **882.0** (Wound, hand)

2. **13101** for complex repair of abdomen (Repair, Wound, Complex); **12004-51** for 12-cm simple repair of back, forearm, and neck added together (Repair, Wound, Simple). (Note that the same types of repair are combined—back (trunk), forearm (extremities), and neck are all included in the code description for 12004.)

3. **12034** for the 10.7-cm intermediate forearm repair (Wound, Repair, Intermediate); **12002-51** for the 3.1-cm scalp repair (Repair, Wound, Simple)

4. Cheek graft: **15120** (Skin Grafts and Flaps, Split Grafts)

    Upper chest: **15100-51, 15101** (Skin Grafts and Flaps, Split Grafts) [no modifier on add-on code 15101]

    Site prep, cheek, 100 cm²: **15004-51** (Skin Grafts and Flaps, Recipient Site Preparation)

    Site prep, chest, 200 cm²: **15002-51, 15003** (Skin Grafts and Flaps, Recipient Site Preparation) [no modifier on add-on code 15003]

    Note: If this claim were submitted to Medicare, modifier -51 would not be appended on the site preparation codes.

5. **14041** (Skin, Adjacent Tissue Transfer)

6. **14040** (Skin, Adjacent Tissue Transfer) (Note that a Z-plasty is a form of adjacent tissue transfer. The excision is included in the adjacent tissue transfer code.)

7. **15732** (Skin, Myocutaneous) (Note that modifier -58 may also be used if the procedure was a staged procedure.)

8. Week 1: **16025 × 5** (Burns, Debridement/Dressing)

    Weeks 2 and 3: **16025 × 6** (Burns, Debridement/Dressing) (Some payers would allow you to submit all treatments together with **16025 × 11**.)

Exercise 13-3

1. **17110** (Destruction, Skin, Lesion, Benign) (If a specific anatomic area was indicated, you could report the destruction with a more specific code. For example, 56501 for destruction of a lesion of the vulva.)

2. **17000** (Destruction, Skin, Benign), **17003 × 13** (Destruction, Skin, Benign); **702.0** (Keratitis, actinic)

3. **17311** (Mohs' Micrographic Surgery)

Exercise 13-4

1. **19000** (Breast, Cyst, Puncture Aspiration)

2. **19303** and **19303-50** or **19303-50** or **19303-RT** and **19303-LT** (Breast, Removal, Simple, Complete)

3. **19307-RT** (Breast, Removal, Modified Radical)

4. **19290-LT** (Breast, Needle Wire Placement)

5. **19350-RT** (Breast, Reconstruction, Nipple, Areola)

CHAPTER 14

Exercise 14-1

1. **21310** (Nasal Bone, Fracture, Closed Treatment)

2. **21800** (Rib, Fracture, Closed Treatment)

3. **28675** (Dislocation, Interphalangeal Joint, Toe, Open Treatment)

4. **27792** (Fracture, Fibula, Open Treatment)

5. **27500** (Fracture, Femur, Closed Treatment)

6. **27235** (Fracture, Femur, Percutaneous Fixation)

7. **23670** (Fracture, Humerus, with Dislocation, Open Treatment); **812.03** (Fracture, humerus, great tuberosity). According to Coding Clinic, 3rd Quarter 1990, p. 13: "For purposes of classification, ICD-9-CM assigns only the fracture code to fracture-dislocations of the same site. It is incorrect to also code the dislocation."

    ICD-10-CM: **S42.256A** (Fracture, humerus, great tuberosity, unspecified humerus, initial encounter for closed fracture)

8. **21453** (Fracture, Mandible, Closed Treatment, Interdental Fixation); **802.20** (Fracture, mandible [closed])

   ICD-10-CM: **S02.60XA** (Fracture, mandible [closed], unspecified site, initial encounter for closed fracture)

9. **25606** (Fracture, Radius, Percutaneous Fixation); **813.81** (Fracture, radius [closed])

   ICD-10-CM: **S52.509A** (Fracture, radius [closed], unspecified site, initial encounter for closed fracture)

10. **27840** (Ankle, Dislocation, Closed Treatment); **837.0** (Dislocation, ankle, closed)

    ICD-10-CM: **S93.06XA** (Dislocation, ankle, closed, unspecified ankle, initial encounter)

Exercise 14-2

1. **20103** (Wound, Exploration, Penetrating Extremity)
2. **20838** (Replantation, Foot)
3. **21015** (Tumor, Resection, Face)
4. **20974** (Electrical Stimulation, Bone Healing, Noninvasive)
5. **20206** (Biopsy, Muscle); **359.22** (Dystrophy, muscular, congenital, myotonic)

   ICD-10-CM: **G71.2** (Dystrophy, muscular, congenital, myotonic)
6. **20600** (Aspiration, Joint); **716.94** (Arthritis, hand)

   ICD-10-CM: **M13.849** (Arthritis, hand, unspecified hand)

Exercise 14-3

1. **29065** (Cast, Long Arm); **99070** or A4580-A4590 or O4005-O4008 (Supply, Materials)
2. **29425** (Cast, Walking)
3. **29705** (Cast, Removal)
4. **29530** (Strapping, Knee)
5. **29345** (Cast, Long Leg); **99070** or A4580-A4590 or O4005-O4008 (Supply, Materials)

Exercise 14-4

1. **29898** (Arthroscopy, Surgical, Ankle)
2. **29870** (Arthroscopy, Diagnostic, Knee)
3. **29805** (Arthroscopy, Shoulder)
4. **29850** (Fracture, Knee, Arthroscopic Treatment)
5. **29891** (Arthroscopy, Surgical, Ankle)

CHAPTER 15

Exercise 15-1

1. **31256** (Antrostomy, Sinus, Maxillary)
2. **31530** (Laryngoscopy, Direct)
3. **31628** (Bronchoscopy, Biopsy)
4. **32605** (Thoracoscopy, Diagnostic, without Biopsy)
5. **32663** (Thoracoscopy, Surgical, with Lobectomy)

Exercise 15-2

1. **30100** (Biopsy, Nose, Intranasal); **478.19** (Lesion, intranasal)

   ICD-10-CM: **J34.89** (Lesion, nose [internal])

2. **30420** (Rhinoplasty, Primary); **470** (Deviation, nasal septum)

ICD-10-CM: **J34.2** (Deviation [in], nasal septum)

3. **30901** (Epistaxis); **784.7** (Hemorrhage, nose)

ICD-10-CM: **R04.0** (Hemorrhage, nose)

4. **30520** (Septoplasty)

5. **30300** (Removal, Foreign Bodies, Nose)

Exercise 15-3
1. **31000** and **31000-50** (Sinuses, Maxillary, Irrigation)

2. **31070** (Sinusotomy, Frontal Sinus, Exploratory)

3. **31090** (Sinusotomy, Combined)

4. **31030** (Sinusotomy, Maxillary)

5. **31040** (Ptergomaxillary Fossa, Incision); **473.0** (Sinusitis, chronic, maxillary)

ICD-10-CM: **J32.0** (Sinusitis, chronic, maxillary)

Exercise 15-4
1. **31320** (Laryngotomy, Diagnostic)

2. **31580** (Laryngoplasty, Laryngeal Web)

3. **31500** (Endotracheal Tube, Intubation)

4. **31368** (Laryngectomy, Subtotal); **146.4** (Neoplasm, glossoepiglottic folds, Malignant, Primary)

ICD-10-CM: **C10.1** (Neoplasm, glosso-epiglottic folds, Malignant Primary)

5. **31390** (Pharyngolaryngectomy); **149.0** (Neoplasm, pharynx region, Malignant, Primary)

ICD-10-CM: **C14.0** (Neoplasm, pharynx region, Malignant Primary)

Exercise 15-5
1. **31605** (Tracheostomy, Emergency)

2. **31785** (Excision, Tumor, Trachea, Cervical)

3. **31715** (Bronchography, Injection, Transtracheal)

4. **31600** (Tracheostomy, Planned); **518.81** (Failure, respiratory, acute)

ICD-10-CM: **J96.0** (Failure, respiratory, acute)

5. **31717** (Bronchial Brush Biopsy, with Catheterization); **466.19** (Bronchiolitis, acute)

ICD-10-CM: **J21.9** (Bronchiolitis, acute)

Exercise 15-6
1. **32095** (Biopsy, Lung, Thoracotomy)

2. **32405** (Biopsy, Lung, Needle)

3. **32480** (Lobectomy, Lung), **32501** (Bronchoplasty) (Note that code 32501 is an add-on code and does not require modifier -51.)

4. **32503** (Resection, Lung); **162.9** (Neoplasm, lung, Malignant, Primary)

ICD-10-CM: **C34.90** (Neoplasm, lung Malignant Primary)

5. **32200** (Pneumonostomy); **513.0** (Abscess, lung)

ICD-10-CM: **J85.2** (Abscess, lung)

CHAPTER 16

Exercise 16-1

1. invasive
2. internal
3. Medicine, Surgery, Radiology (any order)
4. invasive
5. electrophysiology
6. Angiography or Angiogram

Exercise 16-2

1. **33207** (Pacemaker, Heart, Insertion)
2. **33216-78** (Pacemaker, Heart, Insertion, Electrode). Note that -78 is appended because the patient is in a postoperative period. The patient had a single-chamber pacemaker implanted. The replacement of the lead wire is reported as insertion of a new electrode, the removal of the defective electrode is not separately reported.
3. **33214** (Pacemaker, Conversion) also known as an upgrade
4. **33010** (Pericardiocentesis); **518.4** (Edema, pulmonary, lung, acute), **420.90** (Effusion, pericardium, acute)

   ICD-10-CM: **J81.0** (Edema, lung, acute), **I30.8** (Pericarditis, acute)
5. **33120** (Tumor, Heart, Excision); **164.1** (Neoplasm, heart, endocardium, Malignant, Primary)

   ICD-10-CM: **C38.0** (Neoplasm, heart)

Exercise 16-3

1. **33430** (Mitral Valve, Replacement)
2. **33405** (Aorta, Valve, Replacement) (Note that a prosthetic valve, and not a homograft valve, is used.)
3. **33251** (Heart, Arrhythmogenic Focus, Destruction); **427.89** (Arrhythemia, bigeminal rhythm)

   ICD-10-CM: **I49.8** (Arrhythmia, specified NEC)
4. **33282** (Implantation, Cardiac Event Recorder); **785.1** (Palpitation (heart)); **780.4** (Dizziness)

   ICD-10-CM: **R00.2** (Palpitations [heart]), **R42** (Dizziness)

Exercise 16-4

1. **33511** (Bypass Graft, Coronary Artery, Venous Graft)
2A. **33534** (Coronary Artery Bypass Graft, Arterial)
2B. **33519** (Coronary Artery Bypass Graft, Arterial-Venous); **414.01** (Disease, heart, artery, *see* arteriosclerosis, coronary artery native artery)

   ICD-10-CM: **I25.10** (Disease, heart, ischemic, atherosclerotic)
3. **33533** (Bypass Graft, Coronary Artery, Arterial) and **33519** (Coronary Artery, Bypass Graft, Arterial-Venous); **414.01** (Disease, heart, artery, *see* arteriosclerosis, coronary artery native artery), **402.10** (Hypertension, with heart disease, benign)

   ICD-10-CM: **I25.10** (Disease, heart, ischemic, atherosclerotic), **I11.9** (Hypertensive, heart, due to, hypertension)

Exercise 16-5

1. **34201** (Thrombectomy, Aortoiliac Artery)
2. **34001** (Embolectomy, Carotid Artery)
3. **35875** (Thrombectomy, Bypass Graft, Other Than Hemodialysis Graft or Fistula); **996.74** (Complication, vascular device, implant, graft)

   ICD-10-CM: **T82.868** (Complication[s], cardiac, thrombosis)

Exercise 16-6
1. **35506** (Bypass Graft, Carotid Artery)
2. **35556** (Bypass Graft, Femoral Artery)
3. **35650** (Bypass Graft, Axillary Artery)
4. **35141** (Aneurysm Repair, Femoral Artery); **442.3** (Aneurysm, femoral artery)

   ICD-10-CM: **I72.4** (Aneurysm, femoral [artery])
5. **36246-RT** or **36246-59-LT** (Catheterization, Legs), **75716-26** (Angiography, Leg Artery); **443.9** (Disease, peripheral, vascular)

   ICD-10-CM: **I73.9** (Disease, peripheral, vascular)

Exercise 16-7
1. **92950** (CPR)
2. **93015** (Stress Tests, Cardiovascular)
3. **92982-RC, 92984 × 2** (Angioplasty, Percutaneous Transluminal, Angioplasty)
4. **93278-26** (Electrocardiography, Signal-Averaged); **427.1** (Tachycardia, ventricular)

   ICD-10-CM: **I47.2** (Tachycardia, ventricular)

Exercise 16-8
1. Catheterization procedure **93501-26** (Catheterization, Cardiac, Right Heart); Injection procedure **93542-51** (Catheterization, Cardiac, Injection); Supervision, interpretation, and report for injection procedure **93555-26** (Catheterization, Cardiac, Imaging)
2. **93511** (Catheterization, Cardiac, Left Heart); **93543-51** (Catheterization, Cardiac, Injection); **93555** (Catheterization, Cardiac, Imaging); **414.01** (Arteriosclerosis, coronary (artery), native artery), **411.1** (Angina, unstable)

   ICD-10-CM: **I25.110** (Arteriosclerosis, coronary artery, native, with angina pectoris, unstable)
3. False; they are already bundled into the codes.
4. True
5. False; some codes are modifier -51-exempt.

Exercise 16-9
1. **93600** (Electrophysiology Procedure)
2. **93620, 93622** (Electrophysiology Procedure); **780.2** (Syncope, vasovagal)

   ICD-10-CM: **R55** (Syncope, vasovagal)
3. **93720** (Plethysmography, Total Body)

Exercise 16-10
1. Injection procedure for angiography **36215** (Catheterization, Brachiocephalic Artery), angiography **75658** (Angiography, Brachial Artery); contrast material **99070** (Supply, Materials) or **A9521**
2. **36215-LT** (Artery, Carotid, Catheterization), **75660** (Angiography, Carotid Artery)
3. **36216** (Artery, Carotid, Catheterization), **75660** (Angiography, Carotid Artery)
4. **75563** (MRI, Heart); **428.0** (Failure, heart, congestive); **427.69** (Premature beats, ventricular)

   ICD-10-CM: **I50.9** (Failure, heart, congestive), **I49.3** (Premature beats, ventricular)

CHAPTER 17

Exercise 17-1

1. **38550** (Lymph Nodes, Hygroma Cystic Axillary/Cervical, Excision); **228.1** (Hygroma)
   ICD-10-CM: **D18.1** (Hygroma)

2. **38100** (Splenectomy, Total); **272.7** (Gaucher's splenomegaly)
   ICD-10-CM: **E75.22** (Splenomegaly, Gaucher's)

3. **38200** (Splenoportography, Injection Procedure)

4. **38241** (Transplantation, Bone Marrow)

Exercise 17-2

1. **39502** (Diaphragm, Repair, Hernia), **553.3** (Hernia, hiatal)
   ICD-10-CM: **K44.9** (Hernia, hiatal)

2. **39000** (Mediastinum, Exploration), **164.9** (Neoplasm, mediastinum, mediastinal, Malignant, Primary)
   ICD-10-CM: **C38.3** (Neoplasm, mediastinum, mediastinal, Malignant, Primary)

3. **39220** (Mediastinum, Tumor, Excision), **212.5** (Neoplasm, mediastinum, mediastinal, Benign)
   ICD-10-CM: **D15.2** (Neoplasm, mediastinum, mediastinal, Benign)

4. **39520** (Diaphragm, Repair, Hernia)

CHAPTER 18

Exercise 18-1

1. vermilionectomy
2. gallbladder
3. 10.2 (4 × 2.54)
4. **40527** (Repair, Cleft Lip); **749.11** (Cleft, lip)
   ICD-10-CM: **Q36.9** (Cleft, lip)
5. **40650** (Repair, Lip); **140.9** (Neoplasm, lip, Malignant, Primary)
   ICD-10-CM: **C00.9** (Neoplasm, lip, Malignant, Primary)
6. **40800** (Mouth, Hematoma, Incision and Drainage)
7. **41252** (Tongue, Repair, Laceration). Note that the measurement of the laceration was stated in inches and must be converted to centimeters (1.5 in × 2.54 = 3.8 cm).

Exercise 18-2

1. **42826** (Tonsillectomy); **474.00** (Tonsillitis, hypertropic, chronic)
   ICD-10-CM: **J35.01** (Tonsillitis, hypertrophic)
2. **42900** (Suture, Pharynx, Wound)
3. **43045** (Esophagotomy)
4. **43101** (Esophagus, Lesion, Excision)
5. **43450** (Dilation, Esophagus)

Exercise 18-3

1. surgical communication from the colon to the rectum
2. surgical communication from the ileum to the body surface
3. surgical communication from the large intestine to the body surface
4. surgical communication between segments of intestine

5. **44141** (Colon, Excision, Partial); **153.9** (Neoplasm, intestine, colon, Malignant, Primary)

ICD-10-CM: **C26.0** (Neoplasm, intestine, colon, Malignant Primary)

6. **44120** (Enterectomy)

Exercise 18-4

1. **44960** (Excision, Appendix); **540.0** (Appendicitis, acute, with, perforation, peritonitis, or rupture)

ICD-10-CM: **K35.01** (Appendicitis, acute, with, perforation, peritonitis, or rupture)

2. **45331** (Sigmoidoscopy, Biopsy). The description states biopsy, single or multiple, so only one code is used for multiple (three) biopsies.

3. **45385** (Colonoscopy, Removal, Polyp)

4. **45331** (Endoscopy, Colon-Sigmoid, Biopsy)

Exercise 18-5

1. **47562** (Cholecystectomy). Note that the exploratory laparotomy is not coded, as it turns into the surgical approach once the cholecystectomy is performed.

2. **47480** (Cholecystotomy)

3. **49565** (Hernia Repair, Abdominal, Recurrent), **49568** (Implantation, Mesh, Hernia Repair). Note that the mesh code can be used only with incisional hernias, and it is stated to "list separately," so a -51 modifier is not necessary.

4. **49507** (Hernia Repair, Inguinal, Incarcerated)

5. **48155** (Pancreatectomy, Total)

6. **46257** (Hemorrhoidectomy, Simple, with Fissurectomy). Note that 46220 (Papillectomy) and 46080 (Sphincterotomy, Anal) are not reported as they are both bundled into code 46257.

CHAPTER 19

Exercise 19-1

1. **50065** (Nephrolithotomy). Note that the term "secondary" means that the procedure is being repeated. Some may code this 50060-76, but this would not be correct because there is a more accurate code to assign.

2. **50398-LT** (Nephrostomy, Change Tube)

3. **50590-RT** (Lithotripsy, Kidney), **52310-RT** (Cystourethroscopy, Removal, Urethral Stent)

Exercise 19-2

1. **50630-LT** (Ureterolithotomy)

2. **50780-50** (Ureteroneocystostomy) Modifier -50 indicates a bilateral procedure.

3. **50955-RT** (Ureter, Endoscopy, Biopsy), **50684-RT** (Ureter, Injection, Radiologic), **74425** (X-Ray, Urinary Tract)

Exercise 19-3

1. **51100** (Aspiration, Bladder)

2. **52332-RT** (Cystourethroscopy, Insertion, Indwelling Ureteral Stent)

3. **52332-LT** (Ureter, Endoscopy, Insertion, Stent), **74420-26** (Urography, Retrograde)

4. **51840** (Urethropexy)

5. **52320-LT** (Ureter, Endoscopy, Removal Calculus), **74420-50-26** or **74420-26-LT, 74420-26-RT** (Urography, Retrograde)

Exercise 19-4
1. **53520** (Urethra, Repair, Fistula)
2. **53405** (Urethra, Repair, Fistula)

Exercise 19-5
1. **54065** (Penis, Lesion, Destruction, Extensive); **078.19** (Condyloma, genital)
   ICD-10-CM: **A63.0** (Condyloma, genital)
2. **54415** (Removal, Prosthesis, Penis)

Exercise 19-6
1. **54520-50** (Orchiectomy, Simple) (Note that the terms "simple" and "radical" are based on the interpretation of the physician.)
2. **54505-50** (Biopsy, Testes)

Exercise 19-7
1. **54865** (Epididymis, Exploration, Biopsy); **608.9** (Pain, genital, male) (Note that even though the question states without biopsy, the CPT code states with or without biopsy, so this would be the correct code to assign.)
   ICD-10-CM: **N50.9** (Pain, genital, male)
2. **55000** (Tunica Vaginalis, Hydrocele, Aspiration)
3. **55400-50** (Vas Deferens, Repair, Suture), **69990** (Operating Microscope)

Exercise 19-8
1. **55845** (Prostatectomy, Retropubic, Radical); **185** (Neoplasm, prostate Malignant, Primary)
   ICD-10-CM: **C61** (Neoplasm, prostate, Malignant, Primary)
2. **53852** (Transurethral Procedure, Prostate, Radiofrequency)

CHAPTER 20

Exercise 20-1
1. **57061** (Destruction, Lesion, Vagina, Simple)
2. **56605, 56606 × 2** (Vulva, Perineum, Biopsy) (Note that the code 56605 is for the first lesion, and 56606 is for *each* additional lesion.)
3. **57305** (Vagina, Repair, Fistula, Rectovaginal)
4. **57520** (Cervix, Conization) (Note that dilation and curettage is not coded separately because it is included in the description of the conization.)
5. **58661** (Cystectomy, Ovarian, Laparoscopic)
6. c
7. b
8. d
9. a

Exercise 20-2
1. **59151** (Laparoscopy, Ectopic Pregnancy with Salpingectomy and/or Oophorectomy)
2. **59409** (Vaginal Delivery, Delivery only); **59412** (External Cephalic Version) (Note that the version is stated "list in addition"; therefore, modifier -51 is not necessary.)
3. **59320** (Cerclage, Cervix, Vaginal)

CHAPTER 21

Exercise 21-1
1. **60200** (Thyroid Gland, Cyst, Excision)
2. **60280** (Thyroglossal Duct, Cyst, Excision)
3. **60522** (Thymectomy, Sternal Split/Transthoracic Approach)
4. **60600** (Carotid Body, Lesion, Excision)
5. **60210** (Thyroid Gland, Excision, Partial)
6. **60650** (Laparoscopy, Adrenal Gland)
7. **60505** (Parathyroid, Excision), **60512** (Parathyroid Gland, Autotransplant)
8. **60502** (Parathyroid, Exploration)
9. **60605** (Carotid Body, Lesion, Carotid Artery)

Exercise 21-2
1. **61154** (Burr Hole, Skull, Drainage, Hematoma); **432.1** (Hematoma, subdural, nontraumatic)
   ICD-10-CM: **I62.00** (Hematoma, subdural, nontraumatic)
2. **61312** (Craniectomy, Surgical); **853.00** (Hematoma, brain, unspecified state of consciousness)
   ICD-10-CM: **S06.369A** (Hematoma, brain, unspecified state of consciousness)
3. **61607** (Skull Base Surgery, Middle Cranial Fossa, Extradural), **61605** Definitive procedure (Skull Base Surgery, Middle Cranial Fossa, Extradural), **61590-51** Approach Procedure (Skull Base Surgery, Middle Cranial Fossa, Infratemporal Approach); **191.9** (Neoplasm, cranial, fossa, any, Primary)
   ICD-10-CM: **C71.9** (Neoplasm, cranial, fossa, any, Primary)
4. **62258** (Shunt, Brain, Replacement); **742.3** (Hydrocephalus, congenital)
   ICD-10 CM: **Q03.9** (Hydrocephalus, congenital)

CHAPTER 22

Exercise 22-1
1. **65930-LT** (Eye, Removal, Blood Clot)
2. **67318-RT** (Strabismus, Repair, Superior Oblique Muscle)
3. **67145-LT** (Retina, Repair, Prophylaxis, Detachment)
4. **65772-RT** (Cornea, Repair, Astigmatism)
5. **65105-LT** (Removal, Eye, with Implant, Muscles Attached)

Exercise 22-2
1. **69801-LT** (Labyrinthotomy, with/without Cryosurgery)
2. **69436** and **69436-50** (Tympanostomy)
3. **69950-LT** (Vestibular Nerve, Section, Transcranial Approach)
4. **69310-RT** (Reconstruction, Auditory Canal, External)
5. **69820-RT** (Ear, Inner, Incision)

Exercise 22-3
1. exostosis
2. otoplasty
3. cholesteatoma
4. 69990

CHAPTER 23

Exercise 23-1

1. aorta
2. joint
3. biliary system and pancreas
4. bile ducts
5. urinary bladder
6. lacrimal sac or tear duct sac
7. duodenum or first part of the small intestine
8. heart or heart walls or neighboring tissues
9. subarachnoid space and ventricles of the brain
10. epididymis with contrast material
11. liver
12. uterine cavity and fallopian tubes
13. larynx
14. lymphatic vessels and node
15. spinal cord
16. ureter and renal pelvis
17. salivary duct and branches
18. sinus or sinus tract
19. spleen
20. any part of the urinary system
21. vein and tributaries
22. seminal vesicles

Exercise 23-2

1. position
2. projection
3. anteroposterior
4. posteroanterior
5. right anterior oblique
6. left posterior oblique
7. dorsal
8. ventral
9. right lateral recumbent
10. dorsal decubitus, left lateral

Exercise 23-3

1. separate
2. MUE or Medically Unlikely Edits, or Medically Unbelievable Edits
3. Diagnostic Radiology; Diagnostic Ultrasound; Breast, Mammography; Bone/Joint Studies; Radiation Oncology; or Nuclear Medicine (in any order)

Exercise 23-4

1. **77056** (Mammography)
2. **76499** (Radiology, Diagnostic; Unlisted Services and Procedures)
3. **75605** (Aortography)

Exercise 23-5
1. Head and Neck
2. Chest
3. Abdomen and Retroperitoneum
4. Spinal Canal
5. Pelvis
6. Genitalia
7. Extremities
8. Ultrasonic Guidance Procedures
9. Other Procedures

Exercise 23-6
1. **76800** (Ultrasound, Spine)
2. **76604** (Ultrasound, Chest)
3. **76700** (Ultrasound, Abdomen)
4. **76816** (Ultrasound, Pregnant Uterus); **651.03** (Pregnancy, twin, antepartum)
   ICD-10-CM: **O30.003** (Pregnancy, twin, antepartum)
5. **76818** (Ultrasound, Fetus); **648.03** (Pregnancy complicated by Diabetes Mellitus); **250.01** (Diabetes, no complications, Type 1)
   ICD-10-CM: **O24.019** (Pregnancy, complicated by diabetes (mellitus))

Exercise 23-7
1. **77290** (Radiation Therapy, Field Set-Up)
2. **77261** (Radiation Therapy, Planning)

Exercise 23-8
1. **77333** (Radiation Therapy, Treatment Device)
2. **77326** (Radiation Therapy, Dose Plan, Brachytherapy)
3. **77305** (Radiation Therapy, Dose Plan, Teletherapy); **185** (Neoplasm, prostate, Malignant Primary)
   ICD-10-CM: **C61** (Neoplasm, prostate, Malignant, Primary)

Exercise 23-9
1. **77402** (Radiation Therapy, Treatment Delivery, Single Area)
2. **77401** (Radiation Therapy, Treatment Delivery, Superficial)
3. **77412** (Radiation Therapy, Treatment Delivery, Three or More Areas)
4. **77407** (Radiation Therapy, Treatment Delivery, Two Areas)
5. **77412** (Radiation Therapy, Treatment Delivery, Three or More Areas); **198.5** (Neoplasm, bone, spine); **199.1** (Neoplasm, unknown site or unspecified, Malignant Primary)
   ICD-10-CM: **C79.51** (Neoplasm, bone, spine, secondary), **C80.1** (Neoplasm, unknown, Malignant, Primary)

Exercise 23-10
1. **77427** (Radiation Therapy, Treatment Delivery, Weekly)
2. **77499** (Radiation Therapy, Treatment Management, Unlisted Services and Procedures)

Exercise 23-11
1. **77761** (Brachytherapy)
2. **77776** (Brachytherapy)
3. **77789** (Brachytherapy); **183.0** (Neoplasm, ovary, Malignant, Primary)
   ICD-10-CM: **C56.9** (Neoplasm, ovary, Malignant, Primary)

Exercise 23-12
1. Gastrointestinal System
2. Endocrine System
3. Hematopoietic, Reticuloendothelial, and Lymphatic System
4. Musculoskeletal System
5. Nervous System

CHAPTER 24

Exercise 24-1
1. **80076** (Organ or Disease Oriented Panel, Hepatic Function Panel); **070.32** (Hepatitis, type B, chronic)
   ICD-10-CM: **B18.1** (Hepatitis, type B, chronic)
2. seven
3. yes
4. yes

Exercise 24-2
1. **80102** (Drug, Confirmation)
2. **80162** (Drug Assay, Digoxin)
3. **80150** (Drug Assay, Amikacin); **780.60** (Fever); **288.09** (Neutropenia, immune)
   ICD-10-CM: **R50.9** (Fever), **D70.8** (Neutropenia, immune)
4. **80178** (Drug Assay, Lithium); **296.80** (Depression, manic)
   ICD-10-CM: **F31.9** (Manic-depressive)

Exercise 24-3
1. **81003** (Urinalysis, Automated)
2. **81015** (Urinalysis, Microscopic)
3. **82040** (Albumin, Serum)
4. **82247** (Bilirubin, Total, Direct)
5. **82800** (Blood Gases, pH); **518.81** (Failure, respiratory)
   ICD-10-CM: **J96.9** (Failure, respiratory)
6. **84300** (Sodium, Urine); **428.0** (Failure, heart, congestive)
   ICD-10-CM: **I50.9** (Failure, heart, congestive)
7. **84550** (Uric Acid, Blood); **274.0** (Gout, arthritis, acute)
   ICD-10-CM: **M10.00** (Gout, arthritis, acute)

Exercise 24-4
1. **85027** (Hemogram, Automated)
2. **85025** (Hemogram, Automated); **285.1** (Anemia, blood loss, acute)
   ICD-10-CM: **D62** (Anemia, blood loss, acute)
3. **85041** (Red Blood Cell, Count)
4. **85097** (Bone Marrow, Smear); **208.00** (Leukemia, acute, in remission)
   ICD-10-CM: **C95.01** (Leukemia, acute)

Exercise 24-5
1. **86039** (Antibody, Antinuclear)
2. **86063** (Antibody, Antistreptolysin O)
3. **86156** (Cold Agglutinin); **465.9** (Infection, acute, upper respiratory)
   ICD-10-CM: **J06.9** (Infection, acute, upper respiratory)

Exercise 24-6
1. **86900** (Blood Typing, ABO only); **86901** (Blood Typing, Rh)
2. **86945 × 3** (Blood Products, Irradiation)

Exercise 24-7

1. **87536** (Microbiology)
2. **87651** (Microbiology); **784.0** (Headache); **780.60** (Fever)

   ICD-10-CM: **R51** (Headache), **R50.9** (Fever)
3. **87512** (Microbiology); **87530** (Microbiology); **87482** (Microbiology); **616.10** (Vaginitis, bacterial)

   ICD-10-CM: **N76.0** (Vaginitis, bacterial)
4. **87555** (Microbiology); **87528** (Microbiology); **87490** (Microbiology)
5. **87086** (Microbiology); **788.41** (Frequency, urinary)

   ICD-10-CM: **R35.0** (Frequency, urinary)

Exercise 24-8

1. **88309** (Pathology, Surgical, Gross and Micro Exam Level VI)
2. **88309** (Pathology, Surgical, Gross and Micro Exam Level VI)
3. **88305** (Pathology, Surgical, Gross and Micro Exam Level IV)
4. **88302** (Pathology, Surgical, Gross and Micro Exam Level II)

CHAPTER 25

Exercise 25-1

1. **90712** (Vaccines, Poliovirus, Live, Oral); **90473** (Immunization Administration, One Vaccine/Toxoid), **V04.0** (Vaccination, prophylactic)

   ICD-10-CM: **Z23** (Immunization, encounter)
2. **90701** (Vaccines, Diphtheria, Tetanus, Whole Cell Pertussis); **90712** (Vaccines, Polio Virus, Live, Oral); **90471** for first injection; and **90474** for the administration service (Immunization Administration), **V06.3** (Vaccination, prophylactic)

   ICD-10-CM: **Z23** (Immunization, encounter)
3. **99392-25** (Preventive Medicine); **90713** (Vaccines, Poliovirus, Inactivated, Intramuscular or Subcutaneous); **90702** (Vaccines, Diphtheria, Tetanus); **90465** for the first injection; and **90466** for the second injection (Immunization Administration, with Counseling); **V20.2** (Examination, child care, routine), **V06.5** (Vaccination, tetanus toxoid, with diphtheria), **V04.0** (Vaccination, poliomyelitis) (Admission for: well baby and child care; and, admission for vaccination). Note that E/M code 99392 is used here because the well-baby checkup service provided is significant and separate from the injection service.

   ICD-10-CM: **Z00.10** (Evaluation, infant or child), **Z23** (Immunization, encounter)
4. **90658** (Vaccines, Influenza); **90471** (Immunization Administration, One Vaccine/Toxoid), **V04.81** (Vaccination, influenza)

   ICD-10-CM: **Z23** (Immunization, encounter)
5. **99202-25** (Office and/or Other Outpatient Services, New Patient); **90720**, combination code for DTP and Hib (Vaccines, Diphtheria); and **90471** (Immunization Administration); **244.9** (Hypothyroidism); **V03.81** (Vaccination, Haemophilus influenza, Type B [HIB]); **V06.1** (Vaccination, prophylactic). Note: E/M code 99202 is used here because the E/M service provided was significant and separate from the injection service.

   ICD-10-CM: **Z23** (Immunization, encounter)
6. **99392-25** (Preventive Medicine, Established Patient); **90702** (Vaccines, Diphtheria, Tetanus); **90465** (Immunization Administration, One Vaccine/Toxoid); **V20.2** (Admission for: well baby and child care); **V06.5**

(Vaccination, prophylactic). Note that an E/M code, 99392, is used here because the E/M service provided was significant and was separate from the injection service.

ICD-10-CM: **Z00.10** (Encounter, routine health examination), **Z23** (Immunization, encounter)

7. **90658** (Vaccines, Influenza), **90471** (Administration, One Vaccine/ Toxoid); **V04.81** (Vaccination, prophylactic)

ICD-10-CM: **Z23** (Immunization, encounter)

Exercise 25-2

1. **90804** (Psychiatric Treatment, Individual Insight-Oriented, Office or Outpatient); **297.1** (Psychosis, paranoid, chronic)

ICD-10-CM: **F22** (Psychosis, paranoid, chronic)

2. **96101** × 2 (Psychiatric Diagnosis, Psychological Testing); **312.02** (Disturbance, conduct, undersocialized, aggressive)

ICD-10-CM: **F91.1** (Disturbance, conduct, undersocialized, aggressive)

3. **90885** (Psychiatric Diagnosis, Evaluation of Records or Reports); **313.0** (Disturbance, emotions specific to childhood, with anxiety and fearfulness)

ICD-10-CM: **F93.8** (Disturbance, emotions specific to childhood, with anxiety and fearfulness)

4. **90801** (Psychiatric Diagnosis, Interview and Evaluation); **311** (Depression), **781.0** (Tremor)

ICD-10-CM: **F32.9** (Depression), **R25.1** (Tremor)

Exercise 25-3

1. **90875** (Biofeedback, Psychiatric Treatment); **300.02** (Anxiety, generalized); **307.42** (Insomnia, idiopathic); **305.1** (Dependence, nicotine)

ICD-10-CM: **F41.1** (Anxiety, generalized), **F51.01** (Insomnia, idiopathic), **F17.200** (Dependence, nicotine)

2. **90901** (Training, Biofeedback); **402.90** (Hypertension, with heart involvement)

ICD-10-CM: **I11.9** (Hypertension, with heart involvement)

Exercise 25-4

1. **90955** (Dialysis, End-Stage Renal Disease); **585.6** (Disease, kidney, chronic, dialysis)

ICD-10-CM: **N18.6** (Disease, kidney, chronic, dialysis)

2. **90935** (Dialysis, Hemodialysis); **584.9** (Failure, renal, acute)

ICD-10-CM: **N17.9** (Failure, renal, acute)

3. **90947** (Dialysis, Peritoneal); **584.5** (Failure, renal: with, tubular necrosis)

ICD-10-CM: **N17.0** (Failure, renal: with, tubular necrosis)

4. within the lining of the abdominal cavity

5. filtration of blood and waste products through a filter outside the body

6. end stage renal disease

Exercise 25-5

1. **91038** (Esophagus, Acid Reflux Tests); **530.81** (Reflux, gastroesophageal)

ICD-10-CM: **K21.9** (Reflux, gastroesophageal)

2. **91105** (Intubation, Gastric)

3. **91055** (Intubation, Specimen Collection, Stomach); **789.00** (Pain, abdominal), **783.0** (Appetite, loss)

ICD-10-CM: **R10.9** (Pain, abdominal), **R63.0** (Appetite, loss)

4. spontaneous movement study

5. pressure measurements

Exercise 25-6

1. **92014** (Ophthalmology, Diagnostic; Eye Exam; Established Patient)

2. **92070** (Contact Lens Services, Fitting and Prescription)

3. **92120** (Ophthalmology, Diagnostic; Tonography); **365.00** (Glaucoma, borderline)

    ICD-10-CM: **H40.0** (Glaucoma, borderline)

4. **92004** (Ophthalmology, Diagnostic; Eye Exam, New Patient); **250.51, 362.02** (Diabetes, with ophthalmic manifestations); **250.61** (Diabetes, retinopathy, proliferative)

    ICD-10-CM: **E10.359** (Type 1 diabetes mellitus with proliferative diabetic retinopathy), **E10.43** (Type 1 diabetes mellitus with diabetic autonomic (poly) neuropathy)

Exercise 25-7

1. **92592** (Hearing Aid, Check)

2. **92551** (Audiologic Function Tests, Screening)

3. **92511** (Nasopharyngoscopy); **786.3** (Sputum, bloody)

    ICD-10-CM: **R04.2** (Sputum, bloody)

4. **92512** (Nasal Function Study); **786.09** (Inadequate, respiration)

    ICD-10-CM: **R06.9** (Inadequate, respiration)

Exercise 25-8

1. **93965** (Plethysmography, Extremities, Veins); **443.9** (Claudication, intermittent)

    ICD-10-CM: **I73.9** (Claudication, intermittent)

2. **93980** (Vascular Studies, Penile Vessels); **607.84** (Impotence, organic)

    ICD-10-CM: **N52.9** (Impotence, organic)

Exercise 25-9

1. **94620** (Pulmonology, Diagnostic; Stress Test, Pulmonary)

2. **94150** (Vital Capacity Measurement)

3. **94060** (Pulmonology, Diagnostic; Spirometry); **786.2** (Cough); **305.1** (Dependence, nicotine)

    ICD-10-CM: **R05** (Cough), **F17.200** (Dependence, nicotine)

Exercise 25-10

1. **95065** (Allergy Tests, Nose Allergy)

2. **95004 × 10** (Allergy Tests, Skin Tests, Allergen Extract) (Note that one unit is used for each test.)

3. **95115** (Allergen Immunotherapy, Allergen, Injection); **477.0** (Allergy, ragweed)

    ICD-10-CM: **J30.1** (Allergy, ragweed)

4. **95165 × 10; 95115** (one injection code)

Exercise 25-11

1. nasal continuous positive airway pressure

2. electroencephalogram

3. electromyogram

4. electro-oculogram

5. **95816** (Electroencephalography); **780.57** (Apnea, sleep)

    ICD-10-CM: **G47.30** (Apnea, sleep)

6. **95863** (Electromyography, Needle; Extremities); **782.0** (Numbness)

    ICD-10-CM: **R20.0** (Numbness)

7. **95851 × 2** (both legs) (Range of Motion Test, Extremities or Trunk); **781.3** (Incoordination, muscular)

ICD-10-CM: **R27.8** (Incoordination, muscular)

Exercise 25-12

1. **96110** (Developmental Testing); **312.9** (Disturbance, conduct)

ICD-10-CM: **F91.9** (Disturbance, conduct)

2. **96101** (MMPI); **V70.5** (Examination, pre-employment)

ICD-10-CM: **Z02.1** (Examination, pre-employment)

3. **96116** (Cognitive Function Tests); **780.79** (lethargy)

ICD-10-CM: **R53.83** (lethargy)

Exercise 25-13

1. **96440** (Chemotherapy, Pleural Cavity); **162.9** (Cancer, see neoplasm chart, lung, Malignant, Primary)

ICD-10-CM: **C34.90** (Cancer, see neoplasm chart, lung, Malignant Primary)

2. **96521** (Chemotherapy, Pump Services, Portable); **153.9** (Neoplasm, intestine Malignant, Primary)

ICD-10-CM: **C26.0** (Neoplasm, intestine Malignant Primary)

3. **96401** (Chemotherapy, Subcutaneous); **173.5** (Melanoma, skin, chest wall, Malignant, Primary)

ICD-10-CM: **C43.59** (Melanoma, skin, chest wall, Malignant Primary)

4. **96413** (Chemotherapy, Intravenous); **174.9** (Neoplasm, breast, Malignant, Primary); **198.5** (Neoplasm, bone, spine, Malignant, Secondary)

ICD-10-CM: **C50.919** (Neoplasm, breast, Malignant Primary), **C79.51** (Neoplasm, bone, spine, Malignant Secondary)

5. **96450** (Chemotherapy, CNS); **191.9** (Neoplasm, brain, Malignant, Primary)

ICD-10-CM: **C71.9** (Neoplasm, brain, Malignant Primary)

6. **96372** (Injection, Intramuscular, Therapeutic); **J3420** (Vitamin B12)

Exercise 25-14

1. **99241-25** (Consultation, Office and/or Other Outpatient); **96900** (Ultraviolet Light Therapy, for Dermatology); **706.1** (Acne)

ICD-10-CM: **L70.9** (Acne)

2. **99244-25** (Consultation, Office and/or Other Outpatient); **96913** (Photochemotherapy); **694.9** (Dermatosis, bullous)

ICD-10-CM: **L13.9** (Dermatosis, bullous)

Exercise 25-15

1. **97010** (Physical Medicine/Therapy/Occupational Therapy, Modalities, Hot or Cold Pack)

2. **97761 × 2** (Physical Medicine/Therapy/Occupational Therapy, Prosthetic Training)

3. **97116 × 2** (Physical Medicine/Therapy/Occupational Therapy, Procedures, Gait Training); **438.89** (Late effect, CVD). (Note that the stand-alone code 97110 specifies "each 15 minutes.")

ICD-10-CM: **169.059** (Hemiplegia/hemiparesis following nontraumatic subarachnoid hemorrhage)

Exercise 25-16

1. **98940** (Chiropractic Treatment, Spinal, Extraspinal); **719.45** (Pain, joint, hip)

ICD-10-CM: **M25.552** (Pain, joint, hip, left)

2. **98925** (Osteopathic Manipulation); **724.2** (Pain, lumbar region)

ICD-10-CM: **M54.5** (Pain, lumbar region)

Exercise 25-17   1. **99050** (Special Services, After Hours Medical Services)
2. **99000** (Special Services, Specimen Handling)
3. **99070** (Special Services, Supply of Materials)

CHAPTER 26

Exercise 26-1   1. No answer required.
2. a. Pyelonephritis, acute
  b. **590.10**
     ICD-10-CM: **N10**
  c. **590,** Infections of kidney
  d. no
  e. **590.10**
     ICD-10-CM: **N10**
  f. because flank pain and hematuria are symptoms of pyelonephritis

Exercise 26-2   1. No answer required.
2. a. open fracture of the right humerus and distal femur
  b. Fracture
  c. humerus
  d. (closed); **812.30**
     ICD-10-CM: **S42.301A**
  e. Yes, because the patient record did not specify the exact location of the fracture of the humerus, so the "unspecified part of the humerus, open" is as specific as you can get with the information that you have available.
  f. femur
  g. (closed)
  h. distal or distal end
  i. *see* Fracture, femur, lower end
  j. open
  k. **821.30**
     ICD-10-CM: **S42.301A**
  l. yes

Exercise 26-3   1. No answer necessary.
2. a. menorrhagia
  b. **626.2**
     ICD-10-CM: **N92.0**
  c. anemia
  d. **285.1**
     ICD-10-CM: **D62**

Exercise 26-4   1. No answer necessary.

2. a. Fracture

b. *see also* Fracture, by site

c. **198.5**

ICD-10-CM: **C79.51**

Exercise 26-5   1. a. **719.46**

ICD-10-CM: **M25.569**

b. **717.0**

ICD-10-CM: **M23.202**

c. **717.6**

ICD-10-CM: **M23.40**

Exercise 26-6   1. a. **574.10** (Cholelithiasis with cholecystitis, chronic with calculus of gallbladder)

ICD-10-CM: **K80.12** (Cholelithiasis with cholecystitis, chronic with calculus of gallbladder)

b. **486** (Pneumonia)

ICD-10-CM: **J18.9** (Pneumonia)

c. Contraindicated

d. **V64.1** (Procedure not done because of, contraindication)

ICD-10-CM: **Z53.09** (Procedure not done because of, contraindication)

2. a. 2; sterilization and surgery not done

b. **V25.2** (Admission for sterilization)

ICD-10-CM: **Z30.2** (Admission for sterilization)

c. **V64.2** (Procedure, not done, because of, patient's decision)

ICD-10-CM: **Z53.29** (Refusal of, treatment [because of], patient's decision NEC)

Exercise 26-7   1. a. Postoperative ileus

b. **997.4** (Complication, digestive system)

ICD-10-CM: **K91.89** (Complication, digestive system)

c. yes

d. **560.1** (Ileus, paralytic)

ICD-10-CM: **K56.0** (Ileus, paralytic)

e. yes, **153.9** (Neoplasm, malignant, colon, unspecified), **E878.2,** (Reaction, anastomosis)

ICD-10-CM: **C96.9** (Neoplasm, malignant, colon, unspecified), **Y83.2** (Reaction, anastomosis)

2. a. Malfunction insulin pump; **996.57**

ICD-10-CM: **T86.614** (Malfunction insulin pump)

b. **V58.67**

c. **250.01** (Diabetes without complication, type I, not specified as uncontrolled); **E879.8** (Abnormal reaction to other procedure)

ICD-10-CM: **E10.9** (Diabetes without complication, type I, not specified as uncontrolled), **Y84.9**

Exercise 26-8   1. a. Probable aspiration pneumonia

b. **507.0**

ICD-10-CM: **J69.0**

c. yes, **438.82** (Late effect, CVA, dysphagia); **787.20** (Dysphagia, unspecified); **401.9** (Hypertension, unspecified)

ICD-10-CM: **J69.321** (Late effect, CVA, dysphagia), **I69.391** (Dysphagia, unspecified), **I10** (Hypertension, unspecified)

2. a. Suspected malignancy, right kidney

b. **189.0** (Neoplasm, malignant, kidney, unspecified)

ICD-10-CM: **C64.9** (Neoplasm, malignant, kidney, unspecified)

c. yes, **599.70** (Hematuria, unspecified)

ICD-10-CM: **R31.9** (Hematuria, unspecified)

Exercise 26-9   1. a. Postoperative atrial fibrillation

b. **997.1** (Complication, procedure, cardiac)

ICD-10-CM: **I97.190** (Complication, procedure, cardiac)

c. **427.31** (fibrillation, atrial); **710.0** (Lupus); **583.81** (Nephritis due to lupus)

ICD-10-CM: **I48.0** (Fibrillation, atrial), **M32.14** (Lupus), **N08** (Nephritis)

d. yes, **55.23** (biopsy, kidney, percutaneous needle)

e. **E878.8** (Complication other surgical operation); **E849.7** (Place of occurrence, facility)

ICD-10-CM: **Y83.8** (Complication other surgical operation), **Y92.238** (Place of occurrence, facility)

Exercise 26-10   1. History of hysterectomy

2. History of peptic ulcer disease

3. Remote history of appendectomy

Exercise 26-11   1. Yes

2. No

SpeedECoder Exercises

Note: It is recommended that you wait to access this feature until you've finished working through the main text.

As an additional bonus feature, we have included 30-day access to *SpeedECoder* online code editor.

CASES 1 THROUGH 15

Your supervisor has asked you to use the *SpeedECoder* to check the accuracy of several cases that were coded by another coder.

CASES 16 THROUGH 20

For Cases 16 through 20, you are to assign the correct CPT and ICD-9-CM codes. Be sure to check the codes you assign with *SpeedECoder*. Once you have finished, your instructor will provide you with answers for Cases 16-20 so you can check your work.

USING *SPEEDECODER* ONLINE CODE EDITOR

Note: The User Name and Password will only be valid during the current coding year.

Here are some easy steps to start using your free trial of *SpeedECoder*.

1. Start by logging into your Evolve Learning Resources, or registering for FREE at **http://evolve.elsevier.com/Buck/step.** Access your "Step-by-Step Medical Coding 2010 Edition" course, then:
   a. Click "Student Resources"
   b. Click "Chapter 26 - Inpatient Coding"
   c. Click on the **Reference - SpeedECoder** section, then click on the **SpeedECoder** login link to be connected to the **SpeedECoder** site.
2. Once on the *SpeedECoder* site, click "Log In," then enter your **User Name** and **Password** from the card you received with your textbook.
3. The first page that opens in *SpeedECoder* is the main page. Click on **SpeedESearch.** This will take you to the settings page.
4. Below **Include these Datasets,** make sure green checkmarks appear next to the type of services that you are checking (CPT®, ICD-9-CM Vol 1, HCPCS, etc.).
5. You can search for codes using key terms by entering them in the appropriate **Find Records** blanks, then clicking **Search.**

For example, if you enter the word "pneumonia" in the first blank, SpeedECoder *will show several choices of ICD-9-CM, CPT, or HCPCS codes that are related to pneumonia.* When you use key terms to locate codes, keep in mind that you may have to research several of the code results to confirm your code choice is correct. *Again if you search for the word "pneumonia," and the patient's diagnosis was "Pneumonia due to Pseudomonas" you would need to scroll down the list until you located the ICD-9-CM code 482.1. Click on "482.1" for the code details and to confirm this is correct.*

6. Also on the main page is a **Code Search** option. Type a code in the **Enter Code** blank, and *SpeedECoder* will provide the code details.

7. You can save specific codes to a **CodeList** for easy reference. When viewing a particular code's details, click the red **Add to CodeList** link at the top or bottom of the screen. Next click **Manage CodeList** on the left column of the screen for your comprehensive list.

8. You can add notes for your reference within the code details. Click the **Add CodeNote** box at the bottom of the screen, enter your note, and click **Add.** Your note will be saved for future reference.

CASE 1

Cases 1 and 2 are ongoing services provided to the same patient by the same physician.

PREOPERATIVE DIAGNOSIS: Pyogenic granuloma, sinus tract, buttock.

POSTOPERATIVE DIAGNOSIS: Multiple sinus tracts, one extending inferiorly about 7 × 3 cm in diameter, one extending to the right approximately 4 × 3 cm, and one extending to the left for about 3 cm.

SURGICAL FINDINGS: As above, plus granulation tissue present in a capsule of multiple sinus tracts. Sinus tracts measured a total of about 15 × 8 cm in their total dimensions.

SURGICAL PROCEDURE: Partial unroofing (debridement) of sinus tracts.

SURGEON: Tony Wellbed, MD

ANESTHESIA: General endotracheal.

DESCRIPTION OF PROCEDURE: The patient was intubated and turned in the prone position. A probe was inserted in the sinus cavity, and dissection debridement was carried down to full thickness. I encountered a piece of chronically infected granulation tissue coming out of a hole, in which I stuck the probe, but this continued for a distance longer than the probe and accordingly, I put my finger in this and this extended down the length of my index finger (about 7-8 cm by about 3 cm in width). I left this intact, because this would necessitate extensive dissection and we have no blood on this patient at this time. We then unroofed two other sinus cavities, and packed this opened with 2-inch vaginal packing and applied a dressing and Kerlix plus an Elastoplast. Estimated blood loss: 25 cc. The patient seemed to tolerate the procedure well and left the operating room in good condition.

Procedure Key Terms:	debridement, fistula, extensive dissection
ICD-9-CM Key Terms:	granuloma, pyogenic

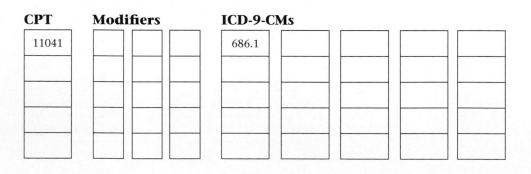

CPT   **Modifiers**   **ICD-9-CMs**

| 11041 | | | | 686.1 | | | | |

CASE 2

PREOPERATIVE DIAGNOSIS: Postop bleeding from sacral wound.

POSTOPERATIVE DIAGNOSIS: Same.

SURGICAL FINDINGS: One very active bleeder and one less active bleeder along the wound margin.

SURGICAL PROCEDURE: Wound exploration and cauterization of two bleeders of the wound edge.

SURGEON: Tony Wellbed, MD

ANESTHESIA: Local with plain 1% Xylocaine, approximately 10 cc along each suture line.

Following her unroofing of the sinus tracts yesterday, I was called by the Recovery Room nurse for a large spot of blood on the dressing. She also incidentally had this on the bed. I took the dressing down and called for some silver nitrate because the patient had a very active bleeder coming from the edge of the wound. I asked for some sterile Kerlix fluffs and light. Because we could not adequately visualize everything that was going on at the time, I took the patient back to the Operating Room where the bleeder was easily identified and cautery was used to stop the bleeding. There was also one other small bleeder cauterized. No other bleeders were noted. I sprayed the bed with topical thrombin and packed some Surgicel in the more proximal aspect of the wound and then packed thrombin-soaked 2-inch vaginal packing in the wound followed by Kerlix fluffs and a snug dressing covered by Elastoplast. The bleeding appeared to be controlled.

DESCRIPTION OF PROCEDURE: The patient was turned in the prone position and we injected more local anesthesia (1% Xylocaine and 1:100,000 epinephrine, having injected some in the Recovery Room). I cauterized the very active bleeder that was noted, and saw one more less-active bleeder along the suture line. Surgicel was in place at the depths of the wound in a pool of topical thrombin that we had placed in the proximal aspect of the wound from where the bleeding came. I then saturated a 2-inch vaginal gauze packing with topical thrombin and packed this in the wound followed by one box of Kerlix fluffs. The wound was then dressed with Elastoplast.

Coincidentally noted at the time of her surgery with the wound exploration was conversion of her electrocardiogram to a Mobitz Type I heart block. I did consult the cardiologist at the same time.

Procedure Key Terms:	hemorrhage, hematoma, complicating procedure
ICD-9-CM Key Terms:	postoperative hemorrhage, complication, Mobitz Type I

CPT   **Modifiers**   **ICD-9-CMs**

17999 | | | | 998.11

CASE 3

Cases 3 and 4 are a continuation of care provided to the same patient by the same physician. The previous decompression fasciotomy was performed 1 day prior to Case 3.

PREOPERATIVE DIAGNOSIS: Status post-fasciotomy, lateral aspect of the right lower extremity.

POSTOPERATIVE DIAGNOSIS: Same.

SURGICAL PROCEDURE: Extension of fasciotomy (repeat procedure), lateral aspect, right thigh and dressing change.

SURGEON: George M. Pathfinder, MD

ANESTHESIA: General endotracheal.

SURGICAL FINDINGS: Open wound, right thigh, with compression of the vastus lateralis laterally.

DESCRIPTION: The dressings were removed. The wound was inspected, and the muscle was quite clean. However, there was some constriction of the vastus lateralis by the tensor fascia lata laterally. The fasciotomy was further incised to extended beyond the original fasciotomy. Dressing of Xeroform, Kerlix fluffs, and a splint was then reapplied.

ESTIMATED BLOOD LOSS: 25 cc.

The patient tolerated the procedure well and left the operating room in good condition.

ADDENDUM: This patient was scheduled originally for skin graft, but we elected at this point to attempt wound vacuum suction on the thigh to see if it could be closed without a skin graft.

Procedure Key Terms:	fasciotomy, decompression
ICD-9-CM Key Terms:	compartment syndrome

CPT	Modifiers			ICD-9-CMs				
27496	RT			958.8				
15852				V58.31				

CASE 4

The same physician completes the decompression fasciotomy 3 days later.

PREOPERATIVE DIAGNOSIS: Status post-fasciotomy, right thigh, for compartment syndrome.

POSTOPERATIVE DIAGNOSIS: Same.

PROCEDURE PERFORMED: Secondary closure, right thigh wound.

SURGEON: George M. Pathfinder, MD

ANESTHESIA: General.

FINDINGS: The wound vac seems to have reduced the volume of the thigh fairly nicely and we were able to close the skin without any undue tension. The wound itself looked clean and there was no evidence of any purulent material at all.

PROCEDURE: While under a general anesthetic, the patient was placed in the supine position on the operating room table. The wound vac was removed from the patient's thigh and the wound appeared to be very clean without any purulent material at all. We then prepped the patient's right leg with Betadine and draped it in a sterile fashion.

We then initially used a Surgilav device with saline and a sponge to scrub the incision and irrigated very thoroughly. After this, we attempted to see if the quadriceps would contract by pinching it with a forceps. We were able to pinch the quadriceps in several areas and it seemed to respond quite nicely.

We then began the extensive closure of the wound from each end using 2-0 Vicryl suture. We were actually able to pull the wound together quite nicely without any undue tension. We were then able to close the skin using skin staples. With the wound closed, we could flex the knee approximately 90 degrees.

We then dressed the wound with Xeroform gauze dressings under 4 × 4s, ABD pads, and an ACE wrap. The dorsalis pedis pulse was strong at the end of the procedure. He was taken from the operating room in good condition and breathing spontaneously. He was given IV Kefzol preoperatively and will be continued on IV Kefzol postoperatively as well. He tolerated the procedure very well.

Procedure Key Terms:	closure, secondary, extensive
ICD-9-CM Key Terms:	compartment syndrome

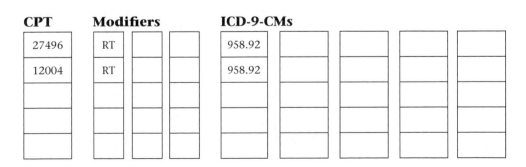

CPT   **Modifiers**   **ICD-9-CMs**

CPT	Modifiers			ICD-9-CMs				
27496	RT			958.92				
12004	RT			958.92				

CASE 5

PREOPERATIVE DIAGNOSIS: Gunshot wound to left thigh.

POSTOPERATIVE DIAGNOSIS: Gunshot wound to left thigh with transection of superficial femoral artery and veins.

PROCEDURE PERFORMED: Exploratory laparotomy with control of left external iliac artery. Debridement of left thigh wound. Repair of left superficial femoral artery using a right greater saphenous vein interposition vein graft. Repair of left superficial femoral vein. Ligation of branch of left profunda femoris artery. Fasciotomy left lower leg.

SURGEON: Marsha Petros, MD

ANESTHESIA: General anesthesia.

INDICATIONS FOR SURGERY: This patient is a 27-year-old Caucasian male who was shot in the left thigh. The exact cause or how the accident occurred is unknown. The patient was initially seen in Anytown and was transferred to Central Hospital for treatment.

DESCRIPTION OF PROCEDURE: The patient was bleeding from the left thigh. The prep was just Betadine solution splashed on the skin. An abdominal incision was then made and the iliac artery on the left side was isolated with a vessel loop and clamp. This controlled the bleeding. The left thigh incision was then opened from the gunshot wound to the groin area. There was a large clot in this area and this whole area was opened. Upon examination there was oozing and bleeding from the torn muscle. The proximal and distal end of the superficial femoral artery was found. There was a large segment missing. The superficial femoral vein was also found and this was repaired. The holes that were in the vein were found and repaired. The nerves of the left thigh were not seen. A repair of the left superficial femoral artery was then done. The right groin area was dissected and the right greater saphenous vein on the upper thigh was excised. The branches of the vein were ligated with 3-0 silk sutures and divided. At the junction of the right femoral vein a vascular clamp was then placed across the saphenous vein. The saphenous vein was then transected. The saphenous vein was then oversewn with a running 4-0 Prolene suture. Clamp was then removed. The dissection was then carried out distally for at least 8 inches. The saphenous vein was then harvested. The distal end was tied with a 2-0 silk suture, and the vein was then removed. The vein was irrigated and was brought into the left wound area. The proximal end of the left superficial femoral artery was then trimmed back to normal tissue. The saphenous vein was then spatulated and sewn end-to-end to the artery using running 5-0 Prolene sutures. After this was completed the distal anastomosis was then done and again the vein in the artery was debrided back to normal tissue. The vein was cut to length and sutured end-to-end to the artery using 5-0 Prolene sutures. Just prior to completion of the closure the clamp on the artery was removed to allow the vein to be flushed, this was done and the closure was then completed. After examination it was noted that the vein was in spasm and even though it was reversed, the flow through the vein was marginal. Because of this the superficial femoral artery was clamped. An arteriotomy was then made in the proximal artery. The catheter was passed down through the graft. A LeMaitre valvulotome was also passed down through the graft and then opened and then all the valves were lysed. After this was completed the opening in the artery was closed with a running 5-0 Prolene suture. This allowed for excellent flow through the graft in the distal artery. Also, before the initial anastomosis of the superficial femoral artery there was some clotting present and so therefore a Fogarty catheter was passed down distally and all that clot was removed. Then the artery was flushed with heparinized saline. The patient did not receive any systemic heparin because his INR was elevated because of the transfusions and because of his extensive blood loss, which required multiple units of transfusion. After the anastomosis was completed and repairs were completed the operative area was irrigated. A small branch of the left profunda femoris artery was found and this was doubly ligated with 2-0 silk sutures. A JP drain was then left in the operative area and the fascia was closed over the drain and also covering the graft. The right groin incision and tissue thigh incision were also closed with a running 3-0 Vicryl suture and skin clips for the skin. The vessel loop on the external iliac artery in the abdomen was then removed and the abdominal incision was closed with a running looped #1 PDS suture. Subcutaneous tissue was irrigated and skin was closed with skin clips. The left thigh incision was then closed with initially figure-of-eight #1 Prolene sutures. After this was completed the left lower leg fasciotomy was then done. The left lower leg was then prepped and draped in the usual manner and fasciotomy was then done opening all compartments. There was marked venous hypertension noted and the muscle did protrude through the fascia indicating swelling. After this was completed the dressings were applied. By this time it was noted that the groin incision was leaking and oozing blood; because of this the incision was prepped and draped again and reopened. Upon reopening it was noted that the patient had pooled blood in the cavity, which was created by the gunshot wound. This area was then irrigated and no obvious bleeding site could be found. There was some generalized oozing from the muscle. This space was then obliterated with figure-of-eight 0 Vicryl sutures. The JP drain was then left in the operative area again and the muscle was again closed around the drain using figure-of-eight 0 Vicryl sutures. Again, the fascia on the anterior layer was closed with interrupted 0 Vicryl sutures. A dressing was then applied. The oozing was now minimal and the patient was transferred to the intensive care unit in critical condition.

This patient is a 27-year-old Caucasian male who was shot in the left thigh. How the accident occurred I am not sure. He was sent from his hometown hospital to this hospital. Upon arriving, the patient was hypotensive with a systolic pressure of 60. He had bleeding from his left thigh wound. His lungs were clear. Heart was tachycardic.

IMPRESSION: Gunshot wound to left thigh.

PLAN: The patient was taken immediately to the operating room for control of his bleeding and exploration of his left thigh. The patient was in critical condition.

Procedure Key Terms:	laparotomy, blood vessel repair, fasciotomy
ICD-9-CM Key Terms:	injury blood vessel, compartment syndrome

CPT	Modifiers			ICD-9-CMs				
35256				890.1	958.8	E922.9		
35218				890.1	958.8	E922.9		
35226				890.1	958.8	E922.9		
27496				958.8	E922.9			

CASE 6

Cases 6 and 7 are ongoing care provided by the same physician.

PREOPERATIVE DIAGNOSIS: Desmoplastic malignant melanoma, submucosal, left side of upper lip.

POSTOPERATIVE DIAGNOSIS: Same.

SURGICAL PROCEDURES:
1. Sentinel node biopsy, left submandibular region.
2. Wide V-excision (1 centimeter) of desmoplastic malignant melanoma, left side of upper lip with through-and-through excision and 1 centimeter margins on all sides.

SURGEON: Brian Wilson, MD

ANESTHESIA: General endotracheal with supplementary 2 cc of 1% Xylocaine and 1:800,000 epinephrine.

SURGICAL FINDINGS: The patient had a scar of the upper lip and a 5 millimeter linear, pigmented lesion near the mucosal junction. There was one submandibular lymph node identified that appeared to be benign. No occipital or posterior submandibular lymph nodes were identified despite assiduous search.

DESCRIPTION OF PROCEDURE: Following injection of radioactive dye in the Radiology Department, the patient was sent to the operating room where the face and neck were prepped with Betadine scrub and solution and draped in a routine sterile fashion.

Sentinal node biopsy: The sites that had been identified in Radiology were noted, and on the mastoid area, I detected 100 on the probe externally. I explored this, but when I got inside, I was unable to reproduce the external reading despite a vigorous exploration of the mastoid area and splitting of the sternocleidomastoid muscle over the site where most of the probe activity was evident. We made about a 3-centimeter incision in this area and explored it thoroughly in all areas indicated. I thought on occasion I palpated a lymph node, but upon deep dissection, it was noted that this was simply another fiber of the sternocleidomastoid muscle, and we abandoned this after a search of about 15 minutes. In the submandibular area, an incision was made, and activity was evident. The skin in the posterior mandibular area had a reading of 13 with an in vivo reading of 63. However, the ex vivo was only approximately 7 on the specimen itself. It may have been too small to have caused any reactivity. The background was 26 following removal of a small lymph node that was less than 1 centimeter in diameter. No anterior mandibular lymph node was ever identified. Also, it should be noted that at no time did I, other than the small lymph node we removed, palpate lymphadenopathy in the mesenteric muscle region nor in the region of the external maxillary artery which crossed the marginal mandibular nerve.

Wide V-excision, left upper lip: I then marked out a margin of 1 centimeter around the previous scar, and in so doing, I noted that included within this resection was a 5-millimeter linear pigmented lesion. This was a wedge resection of the lip, and bleeding of the coronal arteries were clamped and ligated with 4-0 Vicryl. I then began closure of the mucosa, lining up the mucocutaneous junction and lining up the vermilion where it meets the white roll. After completion of the mucosal closure, the musculature was brought together. The orbicularis oculi musculature was brought together with 4-0 Vicryl suture, and interrupted 5-0 Prolene was used to reapproximate the skin. There was no evidence of residual tumor within the specimen submitted. A silk suture tagged the lip side of the specimen. Antibiotic ointment was applied, and 4 × 4 was used to cover the incision. The patient tolerated the procedure well and left the area in good condition.

Pathology report later indicated: Melanocarcinoma.

Procedure Key Terms:	excision, biopsy, excision skin (lip)
ICD-9-CM Key Terms:	melanoma skin, malignant melanoma

CPT	Modifiers			ICD-9-CMs				
38500				172.0				
40520				172.0				

CASE 7

PREOPERATIVE DIAGNOSIS: Residual desmoplastic malignant melanoma, left side of upper lip.

POSTOPERATIVE DIAGNOSIS: Same.

SURGICAL FINDINGS: 1.5 cm healed incision, left side of upper lip through-and-through. No residual tumor seen in resected specimen.

PROCEDURE PERFORMED: Excision of residual malignant melanoma, left side upper lip, with 1 cm margins with reconstruction by flaps created by perialar crescentic incisions producing flaps of 4 × 4 cm and 2.5 × 2 cm.

SURGEON: Brian Wilson, MD

ANESTHESIA: General endotracheal anesthesia plus 7 cc of 1% Xylocaine with 1:800,000 epinephrine.

ESTIMATED BLOOD LOSS: 25 cc.

COMPLICATIONS: None.

SPONGE AND NEEDLE COUNTS: Correct

FINDINGS: It's been 3 weeks since I performed a wide excision of the malignant melanoma of the upper lip. This patient is back today for residual excision and flap creation.

DESCRIPTION: The patient's face was prepped with Betadine scrub and solution and draped in routine sterile fashion. I infiltrated the potential areas of resection with a total of 7 cc of 1% Xylocaine with 1:800,000 epinephrine, and made a left perialar crescentic incision that I excised in continuity with the specimen, which I excised by taking a cm margin on either side of it and up to the nostril sill, taking a block of tissue out through-and-through by using a #11 knife blade from the skin through the mucosa. The top of the crescent was tagged with a silk suture and submitted for frozen section. Dr. Cooley examined the specimen and found no residual tumor at the site that it would be most likely to be located. After assurance there was no tumor in this area I returned to the operating room, and resected a little bit of apparent scar tissue more inferiorly in the wound than the specimen that had been tagged for microscopic examination. After resection of that tissue, I did a right perialar crescentic excision, creating a flap of about 4 × 4 cm, and on the left the resultant perialar crescentic excision resulting in a flap of about 2.5 × 2 cm. Mucosal incisions were made about 5 mm away from the gingival margin, and the mucosa was advanced. I sutured the mucosa with interrupted 4-0 Vicryl, sutured the orbicularis oculi with 4-0 Vicryl and one 4-0 Monocryl, following which I closed the skin with interrupted 4-0 Prolene. Steri-Strips were applied to the lip. The patient tolerated the procedure well and left the operating room in good condition.

Procedure Key Terms:	re-excision, skin (lip)
ICD-9-CM Key Terms:	melanoma skin

CPT   **Modifiers**   **ICD-9-CMs**

CPT	Modifiers			ICD-9-CMs				
40525				172.0				

CASE 8

PREOPERATIVE DIAGNOSIS: Anal fissure.

POSTOPERATIVE DIAGNOSIS: Same.

PROCEDURE PERFORMED:
1. Sphincterotomy.
2. One quadrant hemorrhoidectomy.

SURGEON: Meridian Casha, MD

ANESTHESIA: Spinal.

INDICATION: The patient is a pleasant 46-year-old female who is 120 days post three quadrant hemorrhoidectomy for severe external hemorrhoids. She has an anal fissure as well as the external hemorrhoid and that is quite tender. She presents today for elective sphincterotomy, excision of the external hemorrhoid, understands surgery and the risks of bleeding and infection, possible damage to the sphincter muscles and wishes to proceed.

DESCRIPTION OF PROCEDURE: The patient was brought to the operating room, given spinal anesthesia, and placed in a jackknife position. We could see the enlarged hemorrhoid/sentinel tag at the 10-o'clock position and the fissure right at the base of this. Anoscope was placed and we placed a Kelly clamp behind the hypertrophied scarred band of muscle and divided the muscle. We then excised the external hemorrhoid and then closed the defect with interrupted 3-0 chromic sutures and running locked 3-0 chromic. There were no other hemorrhoids and there were no other fissures. We infiltrated the area with a total of 30 cc of 0.5% Sensorcaine with epinephrine solution, placed four gauze dressings in the area that we will remove in 30 minutes and she was taken to recovery in stable condition.

Procedure Key Terms:	post 120 days, anal fissure, hemorrhoid
ICD-9-CM Key Terms:	hemorrhoid, external

CPT	Modifiers			ICD-9-CMs				
46250				565.0				

CASE 9

PREOPERATIVE DIAGNOSES:
1. Respiratory failure.
2. Morbid obesity.
3. Excess cervical skin and adipose tissue.

POSTOPERATIVE DIAGNOSES:
1. Respiratory failure.
2. Morbid obesity.
3. Excess cervical skin and adipose tissue.

PROCEDURE PERFORMED:
1. Flap tracheostomy.
2. Bilateral cervical lipectomy.
3. Bilateral cervical skin resection, with intermediate closure, 10 cm.

SURGEON: Eda Seekong, MD

ANESTHESIA: General endotracheal anesthesia.

INDICATION: 68-year-old female, with respiratory failure, requiring ventilator support. She also has pancreatitis that will require long-term treatment, as well as ventilator therapy. She has morbid obesity. The patient is now prepared for tracheostomy placement for long-term ventilatory support. Due to her morbid obesity and excessive cervical adipose tissue and skin, lipectomy and skin resection are also necessary.

DESCRIPTION OF PROCEDURE: After written consent was obtained, the patient was taken to the operating room and placed on the operating room table in the supine position. The patient's neck was then prepped with Betadine prep and then draped in a sterile manner. An omega-shaped inferior flap was marked. The area was then infiltrated with 1% Xylocaine with 1:100,000 units epinephrine. After several minutes, sharp dissect was carried down through the skin and subcutaneous tissue. The platysma was identified. Excessive fat from the dermis down to the sternocleidomastoid muscle was removed bilaterally. Additional fat was removed off of the strap muscles. This was done from a level of the thyroid notch to the clavicle. Subsequently, the strap muscles were divided in the midline and retracted laterally. The thyroid was divided in the midline and then retracted laterally. Suture ligatures of 4-0 silk were used for the thyroid. The thyroid was then entered between the second and third tracheal rings. Superior and inferior tracheal cartilage flaps were then made. A #8 Shiley cuff tracheostomy tube was then placed. The superior and inferior skin flaps were secured to the cartilage flaps with 4-0 Vicryl suture in a half vertical mattress closure. Subsequently, the skin and adipose tissue excision was then marked in the submental and upper cervical region bilaterally. This area was then infiltrated with local solution. Sharp dissection was then carried down through the skin and subcutaneous tissue. This skin and excess adipose tissue were then removed. Hemostasis was achieved with the Bovie cautery. The wound was closed by reapproximating the subcutaneous tissue and dermis with interrupted 4-0 Vicryl suture. The skin was then approximated with skin staples. The tracheostomy tube was secured both with sutures and ties. Bacitracin ointment was applied to the upper incision. A dressing of 4 × 4s and Elastoplast was then placed over the submental area. The patient tolerated the procedure well, there was no break in technique, and the patient was taken back to the medical critical care unit in stable condition.

FLUIDS ADMINISTERED: 1800 cc of RL.

ESTIMATED BLOOD LOSS: 100 cc.

URINE OUTPUT: 175 cc.

Procedure Key Terms:	tracheostomy, respiratory failure, excision adipose tissue
ICD-9-CM Key Terms:	respiratory failure, morbid obesity

CPT

| 31610 |
| 15838 |
| |
| |
| |

Modifiers

ICD-9-CMs

| 278.01 |
| 278.01 |
| |
| |
| |

CASE 10

PREOPERATIVE DIAGNOSIS: Torn left lateral meniscus.

POSTOPERATIVE DIAGNOSES:
1. Torn left lateral meniscus.
2. Chondromalacia, left knee.

PROCEDURE PERFORMED:
1. Examination of left knee under anesthesia.
2. Arthroscopy of left knee with partial lateral meniscectomy and debridement of chondromalacia.

SURGEON: Pita Hortaga, MD

ANESTHESIA: General.

FINDINGS: The patient was found to have significant chondromalacia in all three compartments of her left knee. She has bare bone exposed on the weight-bearing surface of the medial and lateral femoral condyles and she has significant chondromalacia on the articular surface of the patella almost down to subchondral bone. She had a degenerative tear involving the lateral meniscus. The medial meniscus appeared to be intact. The anterior cruciate ligament was intact.

PROCEDURE: While under a general anesthetic, the patient's left knee was examined. The collateral ligaments were intact and Lachman's test was negative, as was pivot shift. McMurray's test was negative.

We then prepped the patient's left leg with Betadine and draped it in a sterile fashion. An Esmarch bandage was used to exsanguinate the leg and a tourniquet on the thigh was inflated to 300 mmHg. We ended up deflating this tourniquet after about 5-10 minutes as the bleeding was not controlled. The total tourniquet time including the first and second tourniquet times was about 43 minutes.

We created three portals. The first was placed along the superior anterolateral aspect. The second was placed along the inferior anteromedial aspect and the third along the inferior anterolateral aspect of the knee. We distended the knee with lactated Ringer's solution. We examined the suprapatellar pouch and the medial and lateral gutters. She appeared to have somewhat hypertrophic synovium and was somewhat reddish and angry in appearance. We then examined the articular surface of the patella and found that she had significant chondromalacia characterized by fraying almost down to subchondral bone. We used a shaver to trim this area. The adjacent surface of the trochlea, however, appeared to be in relatively good condition.

We then examined the medial compartment and the medial meniscus appeared to be in relatively good condition with only minor fraying. We then examined the articular surface of the medial femoral condyle and noticed that she had a raised blister of articular cartilage. There was fissure over this and we could pass a probe underneath the articular cartilage. We gave some consideration to leaving this alone; however, we eventually elected to unroof this blister. This left an area of bare bone on the weight-bearing surface of the medial femoral condyle. This blister was therefore made up of cartilage that had no attachment to the subchondral bone and was fairly easily debrided with a shaver. We tried to smooth this area as best as possible with the shaver and soften the edges around this area.

We then turned our attention to the notch area and probed the anterior cruciate ligament. It was intact. There was an obvious tear of the lateral meniscus as there was a fragment of the meniscus laying against the anterior cruciate ligament, which we removed. She had a degenerative tear involving the entire length of the lateral meniscus. We used a combination of basket forceps and the shaver to trim the lateral meniscus back to a stable rim. The lateral compartment has significant chondromalacia in both the femur and the tibia. The articular surface on the lateral femoral condyle has worn almost down to subchondral bone and subchondral bone actually could be seen through the thin layer of articular cartilage. We used the shaver to trim the chondromalacia as best as possible.

At this point, then, we would look for any remaining loose fragments and drain the knee. We then injected 80 mg of Depo-Medrol with 2 ml of 1% Xylocaine. The skin incisions were closed using 4-0 nylon suture and sterile dressings were applied under ABD pads and an ACE wrap. She was taken from the operating room in good condition breathing spontaneously. The final sponge and needle counts were correct. The prognosis for her left knee is only fair since she does have significant chondromalacia in all three compartments.

Procedure Key Terms:	meniscectomy, arthroscopy
ICD-9-CM Key Terms:	meniscus tear, chondromalacia

CPT	Modifiers			ICD-9-CMs				
29877	LT			733.92				

CASE 11

PREOPERATIVE DIAGNOSIS: Right knee medial meniscus old bucket handle tear.

POSTOPERATIVE DIAGNOSIS: Same.

PROCEDURES PERFORMED:
1. Diagnostic arthroscopy.
2. Right knee arthroscopy with partial medial meniscectomy.

SURGEON: Dennis M. Schaffer, MD

ANESTHESIA: General anesthesia.

DRAINS: None.

FINDINGS: 40-year-old male suffering with persistent pain in his knee following medial meniscus repair and ACL reconstruction of 1 year. He is taken back to surgery. After appropriate level of anesthesia was achieved the right knee was prepped and draped in an orthopedic manner. We went through the previous portal sites. Sharp dissection was carried through the skin; blunt dissection was carried into the joint space. The patient had some scar tissue in the notch area and we went ahead and debrided this. The hamstring was probed and felt to be intact and functioning nicely. Immediately the patient's old meniscus repair was not functioning. The patient's meniscus was a little bit more complexly torn. I went ahead and debrided it. This was an essential bucket handle that would have been previously repaired. We debrided back to stable tissue. We explored the lateral compartment and it was felt to be intact. No loose bodies were noted. We explored the medial and lateral gutters, suprapatellar pouch, and no loose bodies were noted.

The articular surface was noted to be in good shape. There was some minimal grade two chondromalacia involving the medial femoral condyle area. The knee was irrigated copiously. 20 cc of 0.25% Marcaine was injected into the joint space and portal sites. We repaired the wounds with interrupted nylon sutures. We dressed the wound sterilely and the patient was placed in a knee immobilizer. The patient tolerated the procedure well and left the operating room in good condition.

Procedure Key Terms:	arthroscopy, meniscectomy
ICD-9-CM Key Terms:	tear meniscus, old bucket handle tear

CPT	Modifiers			ICD-9-CMs				
29881	59	RT		717.0				

CASE 12

PREOPERATIVE DIAGNOSES: Persistent hemoptysis and pneumonia and changes on x-ray.

POSTOPERATIVE DIAGNOSES: Same.

PROCEDURE: Transbronchial biopsy, bronchial biopsy, bronchoalveolar lavage, bronchial washings, and bronchial brushings.

PHYSICIAN: Hurada Maltose, MD

FINDINGS: The patient was sedated and preop'd while he was on the ventilator (status, ventilator dependent is reported with a V code), which did not really require much additional drug at all. Please see the drug sheet for further information.

PROCEDURE: The patient was monitored throughout the procedure with usual monitoring. There were no significant changes in blood pressure, oxygen saturation, or pulse rate, nor did any arrhythmias develop. No pneumothorax was discovered postprocedure by chest x-ray or by auscultation.

Once the patient was sedated, more than usual since he was maintained on a ventilator in the first place, the bronchoscope was introduced with a #9 endotracheal tube so it fit quite easily, and we were able to see the distal 2 centimeters of trachea, which was red and swollen, and the carina, which was red and swollen, and all the airways were red and swollen and with white plaquing consistent with candidiasis on the left mainstem and going down toward the lower lobe. The area in question was biopsied, brushed, and washed and subjected to bronchioalveolar lavage as well as bronchial brushings with sheath and non-sheath brushes as well as bronchial biopsies and transbronchial biopsies performed in that area. There were no complications. There was some blood seen in the left lower lobe, which was where most of the secretions were, and they were bloody. There were excess secretions everywhere but most were in the left lower lobe. The specimens were sent for appropriate pathological, cytological, and bacteriological studies, including a tissue sample, which was sent for bacteriological studies. Followup will be done in the Intensive Care Unit when we get the information back from the Lab.

Procedure Key Terms:	bronchoscopy, lung biopsy, bronchoalveolar lavage
ICD-9-CM Key Terms:	hemoptysis, pneumonia

CPT	Modifiers			ICD-9-CMs				
31624				786	486	V46.11		
31623				786	486	V46.11		
31628				786	486	V46.11		

CASE 13

SAME-DAY SURGERY

PREOPERATIVE DIAGNOSIS: Basal cell carcinoma, right side of nose.

POSTOPERATIVE DIAGNOSIS: Same.

SURGICAL FINDINGS: Healing 5-mm ulcer, right side of nose, with surrounding inflammatory response.

SURGICAL PROCEDURE: Excision of a 0.5 cm basal cell carcinoma, right side of nose, with reconstruction by 3 × 2.5 centimeter bilobed flap.

SURGEON: Bella Donald, MD

ANESTHESIA: Standby sedation with 5 cc of 1% Xylocaine with 1:100,000 epinephrine.

DESCRIPTION OF PROCEDURE: The patient's face was prepped with Betadine scrub and solution, and draped in a routine sterile fashion. The lesion and the surrounding tissue for the flap were both anesthetized with a total of 5 cc of 1% Xylocaine with 1:100,000 epinephrine. The lesion was excised circumferentially with a 5-mm margin. It was submitted for frozen section with a tag on the inferior aspect. The lesion was clear on all margins. Bleeding was electrocoagulated. We developed a 3 × 2.5 cm bilobed flap based on the left side, rotating it in place, and insetting it with 5-0 Prolene. Antibiotic ointment and Surgicel were applied followed by a 4 × 4. The patient tolerated the procedure well and left the area in good condition.

Pathology report later indicated: Carcinoma, basal cell.

Procedure Key Terms:	tissue transfer, tissue rearrangement, excision
ICD-9-CM Key Terms:	malignant lesion, basal cell carcinoma, neoplasm nose

CPT	Modifiers			ICD-9-CMs				
14060	52			173.3				

CASE 14

The procedures in Cases 14 and 15 are provided on the same day, to the same patient, by the same physician.

PREOPERATIVE DIAGNOSIS: Hematochezia.

POSTOPERATIVE DIAGNOSIS: Numerous diverticula in the descending sigmoid colon, burgundy and *slight* fresh blood present, but no active bleeding.

PROCEDURE PERFORMED: Flexible sigmoidoscopy.

SURGEON: Mohammad Kang, MD

INDICATION: 62-year-old white male, who was admitted with five episodes of dark red blood per rectum and then some melanotic stool. His hemoglobin was 14 on admission, dropped to 10.5 by *yesterday* evening, and now is 10.0. He had a colonoscopy at the hospital. The report was reviewed, and there were numerous diverticula. He had previous radiation for prostate carcinoma. There was no mention of radiation proctitis.

PREOPERATIVE MEDICATIONS: Fentanyl 100 mcg IV with Versed 3 mg IV.

FINDINGS: The Pentax video colonoscope was inserted without difficulty to the mid descending colon. Inspection in the descending sigmoid revealed numerous diverticula and many that had wide openings. There was blood clot and burgundy throughout, but no active bleeding. The rectum was normal. Only a small amount of the rectal surface was visualized, and it was questionable whether there was any radiation proctitis. The patient tolerated the procedure well.

IMPRESSION: Burgundy and some fresh blood throughout the colon, numerous diverticula in the descending sigmoid colon, questionable radiation proctitis.

PLAN: The patient's bleeding is likely from diverticular disease, and it is certainly not due to radiation proctitis. Because of the melena, we are going to do an upper endoscopy. We would recommend a technetium RBC scan if he continues bleeding requiring further transfusion.

Procedure Key Terms:	hematochezia, history of prostate cancer
ICD-9-CM Key Terms:	flexible sigmoidoscopy

CPT	**Modifiers**			**ICD-9-CMs**				
45330				562.10				

CASE 15

PREOPERATIVE DIAGNOSIS: Question of melena.

POSTOPERATIVE DIAGNOSIS: Gastritis with erosions, duodenitis—mild, biopsy for *H. pylori.*

PROCEDURE PERFORMED: Esophagogastroduodenoscopy.

SURGEON: Mohammad Kang, MD

INDICATION: 62-year-old white male, who was admitted with five episodes of dark red blood per rectum and then some melanotic stool. His hemoglobin was 14 on admission, dropped to 10.5 by yesterday evening, and now is 10.0. He had a colonoscopy at the hospital. The report was reviewed, and there were numerous diverticula. He has had previous radiation for prostate carcinoma. There was no mention of radiation proctitis.

PREOPERATIVE MEDICATION: Fentanyl 100 mcg IV, Versed 3 mg IV

FINDINGS: The Pentax video pediatric endoscope was passed without difficulty into the oropharynx. The gastroesophageal junction was seen at 42 cm. Inspection of the esophagus revealed no erythema, ulceration, exudate, friability, stricture, varices, or other mucosal abnormalities. The stomach proper was entered. The endoscope was advanced to the second duodenum. Inspection of the second duodenum and first duodenum revealed no abnormalities. The duodenal bulb revealed some mild erythema. The antrum revealed several small erosions, not bleeding. Biopsies were obtained for *H. pylori.* There was no active ulceration. No bleeding. Retroflexion revealed no lesions along the cardia or fundus. Inspection of the body revealed no abnormalities. The patient tolerated the procedure well.

IMPRESSION: Gastritis with erosions, duodenitis—mild, biopsy for *H. pylori.*

PLAN: The patient will be on Protonix and will be observed carefully and given a technetium RBC scan if he has continued lower GI bleeding.

Procedure Key Terms:	endoscopy
ICD-9-CM Key Terms:	gastritis, duodenitis

CPT	Modifiers			ICD-9-CMs				
43239	58			535.40	535.60			

CASE 16

PREOPERATIVE DIAGNOSES:
1. Fat atrophy of the latissimus dorsi flap of right breast.
2. Asymmetry of the breasts.
3. Scar tissue, right side of back incision.

POSTOPERATIVE DIAGNOSES: Same.

INDICATIONS: 56 year old who is now 4 months post mastectomy of the right breast.

SURGICAL FINDINGS:
1. There was a clean and relatively avascular pectoralis submuscular pocket on the right side.
2. There was what appeared to be scar tissue mass with fat necrosis, also a cutaneous scar, of the more lateral aspect of the donor site from the previous latissimus dorsi flap.

SURGICAL PROCEDURES:
1. Insertion of submuscular breast implant, right breast. 150 cc implant was used.
2. Excision of scar tissue, donor area on latissimus dorsi flap, right side of back.

SURGEON: Mary Hallowell, MD

ANESTHESIA: Approximately 5 cc of 1% Xylocaine, 1:100,000 epinephrine.

DESCRIPTION OF PROCEDURE: The patient's chest and right side of the back were prepped with Betadine scrub and solution and draped in a routine sterile fashion. I injected a total of about 5 cc of 1% Xylocaine, 1:100,000 epinephrine in both the incision site of the medial aspect of the right breast and the back incision. The scar was excised from the lower aspect of the right breast, and a right pectoralis submuscular pocket was created using the balloon dissector to aid in dissection. Hemostasis was satisfactory, and following insertion of the balloon dissector, which we inflated to about 300 cc, I inserted a 230 cc Pfizer. This obviously was too large compared to the left side. In accordance with the patient's wishes, we put a 150 cc implant in, which made the right breast appear to be somewhat larger than the left, although they appeared the same with the patient in the recumbent position. The patient had expressly told us that she wished to have the right breast to be somewhat larger than the left breast and we tried to comply with the patient's wishes by insertion of the 150 cc implant. I felt that 100 cc would perhaps be too small, but the 150 cc did make the right breast larger than the left, although this may equilibrate more with the patient in the standing position. After insertion of the implant, I closed the wound with fascial sutures of 3-0 Monocryl and used interrupted twists of 5-0 Prolene. I excised the scar on the back in continuity with some scar tissue underneath and then excised a separate nodule of apparent scar tissue and fat necrosis, closing 6.8-cm wound with subcuticular 3-0 Monocryl in interrupted twists using some horizontal mattress twists of 4-0 Prolene. Xeroform and a 4 × 4 were applied to the back, and Kerlix fluffs and a support bra were used to dress the right breast reconstruction. Estimated blood loss was negligible. No drains were inserted. The patient tolerated the procedure well and left the operating room in good condition.

Procedure Key Terms:	breast prosthesis, delayed insertion
ICD-9-CM Key Terms:	atrophy of breast, scar tissue skin

CPT

Modifiers

ICD-9-CMs

CASE 17

Code only Dr. Foxtrot's services.

PREOPERATIVE DIAGNOSES:
1. Bunion with hallux abductovalgus, right foot.
2. Severe diaphysitis with fat pad atrophy, right foot.

POSTOPERATIVE DIAGNOSES: Same.

PROCEDURES:
1. Bunionectomy with distal first metatarsal osteotomy with internal fixation, right foot.
2. Metatarsal head resection, 2 through 5, right foot.

SURGEON: Douglas Foxtrot, MD

ANESTHESIA: General.

HEMOSTASIS: Ankle tourniquet at 250 millimeters of mercury.

ESTIMATED BLOOD LOSS: Less than 20 cc.

MATERIALS: 4-0 Vicryl, 5-0 Prolene, 2.0 millimeter cortical stainless screws × 2.

INJECTABLES: 18 cc of a 1:1 mix of 1% lidocaine plain, 0.5% Marcaine plain in postoperative anesthesia.

INDICATION FOR PROCEDURE: Patient had presented to my office upon consult from Dr. Bowler for complaint of right foot pain. In discussing and evaluating the patient, we discussed the possibility of conservative treatment versus surgical intervention. She would like to forego all conservative treatment at this point and proceed with surgical intervention to her right foot. I explained to her all the risks, benefits, and complications of the procedure with all questions answered to her satisfaction. No guarantees were given. She understands. She was consented for bunionectomy with distal first metatarsal osteotomy, internal fixation of the right foot with metatarsal head resections, 2 through 5, of the right foot secondary to severe long-term diaphysitis. This is going to be done in conjunction with Dr. Mathews' procedure in which he is defatting a flap to her right heel. Her NPO status was confirmed. The surgical consent was signed and in the chart.

SURGERY IN DETAIL: Under mild IV sedation, the patient was brought back to the operating room and placed under general anesthesia and intubated. She was placed in the prone position. Dr. Mathews proceeded with defatting of a flap to the right heel. Following this procedure, in which he did not use a tourniquet, she was replaced on the operating table in the supine position. A well-padded tourniquet was placed about her right ankle. Local anesthesia was infiltrated in the forefoot region, obtaining postoperative anesthesia with a total of 18 cc of a 1:1 mix of 1% lidocaine plain and 0.5 % Marcaine plain. The right foot was then rescrubbed, prepped, and draped in the usual aseptic manner. The right foot was exsanguinated. The ankle tourniquet was elevated to 250 millimeters of mercury. Attention was directed to the dorsum of the right foot where a 2-centimeter linear longitudinal incision was made over the second metatarsophalangeal joint. Dissection was carried down through the subcutaneous tissues. All bleeders were cauterized and ligated. All vital neurovascular structures were identified and retracted. Capsulotomy of the second metatarsophalangeal joint was performed. A periosteal elevator was used to free the capsule and periosteum from the head and neck of the second metatarsal. An oscillating saw was used to resect the head of the second metatarsal just proximal to the articular cartilage, angled in a dorsal distal to planter proximal attitude. The metatarsal head was removed from the operative field through sharp dissection. The wound was irrigated with copious amounts of normal sterile saline. The periosteal and capsular structures were reapproximated with 4-0 Vicryl. The skin was reapproximated with 5-0 Prolene. The identical procedure was performed to the third, fourth, and fifth metatarsophalangeal joints with the same type linear 2 centimeter incision with resection of the metatarsal heads, 3, 4, and 5. All wounds were irrigated in a similar fashion and closed in a similar fashion as that of the second metatarsophalangeal joint. The tourniquet was then released after sterile 4 × 4s and a mildly compressive ACE bandage was placed over all the wounds to aid in re-nourishment of that flap per the request of Dr. Matthews. The tourniquet was deflated and left deflated for 10 minutes. The foot was re-exsanguinated with elevation for 3 minutes, and the ankle tourniquet was then re-elevated to 250 millimeters of mercury. Attention was then directed to the bunion deformity of the right foot where a 6-centimeter linear longitudinal incision was made just medial to the extensor hallucis longus tendon. Dissection was carried down through the subcutaneous tissues. All bleeders were cauterized and ligated. All vital neurovascular structures were identified and retracted. Dissection was carried into the first interspace where the deep transverse intermetatarsal ligament was identified and transected. A lateral capsulotomy of the first metatarsophalangeal joint was performed. The fibular sesamoid was freed of all the soft tissue ligamentous structures proximally, distally and laterally. The conjoined tendon of the adductor hallucis muscle inserts at the base of the proximal phalanx was transected, and flexibility was then noted. Inverted L-capsulotomy of the first metatarsophalangeal joint was made dorsally and medially. The head of the first metatarsal was freed of all of its soft tissue and periosteal structures. Hypertrophic dorsal medial eminence of the first metatarsal head was resected and removed from the operative field. Chevron-style osteotomy was made from medial to lateral in the first metatarsal with the apex at the central most portion of the metatarsal head. Osteotomy exited dorsal-proximal and plantar-proximal, and a dorsal proximal osteotomy was made more proximal to aid in fixation. Capsular fragment was then moved laterally to the correct anatomical position. Utilizing proper AO technique in lag fashion, 2.0 millimeter cortical stainless steel screws × 2 were driven across the osteotomy utilizing proper AO technique in a lag fashion with excellent compression noted. The medial cortical bone shelf was resected and removed from the operative field. All rough edges were smoothed, utilizing back-brushing technique with the oscillating saw. Intraoperative fluoroscopy revealed that anatomical alignment of the first ray had been restored with good position of the screw fixation noted on multiple views. The wound was irrigated with copious amounts of normal sterile saline. Medial capsulorraphy was performed, resecting all redundant medial capsular tissue. The periosteal and capsular structures were reapproximated with 4-0 Vicryl. The skin was reapproximated with 5-0 Prolene. All surgical sites were dressed with Adaptic, sterile 4 × 4s, Kerlix roll, and an ACE bandage. The ankle tourniquet was deflated and prompt hyperemic response was noted to all digits of the right foot. The anatomical alignment of all digits were splinted in place with the soft dressing. The patient tolerated the procedure and anesthesia well with vital signs stable throughout. She was sent to the recovery room with vascular status intact to the right foot. Following a period of postoperative monitoring, she will be admitted under doctor's care for postoperative follow-up for the defatting of the flap to the aspect of her right heel.

I will see her postoperatively in the hospital and will follow-up with her when she is discharged in my office.

Procedure Key Terms:	bunionectomy, chevron-style procedure, ostectomy, metatarsal resection
ICD-9-CM Key Terms:	bunion, diaphysitis

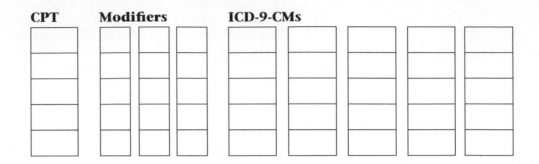

CPT   **Modifiers**   **ICD-9-CMs**

CASE 18

PREOPERATIVE DIAGNOSIS: Urinary retention.

POSTOPERATIVE DIAGNOSIS: Recurrent prostatic hyperplasia.

PROCEDURE PERFORMED: Cystoscopy and transurethral resection of the prostate.

SURGEON: Edith Hopkins, MD

ANESTHESIA: Spinal.

CLINICAL NOTE: This is a 75-year-old gentleman who underwent right hip arthroplasty. Prior to need for hip procedure this gentleman had undergone a right transurethral resection of the prostate for urinary retention and has again developed urinary retention. He has had several trials of voiding with both alpha blockade and bethanechol. Cystoscopy revealed recurrent prostatic hyperplasia. There is a large piece of tissue acting as a ball valve.

PROCEDURE: The patient was given a spinal anesthetic, prepped, and draped in the lithotomy position. A 28-French resectoscope was passed under direct vision. Again, the prostate shows irregular ingrowth and obstruction. The bladder shows mild to moderate trabeculation. The prostate was thoroughly resected on the left and chips evacuated from the bladder and hemostasis achieved. A 22-French three-way catheter was inserted into the bladder and placed at continuous bladder irrigation. The patient tolerated the procedure well and was transferred to the recovery room in good condition.

Procedure Key Terms:	transurethral resection
ICD-9-CM Key Terms:	recurrent hyperplasia, urinary retention

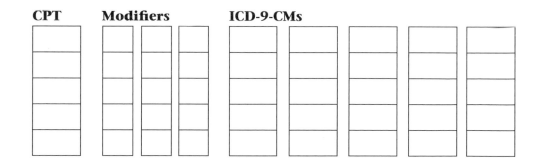

CPT   **Modifiers**   **ICD-9-CMs**

CASE 19

PREOPERATIVE DIAGNOSIS: Dysfunctional uterine bleeding.

POSTOPERATIVE DIAGNOSIS: Same.

PROCEDURE PERFORMED: Hysteroscopy with fractional dilation and curettage and lysis of intrauterine synechiae (adhesions).

SURGEON: Timothy Canterwell, MD

ANESTHESIA: Laryngeal general mask anesthesia.

ESTIMATED BLOOD LOSS: Less than 10 cc.

COMPLICATIONS: None.

PROCEDURE: The patient was prepped and draped in the lithotomy position under general laryngeal mask anesthesia. The bladder was straight cathed. A weighted speculum was placed in the vagina. The anterior lip of the cervix was grasped with a single tooth tenaculum. Kevorkian curet was then used to obtain endocervical curettages. The uterus was then sounded to a depth of 6 cm. The cervical os was then serially dilated to allow passage of the hysteroscope. The hysteroscope was then passed and uterine contents were examined, documented, and photographed. No evidence of polyps or fibroids. There were some adhesions seen. These were broken down easily. The sharp curet was then used to thoroughly sample the endometrial cavity with return of a moderate amount of tissue. The tenaculum was removed from the cervix and the tenaculum site was over-sewn with 3-0 chromic figure-of-eight sutures. The instruments were removed from the vagina. All sponges and needles were accounted for upon completion of the procedure. The patient left the Operating Room in apparent good condition having tolerated the procedure well.

Procedure Key Terms:	hysteroscopy, adhesions
ICD-9-CM Key Terms:	bleeding uterus, synechiae

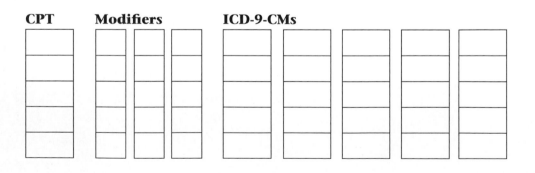

CPT   **Modifiers**   **ICD-9-CMs**

CASE 20

PREOPERATIVE DIAGNOSIS: Phimosis.

POSTOPERATIVE DIAGNOSIS: Same.

PROCEDURE PERFORMED: Lysis of prepuce adhesions, meatotomy, and cystoscopy.

CLINICAL NOTE: This 4-year-old has voiding dysfunction and his urine sprays and goes up rather than down. He had had prior circumcision. There is a minimal amount of redundant foreskin.

SURGEON: Lucama Hitachi

ANESTHESIA: General mask.

PROCEDURE: The patient was given a general mask anesthetic, prepped, and draped in the supine position. There were some adhesions between the glans and the prepuce. These were broken down easily. Meatus was quite stenotic, and I believe this is a result of a congenital atresia of the ureter. Meatotomy was performed at the 6-o'clock position. A clamp was placed, skin divided, and then reapproximating sutures using 5-0 chromic were placed. The patient was then cystoscoped using a 9.2 rigid instrument. There was no evidence of urethral stricture posterior to the urethral valves. Bladder mucosa and ureteric orifices were all normal. Cystoscope was withdrawn. Bacitracin ointment was applied. The patient tolerated the procedure well and was transferred to the recovery room in good condition.

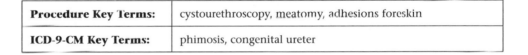

Procedure Key Terms:	cystourethroscopy, meatomy, adhesions foreskin
ICD-9-CM Key Terms:	phimosis, congenital ureter

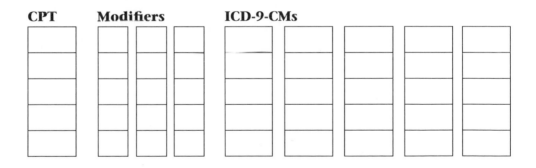

CPT   Modifiers   ICD-9-CMs

A-mode: one-dimensional ultrasonic display reflecting the time it takes a sound wave to reach a structure and reflect back; maps the structure's outline

ablation: removal by cutting

abortion: termination of pregnancy

abscess: localized collection of pus that will result in the disintegration of tissue over time

abuse: misuse of substance

acquired: not genetic

actinotherapy: treatment of acne using ultraviolet rays

acute: of sudden onset and short duration

addiction: dependence on a drug

admission: attention to an acute illness or injury resulting in admission to a hospital

adrenal: glands, located at the top of the kidneys, that produce steroid hormones

AHA: American Hospital Association

AHIMA: American Health Information Management Association

allogenic: a graft that is from the same species, but genetically different

allograft: tissue graft between individuals who are not of the same genotype

allotransplantation: transplantation between individuals who are not of the same genotype

amniocentesis: percutaneous aspiration of amniotic fluid

anastomosis: surgical connection of two tubular structures, such as two pieces of the intestine

aneurysm: is an abnormal weakening of a vessel wall with outpouching beyond the normal confines of the vessel

angiography: taking of x-ray films of vessels after injection of contrast material

angioplasty: surgical or percutaneous procedure in a vessel to dilate the vessel opening; used in the treatment of atherosclerotic disease

angioscopy: studying the capillaries of the eyes

anomaloscope: instrument used to test color vision

anomaly: abnormality

anoscopy: procedure that uses a scope to examine the anus

antepartum: before childbirth

anterior (ventral): in front of

anterior segment: those parts of the eye in the front of and including the lens, orbit, extraocular muscles, and eyelid

anterior synechiae: adhesions of the iris to the cornea

anteroposterior: from front to back

antrum: sinus

aortography: radiographic recording of the aorta

apexcardiography: noninvasive graphic recording of the movement of the chest wall from the cardiac pulsations from the region of the apex of the heart, usually of the left ventricle

APC (Ambulatory Payment Classification): a patient classification that provides a payment system for outpatients

aphakia: absence of the lens of the eye

apicectomy: excision of a portion of the temporal bone

Appendix A: located near the back of the CPT manual; lists all modifiers with complete explanations for use

Appendix B: located near the back of the CPT manual; contains a complete list of additions to, deletions from, and revisions of the previous edition

Appendix C: located near the back of the CPT manual; presents clinical examples of Evaluation and Management (E/M)

Appendix D: located near the back of the CPT manual; contains a list of the CPT add-on codes

Appendix E: located near the back of the CPT manual; contains a list of modifier -51 exempt codes

Appendix F: located near the back of the CPT manual; contains information about modifier -63, Procedures Performed on Infants less than 4-kg

Appendix G: located near the back of the CPT manual; contains information about moderate (conscious) sedation

Appendix H: located near the back of the CPT manual; contains information about performance measures of Category II codes

Appendix I: located near the back of the CPT manual; contains information about Category II modifiers

Appendix J: located near the back of the CPT manual; contains information on sensory, motor, and mixed nerves and the corresponding conduction study code

Appendix K: located near the back of the CPT manual; contains the codes that are pending FDA (Food and Drug Administration) approval

Appendix L: located near the back of the CPT manual; contains the vascular families

Appendix M: located near the back of the CPT manual; contains a crosswalk of deleted CPT codes

arteriovenous fistula: direct communication (passage) between an artery and vein

artery: vessel that generally carries oxygenated blood from the heart to body tissues (pulmonary artery carries un-oxygenated blood)

arthrodesis: surgical immobilization of a joint

arthrography: radiographic recording of a joint

arthroplasty: reshaping or reconstruction of a joint

aspiration: use of a needle and a syringe to withdraw fluid

assignment: Medicare's payment for the service, which participating physicians agree to accept as payment in full

astigmatism: condition in which the refractive surfaces of the eye are unequal

asymptomatic: not showing any of the typical symptoms of a disease or condition

atrium: chamber in the upper part of the heart

attending physician: the physician with the primary responsibility for care of the patient

audi-: prefix meaning hearing

audiometry: hearing testing

aur-: prefix meaning ear

aural atresia: congenital absence of the external auditory canal

autogenous, autologous: from oneself

axillary nodes: lymph nodes located in the armpit

B-scan: two-dimensional display of tissues and organs

backbench work: special preparation of an organ before organ transplantation

bariatric surgery: gastric restrictive procedures that are used to treat morbid obesity and are accomplished by placing a restrictive device around the stomach to decrease its functional size

barium enema: radiographic contrast medium–enhanced examination of the colon

benign: not progressive

benign hypertension: hypertensive condition with a continuous, mild blood pressure elevation

bifocal: two focuses in eyeglasses, one usually for close work and the other for improvement of distance vision

bilateral: occurring on two sides

bilobectomy: surgical removal of two lobes of a lung

biofeedback: process of giving a person self-information

biometry: application of a statistical measure to a biologic fact

biopsy: removal of a small piece of living tissue for diagnostic purposes

blephar(o)-: prefix meaning eyelid

block: frozen piece of a sample

blood patch: a procedure in which a cerebrospinal fluid leak is closed by means of an injection of the patient's blood into the area used during spinal anesthesia

brachytherapy: therapy using radioactive sources that are placed inside the body

bronchography: radiographic recording of the lungs

bronchoplasty: surgical repair of the bronchi

bronchoscopy: inspection of the bronchial tree using a bronchoscope

bulbocavernosus: muscle that constricts the vagina in a female and the urethra in a male

bulbourethral gland: rounded mass of the urethra

bypass: to go around

calculus: concretion of mineral salts, also called a stone

calycoplasty: surgical reconstruction of a recess of the renal pelvis

calyx: recess of the renal pelvis

cannulation: insertion of a tube into a duct or cavity

carcinoma in situ: a cancerous tumor in its original place that has not invaded neighboring tissues

cardiopulmonary: refers to the heart and lungs

cardiopulmonary bypass: blood bypasses the heart through a heart-lung machine during open-heart surgery

cardioversion: electric shock to the heart to restore normal rhythm

cardioverter-defibrillator: surgically placed device that directs an electric current shock to the heart to restore rhythm

cataract: opaque covering on or in the lens

Category I: CPT codes approved by the FDA and representing widely used services and procedures

Category II: Supplemental codes that can be used for performance measurements

Category III: Temporary CPT codes

catheter: tube placed into the body to put fluid in or take fluid out

caudal: away from the head, or the lower part of the body; same as inferior

cauterization: destruction of tissue by the use of cautery

cavernosa–corpus spongiosum shunt: creation of a connection between a cavity of the penis and the urethra

cavernosa–glans penis fistulization: creation of a connection between a cavity of the penis and the glans penis, which overlaps the penis cavity

cavernos–saphenous vein shunt: creation of a connection between the cavity of the penis and a vein

cavernosography: radiographic recording of a cavity, e.g., the pulmonary cavity or the main part of the penis

cavernosometry: measurement of the pressure in a cavity, e.g., the penis

-centesis: suffix meaning puncture of a cavity

central nervous system (CNS): brain and spinal cord

cervical: pertaining to the neck or to the cervix of the uterus

cervix uteri: rounded, cone-shaped neck of the uterus

cesarean: surgical opening through abdominal wall for delivery

CF (conversion factor): national dollar amount that is applied to all services paid on the Medicare Fee Schedule basis

cholangiography: radiographic recording of the bile ducts

cholangiopancreatography (ERCP): radiographic recording of the biliary system and pancreas

chole-: prefix meaning bile

cholecystectomy: surgical removal of the gallbladder

cholecystoenterostomy: creation of a connection between the gallbladder and intestine

cholecystography: radiographic recording of the gallbladder

chordee: condition resulting in the penis' being bent downward

chorionic villus sampling (CVS): biopsy of the outermost part of the placenta

chromotubation: surgical procedure to open obstructed fallopian tubes

chronic: of long duration

Cloquet's node: also called a gland; it is the highest of the deep groin lymph nodes

closed treatment: fracture site that is not surgically opened and visualized

CMS: Centers for Medicare and Medicaid Services, formerly HCFA, Health Care Financing Administration

colonoscopy: fiberscopic examination of the entire colon that may include part of the terminal ileum

colostomy: artificial opening between the colon and the abdominal wall

combination code: single ICD-9-CM code used to identify etiology and manifestation of a disease

combination coding: a code from the Radiology section as well as a code from one of the other sections must be used to fully describe the procedure

communicable disease: disease that can be transmitted from one person to another or one species to another

comparative conditions: patient conditions that are documented as "either/or" in the medical record

component: part

component coding: a code from the Radiology section as well as a code from one of the other sections must be used to fully describe the procedure

computed axial tomography (CAT or CT): procedure by which selected planes of tissue are pinpointed through computer enhancement, and images may be reconstructed by analysis of variance in absorption of the tissue

concurrent care: the provision of similar services (e.g., hospital visits) to the same patient by more than one physician on the same day. Each physician provides services for a separate condition, not reasonably expected to be managed by the attending physician. When concurrent care is provided, the diagnosis must reflect the medical necessity of different specialties

congenital: existing from birth

conjunctiva: the lining of the eyelids and the covering of the sclerae

conscious sedation: a decreased level of consciousness in which the patient is not completely asleep

constitutional examination element: assessment of the patient's general condition and the recording of the vital signs

consultation: includes those services rendered by a physician whose opinion or advice is requested by another physician or agency concerning the evaluation and/or treatment of a patient; a consultant is not an attending physician

contralateral: the opposite side

contributory factors: counseling, coordination of care, nature of the presenting problem, and time of an E/M service

cordectomy: surgical removal of the vocal cord(s)

cordocentesis: procedure to obtain a fetal blood sample; also called a percutaneous umbilical blood sampling

corneosclera: cornea and sclera of the eye

corpora cavernosa: the two cavities of the penis

corpus uteri: uterus

counseling: a discussion with a patient and/or family concerning one or more of the following areas: diagnostic results, impressions, and/or recommended diagnostic studies; prognosis; risks and benefits of treatment; instructions for treatment; importance of compliance with treatment; risk factor reduction; and patient and family education

CPT (Current Procedural Terminology): a coding system developed by the American Medical Association (AMA) to convert widely accepted, uniform descriptions of medical, surgical, and diagnostic services rendered by health care providers into five-digit codes

cranium: that part of the skeleton that encloses the brain

critical care: the care of critically ill patients in medical emergencies that requires the constant attendance of the physician (e.g., cardiac arrest, shock, bleeding, respiratory failure); critical care is usually, but not always, given in a critical care area, such as the coronary care unit (CCU) or the intensive care unit (ICU)

CRNA: certified registered nurse anesthetist

Crohn's disease: regional enteritis

cryosurgery: destruction of lesions using extreme cold

curettage: scraping of a cavity using a spoon-shaped instrument

cycl/o-: prefix meaning ciliary body or eye muscle

cyst: closed sac containing matter or fluid

cystic hygroma: congenital deformity or benign tumor of the lymphatic system

cystocele: herniation of the bladder into the vagina

cystography: radiographic recording of the urinary bladder

cystolithectomy: removal of a calculus (stone) from the urinary bladder

cystolithotomy: cystolithectomy

cystometrogram (CMG): measurement of the pressures and capacity of the urinary bladder

cystoplasty: surgical reconstruction of the bladder

cystorrhaphy: suture of the bladder

cystoscopy: use of a scope to view the bladder

cystostomy: surgical creation of an opening into the bladder

cystotomy: incision into the bladder

cystourethroplasty: surgical reconstruction of the bladder and urethra

cystourethroscopy: use of a scope to view the bladder and urethra

cytopathology: study of the diseases of cells

dacry/o-: prefix meaning tear or tear duct

dacryocyst/o-: prefix meaning pertaining to the lacrimal sac

dacryocystography: radiographic recording of the lacrimal sac or tear duct sac

debridement: cleansing of or removal of dead tissue from a wound

delivery: childbirth

Demerol: a narcotic analgesic

dermatoplasty: surgical repair of the skin

dermis: second layer of skin, holding blood vessels, nerve endings, sweat glands, and hair follicles

destruction: killing of tissue by means of electrocautery, laser, chemicals, or other means

DHHS: Department of Health and Human Services

diagnostic: that done to identify the cause, origin, or extent of a condition

diaphragm: muscular wall that separates the thoracic and abdominal cavities

diaphragmatic hernia: hernia of the diaphragm

dilation: expansion (of the cervix)

diskography: radiographic recording of an intervertebral joint

dislocation: placement in a location other than the original location

displacement therapy: procedure in which the physician flushes saline solution into the sinuses to remove mucus or pus

distal: farther from the point of attachment or origin

distinct procedure: one service or procedure that has no relationship to another service or procedure

Doppler: ultrasonic measure of blood movement

dosimetry: scientific calculation of radiation emitted from various radioactive sources

drainage: free flow or withdrawal of fluids from a wound or cavity

DRGs (Diagnosis Related Groups): a disease classification system that relates the type of inpatients a hospital treats (case mix) to the costs incurred by the hospital (now MS-DRGs)

dual-chamber pacemaker: electrodes of the pacemaker are placed in both the atria and the ventricle of the heart

duodenography: radiographic recording of the duodenum, or first part of the small intestine

E Codes: alphanumeric designations preceded by the letter "E," used to classify external causes

ear, parts of the external: auricle, pinna, external acoustic, meatus, and tympanic membrane

ear, parts of the inner: vestibule, semicircular canals, and cochlea

ear, parts of the middle: malleus, incus, and stapes

ECG: *see* electrocardiogram

echocardiography: radiographic recording of the heart or heart walls or surrounding tissues

echoencephalography: ultrasound of the brain

echography: ultrasound procedure in which sound waves are bounced off an internal organ and the resulting image is recorded

-ectomy: suffix meaning removal of part or all of an organ of the body

ectopic: pregnancy outside the uterus (i.e., in the fallopian tube)

EEG: *see* electroencephalogram

electrocardiogram (ECG): written record of the electrical activity of the heart

electrocochleography: stimulation of the cochlea to measure electrical activity

electrode: lead attached to a generator that carries the electric current from the generator to the atria or ventricles

electrodesiccation: destruction of a lesion by the use of electric current radiated through a needle

electroencephalogram (EEG): written record of the electrical activity of the brain

electrohydraulic fragmentation: use of a probe containing two electrodes that are applied, one on each side, of the calculus

electromyogram (EMG): written record of the electrical activity of the skeletal muscles

electromyography (EMG): recording of the electrical impulses of muscles

electro-oculogram (EOG): written record of the electrical activity of the eye

electrophysiology: the study of the electrical system of the heart, including the study of arrhythmias

embolectomy: removal of blockage (embolism) from vessels

embolism: blockage of a blood vessel by a blood clot or other matter that has moved from another area of the body through the circulatory system

emergency care services: services that are provided by the physician in the emergency department for unplanned patient encounters; no distinction is made between new and established patients who are seen in the emergency department

encephalography: radiographic recording of the subarachnoid space and ventricles of the brain

endarterectomy: incision into an artery to remove the inner lining so as to eliminate disease or blockage

endomyocardial: pertaining to the inner and middle layers of the heart

endopyelotomy: procedure involving the bladder and ureters, including the insertion of a stent

endoscopy: inspection of body organs or cavities using a lighted scope that may be inserted through an existing opening or through a small incision

endotracheal tube: can be inserted through the nose or mouth and passed into the trachea for ventilation

endovascular aneurysm repair (EVAR): an emerging technology that involves placing a stent graft, or a fabric tube, inside the affected area of the blood vessel by access through an artery

enterocystoplasty: surgical reconstruction of the small intestine after the removal of a cyst and usually including a bowel anastomosis

enucleation: removal of an organ or organs from a body cavity

epicardial: over the heart

epidermis: outer layer of skin

epididymectomy: surgical removal of the epididymis

epididymis: tube located at the top of the testes that stores sperm

epididymography: radiographic recording of the epididymis

epididymovasostomy: creation of a new connection between the vas deferens and epididymis

epidural anesthesia: injection of an anesthesia agent into the spaces between the vertebrae. Also known as peridural anesthesia, epidural, epidural block, and intraspinal anesthesia

epiglottidectomy: excision of the covering of the larynx

eponym: disease, structure, or procedure that is named after a person

ESRD: end-stage renal disease

established patient: a patient who has received face-to-face professional services from the physician or another physician of the same specialty in the same group within the past 3 years

etiology: study of causes of diseases

eventration: protrusion of the bowel through the viscera of the abdomen

evisceration: pulling the viscera outside of the body through an incision

exacerbation: worsening or increase of severity of a condition or disease

excision: it is full-thickness removal of a lesion that may include simple closure

excisional: removal of an entire lesion for biopsy

Exclusive Provider Organization (EPO): similar to a Health Maintenance Organization except that the providers of the services are not prepaid, but rather are paid on a fee-for-service basis

exenteration: removal of an organ all in one piece

exostosis: bony growth

exstrophy: condition in which an organ is turned inside out

exteriorization: developing an artificial opening through the abdominal wall to take out a diseased portion of the intestine

extirpation: taking or cutting out solid matter from a body part

false aneurysm: sac of clotted blood that has completely destroyed the vessel and is being contained by the tissue that surrounds the vessel

fascia lata grafts: a graft of fibrous tissue that is found beneath the skin

fasciectomy: excision of fascia

FDA (Food and Drug Administration): responsible for the safety of food and drugs in America; is an agency within the U.S. Public Health Service, which is part of the Department of Health and Human Services

Federal Register: official publication of all "Presidential Documents," "Rules and Regulations," "Proposed Rules," and "Notices"; government-instituted national changes are published in the Federal Register

fenestration: creation of a new opening in the inner wall of the middle ear

fimbrioplasty: surgical repair of the fringe of the uterine tube

first-listed diagnosis: outpatient diagnosis

Fiscal Intermediary (FI): handles administration of Medicare claims but will be phased out by 2011 into MACs

fistula: abnormal opening from one area to another area or to the outside of the body

fluoroscopy: procedure for viewing the interior of the body using x-rays and projecting the image onto a television screen

forensic examination: a head to toe examination performed when an injury occurs that was not the result of natural causes; involves legal investigation

fracture: break in a bone

fulguration: use of electric current to destroy tissue

fundoplasty: repair of the bottom of an organ or muscle

gastro-: prefix meaning stomach

gastrointestinal: pertaining to the stomach and intestine

gastroplasty: operation on the stomach for repair or reconfiguration

gastrostomy: artificial opening between the stomach and the abdominal wall

general anesthesia: a state of unconsciousness produced by the administration of a drug; it can be administered by inhalation or intramuscularly, rectally, or intravenously

gloss(o)-: prefix meaning tongue

gonioscopy: use of a scope to gain a view of the iridocorneal angle, or the anatomical angle formed between the eye's cornea and iris

Group Practice Model: an organization of physicians who contract with a Health Maintenance Organization to provide services to the enrollees of the HMO

grouper: computer used to input the principal diagnosis and other critical information about a patient and then provide the correct MS-DRG code

Guidelines: provide specific instructions about coding for each section of the CPT manual; the Guidelines contain definitions of terms, applicable modifiers, explanation of notes, subsection information, unlisted services, special reports information, and clinical examples

HCFA: Health Care Financing Administration, now known as Centers for Medicare and Medicaid Services (CMS)

Health Maintenance Organization (HMO): a health care delivery system in which an enrollee is assigned a primary care physician who manages all the health care needs of the enrollee

hemodialysis: cleansing of the blood outside of the body

hepat(o)-: prefix meaning liver

hepatography: radiographic recording of the liver

hernia: organ or tissue protruding through the wall or cavity that usually contains it

histology: study of the minute structures, composition, and function of tissues

Hodgkin's disease: malignant lymphoma

hydrocele: sac of fluid

hypertension, uncontrolled: untreated hypertension or hypertension that is not responding to the therapeutic regimen

hypertensive heart disease: secondary effects on the heart of prolonged, sustained systemic hypertension; the heart has to work against greatly increased resistance, causing increased blood pressure

hypogastric: lowest middle abdominal area

hyposensitization: decreased sensitivity

hypospadias: congenital deformity of the urethra in which the urethral opening is on the underside of the penis rather than at the end

hypotension: abnormally low blood pressure; sometimes induced during surgical procedures

hypothermia: low body temperature; sometimes induced during surgical procedures

hysterectomy: surgical removal of the uterus

hysterorrhaphy: suturing of the uterus

hysterosalpingography: radiographic recording of the uterine cavity and fallopian tubes

hysteroscopy: visualization of the canal of the uterine cervix and cavity of the uterus using a scope placed through the vagina

hysterotomy: incision into the uterus

ileostomy: artificial opening between the ileum and the abdominal wall

imbrication: overlapping

immunotherapy: therapy to increase immunity

incarcerated: regarding hernias, a constricted, irreducible hernia that may cause obstruction of an intestine

incision: surgically cutting into

incision and drainage: to cut and withdraw fluid

incisional: *see* incision

Individual Practice Association (IPA): an organization of physicians who provide services for a set fee; Health Maintenance Organizations often contract with the IPA for services to their enrollees

infectious disease carrier: person who has a communicable disease but is symptom free despite having the disease

infectious disease contact: encounter with a person who has a disease that can be communicated or transmitted

inferior: away from the head or the lower part of the body; also known as caudal

inguinofemoral: referring to the groin and thigh

injection: introduction of fluid into a tissue, vessel, or cavity

inpatient: one who has been formally admitted to a health care facility

in situ: malignancy that is within the original site of development and has not invaded neighboring tissue

internal/external fixation: application of pins, wires, screws, and so on to immobilize a body part; they can be placed externally or internally

intracardiac: inside the heart

intramural: within the organ wall

intramuscular: into a muscle

intraoperative: period of time during which a surgical procedure is being performed

intravascular ultrasound: a test that uses sound waves to examine coronary vessels of the heart

intravenous: into a vein

intravenous pyelography (IVP): radiographic recording of the urinary system

introitus: opening or entrance to the vagina

intubation: insertion of a tube

invasive: entering the body, breaking the skin

iontophoresis: introduction of ions into the body

ischemia: deficient blood supply due to obstruction of the circulatory system

isthmus: connection of two regions or structures

isthmus, thyroid: tissue connection between right and left thyroid lobes

isthmusectomy: surgical removal of the isthmus

italicized code: an ICD-9-CM code that can never be sequenced as the principal or primary diagnosis

jejunostomy: artificial opening between the jejunum and the abdominal wall

joint movement:

  abduction: movement of a limb away from the midline of the body

  adduction: movement of a limb toward the midline of the body

circumduction: circular movement of a limb

extension: movement by which two parts are drawn away from each other

flexion: movement by which two parts are drawn toward each other

hyperextension: excessive extension of a limb

pronation: applied to the hand, the act of turning the palm down

supination: applied to the hand, the act of turning the palm up

jugular nodes: lymph nodes located next to the large vein in the neck

kerat/o-: prefix meaning cornea

keratoplasty: surgical repair of the cornea

key components: the history, examination, and medical decision-making complexity of an E/M service

Kock pouch: surgical creation of a urinary bladder from a segment of the ileum

kyphosis: humpback, the abnormal curvature of the spine

labyrinth: inner connecting cavities, such as the internal ear

laminectomy: surgical excision of the lamina

laparoscopy: exploration of the abdomen and pelvic cavities using a scope placed through a small incision in the abdominal wall

laryngeal web: congenital abnormality of connective tissue between the vocal cords

laryngectomy: surgical removal of the larynx

laryngo-: prefix meaning larynx

laryngography: radiographic recording of the larynx

laryngoplasty: surgical repair of the larynx

laryngoscope: an endoscope used to view the inside of the larynx

laryngoscopy: viewing of the larynx using a fiberoptic scope

laryngotomy: incision into the larynx

late effect: residual effect (that a condition produced) after the acute phase of an illness or injury has terminated

lateral: away from the midline of the body (to the side)

lavage: washing out of an organ

lesion: abnormal or altered tissue, e.g., wound, cyst, abscess, or boil

ligament: a band of fibrous tissue that connects cartilage or bone and supports a joint

ligation: binding or tying off, as in constricting the bloodflow of a vessel or binding fallopian tubes for sterilization

litholapaxy: lithotripsy

lithotomy: incision into an organ or a duct for the purpose of removing a stone

lithotripsy: crushing of a gallbladder or urinary bladder stone followed by irrigation to wash the fragment out

lobectomy: surgical excision of a lobe of the lung

lymph node: station along the lymphatic system

lymphadenectomy: excision of a lymph node or nodes

lymphadenitis: inflammation of a lymph node

lymphangiography: radiographic recording of the lymphatic vessels and nodes

lymphangiotomy: incision into a lymphatic vessel

lysis: releasing

M-mode: one-dimensional display of movement of structures

MAAC (Maximum Actual Allowable Charge): limitation on the total amount that can be charged by physicians who are not participants in Medicare

MAC (Medicare Administrative Contractor): an entity that manages the process claims for CMS

magnetic resonance imaging (MRI): procedure that uses nonionizing radiation to view the body in a cross-sectional view

malignancy: used in reference to a cancerous tumor

malignant: used to describe a cancerous tumor that grows worse over time

malignant hypertension: accelerated, severe form of hypertension, manifested by headaches, blurred vision, dyspnea, and uremia; usually causes permanent organ damage

mammography: radiographic recording of the breasts

Managed Care Organization (MCO): a group that is responsible for the health care services offered to an enrolled group of persons

mandated service: a service required by an agency or organization to be performed for a patient; usually the agency or organization pays all or a portion of the patient's medical bills

manifestation: sign of a disease

manipulation or reduction: words used interchangeably to mean the attempted restoration of a fracture or joint dislocation to its normal anatomic position

marsupialization: surgical procedure that creates an exterior pouch from an internal abscess

mast-: prefix meaning breast

mastoid-: prefix meaning posterior temporal bone

MDC (Major Diagnostic Categories): the division of all principal diagnoses into 25 mutually exclusive principal diagnosis areas within the MS-DRG system

meatotomy: surgical enlargement of the opening of the urinary meatus

medial: toward the midline of the body

mediastinoscopy: use of an endoscope inserted through a small incision to view the mediastinum

mediastinotomy: cutting into the mediastinum

mediastinum: area between the lungs that contains the heart, aorta, trachea, lymph nodes, thymus gland, esophagus, and bronchial tubes

Medicare Administrative Contractor (MAC): handles the administration of Medicare claims and will be the only administrators by 2011

Medicare Risk HMO: a Medicare-funded alternative to the standard Medicare supplemental coverage

MEI (Medicare Economic Index): government-mandated index that ties increases in the Medicare prevailing charges to economic indicators

MeV: megaelectron volt

MFS (Medicare Fee Schedule): schedules that list the allowable charges for Medicare services

modality: treatment method

moderate (conscious) sedation: a decreased level of consciousness in which the patient is not completely asleep

modifiers: added to codes to supply more specific information about the services provided

monofocal: eyeglasses with one vision correction

morbidity: condition of being diseased or morbid

morphine: a narcotic analgesic

morphology: the science of the form and structure of organisms

mortality: death

MS-DRG (Medicare Severity Diagnosis Related Groups): a system of classifying patient groups by related diagnoses

MSLT: multiple sleep latency testing

multiple coding: also known as dual coding, use of more than one ICD-9-CM code to identify both etiology and manifestation of a disease, as contrasted with combination coding

muscle: fibrous structures that can contract and facilitate movement of the body. There are three types of muscles: smooth, skeletal, and cardiac

MVPS (Medical Volume Performance Standards): government's estimate of how much growth is appropriate for nationwide physician expenditures paid by the Part B Medicare program

myasthenia gravis: syndrome characterized by muscle weakness

myelography: radiographic recording of the subarachnoid space of the spine

myocardial infarction (MI): necrosis of the myocardium resulting from interrupted blood supply

myring-: prefix meaning eardrum

nasal button: a synthetic circular disk used to cover a hole in the nasal septum

nasopharyngoscopy: use of a scope to visualize the nose and pharynx

NCPAP: nasal continuous positive airway pressure

NEC: not elsewhere classifiable

neoplasm: new tumor growth that can be benign or malignant

nephrectomy, paraperitoneal: surgical removal of a kidney by a cut through the side along the twelfth rib

nephro-: prefix meaning kidney

nephrocutaneous fistula: a channel from the kidney to the skin

nephrolithotomy: removal of a kidney stone through an incision made into the kidney

nephrorrhaphy: suturing of the kidney

nephrostolithotomy: procedure to establish an artificial channel between the skin and the kidney

nephrostomy: creation of a channel into the renal pelvis of the kidney

nephrostomy, percutaneous: creation of a channel from the skin to the renal pelvis

nephrotomy: incision into the kidney

new patient: a patient who has not received any face-to-face professional services from the physician or another physician of the same specialty in the same group within the past 3 years

newborn care: the evaluation and determination of care management of a newly born infant

noninvasive: not entering the body, not breaking the skin

nonselective catheter placement: catheter or needle that is not manipulated and is placed directly into an artery or vein or is placed only into the aorta from any approach

NOS: not otherwise specified

nuclear cardiology: diagnostic specialty that uses radiopharmaceuticals to aid in the diagnosis of cardiologic conditions

nystagmus: rapid involuntary eye movements

objective information: findings observed by the physician during an examination

OBRA (Omnibus Budget Reconciliation Act of 1989): act that established new rules for Medicare reimbursement

ocul/o-: prefix meaning eye

ocular adnexa: orbit, extraocular muscles, and eyelid

office visit: a face-to-face encounter between a physician and a patient in the physician's private office to allow for primary management of a patient's health care status

Official Guidelines for Coding and Reporting: rules of coding diagnosis codes (ICD-9-CM) published by the Editorial Advisory Board of Coding Clinic

omentum: peritoneal connection between the stomach and other internal organs

oophor-: prefix meaning ovary

oophorectomy: surgical removal of the ovary(ies)

opacification: area that has become opaque (milky)

open treatment: fracture site that is surgically opened and visualized

ophthalmodynamometry: test of the blood pressure of the eye

ophthalmology: body of knowledge regarding the eyes

optokinetic: movement of the eyes to objects moving in the visual field

orchiectomy: castration

orchiopexy: fixation or suturing of an undescended testicle to secure it in the scrotum

orthoptic: corrective; in the correct place

osteotomy: cutting into bone

ostomy: artificial opening

oto-: prefix meaning ear

-otomy: suffix meaning incision into

outpatient: a patient who receives services in an ambulatory health care facility and is currently not an inpatient

overdose: excessive dose

oviduct: fallopian tube

pacemaker: electrical device that controls the beating of the heart by electrical impulses

paraesophageal hiatal hernia: hernia that is near the esophagus

parathyroid: produces a hormone to mobilize calcium from the bones to the blood

paring: removal of thin layers of skin by peeling or scraping

Part A: Medicare's Hospital Insurance; covers hospital/facility care

Part B: Medicare's Supplemental Medical Insurance; covers physician services and durable medical equipment that are not paid for under Part A

Part C: Medicare Advantage is a set of health care options from which beneficiaries choose health care providers

Part D: Medicare's prescription drug program

participating provider program: Medicare providers who have agreed in advance to accept assignment on all Medicare claims; now termed QIO

pathologic fracture: fracture due to a bone disease or a change surrounding the bone tissue that makes the bone weak

patient-controlled analgesia (PCA): a system that allows the patient to self-administer an analgesic drug, such as morphine, to control pain. A hand-held device is attached to a pump holding the drug and the patient can depress a button to administer a dose of the drug. In this way, the patient can control the amount of the drug, frequency of administration, and manage postoperative pain. The system is used with patients with chronic pain.

pelviolithotomy: pyeloplasty

penoscrotal: referring to the penis and scrotum

percutaneous: through the skin

percutaneous skeletal fixation: considered neither open nor closed; the fracture is not visualized, but fixation is placed across the fracture site under x-ray imaging

pericardiocentesis: procedure in which a surgeon withdraws fluid from the pericardial space by means of a needle inserted percutaneously into the space

pericarditis: inflammation of the sac surrounding the first few centimeters of great vessels and the heart

pericardium: membranous sac enclosing the heart and the ends of the great vessels

perineal approach: surgical approach in the area between the thighs

perinephric cyst: cyst in the tissue around the kidney

perineum: area between the vulva and anus; also known as the pelvic floor

peripheral nerves: 12 pairs of cranial nerves, 31-pairs of spinal nerves, and autonomic nervous system; connects peripheral receptors to the brain and spinal cord

perirenal: around the kidney

peritoneal: within the lining of the abdominal cavity

peritoneoscopy: visualization of the abdominal cavity using one scope placed through a small incision in the abdominal wall and another scope placed in the vagina

perivesical: around the bladder

perivisceral: around an organ

pharyngolaryngectomy: surgical removal of the pharynx and larynx

phlebotomy: cutting into a vein

phonocardiogram: recording of heart sounds

photochemotherapy: treatment by means of drugs that react to ultraviolet radiation or sunlight

physical status modifiers: modifying units in the Anesthesia section of the CPT manual that describe a patient's condition at the time anesthesia is administered

physics: scientific study of energy

-plasty: suffix meaning technique involving molding or surgically forming

plethysmography: determining the changes in volume of an organ part or body

pleura: covering of the lungs and thoracic cavity that is moistened with serous fluid to reduce friction during respiratory movements of the lungs

pleurectomy: surgical excision of the pleura

pneumo-: prefix meaning lung or air

pneumoncentesis: surgical puncturing of a lung to withdraw fluid

pneumonolysis: surgical separation of the lung from the chest wall to allow the lung to collapse

pneumonostomy: surgical procedure in which the chest cavity is exposed and the lung is incised

pneumonotomy: incision of the lung

pneumoplethysmography: determining the changes in the volume of the lung

polyp: tumor on a pedicle that bleeds easily and may become malignant

polysomnography: measurement of the brain waves and various stages of sleep during sleep

posterior (dorsal): in back of

posterior segment: those parts of the eye behind the lens

posterior synechiae: adhesions of the iris to the lens of the eye

posteroanterior: from back to front

postoperative: period of time after a surgical procedure

postpartum: after childbirth

Preferred Provider Organization (PPO): a group of providers who form a network and who have agreed to provide services to enrollees at a discounted rate

preoperative: period of time prior to a surgical procedure

priapism: painful condition in which the penis is constantly erect

primary diagnosis: first-listed diagnosis, used in the outpatient setting to identify the reason for the encounter

primary site: site of origin or where the tumor originated

principal diagnosis: defined in the Uniform Hospital Discharge Data Set (UHDDS) as "that condition established after study to be chiefly responsible for occasioning the admission of the patient to the hospital for care"; the principal diagnosis is sequenced first

proctosigmoidoscopy: fiberscopic examination of the sigmoid colon and rectum

professional component: term used in describing physician's services in radiology or pathology

prognosis: probable outcome of an illness

prophylactic: substance or agent that offers some protection from disease

PROs (Peer Review Organizations): groups established to review hospital admission and care; now termed QIO

prostatotomy: incision into the prostate

PSRO (Professional Standards Review Organization): voluntary physicians' organization designed to monitor the necessity of hospital admissions, treatment costs, and medical records of hospitals

punch: use of a small hollow instrument to puncture a lesion

pyelo-: prefix meaning renal pelvis

pyelocutaneous: from the renal pelvis to the skin

pyelography: radiographic recording of the kidneys, renal pelvis, ureters, and bladder

pyelolithotomy: surgical removal of a kidney stone from the renal pelvis

pyeloplasty: surgical reconstruction of the renal pelvis

pyeloscopy: viewing of the renal pelvis using a fluoroscope after injection of contrast material

pyelostolithotomy: removal of a kidney stone and establishment of a stoma

pyelostomy: surgical creation of a temporary diversion around the ureter

pyelotomy: incision into the renal pelvis

pyloroplasty: inision and repair of the pyloric channel

QIO (Quality Improvement Organization): consists of a national network of 53 entities that work with consumers, physicians, hospitals, and caregivers to refine care delivery systems

qualifying circumstances: five-digit CPT codes that describe situations or conditions that affect the administration of anesthesia

qualitative: measuring the presence or absence of

quantitative: measuring the presence or absence of and the amount of

rad: radiation absorption dose, the energy deposited in patients' tissues

radiation oncology: branch of medicine concerned with the application of radiation to a tumor site for treatment (destruction) of cancerous tumors

radiograph: film on which an image is produced through exposure to x-radiation

radiologist: physician who specializes in the use of radioactive materials in the diagnosis and treatment of diseases and illnesses

radiology: branch of medicine concerned with the use of radioactive substances for diagnosis and therapy

RBRVS (Resource-Based Relative Value Scale): scale designed to decrease Medicare expenditures, redistribute physician payment, and ensure quality health care at reasonable rates

real time: two-dimensional display of both the structures and the motion of tissues and organs, with the length of time also recorded as part of the study

reanastomosis: reconnection of a previous connection between two places, organs, or spaces

rectocele: herniation of the rectal wall through the posterior wall of the vagina

reducible: able to be corrected or put back into a normal position

referral: the transfer of the total or a specific portion of care of a patient from one physician to another that does not constitute a consultation

regional anesthesia: the interruption of the sensory nerve conductivity in a region of the body, which is produced by field block (forming a wall of anesthesia around the site by means of local injections) or by nerve block (injection of the area close to the major sensory nerve supplying a field); also known as block anesthesia, block, or conduction anesthesia

Relative Value Guide: comparison of anesthesia services; published by the American Society of Anesthesiologists (ASA)

renal pelvis: funnel-shaped sac in the kidney where urine is received

repair: to remedy, replace, or heal (in the Integumentary subsection pertains to suturing a wound)

residual: that which is left behind or remains

resource intensity: refers to the relative volume and type of diagnostic, therapeutic, and bed services used in the management of a particular illness

retrograde: moving backward or against the usual direction of flow

retroperitoneal: behind the sac holding the abdominal organs and viscera (peritoneum)

rhino-: prefix meaning nose

rhinoplasty: surgical repair of the nose

-rrhaphy: suffix meaning suturing

rubric: heading used as a direction or explanation as to what follows and the way in which the

information is to be used. In ICD-9-CM coding, the rubric is the three-digit code that precedes the four- and five-digit codes

rule of nines: rule used to estimate burned body surface area in burn patients

RUQ: right upper quadrant

RVU (Relative Value Unit): unit value that has been assigned for each service

salpingectomy: surgical removal of the uterine tube

salping(o)-: prefix meaning tube

salpingostomy: creation of a fistula into the uterine tube

scan: mapping of emissions of radioactive substances after they have been introduced into the body; the density can determine normal or abnormal conditions

sclera: the white, outer covering of the eye

scoliosis: abnormal lateral curvature of the spine

secondary site: place to which a malignant tumor has spread; metastatic site

section: slice of a frozen block

sections: the six major areas into which all CPT codes and descriptions are categorized

See: a cross-reference term within the index of the CPT manual used to direct the coder to another term or other terms. The *See* indicates that the correct code will be found elsewhere

segmentectomy: surgical removal of a portion of a lung

selective catheter placement: catheter must be moved, manipulated, or guided into part of the arterial system other than the aorta or the vessel punctured, generally under fluoroscopic guidance

seminal vesicle: gland that secretes fluid into the vas deferens

sentinel node: the first lymph node to receive drainage from a tumor; used to determine whether there is a lymphatic metastasis in certain types of cancer

separate procedures: minor procedures that when done by themselves are coded as a procedure, but when performed at the same time as a major procedure are considered incidental and not coded separately

septoplasty: surgical repair of the nasal septum

sequela: a condition that follows an illness

severity of illness: refers to the levels of loss of function and mortality that may be experienced by patients with a particular disease

shaving: horizontal or transverse removal of dermal or epidermal lesions, without full-thickness excision

shunt: divert or make an artificial passage

sialography: radiographic recording of the salivary duct and branches

sigmoidoscopy: fiberscopic examination of the rectum and sigmoid colon that may include a portion of the descending colon

signal-averaged electrocardiography (SAECG): type of electrocardiography that can help physicians predict certain tendencies to abnormalities such as ventricular tachycardia

signal node: the first lymph node that may "signal" a malignant neoplasm's presence

single chamber pacemaker: the electrode of the pacemaker is placed only in the atrium or only in the ventricle, but not placed in both

sinography: radiographic recording of the sinus or sinus tract

sinus tract injection: a cyst or abscess inside the body with a tract (otherwise known as a fistula)

sinuses: cavities within the facial bones (maxillary, frontal, sphenoid, and ethmoid)

sinusotomy: surgical incision into a sinus

skin graft: transplantation of skin tissue

skull: entire skeletal framework of the head

slanted brackets: indicate that the ICD-9-CM code can never be sequenced as the principal or primary diagnosis

soft tissue: tissues (fascia, connective tissue, muscle, and so forth)

somatic nerve: sensory or motor nerve that supplies a dermatome

special reports: detailed reports that include adequate definitions or descriptions of the nature, extent, and need for the procedure and the time, effort, and equipment necessary to provide the services

specimen: sample of tissue or fluid

spermatocele: cyst filled with spermatozoa

spirometry: measurement of breathing capacity

splenectomy: excision of the spleen

splenography: radiographic recording of the spleen

splenoportography: radiographic procedure to allow visualization of the splenic and portal veins of the spleen

spontaneous fracture: fracture due to a bone disease or a change surrounding the bone tissue that makes the bone weak

Staff Model: a Health Maintenance Organization that directly employs the physicians who provide services to enrollees

stem cell: immature blood cell

stent: mold that is surgically placed to reinforce or hold open an area

stereotaxis: method of identifying a specific area or point in the brain

strabismus: extraocular muscle deviation resulting in unequal visual axes

strangulated hernia: blood supply is cut off to hernia

subcutaneous: tissue below the dermis, primarily fat cells that insulate the body

subjective information: complaint or problem in the history portion of the encounter that is usually described by the patient

subsections: the further division of sections into smaller units, usually by body systems

superior: toward the head or the upper part of the body; also known as cephalic

supine: lying on the back

surgical package: bundling together of time, effort, and services for a specific procedure into one code instead of reporting each component separately

suture: to unite parts by stitching them together

Swan-Ganz catheter: central venous catheter

symbols: special guides that help the coder compare codes and descriptors with the previous edition. A <u>bullet</u> (•) is used to indicate a new procedure or service code added since the previous edition of the CPT manual. A <u>solid triangle</u> (▲) placed in front of a code number indicates that the code has been changed or modified since the last edition. A <u>plus</u> (+) is used to indicate an add-on code. A <u>circle with a line through it</u> (⊘) is used to identify a modifier -51 exempt code. <u>Right and left triangles</u> (►◄) indicate the beginning and end of the text changes. A <u>bullseye</u> (⊙) indicates procedures that include moderate sedation. A <u>lightning bolt symbol</u> (⚡) identifies codes that are being tracked by the AMA to monitor FDA status for approval of a drug.

sympathetic nerve: part of the peripheral nervous system that controls automatic body function and sympathetic nerves activated under stress

symphysiotomy: cutting of the pubic cartilage to help in birthing

systemic: affecting the entire body

tarsorrhaphy: suturing together of the eyelids

technical component: term used in describing the services provided by the facility

TEFRA (Tax Equity and Fiscal Responsibility Act): act that contains language to reward costconscious health care providers

tenodesis: suturing the end of a tendon to a bone

tenorrhaphy: suturing together two parts of a tendon

term location methods: service/procedure, anatomic site/body organ, condition/disease, synonym, eponym, and abbreviation

thermogram: written record of temperature variation

thoracentesis: surgical puncture of the thoracic cavity, usually using a needle, to remove fluids

thoracic duct: collection and distribution point for lymph, and the largest lymph vessel located in the chest

thoracoplasty: surgical procedure that removes rib(s) to allow the collapse of a lung

thoracoscopy: use of a lighted endoscope to view the pleural spaces and thoracic cavity or perform surgical procedures

thoracostomy: surgical incision into the chest wall and insertion of a chest tube

thoracotomy: surgical incision into the chest wall

thrombosis: blood clot

thrombus: blood clot that occludes, or shuts off, a vessel

thymectomy: surgical removal of the thymus

thymus: gland that produces hormones important to the immune response

thyroglossal duct: a duct in the embryo between the thyroid primordium and the posterior tongue

thyroglossal duct cyst: a cyst of the neck caused by persistence of portions of or by the lack of closure of the primitive thyroglossal duct

thyroid: part of the endocrine system that produces hormones that regulate metabolism

thyroidectomy: surgical removal of the thyroid

thyroiditis: a thyroid gland inflammation

tissue transfer: piece of skin for grafting that is still partially attached to the original blood supply and is used to cover an adjacent wound area

tocolysis: repression of uterine contractions

tomography: procedure that allows viewing of a single plane of the body by blurring out all but that particular level

tonography: recording of changes in intraocular pressure in response to sustained pressure on the eyeball

tonometry: measurement of pressure or tension

total pneumonectomy: surgical removal of an entire lobe of a lung

tracheostomy: creation of an opening into the trachea

tracheotomy: incision into the trachea

traction: application of force to a limb

transabdominal: across the abdomen

transcutaneous: entering by way of the skin

transesophageal echocardiogram (TEE): echocardiogram performed by placing a probe down the esophagus and sending out sound waves to obtain images of the heart and its movement

transfer order: official document that transfers the care of a patient from one physician to another; often required by third-party payers to legally transfer the care of a patient

transglottic tracheoplasty: surgical repair of the vocal apparatus and trachea

transhepatic: across the liver

transmastoid antrostomy: called a simple mastoidectomy, it creates an opening in the mastoid for drainage

transplantation: grafting of tissue from one source to another

transseptal: through the septum

transthoracic: across the thorax

transtracheal: across the trachea

transureteroureterostomy: surgical connection of one ureter to the other ureter

transurethral resection, prostate: procedure performed through the urethra by means of a cystoscopy to remove part or all of the prostate

transvenous: across a vein

transverse: horizontal

transvesical ureterolithotomy: removal of a ureter stone (calculus) through the bladder

trocar needle: a sharp-pointed instrument equipped with a cannula, used to puncture the wall of a body cavity and withdraw fluid

tumescence: state of being swollen

tumor: swelling or enlargement; a spontaneous growth of tissue that forms an abnormal mass

tunica vaginalis: covering of the testes

tympanic neurectomy: excision of the tympanic nerve

tympanometry: procedure for evaluating middle ear disorders

UHDDS: Uniform Hospital Discharge Data Set

ultrasound: technique using sound waves to determine the density of the outline of tissue

unbundling: assigning multiple CPT codes when one CPT code would fully describe the service or procedure

uncertain behavior: refers to the behavior of a neoplasm as being neither malignant nor benign but having characteristics of both kinds of activity

uncertain diagnosis: diagnosis documented at the time of discharge as "probable," "suspected," "likely," "questionable," "possible," or "rule out"

unilateral: occurring on one side

unlisted procedures: procedures that are considered unusual, experimental, or new and do not have a specific code number assigned; unlisted procedure codes are located at the end of the subsections or subheadings and may be used to identify any procedure that lacks a specific code

unspecified hypertension: hypertensive condition that has not been specified as either benign or malignant hypertension

unspecified nature: when the behavior or histology of a neoplasm is not known or is not specified

uptake: absorption of a radioactive substance by body tissues; recorded for diagnostic purposes in conditions such as thyroid disease

urachal cyst: between the umbilicus and bladder dome, often diagnosed in young children when the cyst becomes infected

urachal sinus: congenital abnormality in which prenatal tissue remains, causes drainage to the umbilicus, and results in infection and umbilicus drainage

ureterectomy: surgical removal of a ureter, either totally or partially

ureterocolon: pertaining to the ureter and colon

ureterocutaneous fistula: the channel from the ureter to the exterior skin

ureteroenterostomy: creation of a connection between the intestine and the ureter

ureterolithotomy: removal of a stone from the ureter

ureterolysis: freeing of adhesions of the ureter

ureteroneocystostomy: surgical connection of the ureter to a new site on the bladder

ureteroplasty: surgical repair of the ureter

ureteropyelography: ureter and bladder radiography

ureteropyelonephrostomy: surgical connection of the ureter to a new site on the kidney

ureteropyelostomy: ureteropyelonephrostomy

ureterosigmoidostomy: surgical connection of the ureter into the sigmoid colon and out through a new opening in the skin

ureterotomy: incision into the ureter

ureterovisceral fistula: surgical formation of a connection between the ureter and the bladder

urethrocutaneous fistula: surgically created channel from the urethra to the skin surface

urethrocystography: radiography of the bladder and urethra

urethromeatoplasty: surgical repair of the urethra and meatus

urethroplasty: surgical repair of the urethra

urethrorrhaphy: suturing of the urethra

urethroscopy: use of a scope to view the urethra

urography: same as pyelography; radiographic recording of the kidneys, renal pelvis, ureters, and bladder

uveal: vascular tissue of the choroid, ciliary body, and iris

V codes: numeric designations in the ICD-9-CM preceded by the letter "V"; used to classify persons who are not currently sick when they encounter health services

vagina: canal from the external female genitalia to the uterus

vagotomy: surgical separation of the vagus nerve

Valium: a sedative

varicocele: swelling of a scrotal vein

vas deferens: tube that carries sperm from the epididymis to the urethra

vasogram: recording of the flow in the vas deferens

vasotomy: creation of an opening in the vas deferens

vasovasorrhaphy: suturing of the vas deferens

vasovasostomy: reversal of a vasectomy

VBAC: vaginal delivery after a previous cesarean delivery

vectorcardiogram (VCG): continuous recording of electrical direction and magnitude of the heart

vein: vessel that carries unoxygenated blood to the heart from body tissues; pulmonary veins carry oxygenated blood back to the heart

vena caval thrombectomy: removal of a blood clot from the blood vessel (inferior vena cava or superior vena cava)

venography: radiographic recording of the veins and tributaries

ventricle: chamber in the lower part of the heart

version: turning of the fetus from a presentation other than cephalic (head down) to cephalic for ease of birth

vesicostomy: surgical creation of a connection of the bladder mucosa to the skin

vesicovaginal fistula: creation of a tube between the vagina and the bladder

vesiculectomy: excision of the seminal vesicle

vesiculography: radiographic recording of the seminal vesicles

vesiculotomy: incision into the seminal vesicle

vitre/o-: prefix meaning pertaining to the vitreous body of the eye

vulva: external female genitalia including the labia majora, labia minora, clitoris, and vaginal opening

World Health Organization (WHO): group that deals with health care issues on a global basis

wound repair, complex: involves complicated wound closure, including revision, debridement, extensive undermining, and more than layered closure

wound repair, intermediate: requires closure of one or more subcutaneous tissues and superficial fascia, in addition to the skin closure

wound repair, simple: superficial wound repair, involving epidermis, dermis, and subcutaneous tissue, requiring only simple, one-layer suturing

xeroradiography: photoelectric process of radiographs

CODER'S INDEX

References are to pages. Current Procedural Terminology (CPT) codes begin on page 853; ICD-9-CM and ICD-10 codes begin on page 862; HCPCS codes begin on page 866.

CURRENT PROCEDURAL TERMINOLOGY (CPT) CODES

00100-01999: 218, 252
00142: 358
00400: 360
00740: 364
00810: 364
0090T: 372
01916-01936: 350
01922: 350
01925: 350
01951-01953: 350
01958-01969: 350
01990-01999: 350
01996: 637
01999: 362
10021: 368, 378, 594
10021-10022: 378
10021-69990: 218, 264
10022: 378, 463, 594
10040-10180: 383
10040-19499: 270
10080: 375
10081: 375
10160: 383
11000: 215, 384
11000-11044: 384, 385, 401
11004-11006: 384
11040-11044: 384, 739
11042: 385
11055-11057: 388
11100: 260, 390, 417, 452
11101: 260, 390, 417
11200: 391
11201: 391
11300-11313: 391
11400-11471: 392
11401: 261
11402: 258
11406: 257
11420-11426: 602
11423: 258

11440-11444: 528
11446: 528
11450-11471: 392
11600-11646: 393
11620-11626: 602
11640-11644: 528
11646: 528
11719: 394
11719-11765: 394
11720: 394
11730: 395
11732: 395
11740: 395
11750-11752: 396
11755: 396
11770-11772: 396
11900: 397
11900-11983: 396
11901: 397
11920-11922: 397
11950-11954: 397
11960-11971: 397
11975-11977: 397
11980: 398
12001: 401
12001-12021: 399
12004: 377
12014: 377
12020: 377
12031-12057: 399
12031-13160: 392
12032: 257
12042: 254
13100-13160: 399
13131-13153: 528
14000-14350: 402
14040-14302: 533
15002-15005: 403
15002-15431: 403
15050: 404
15110-15116: 404
15120: 646, 653
15121: 646, 653
15130-15136: 405

15150-15157: 405
15170-15176: 405
15260: 646
15261: 646
15300-15321: 405
15300-15366: 405
15400-15431: 405
15501: 262
15570-15738: 407, 410
15740-15750: 407
15740-15776: 407
15780-15783: 408
15780-15879: 408
15783: 408
15786: 408
15787: 408
15788-15793: 408
15819: 408
15820-15823: 408
15824-15829: 408
15830: 410
15830-15839: 410
15840-15845: 410
15847: 410
15850-15852: 410
15876-15879: 410
15920-15999: 410
15946: 262
16000-16036: 384, 414
16020-16030: 413
16035: 414
16036: 414
17000: 416
17000-17004: 415
17000-17250: 392
17000-17286: 415
17004: 416
17260-17286: 393
17311: 417
17311-17315: 416, 417, 644
19000-19499: 417
19100: 373
19101: 378
19102: 418

19103: 418
19120: 373
19290: 260, 417
19291: 260
19295: 418
19301: 418
19302: 418
19303: 256, 264, 418
19304: 373, 418
19305: 418
19306: 418
19307: 373
19316-19396: 419
19318: 419
19324: 419
19342: 397
19357: 397, 419
19499: 270
20000: 430, 431
20000-69990: 270
20005: 431
20100-20103: 432
20150-20251: 433
20206: 433
20520: 222
20520-20525: 433
20525: 222
20550: 434
20551: 434
20553: 434
20600-20610: 434
20612: 434
20650: 435
20665: 435
20670: 435
20680: 435
20690: 435
20692: 435
20693: 436
20694: 436
20900-20938: 437
20920: 437
20922: 437
20930-20938: 437
20950: 438
20950-20999: 438
20955-20962: 438
20962: 438
20969-20973: 438
20974-20979: 438
20985: 438
21182: 212
21320: 426
21451: 256
22010-22899: 438

22210-22216: 438
22305-22325: 229
22590-22600: 438
22600-22612: 439
22612: 258
22614: 439
22840-22848: 439
22851: 439
22856: 372
23065-23066: 444
23100-23101: 444
23630: 427
24071: 433
25500: 426
25545: 436
25999: 371
26010: 222, 383
26011: 222, 383
26645: 229
26650: 229
26756: 260
27130: 425
27236: 426
27395: 257
27435: 443
27447: 256, 257
27506: 427, 446
27507: 427
27658: 259
27705: 222
27707: 222
27709: 222
27784: 427
27792: 427
28285: 262
28290-28299: 440
28292: 440
28496: 427
29000-29799: 426, 440
29800-29999: 443
29805: 444
29806: 444
29877: 443
29881: 443
30000: 451
30020: 451
30100: 452
30100-30160: 452
30115: 452
30140: 455
30200: 453
30200-30220: 453
30210: 453
30220: 454
30300: 454

30310: 454
30400: 448
30400-30630: 454
30420: 448
30460: 529
30462: 529
30520: 455
30801: 455
30802: 455
30901-30999: 455
31000: 457
31002: 457
31038: 761
31231-31294: 449
31255: 260
31276: 449
31300-31599: 458
31360: 537
31500: 323, 459
31502: 459
31505: 222, 450
31510: 222, 535
31511: 222
31512: 222
31513: 222
31515: 449, 450
31535: 535
31536: 535
31600-31899: 460
31603: 460
31605: 460
31622: 449
31715: 462
31715-31730: 462
31750-31830: 462
31770: 462
32035-32999: 463
32141: 449
32201: 217
32310: 463
32405: 463
32501: 464
32655: 449
32905: 465
32960: 465
32999: 225
33010: 474, 475, 486
33010-33050: 476
33010-33999: 473, 474
33010-37799: 473
33011: 474, 475
33015: 475
33020-33050: 475
33120: 476
33130: 476

33140: 476
33141: 476
33202-33249: 472, 476
33206-33208: 349
33207: 477
33208: 477
33250: 472
33250-33261: 506, 507
33250-33266: 472, 480
33265: 480
33266: 480
33282: 480
33284: 480
33400-33496: 481
33500-33507: 481
33510: 272
33510-33516: 483
33517-33523: 483, 484
33533-33536: 483, 484
33935: 271
34001-34490: 488
34001-37799: 473, 484
34501-34530: 489
34800-34834: 489
34900: 489
35001-35152: 489
35180-35190: 489
35188: 490
35400: 490
35450-35476: 490
35480-35495: 490
35500-35671: 490
35506: 490
35820: 272
36000: 486
36000-36522: 491
36012: 486
36215: 488, 511
36217: 487, 492
36218: 487, 492
36245: 488
36415: 690
36430: 698
36440: 334
37201: 495
38100: 518
38100-38200: 518
38100-38999: 517
38101: 518
38115: 229, 518
38120: 518
38129: 518
38200: 518
38204-38242: 697
38205-38206: 519

38207-38215: 519
38220: 378, 518
38221: 518
38230: 518
38240-38242: 519
38500: 519
38500-38555: 519
38510-38530: 519
38562-38564: 519
38570: 519
38571: 519
38571-38589: 519
38572: 519
38700: 520
38700-38780: 519, 520
38720: 520
38724: 520
38790: 520
38792: 522
39000: 523
39000-39599: 522
39010: 523
39200: 523
39400: 523
39501-39599: 523
40490-40799: 527
40490-49999: 527
40500: 527, 528
40510: 527, 528
40510-40527: 527
40520: 528
40525: 527, 528
40527: 528
40530: 528
40650: 529
40650-40654: 529
40652: 529
40654: 529
40700: 529
40700-40761: 529
40701: 529
40702: 529
40720: 529
40800-40899: 529
40818: 533
41000-41009: 530
41000-41599: 529, 530
41010: 530
41015-41018: 530
41100-41108: 530
41100-41155: 530
41114: 530
41115: 530
41250-41252: 531
41520: 530

41800: 531
41800-41899: 529, 531
41820: 531
41826: 531
41828: 531
42000-42299: 533
42120: 370
42145: 533
42200: 529
42200-42225: 533
42205: 529
42225: 536
42300-42699: 534
42400: 533, 534
42405: 533
42410: 534
42440: 534
42450: 534
42508: 534
42509: 534
42550: 534
42700-42725: 535
42700-42999: 535
42800-42806: 535
42810: 535
42815: 535
42820-42836: 535
42950: 536
42955: 536
42955-42999: 536
42960-42972: 536
43020: 537
43020-43499: 537
43045: 537
43100: 537
43100-43135: 537
43101: 537
43107: 537
43116: 537
43124: 537
43200: 373, 537, 538
43200-43228: 537
43200-43232: 543
43201: 538
43201-43232: 538
43215: 538
43216: 538
43217: 538
43220: 537
43231: 537
43234-43259: 538
43236: 538
43239: 539
43245: 539
43259: 539

43260: 504
43260-43272: 539
43279-43289: 540
43405: 539
43450: 538
43453: 538
43456: 538
43458: 538
43460: 538
43500: 541
43500-43999: 541
43621: 541
43644: 541
43653: 541
43752: 324
43770: 541
43770-43775: 541
43820: 223
44005-44799: 543
44141: 543
44388-44397: 548
44800: 545
44900: 546
44901: 546
44950: 546
44955: 546
44960: 546
44970: 546
45000-45999: 546
45126: 547
45300: 547, 548
45300-45327: 547
45303-45327: 547
45330-45345: 547
45331: 550
45331-45345: 547
45332: 550
45333: 550
45335: 538
45338: 550
45339: 550
45355: 548
45355-45392: 548
45378: 264, 548, 549, 550
45378-45392: 548
45379-45392: 549
45380: 548
45381: 538, 551
45382: 551
45384: 268
45385: 268, 548
45900: 554
45905: 554
45910: 554
45915: 554

46020: 553
46020-46999: 553
46030: 553
46040: 554
46080: 554
46200: 553, 554
46220: 554
46221: 554
46230: 554
46250: 554, 555
46257: 554
46258: 554
46260: 555
46260-46262: 554
46270: 554
46270-46285: 553
46275: 554
46280: 554
46285: 554
46288: 553, 554
46500: 555
46600: 554, 554
46600-46615: 554
46900: 555
46900-46942: 555
46910: 555
46916: 555
46940: 554
46942: 554
47000: 556, 676
47001: 556
47100: 556
47133-47147: 556
47400: 556
47400-47490: 556
47500: 510, 557
47505: 557
47511: 557
47525: 557
47530: 557
47560-47579: 557
47562: 557
47563: 557
47600: 557
47605: 557
48000: 557
48000-48999: 627
48001: 557
48020: 557
48100: 557
48102: 557
48140-48160: 557
48400: 557
48550-48554: 557
49000: 545

49010: 564
49060: 564, 565
49203-49205: 564
49320: 518, 519, 557, 612, 613
49323: 557
49491-49496: 270
49491-49611: 557, 562
49495-49501: 588
49650-49659: 557, 562
50010: 564
50010-50135: 564
50010-50593: 564
50010-53899: 564
50020: 565
50020-50290: 571
50021: 565
50040: 565
50045: 565
50060: 265, 266, 565
50065: 565
50070: 565
50075: 565
50080: 567
50081: 567
50200: 567
50205: 567
50220-50240: 567
50250: 567, 571
50300: 568
50320: 568
50323: 568
50325: 568
50327-50329: 568
50340: 568
50360: 568
50380: 568
50382-50389: 568
50390: 569
50390-50405: 571
50400: 569
50400-50540: 569
50405: 569
50520: 570
50520-50526: 570
50525: 570
50526: 570
50541: 571
50541-50548: 571
50541-50549: 571
50542: 567, 571
50543: 567
50545-50548: 567
50547: 568
50551-50562: 571, 573
50551-50580: 571

50555: 571
50570-50580: 565
50574: 571
50590: 567, 571, 579
50593: 567, 571
50600: 572
50600-50630: 572
50600-50980: 572
50605: 572
50605-50630: 575
50610: 572
50610-50630: 572
50650: 572
50660: 572, 573
50684: 573, 574
50684-50690: 573
50686: 573
50700-50940: 573
50740-50760: 575
50780-50840: 575
50860-50940: 575
50945: 572
50945-50980: 575
50947: 573
50948: 573
50951: 573, 574
50951-50961: 573
50951-50980: 573
50955: 574
50970: 573
50970-50980: 573
51020-51045: 575
51020-52700: 575
51050: 576
51060: 576
51065: 576
51102: 576
51500: 576
51520-51596: 576
51575: 270
51597: 576
51600: 689
51600-51610: 576, 581
51701: 577, 578
51702: 577
51703: 577
51720: 577
51725-51798: 577
51727: 577
51800-51980: 577
51840: 577
51841: 577
51900: 606
51990: 577
51992: 577

52000: 578, 579
52000-52010: 578
52000-52700: 581
52005: 578
52005-52010: 580
52007: 578
52204: 579
52204-52318: 576, 579
52204-52355: 579
52214: 579
52224: 579
52234-52240: 579
52276: 580
52282: 591
52310: 579, 580
52315: 579, 580
52320: 579, 580
52320-52355: 579, 580
52332: 579
52352: 565
52353: 567
52400-52700: 580
52450: 580, 592
52500: 580
52601: 591
52630: 591
52647: 592
52648: 592
53000-53899: 581
53020: 581
53025: 581
53060: 581, 601
53200-53275: 581
53210: 581
53215: 581
53220: 581
53270: 581, 601
53400-53431: 581
53415: 581
53420: 581
53425: 581
53431-53442: 577
53444: 581
53446-53448: 581
53449: 581
53450: 581
53460: 581
53600-53665: 581
53850: 591
53852: 591
53855: 591
54000-54015: 582
54000-55899: 582
54015: 582
54050-54065: 583

54100: 583
54100-54164: 583
54105: 583
54110: 584
54110-54112: 584
54111: 584
54112: 584
54115: 585
54120: 584
54125: 584
54130: 584
54135: 584
54150: 584
54150-54161: 584
54160: 584
54161: 584
54200: 585
54200-54250: 584
54205: 585
54220: 585
54300-54440: 585
54304: 585
54380: 585
54400: 585
54400-54417: 585
54401: 585
54406: 585
54410: 585
54411: 585
54416: 585
54417: 585
54500: 586
54500-54535: 586
54500-54560: 587
54505: 586, 589
54512: 586
54520: 586
54520-54535: 586
54530: 586
54550: 586
54560: 586
54640: 586
54640-54680: 587
54650: 586
54690-54692: 587
54692: 586
54700: 587, 588
54700-54840: 588
54800-54861: 588
54840: 588
54900: 588
54901: 588
55000: 588
55040: 588
55041: 588

55060:	588	
55100:	588	
55175:	588	
55180:	588	
55200:	588	
55250:	589	
55300:	589	
55400:	589	
55500:	589	
55500-55550:	590	
55530:	589	
55535:	589	
55550:	590	
55600:	590	
55600-55680:	590	
55605:	590	
55650:	591	
55680:	591	
55700:	593, 594	
55705:	593, 594	
55706:	594	
55720:	594	
55725:	594	
55801-55865:	592	
55812:	593	
55812-55815:	593	
55815:	593	
55842:	593	
55842-55845:	593	
55845:	593	
55860:	595	
55860-55865:	594	
55862:	595	
55865:	595	
55866:	593	
55875:	595, 600	
55920:	600	
55970:	600	
55980:	600	
56405-56821:	601	
56405-58999:	600	
56605:	602	
56606:	602	
56620-56640:	602	
56800-56810:	603	
56970:	574	
57000-57010:	604	
57000-57425:	604	
57020:	604	
57061:	604	
57065:	604	
57100-57135:	604	
57150-57180:	605	
57155:	600	
57200-57335:	606	

57240:	606	
57250:	606	
57268:	606	
57270:	606	
57287-57289:	577	
57288:	577	
57289:	577	
57330:	606	
57400-57415:	606	
57409:	617	
57410:	617	
57420-57426:	606	
57421:	607	
57452-57461:	607	
57452-57800:	607	
57460:	608	
57461:	608	
57700:	609	
57720:	609	
57800:	609	
58100:	609	
58100-58579:	609	
58110:	609	
58120:	609	
58140:	610	
58145:	610	
58150:	373, 601	
58150-58240:	610	
58150-58294:	609	
58200:	257	
58240:	576	
58260:	610	
58260-58294:	610	
58290:	610	
58300:	611	
58300-58356:	610	
58301:	611	
58340:	611	
58345:	611	
58346:	600	
58350:	611	
58541-58579:	611	
58545:	610	
58546:	610	
58600-58770:	612	
58611:	613	
58660:	613	
58660-58679:	613	
58670:	613	
58720:	373	
58740:	613	
58800-58960:	614	
58950-58956:	614	
58951:	624	
58953:	624	

58954:	624	
58956:	624	
58970:	614	
58970-58976:	611	
59000:	618	
59000-59899:	615	
59001:	618	
59012:	618	
59015:	678	
59100:	618	
59120-59150:	618	
59160:	609	
59200:	620	
59400:	617	
59400-59622:	620	
59409:	617	
59510:	617	
59514:	617	
59610:	617	
59612:	617	
59618:	617	
59620:	617	
59812:	620	
59812-59857:	620	
59820-59821:	620	
59830:	620	
59840:	620	
59840-59857:	621	
59841:	620	
59855-59857:	620	
59857:	621	
60000-60300:	626, 627	
60000-60699:	626	
60210:	628	
60212:	628	
60220:	628	
60225:	628	
60240:	628	
60252:	628	
60254:	628	
60270:	523	
60300:	629	
60500-60512:	626	
60500-60699:	627	
60520:	523	
60520-60522:	626	
60540-60545:	626	
60600:	627	
60605:	627	
60650:	626	
61000-61070:	632	
61000-64999:	631	
61020-61026:	632	
61050:	632	
61055:	632	

61105-61253: 632
61304-61576: 632
61312: 632
61330-61334: 650
61580: 632, 633
61580-61598: 632
61580-61619: 632
61600: 632, 633
61600-61616: 632
61613: 633
61615: 633
61616: 633
61618: 633
61619: 633
61680-61711: 633
62180-62258: 633
62223: 633
62263-63746: 635
62270: 636
62273: 366
62280: 637
62280-62282: 637
62281: 637
62282: 637
62310-62319: 637
62318: 637
62319: 637
63030: 258
64400-64530: 638, 642
64400-64907: 638
64400-64999: 638
64490-64495: 639
64600-64640: 638
64600-64681: 642
64612: 638
64680-64681: 638
64702-64727: 639
64721: 639
64831-64876: 639
64885-64911: 639
65091: 644
65091-65114: 644
65091-68899: 644
65093: 644
65101-65105: 644
65110-65114: 644
65125-65155: 646
65175: 646
65205: 646
65205-65265: 644
65220: 647
65222: 647
65286: 647
65400: 648
65410: 648

65710: 648
65710-65756: 648
65730-65755: 648
65800: 648
65800-65880: 648
65805-65815: 648
65820: 648
65850: 649
65860-65880: 648
65900-65930: 648
66020: 648
66020-66030: 648
66030: 648
66130: 648
66150: 649
66155: 649
66160: 649
66170: 649
66172: 649
66600: 649
66625: 649
66630: 649
66761: 649
66762: 649
66830-66990: 649
66983: 649
66984: 649
67141: 267, 644
67145: 267, 644
67311: 649
67312: 649
67314: 649
67316: 649
67331: 644
67400-67414: 649
67415: 650
67420-67450: 650
67424: 653
67550: 646
67800-67850: 393
67850: 644
67914-67917: 650
67921-67924: 650
67930: 646
67935: 646
68020-68040: 650
68200: 651
68320-68340: 651
68326-68328: 651
68400-68850: 651
68810: 651
68811: 651
69000: 653
69000-69979: 651
69005: 653

69020: 653
69100: 653
69105: 653
69110: 653
69120: 653
69140: 653
69200: 653
69205: 653
69210: 653
69300: 653
69310: 653
69320: 653
69400: 653
69401: 653
69420: 653
69421: 653
69424: 653
69433: 653
69436: 653
69502-69511: 654
69530: 654
69540: 654
69550-69554: 654
69601: 654
69604: 654
69631-69633: 655
69631-69646: 653
69632: 655
69633: 655
69637: 655
69641-69646: 655
69642: 655
69801: 655
69802: 655
69905: 655
69910: 655
69930: 656
69950: 656
69950-69970: 651
69955: 656
69960: 656
69970: 656
69990: 368, 438, 588, 589,
   651, 656
70010-76499: 672
70010-79999: 218
70390: 534
71030: 688
71040: 462
71090: 477, 478
72010-72295: 672
72192: 672
72195: 672
72198: 672
73000: 255

74000:   670
74010:   670
74210:   670
74220:   670
74235:   538
74240:   670
74241:   670
74245:   670
74249:   670
74320:   510
74328:   504
74329:   504
74330:   504
74360:   537, 538
74425:   573, 574
74430:   581
74440:   589
74450:   581
74455:   581, 689
74740:   611
74742:   611
75557-75574:   473, 511
75600:   473
75600-75791:   473, 511
75659:   509
75710:   511
75801-75807:   520
75801-75893:   473
75810:   518
75989:   565
76000:   567
76001:   567
76506-76999:   675
76805:   675
76810:   688
76831:   611
76872:   595
76873:   595
76930:   475
76930-76999:   678
76941:   618
76942:   534, 576
76945:   678
76946:   618
76965:   595
76975:   539
77002:   534, 576
77012:   534, 576, 676
77021:   534
77051-77059:   674
77055:   674
77056:   674
77057:   674, 675
77261-77263:   506, 679
77261-77799:   679

77263:   682
77280-77295:   506
77280-77299:   679
77300:   682
77300-77370:   506, 680
77336:   682
77371-77373:   681
77399:   680
77401-77423:   681
77417:   682
77427:   682
77427-77499:   682
77520-77525:   683
77600-77615:   683
77620:   683
77750-77799:   683
77776-77778:   595
77776-77787:   595
78000-78999:   685
78000-79999:   684
79005:   685
79005-79999:   685
79101:   685
79440:   685
79445:   685
80047-80076:   690
80047-89398:   218
80055:   690, 691
80100:   692
80100-80103:   691
80102:   692
80150-80299:   692
80152:   693
80400:   693
80400-80440:   693
80500:   694
80502:   694
81000-81003:   695
81000-81099:   696
81000-84999:   695
82533:   693
84580:   696
85002-85999:   697
85004-85009:   697
85004-85049:   697
85025:   697
85027:   697
85060:   697
85097:   697
85610:   697
86000-86804:   698
86701-86703:   276
86850-86999:   698
86890:   699
87001-87999:   699

88000:   700
88000-88099:   700
88005:   700
88007:   700
88020:   700
88025:   700
88027:   700
88104-88199:   701
88172:   378
88173:   378
88230-88299:   701
88300:   701
88300-88399:   701
88302:   260, 701
88304:   701, 702
88305:   518, 701, 702
88307:   702
88309:   702
88321-88334:   694
88329:   694, 695
88331:   417, 694, 695
88332:   694, 695
90281-90399:   709
90281-99199:   218
90281-99607:   708
90375:   733
90465:   261, 710, 733
90465-90468:   710
90465-90474:   710
90466:   261, 710, 733
90467:   710
90468:   710
90471:   710, 711, 712, 713, 733
90472:   710, 711, 712, 733
90476-90749:   710, 711
90633:   712
90657:   711, 712
90658:   711, 712
90669:   711
90700:   261
90701:   711
90702:   711
90703:   710, 711
90706:   710, 711
90707:   261
90718:   711
90719:   710
90732:   711, 712
90760:   733
90801:   715
90801-90899:   714
90802:   715
90804:   715
90804-90809:   715
90810-90815:   715

90816-90822: 715
90817: 714
90823-90829: 715
90853: 715
90857: 715
90875: 716
90901: 716
90911: 716
90935: 719
90935-90999: 717
90937: 719
90945: 719
90947: 719
90951: 718
90951-90962: 718
90951-90970: 718
90952: 718
90953: 718
90954: 718
90955: 718
90956: 718
90957: 718
90958: 718
90959: 718
90960: 718
90961: 718
90962: 718
90963: 718
90964: 718
90965: 718
90966: 718
90967: 718
90967-90970: 717, 719
90968: 718
90969: 718
90970: 718, 720
91000-91299: 720
91055: 720
91105: 324
92002: 722
92002-92014: 253, 266
92002-92499: 721
92004: 722
92012: 722
92014: 722
92018: 722
92020: 257
92310: 708
92502-92700: 724
92511: 724
92950-92998: 724
92950-93799: 495
92974: 506
92975: 495
92978: 496

92979: 496
92980: 496
92981: 496
92982: 496, 724
92984: 496, 497, 724
92986-92990: 497
93000-93010: 500
93000-93278: 472, 497, 724
93012: 500
93014: 500
93015-93018: 500
93016-93018: 500
93040-93278: 500
93278: 500
93279-93285: 501
93279-93299: 501, 508, 724
93286: 501
93287: 501
93288-93292: 501
93293: 501
93294: 501
93294-93299: 501
93297: 501
93303-93350: 472
93303-93352: 501, 676
93501-93533: 502, 504, 725
93503: 352
93526: 503
93539-93545: 504, 725
93540: 502
93544: 473, 502
93544-93556: 504
93545: 502
93555: 503, 504
93555-93556: 725
93556: 503, 504
93561-93572: 504
93600-93603: 506
93600-93662: 472, 506
93602: 507
93603: 507
93609: 507
93610: 506, 507
93612: 506, 507
93613: 507
93619: 506
93619-93622: 507
93631: 507
93668: 508
93701-93790: 508
93720-93722: 508
93784-93790: 508
93797-93799: 508
93875-93990: 676, 725
94002: 323

94002-94799: 726
94999: 262
95004-95075: 727
95004-95199: 727
95115: 728, 733
95117: 733
95120: 728
95250: 729
95251: 729
95803: 731
95803-96020: 729
95805-95811: 729
95900: 217, 730
95900-95905: 730
95903: 217, 730
95904: 217, 730
95925: 636
95934-95936: 730
95950: 633
96101: 715
96101-96125: 731
96150-96155: 732
96360: 732, 733
96360-96361: 734
96361: 732, 733, 735
96365: 733, 735
96365-96368: 733
96365-96379: 694, 733, 734
96366: 733, 735
96367: 733, 735
96368: 733, 735
96369: 733
96369-96371: 733
96370: 733
96371: 733
96372: 733
96372-96376: 733
96373: 733
96374: 733, 735
96375: 733, 735, 736
96376: 733
96401-96417: 733
96401-96459: 733, 734, 736
96413: 735, 736
96415: 736
96420-96425: 734
96440: 734
96440-96549: 734
96445: 734
96450: 734
96521: 734
96522: 734
96567-96571: 737
96900: 738
96900-96999: 737

97001-97799:   738
97597-97606:   739
97605:   739
97606:   739
97750:   739
97761:   738
97802-97804:   741
98925-98929:   741
98940-98943:   741
98966-98968:   742
98966-98969:   332
98969:   742
99000-99091:   742
99024:   253, 377, 742
99050:   742
99070:   375, 377, 451, 491,
    510, 511, 605, 611, 671, 694,
    708, 742
99100:   358, 360
99100-99140:   218, 358
99143-99145:   349
99143-99150:   349, 743
99148-99150:   349
99170-99199:   743
99190-99192:   743
99201:   226, 304
99201-99205:   280, 305
99201-99350:   331
99201-99499:   218, 266
99203:   232, 303
99205:   299
99211:   307
99211-99215:   280, 307, 315
99212:   298, 328, 329, 377
99212-99215:   310
99213:   310
99214:   283, 303
99215:   310
99217:   280, 309, 310, 326
99218-99220:   280, 309, 310
99219:   310
9921X: 253
99221:   311
99221-99223:   280, 310
99221-99233:   715
99221-99239:   311
99222:   311
99231:   312
99231-99233:   265, 315
99231-99239:   312
99234-99236:   280, 309,
    310, 313
99238:   313, 333
99238-99239:   280, 326
99239:   313, 314, 333

99241-99245:   280, 315, 715
99241-99255:   315, 316
99242:   316
99243:   316
99251-99255:   280, 315, 316
99281-99285:   304, 320
99281-99288:   280, 320
99283:   320
99285:   320, 235
99288:   321
99291:   323
99291-99292:   280, 322
99292:   323
99304-99306:   280, 325, 326
99306:   325
99307-99310:   280, 325
99315:   325
99315-99316:   280
99316:   325
99318:   280, 325
99324-99328:   280
99324-99337:   327
99334-99337:   280
99339:   327
99339-99340:   280
99340:   327
99341-99345:   280
99341-99350:   327
99347-99350:   280
99354:   329
99354-99357:   280
99354-99359:   328
99358-99359:   280
99360:   280, 329, 330
99363:   280, 330
99363-99368:   330
99364:   280, 330
99366-99368:   280, 330
99374-99380:   280, 331
99381-99387:   280
99381-99429:   331
99383:   261
99391-99397:   280
99401-99404:   280
99401-99429:   332
99411-99412:   280
99420-99429:   280
99441-99443:   280, 332
99444:   280, 332
99450-99456:   280, 332
99460:   333
99460-99463:   280
99460-99465:   333
99461:   333
99462:   333

99463:   333
99464:   333
99464-99465:   280
99465:   333
99466:   280, 334
99467:   334
99468-99476:   280, 334
99471-99476:   280
99477-99480:   280, 334
99499:   280, 335
99500-99602:   743
99500-99607:   218
99601:   743
99602:   743
99605-99607:   743

ICD-9-CM AND ICD-10 CODES

10.2-23.6:   547
11:   155
21.1:   35
23.6:   548
27.54:   35, 70
39.21:   64
39.51:   67
39.52:   67
39.61:   64
40.9:   70
42.40-42.42:   64
42.6:   64
43.1:   64
43.19:   65
45.51:   68
57.87:   68
68.49:   61
75.36:   155
78.4:   69
80.00:   68
80.10:   68
80.12:   68
80.17:   68
81.92:   68
82.69:   70
83.86:   70
86.22:   181
86.28:   181
87-99:   61
99.25:   84
C50.4:   38
D51.1:   196
E11.21:   195
F10.150:   195
I25.110:   195
R10.0:   196

S06.336: 195
S50.351: 194
001: 33, 34, 40
001-009: 40
001-139: 49
001-999: 82
001.0: 80
002: 40
003: 40
004: 40
005: 40
006: 40, 49
006.8: 34
007: 40
007.8: 49
008: 40
009: 40
010-018: 49
017.9: 34
034: 109
034.0: 50
038: 163
039.8: 34
041: 105, 106, 118, 150, 158, 163
041.0: 150
041.0-041.9: 56
041.00: 150
041.1: 106, 116, 158
041.10: 106, 158
041.11: 158
041.4: 118, 750
041.7: 56
042: 101, 119, 120, 155, 758
112.0: 118
136.9: 158
137-139: 49
137.0-137.4: 49
140-198: 125
140-239: 38, 123
158: 47
158.8: 47
159: 44
159.0: 44
172.0-172.9: 520
174.0-174.9: 520
174.4: 38, 122, 123
174.9: 84, 91
175: 73
175.0-175.9: 520
196: 123
196.3: 91, 122, 123
198: 127
198.5: 127
199: 127

199.1: 127
200-202: 99
200-203: 125
201: 99
201.9: 99
201.90: 99
201.9X: 99
204.00: 73
236.1: 253
238.4: 91
239.6: 91
242.0: 758
242.00: 87, 758
244: 44
244.8: 34, 44
244.9: 77
245: 108
245.0: 108
245.8: 108
249: 155
249.1: 54
249.2: 54
249.3: 54
249.5: 56
249.5X: 57
249.7: 54
249.8: 54
249.80-249.81: 57
249.9: 54
250: 105, 155
250.0: 54
250.00: 89, 90, 92, 129
250.00-250.09: 227
250.0X: 85
250.1: 54
250.1-250.8: 128
250.2: 54
250.3: 54
250.5: 46, 56, 105, 129
250.51: 105
250.5X: 46, 57
250.7: 54
250.8: 54
250.80-250.83: 57
250.9: 54
250.XX: 128
276.5: 103
276.51: 103
277.4: 59
280.9: 153
281.0: 91
281.1: 196
281.9: 131, 153
285.2: 130
285.22: 124, 130

285.29: 130
285.9: 131, 153
290: 132
290.4: 132, 133
290.40: 132
290.41: 132
294.8: 132
303-305: 132
303.9x: 132
307.9: 41
320: 133
320.1: 133
324: 55
326: 55
331: 73
333.81: 638
333.82: 638
351.8: 638
362: 105
362.0: 105
362.01: 46, 105, 128
362.72: 73
362.81: 46
364.3: 129, 134
364.4: 129
364.42: 129
366.4: 56
366.41: 56, 57
366.9: 92
401.9: 87, 90, 92
401.X: 294
410: 100
410.2: 100
411: 114
411.1: 114
414.00: 90
414.01: 92
420: 108
420.0: 34
420.9: 108
420.90: 108
423: 108
423.8: 108
426.8: 46
426.89: 46
428.0: 90
429.81: 42
430: 101
430-437: 111
433: 100
433.2: 100
433.21: 100
434.9: 100
434.91: 100
437: 132

437.0: 132, 133
438: 110, 111
438.11: 111
440.23: 57
444: 73
459.0: 46, 149
459.11: 57
459.13: 57
459.31: 57
459.33: 57
460-466: 49
461.9: 35
463: 50
472.31: 92
473: 48
474: 54
474.00: 78
478.30: 55
482.8: 5
482.81: 45
482.83: 45
482.84: 45
482.89: 45
484.5: 73
486: 91, 102, 103, 165
487.0-487.8: 49
488.0: 758
488.0-488.1: 49
490: 45, 758
493.90: 89
496: 35
510: 56
510.9: 56
530.81: 538, 539
530.83: 538
531: 103, 149
531.0: 149
531.00-534.91: 148, 149
531.40: 93
531.9: 103, 149
531.90: 103
535.0-535.6: 148
537.83: 148
540.9: 165
550.90: 78, 79, 92
555: 101
555.1: 101
555.9: 101
560.1: 47
562: 148
562.02: 148
562.11: 148
562.12: 148
562.13: 148
564.00: 77

569.85: 148
571.5: 104
574: 109
574.0: 109
574.00: 109
577: 107
577.0: 107
577.1: 107
578: 148, 149
578.9: 93, 149, 148
585.9: 34
586: 34
590.10: 750
591: 73
599.0: 93, 118
601: 150
601.0: 150
601.9: 150
617.0: 61
628: 48
628.4: 48
634: 157
635: 151, 157
635.1: 151
639: 151, 152, 157
639.0: 151
639.1: 151
639.2: 151
639.3: 151
639.4: 151
639.5: 151
639.6: 151
639.8: 151
639.9: 151
640: 114
640.0: 114
640.03: 114
641.1: 152
644.21: 157
646.63: 93
646.9: 153
647.6X: 119, 120, 155
648.00-648.04: 227
648.0x: 155
648.2: 153
648.23: 153
648.8x: 155
648.x: 155
650: 152, 155
655: 154
656: 154
677: 156
681: 157, 158
681.0: 158
682: 101, 106, 157

682.0: 106
682.6: 101
682.9: 158
683: 157
707: 57
707.1: 57
707.10: 57
708: 175
708.0: 175
708.9: 175
710: 159
710.0: 89
711: 159
711.0: 159
711.03: 159
716.9: 159
719: 37, 159
719.0: 37
720: 159
724: 159
730: 159, 160
730.0: 35
730.01: 35
731.8: 54
733.0: 160
733.00: 160
733.1: 160, 186
733.10: 160
733.14: 160
736.89: 101
738.4: 50
754: 101
754.4: 101
754.42: 101
756.12: 50
757: 157
758: 164
758.0: 164
764: 163
765.0: 163
765.1: 163
765.2: 163
771.2: 49
771.81: 163
779.89: 162
780: 178
780.0-799.9: 81
780.01: 174, 178
780.09: 173
780.60: 89, 173, 758
780.79: 77, 87
780.93: 172
781.3: 42
782.4: 87, 89
783.0: 89

783.1: 77
785.4: 54
786.09: 87
786.2: 89, 758
786.50: 299, 758
786.59: 79
787.20: 538
787.24: 42
789.0: 101
789.00: 174
789.01: 101
789.03: 165
789.59: 104
794: 165
794.8: 165
794.9: 165
795.71: 119
796.4: 165
805: 73
819: 186
820.8: 110, 187
822: 187
822.0: 187
828: 186
829.0: 160
861: 49
887.2: 57
887.3: 57
887.4: 57
891.0: 187
891.1: 187
901.0-901.9: 49
905.3: 110
906.5-906.9: 181
935.1: 538
940: 182
941: 184
941.2: 184
941.24: 184
942: 184
942.2: 184
942.24: 184
943: 184
943.3: 184
943.36: 184
946: 181
948: 181, 182
948.0: 182, 184
949: 181, 182
958.3: 181
960.1: 39
965.01: 174
969: 178
969.4: 173, 178
984.0: 172

985.1: 174
995: 177
995.20: 177
995.85: 174
995.9: 167
995.91: 163
995.92: 163
996-999: 756
999: 33
999.9: 82
E800-E999: 32, 40, 171
E806.9: 171
E845: 171
E849: 168
E849.9: 168
E850-E869: 172
E853: 178
E853.2: 178
E861.5: 172
E870-E876: 170
E878-E879: 170
E904.0: 169
E906.8: 171
E910.3: 171
E928.9: 169
E929: 169
E930: 175
E930-E949: 169, 173, 175, 178
E930.0: 175, 177
E949.9: 173
E950-E959: 173
E950.3: 173
E958.9: 169
E959: 169
E960-E968: 169
E960-E969: 170, 174
E962.1: 174
E967: 169
E968.9: 169
E969: 169
E977: 169
E979: 170
E979.9: 170
E980-E989: 169, 174, 178
E980.0: 174
E989: 169
E999.1: 169, 170
M8140/3: 122, 123
M8140/6: 123
M8500/3: 38
M8851/0: 55
V01-V89: 32, 40, 82
V01.0-V89: 81
V01.0-V89.09: 82
V01.2: 83

V02.0-V02.9: 49
V03-V06: 713
V03.82: 711
V04: 83
V04.0: 83
V05.3: 713
V08: 119, 120, 155
V10: 124
V10-V19: 90, 761
V10.00-V10.9: 125
V10.05: 550
V10.06: 550
V11.3: 132
V12.54: 111
V12.72: 550
V14: 84
V14.0: 84
V14.1: 84
V16.0: 550
V18.5X: 550
V22.0: 93, 95, 154
V22.1: 93, 95, 154
V22.2: 153
V23: 154
V24.0: 156
V27: 152
V27.0: 155
V27.0-V27.9: 154
V29: 162, 163
V30: 84, 162, 163, 164
V30-V39: 162, 163
V30.00: 84, 164
V30.01: 164, 165
V45.81: 90
V45.82: 92
V54.0: 186
V54.1: 186
V54.8: 186
V54.9: 186
V58: 94
V58.0: 125
V58.11: 84, 91, 125
V58.12: 125
V58.67: 155
V59: 83
V59.4: 83
V62: 83
V62.3: 83
V64.3: 78
V65.44: 120
V69.8: 120
V71.0-V71.9: 86
V72.5: 90
V72.6: 90
V72.60: 91

V72.8:   92
V72.81:   92
V72.82:   92
V72.83:   92
V72.84:   92
V72.86:   91
V73.89:   120
V76.51:   549, 550, 551
V89:   80
Z12.11:   549, 550, 551
Z80.0:   550
Z83.7X: 550
Z85.04:   550
Z85.3:   550
Z86.010:   550

HCPCS Codes

A4550:   375
A4561:   605
A4580-A4590:   441
A4643:   689
A4918:   237
A9521:   511
E0571:   236
E0572:   236
E0607:   236
G0008:   712
G0009:   711, 712
G0104:   550, 551
G0105:   550, 551
G0106:   550, 551
G0120:   550, 551
G0121:   550, 551
G0122:   550
G0127:   394

G0168:   401
G0308-G0319:   720
G0320-G0327:   720
G0328:   549
J0585:   538
J1100:   736
J1200:   736
J2270:   735
J2469:   736
J7300:   611
J7307:   397
J9310:   736
K0178-K0179:   236
K0180:   236
L0984:   742
L3700-L3766:   738
L8000-L8039:   738
P9010:   699
P9021:   699
V2500-V2599:   709

INDEX

References are to pages. Pages followed by "f" indicate figures; "t," tables.

A

Abbe-Estlander flap, 528, 528f
Abdomen, 557
Abdominal pain, 101
Ablation, 507
  of kidney lesion, 567, 568f
Abnormal investigations, 165
Abortion services, 615, 620–621
  ICD-9-CM codes, 156–157
  threatened abortion, 114
Abscess
  nasal, 451, 452f
  soft tissue, 431
Abuse of persons, 169
Actinotherapy, 738
Adenoidectomy, 535–536
Adenoids, 535–536
  chronic disease of, 54
Adrenal glands, 626f, 627
Adult abuse, 169
AIDS, 101
  see also HIV infection
Allergen immunotherapy, 728
Allergy testing, 727
Allogenic bone marrow, 519
Allografts, 404, 405
Ambulatory surgery, 92
Amebiasis, 49
Amniocentesis, 618
Amputation, 57
Anal fissure, 553, 554f
Anal fistula, 553, 554f
Analgesia, 346
Anastomoses, 544–545, 544f
Anatomic pathology, 700–701
Anemia, 130
  of chronic disease, 130
  chronic simple, 131
  pernicious, 91
  pregnancy, iron deficiency
    anemia complicating, 153
Anesthesia, 346
  ASA's base units, 352, 353f
  basic unit value, 352, 354f
  CMS's base units, 353, 354f
  concurrent care modifiers,
    361–362
  conscious sedation, 348–349
  conversion calculations/factors,
    359–360
  for infant less than 4 kg, 270
  medical records, 356f–357f
  moderate sedation, 348–349
  modifying units, 355, 358–359
  multiple procedures, 360
  payment formula, 351–360
  physical status modifiers,
    358–359, 359f
  qualifying circumstances,
    355, 358, 358f
  Relative Value Guide, 352, 354f
  return to operating room, 364

Anesthesia *(Continued)*
  surgeon, anesthesia by, 256
  time, 354–355
  types of, 346–349
  unlisted procedure code, 363
  unusual, 252–253
Anesthesia section, of the CPT
  manual
  codes and modifiers
    see Anesthesia
  format of, 349–350, 350f
Aneurysmorrhaphy, 67
Aneurysms
  brain, 633
  cardiovascular repairs, 489
Angiography, 472–473, 674, 674f
Angioplasty
  percutaneous transluminal
    coronary angioplasty,
    482, 483f
  transluminal, 490
Angioscopy, 490
Ankyloglossia, 530, 530f
Anoscopy, 554
Antepartum services
  see Maternity care and delivery
Anticoagulant management, 330
Anus, 553–556
Aorta, radiology coding, 511
Aphakia, 648
Aphasia, due to a previous
  cerebrovascular accident, 111
Appendectomy, 546
Appendix, 546
Arteries, 485f
  coronary
    see Coronary artery
  radiology coding, 511
Arthritic wrist, pyogenic, 159
Arthrocentesis, 434–435, 434f
Arthrodesis, 438–439
Arthroscopy, 443
Arthroscopy codes, 443–444
Arthrotomy, 68
Artificial insemination, 611
Artificial urinary sphincter, 581
Ascites due to cirrhosis of the liver,
  104
Asthma, 89
  COPD with, 141
Atherectomy, transluminal, 490
Attending physician, 313
Auditory system, 651, 652f
  external ear procedures, 653
  format of subsection, 651
  inner ear procedures, 655–656
  middle ear procedures, 653–655
  middle fossa approach, 656
  operating microscope, 651, 656,
    656f
  temporal bone, 656
Autografts, 404–405, 405f

Autologous bone marrow, 519
Autonomic nervous system, 638–639

B

Bariatric surgery, 541, 542f
Baroreceptor system, 627f
Basket forceps, 443
Bedsores, 410–411, 411f
Behavior assessment/intervention,
  732
Behavior change intervention, 332
Benign prostatic hyperplasia,
  591–593
Biliary tract, 556–557
Biofeedback, 716
Biometry, 662
  see also Radiology
Biopsies
  arthrocentesis, 434–435, 434f
  bone marrow, 518
  breasts, 417–418
  cervical, 607, 608–609
  corpus uteri, 609
  fine needle, 378, 378f
  fixation devices, codes, 435–436
  grafts, 437
  implants, 437
  injection codes, 434
  laryngoscopic, 535
  liver, 556
  lung or mediastinum,
    percutaneous needle, 463
  nose, skin outside of, 452
  pancreatic, 557
  percutaneous, 433
  pins, insertion of, 435
  prostate, 593–594
  removal codes, 433–434
  sentinel node, 520, 522
  sinus tract injection procedure
    codes, 433
  skin lesions, 389–390, 417
    breast procedures, 417–418
  vagina, 607
  wires, insertion of, 435
Birth control
  abortion services
    see Abortion services
  implantable capsules, 397
  intrauterine devices, 610–611, 610f
Bishop Scoring System of cervical
  ripening, 620f
Bladder, 575, 575f
  cystourethroscopy, 579
  endoscopy, 578
  excision, 576–577
  incision, 575–576
  injection procedures, 576
  laparoscopy, 577–578
  reconstruction of, 68
  removal of, 576
  repair procedures, 577–578

Bladder *(Continued)*
transurethral resection of tumor, 579
transurethral surgery, 579–580
urodynamics, 577
vesical neck and prostate codes, 580
Bladder cancer, instillation procedure, 577
Bladder cuff, 572–573
Bleeding
see Hemorrhage
Blepharoplasty, 408
Blood and blood-forming organs, diseases of, 130–131
Blood coagulation tests, 696–698
Blood patch, 346–347
Blood pressure
ambulatory monitoring, 508
elevated
see Hypertension
Blood typing, 91
Boarding home services, 327
Bone cancer, metastatic, 127
Bone grafts, 438
Bone marrow aspiration, 518
Bone marrow biopsy, 518
Bone marrow harvesting, 518–519
Bone marrow transplants, 519
Bottle type repair, 588
Bowing of femur, 101
BPH treatment procedures, 591–593
Brachiocephalic vascular family, 487f
Brachytherapy
clinical, 683–684, 684f
intracoronary, 505–506
for prostate cancer, 594–595
Brain, 639–640
aneurysm, 633
arteriovenous malformation, 633
vascular disease, 633
Branchial cleft cyst, 535
Breasts/breast cancer
adenocarcinoma of, 122–123
biopsies, 417–418
chemotherapy, 91
mammography, 674–675
mastectomies, 418–419, 418f, 419f, 420f
Bronchi
see Trachea and bronchi
Bronchitis, 45
Bronchoplasty, 462
Bronchoscopy, 449
Bulbourethral gland, 581
Bundle of His recording, 507
Burns, 411–412
classification of, 183f, 412, 413f
coding of, 180–182, 184
first degree, 180f
Lund-Browder chart/classification, 183f, 412f
Rule of Nines, 183f, 412f
second degree, 180f
third degree, 180f
treatment of, 412–414, 413f
Bypass surgery
cardiovascular bypass grafting materials, 490–491
coronary artery bypass, 482–484, 483f
Roux-en-Y gastric bypass, 541, 542f

C
Canaloplasty, 653
Cancer
bladder cancer, instillation procedure, 577
bone cancer, metastatic, 127
breast cancer
see Breasts/breast cancer
chemotherapy
see Chemotherapy
colorectal cancer screening, 549–551
nuclear medicine, 684–685
peritoneum, malignant neoplasm of, 47
prostate
see Prostate cancer
radiation oncology
see Radiation oncology
retroperitoneum, malignant neoplasm of, 47
skin lesions, excision of, 393, 394f
Candidiasis infection of mouth, 118
Cardiac catheterization, 502–504, 725, 725f
catheter insertion, 491–492, 492f
catheter placement, 486–489
Cardiac tumor, 476
Cardiac valves, 481
Cardiography, 497–500
Cardiologists, 471
Cardiovascular system
angiography, 472–473
angioplasty
see Angioplasty
bypass
see Bypass surgery
coding of services, 471
medicine codes, *below*
radiology codes, *below*
surgery codes, *below*
diseases of, 134–140
electrocardiograms
see Electrocardiograms
electrophysiology, 472
intracardiac procedures, 506–507
hypertension
see Hypertension
ICD-9-CM manual, 134–140
invasive cardiology, 471–472
medicine codes, 471f, 495
blood pressure monitoring, ambulatory, 508
cardiac catheterization, 502–504, 725, 725f
cardiography, 497–500
echocardiography, 501–502, 501f, 725
intracardiac electrophysiologic procedures, 506–507
intracoronary stent placement, 496–497, 496f
intravascular ultrasound, 496
noninvasive physiologic studies, 508
other procedures, 508
peripheral arterial disease rehabilitation, 508
plethysmography, 508
stress tests, 497–500
therapeutic services, 495–497, 724
thrombolysis, 495
valvuloplasty, 497

Cardiovascular system *(Continued)*
myocardial infarction
see Myocardial infarction
noninvasive services, 472
radiology coding, 471f
aorta and arteries, 511
contrast material, 510–511
heart coding, 511
interpretation, 509
professional component, 509
supervision, 509
technical component, 509
surgery codes, 471f, 473
aneurysm repair, 489
angioscopy, 490
arteries, 484
bypass grafting, 490–491
cardiac tumor, 476
cardiac valves, 481
catheter placement, 486–489
coronary artery anomalies, 481
coronary artery bypass, 482–484, 483f
electrophysiologic operative procedures, 480
embolectomy, 236f, 488–489
fistula repair, 489
pacemaker/cardioverter-defibrillator, 476–478
patient-activated event recorder, 480
pericardiocentesis, 475, 475f
thrombectomy, 488–489
transluminal angioplasty, 490
transluminal atherectomy, 490
transmyocardial revascularization, 476
vascular access, 491
vascular injection procedures, 491–492, 493f, 494f
vein repairs, 489
veins, 484
Cardioverter-defibrillators, 476–478
Care plan oversight services, 331
Carotid body, 626f, 627–628, 627f
Carpal tunnel release, 639, 640f
Case management services, 330
Casts
codes, 440–442
removal of, 440
CAT scanning, 672, 672f
Cataracts
diabetic cataract, 56
removal and lens replacements, 649
Catheterization
cardiac
see Cardiac catheterization
corpus uteri, 611
Swan-Ganz catheter, 351f, 352
thrombolysis, 495
ureteral, 577
urethral, 581
Caval-pulmonary artery anastomosis, 64
Cellulitis
and abscess of finger and toe, 158
face, staphylococcal, 106
of the upper leg, 101
Central nervous system, 630
assessments/tests, 731
see also Spine and spinal cord
Cerclage, nonobstetric, 609
Cerebral atherosclerosis, 132, 541

Cerebrospinal fluid shunts, 633, 634f
Cerebrovascular disease
 hypertensive, 137
 late effects of, 111
Certificates of medical necessity
 oxygen necessity, 244f
 transcutaneous electrical nerve
  stimulation, 243f
Cervical conization, 608, 608f
Cervicoplasty, 408
Cervix uteri, 601f, 607
 biopsy of, 607, 608–609
 dilation of, 609
 endoscopy, 607
 excision, 607–609
 repair, 609
Cheiloplasty, 529
Chemical peels, 408, 409f
Chemistry, 695–696
Chemotherapy, 84, 733–736
 for breast cancer, 91
Chest tube, 464
Chief complaint, 285
Child abuse, 169
Childbirth
 see Maternity care and delivery
Chiropractic manipulative
  treatment, 741
Cholecystitis with cholelithiasis,
  acute, 109
Cholecystostomy, 557
Choledochotomy, 556
Cholesteatoma, 654
Chordee, 585
Chromotubation, 611
Chronic obstructive pulmonary
  disease, 141
Ciliary body, 649
Circulatory system, diseases of,
  134–140
Circumcision, 584
Cirrhosis of the liver
 ascites due to, 104
 without mention of alcohol, 104
Cisternal puncture, 632
Claim forms
 CMS-1450, 29, 31f
 CMS-1500, 29, 30f, 213f
 skin lesions, treatment of, 390,
  390f, 391
Cleft palate, 529, 529f
Clitoroplasty, 603, 604f
CMS Documentation Guidelines,
  338–340
CMT, 741
CNS
 see Central nervous system
Coagulation tests, 696–698
Cochlear device implant, 655–656,
  655f
Colon, diverticulitis with
  hemorrhage, 148
Colonoscopy, 548–549
 diagnostic, 548
 injection, 551
 measurements, 547f
 multiple procedures, 551–552
 virtual, 552, 552f
Colorectal cancer screening, 549–551
Colpocentesis, 604
Colporrhaphy, 606
Colpotomy, 604
Coma from Valium overdose, 178
Comprehensive examination, 291

Computed tomography, 672, 672f
Computer-assisted surgical
  navigation, 438
Congenital anomalies, 161, 163,
  164
Congestive heart failure, 90
 with benign hypertension, 138
Conization of the cervix, 608, 608f
Conjunctiva, 650–651
Connective tissue diseases, 159–160
Conscious sedation, 348–349
Consultant, 314
Consultation services, 314–315
 clinical pathology, 694–695
 initial inpatient consultations,
  316
 office/outpatient consultations,
  315
 request for, 314
Contraceptives
 see Birth control
Coordination of care, 302
COPD (chronic obstructive
  pulmonary disease), 141
Cordocentesis, 618
Cornea, 648
Coronary artery
 anomalies, 481
 bypass, 482–484, 483f
 disease, 90
Corpus uteri, 601f, 609
 excision, 609
 hysteroscopy, 611–612, 612f
 introduction codes, 610–611
 laparoscopy, 611–612, 612f
Cough, 89
Counseling, 301
 behavior change intervention,
  332
 risk factor reduction, 332
Cowper's gland, 581
CPT coding system, 212
 see also CPT manual
CPT manual
 add-on codes, 215, 215f
 Appendix A, 216
 Appendix B, 216
 Appendix C, 216, 217f
  see also E/M codes
 Appendix D, 215
 Appendix E, 215
 Appendix F, 216
 Appendix G, 217
 Appendix H, 217
 Appendix I, 217
 Appendix J, 217
 Appendix K, 217–218
 Appendix L, 218
 Appendix M, 218
 assistant surgeon, 273
  minimum, 273–274
  when qualified resident
   surgeon not available, 274
 bilateral procedures, 256–257
 categories and subcategories, 219,
  220f
 Category I codes, 227
 Category II codes, 225–227
 Category III codes, 227–228
 changed code symbol, 215f
 changed text symbols, 215f
 code format, 221–222
 decision for surgery, 266
 discontinued procedure, 264

CPT manual (Continued)
 distinct procedural service, 268
 E/M section
  code assignment in
   see E/M codes
  contents of, 280
  levels of E/M service
   see E/M services
 Guidelines, 220, 220f
 increased procedural services,
  251–252
 indented codes, 221–222
 Index, 229
  locating terms, 230–233
  multiple codes, 229
  range of codes, 229–230
  "See" cross-references, 233
  single code, 229
 infants less than 4 kg, procedure
  performed on, 270
 laboratory platform testing,
  alternative, 276
 mandated services, 256
 mastectomies, 264
 modifiers, 215–216, 216f, 223,
  224f, 250–278
 multiple modifiers, 276
 multiple procedures
  CPT modifiers, 257–261
  multiple operation(s), same
   operative session, 258
  procedure performed multiple
   times, 259
  same operation, different site,
   258
 outside laboratory, 275
 postoperative management only,
  265
 postoperative period
  return to the operating room
   for a related procedure
   during, 272
  unrelated procedure or service
   by the same physician
   during, 273
 preoperative management only,
  265–266
 professional component, 254–255
 purpose of, 212
 reduced services, 261–262
 reference laboratory, 275
 repeat clinical diagnostic
  laboratory test, 276
 repeat procedure
  by another physician, 271
  by same physician, 271
 revisions, 212, 214
 sections, 218–219, 220f
  see also specific topics throughout
   this index
 service by the same physician
  during the postoperative
  period, 267
 significant separately identifiable
  E/M service, by the same
  physician on the same day
  of the procedure or other
  service, 254
 special reports, 228
 specific notes, 220f
 staged or related procedure, 267
 stand-alone codes, 221–222
 subheadings, 219, 220f
 subsections, 219, 220f

CPT manual *(Continued)*
  surgeon, anesthesia by, 256
  surgical care only, 264–265
  surgical team, 270–271
  symbols used, 214–215
  two surgeons, 269–270
  unlisted procedures, 224–225, 225f
  unrelated evaluation and
    management service, by the
    same physician during a
    postoperative period, 253
  unusual anesthesia, 252–253
Craniectomy, 632
Craniotomy, 632
Cricothyroid tracheostomy, 460,
  461f, 463f
Critical care services, 322–323
  inpatient neonatal and pediatric
    critical care services, 334
  pediatric critical care patient
    transport, 334
Crohn's disease, 101
Cryoablation, 507
Cryptorchidism, 586
CT scanning, 672, 672f
Current Procedural Terminology
  see CPT manual
Custodial care services, 327
Cystectomy, 576
Cystolithotomy, 576
Cystotomy, 575, 576
Cystourethroscopy, 579
Cysts
  branchial cleft, 535
  pilonidal, 396–398
  renal, 569
  urachal, 576
Cytogenic studies, 701
Cytopathology, 701

D

Decision making
  see Medical decision making
Decubitus ulcers, 410–411, 411f
Dehydration due to pneumonia, 103
Delayed flap, 407
Delivery, 616
  see also Maternity care and
    delivery
Dementia with delirium,
  arteriosclerotic, 132
Dental claim form, 532f
Dentoalveolar structures, 531
Dermabrasion, 408, 409f
Dermatological procedures, special,
  737–738
Detailed examination, 290
Diabetes/diabetes mellitus, 89, 90,
  128–129
  with ophthalmic manifestations,
    105, 129
  in pregnancy, 155
  "with," 54
  without complication mentioned,
    129
Diabetic cataract, 56
Diabetic retinal hemorrhage, 46
Diabetic retinopathy, with type I
  diabetes, 105
Diagnosis-related groups
  see Medicare program
Dialysis, 717–720
Diaphragm, 523

Digestive system, 527
  abdomen, 557
  adenoids, 535–536
  anus, 553–556
  appendix, 546
  biliary tract, 556–557
  diaphragm, 523
  diseases of, 148–149
  esophagus, 537–540
  format of subsection, 527
  ICD-9-CM manual, 148–149
  intestines, 543–545
  lips, 527–529
  liver, 556
  Meckel's diverticulum, 545
  mediastinum, 522–523
    biopsy, 463
  mouth
    see Mouth
  omentum, 557
  pancreas, 557
  peritoneum, 557
  pharynx, 535–536
  rectum, 546–547
  stomach, 541
  tongue, 530–531
  tonsils, 535–536
  uvula, 533
Digital block, 429, 430f
Dilation and curettage, 609, 621
Dilation and evacuation, 621
Direct face-to-face time, 302–303
Dislocations, 429, 430f
Displacement therapy, 453
Diverticulitis of the colon with
  hemorrhage, 148
Documentation Guidelines, 338–340
Domiciliary care services, 327
Doppler ultrasound, 678
Dosimetry, 680
Down's syndrome, 164
DRGs
  see Medicare program
Drug assays, 692–693
Drugs
  adverse effects of, 168, 174–178
  HCPCS table of, 238–239, 239f
  ICD-9-CM manual: Tabular List,
    Volume 1, Appendix C, 39
  Medicare prescription drugs, 6
  National Codes
    routes of administration of
      drugs, 239, 240, 240f
    table of drugs, 238–239, 239f
Drug testing, 691–692
Dual cuff, 581
Durable Medical Equipment (DME)
  MACs, 3–4, 4f
Dyspnea, 87

E

E. coli infection, 118
Ear
  external ear procedures, 653
  inner ear procedures, 655–656
  middle ear procedures, 653–655
Earwax removal, 653
Echocardiography, 501–502, 501f, 725
Ectopic pregnancy, 151, 618–619, 619f
Ectropion, 650, 650f
Eczema, 384
Electrical stimulation of the
  musculoskeletal system, 438

Electrocardiograms, 498–500
  signal-averaged
    electrocardiography, 500
  telephonic transmission, 500
Electromyographic studies, 731
Electronic medical records, 9
Electronic Remittance Advice
  (ERA), 14
Electrophysiologic operative
  procedures, 480
Electrophysiology, 472
  intracardiac procedures,
    506–507
Embolectomy, 488–489
Embolus, 488
E/M codes
  anticoagulant management, 330
  care plan oversight services, 331
  case management services, 330
  choosing the correct code, 301
  consultation services
    see Consultation services
  custodial care services, 327
  Documentation Guidelines,
    338–340
    see also E/M services
  domiciliary care services, 327
  emergency department services,
    320–321
  example, 304–305, 305f
  home care plan oversight services,
    327
  home services, 327
  hospital inpatient services
    see Hospital inpatient services
  hospital observation services
    see Hospital observation
      services
  medical records documentation,
    282–283
  medical team conferences, 330
  newborn care
    see Newborn care
  non-face-to-face physician
    services, 332
  nursing facility services
    see Nursing facilities
  office/outpatient services
    see Office/outpatient services
  online medical evaluations, 332
  other services, 335
  patient status, 281
  physician standby services,
    329–330
  place of service, 280–281
  practice with, 335–336
  preventive medicine services,
    331–332
  prolonged physician services,
    328–330
  rest home services, 327
  special services, 332
  telephone services, 332
  type of service, 281
  using, 305–337
E/M section, of the CPT manual
  code assignment in
    see E/M codes
  contents of, 280
  levels of E/M service
    see E/M services
E/M services
  coding
    see E/M codes

E/M services (Continued)
  contributing factors, 301–303
  coordination of care, 302
  counseling, 301
  Documentation Guidelines, 338–340
  key components, 283
  levels of, 283–305
  medical decision making
    see Medical decision making
  medical examination
    see Examination
  medical records
    see Medical records
  office, new patient, 283–301, 305
  patient history
    see History
  presenting problem, nature of, 302–303
Emergency department services, 320–321
Empyema, 56
Endocardial resection, 507
Endocrine diseases, 128–129
Endocrine system, 626–629, 626f
  glucose monitoring, 728–729
Endometrial sampling, 609
Endoscopic retrograde cholangiopancreatography, 539–540
Endoscopy
  bladder, 578
  cervix uteri, 607
  esophageal, 537–538, 543f
  kidney, 571
  musculoskeletal system, 443–444
  rectal, 547–552
  respiratory system, 448–449
  ureter, 573–575
  vagina, 606–607
Endotracheal anesthesia, 346, 347f
Endotracheal intubation, 459, 459f
Endovascular aneurysm repair (EVAR), 489
End-stage renal disease, 717, 719
Entropion, 650, 650f
Enucleation, 644
Epididymis, 587–588
Epididymovasostomy, 588
Epidural anesthesia, 346
EPOs, 22
Esophagogastroduodenoscopy, 538–539
Esophagus, 537–540
  endoscopy of, 537–538, 543f
ESWL, 565–566, 566f
Ethical Coding, Standards of, 27, 28f
Evaluation and Management section (of the CPT manual)
  code assignment in
    see E/M codes
  contents of, 280
  levels of E/M service
    see E/M services
Evisceration, 644
Evocative/suppression testing, 693–694
Examination, 290–292
  elements of, 291f
  general multi-system, 340f
  laboratory exam without any sign or symptom, 91
  levels of, 290–292
  pre-anesthetic, 364

Exclusive Provider Organizations (EPOs), 22
Exenteration, 644
Exostosis, 653
Expanded problem focused examination, 290
Extracapsular cataract extraction, 649
Extracorporeal shockwave lithotripsy, 565–566, 566f
Extracranial nerves, 638–639
Eye and ocular adnexa, 644, 645f
  anterior chamber, 648
  anterior sclera, 648–649
  anterior segment, 647–651
  ciliary body, 649
  conjunctiva, 650–651
  cornea, 648
  extraocular muscles, 649
  eyeball
    see Eyeball
  eyelids, 645f, 650
  format of subsection, 644
  iris, 649
  lacrimal apparatus, 645f
  lacrimal sac, 645f
  lens, 649
  orbit, 649–650
Eyeball
  foreign bodies, removal of, 646–647
  implants, 646, 647f
  laceration repair, 647
  removal of, 644, 646
Eyelids, 645f, 650

F

Fallopian tubes
  see Oviduct/ovary
Family history, 287–288
Fascia lata grafts, 437
Fatigue, 87
Federal Register, 9–10, 11f
Female genital system, 601f
  cervix uteri
    see Cervix uteri
  corpus uteri
    see Corpus uteri
  diseases of, 150
  format of subsection, 600–601
  ICD-9-CM manual, 150
  intersex surgery, 600
  ovary
    see Oviduct/ovary
  oviduct
    see Oviduct/ovary
  perineum
    see Vulva, perineum, and introitus
  Skene's glands, 5, 581, 601
  vagina
    see Vagina
  in vitro fertilization, 614
  vulva
    see Vulva, perineum, and introitus
Female infertility, 48
Fetuses
  abortion services
    see Abortion services
  conditions complicating, 154–155
  congenital anomalies, 161, 163, 164
  gestational diabetes, 155

Fetuses (Continued)
  growth retardation, 163
  ultrasound showing twins, 676f
  in utero surgery, 154–155
Fever, 89
  scarlet fever and streptococcal pharyngitis, 109
Fine needle biopsies, 378, 378f
Fingernails, 394
Flaps
  Abbe-Estlander, 528, 528f
  free osteocutaneous, 438
  lingual frenum, 530
  rotation flaps, 402, 403f
  skin grafts, 406–408
Fluoroscopy, 662
  see also Radiology
Foot repairs, 440
Forceps, basket, 443
Fractures, 425
  casts
    see Casts
  closed treatment, 425, 426
    with manipulation, 426
    without manipulation, 426
  coding of, 185–187
  hip
    see Hip fracture
  manipulation, 426
  nasal
    see Nasal fractures
  open treatment, 425, 426–427
  percutaneous skeletal fixation, 427, 428f
  repair, 441
  splints
    see Splints
  strapping
    see Strapping
  traction, 427, 428f
  traumatic, 186
Fraud
  see Medicare fraud and abuse
Free osteocutaneous flaps, 438
Frenotomy, 530
F-wave studies, 730

G

Gallbladder
  with acute cholecystitis, 109
  gallstone, ultrasound showing, 676f
Gastric ulcer, 103, 149
Gastroenterology, 720
Gastrointestinal hemorrhage, 148, 149
General anesthesia, 346, 348
Genitourinary system
  female genitals
    see Female genital system
  male genitals
    see Male genital system
  urinary system
    see Urinary system
Gestational diabetes, 155
Global radiology service, 509–510
Global surgery period, 375
Glucose monitoring, 728–729
Goniotomy, 648
Grafting procedures
  see Skin grafts
Grafts
  bone, 438

Grafts *(Continued)*
  cardiovascular bypass grafting
    materials, 490–491
  skin
    see Skin grafts
Graves' disease, 87
Group Practice Model (GPM), 22
Gunshot wounds, 432–433

H
HCPCS
  see Healthcare Common
    Procedure Coding System
Healthcare Common Procedure
    Coding System, 233
  Level I codes, 233
    see also Medicine codes
  Level II codes. National Codes,
    below
  Level III codes (Local Codes), 234
  National Codes, 233, 234–235
    colorectal cancer screening,
      549–551
    durable medical equipment,
      241
    general guidelines, 235–237
    index, 237, 237f, 238f
    national physician fee
      schedule, 241, 245f
    routes of administration of
      drugs, 239, 240, 240f
    table of drugs, 238–239, 239f
Health Insurance Portability and
    Accountability Act (HIPAA), 7
  code sets, 8
  electronic transactions, 8
  National Provider Identification, 9
  privacy requirements, 8
  security requirements, 8–9
Health Maintenance Organizations,
    22–23
Heart
  external view, 474f
  injury to, 49–50
  internal view, 474f
  see also Cardiovascular system
Hematology, 696–698
Hemic and lymphatic systems, 517
  axillary lymph nodes, metastasis
    to, 91
  bone marrow procedures, 518–519
  format of subsection, 517
  lymph nodes and lymphatic
    channels, 519–522
  spleen, 518
Hemodialysis, 490f, 717
Hemophilus influenzae, 141
Hemorrhage, 149
  diabetic retinal, 46
  diverticulitis of the colon with, 148
  gastrointestinal, 148, 149
  ICD-9-CM coding, 101
  nasal hemorrhage control
    see Nose
  subarachnoid, 101
Hemorrhoids, 555, 556f
Hernia repairs, 557–558
Hip fracture, 187
  osteoporosis, due to, 160
HIPAA
  see Health Insurance Portability
    and Accountability Act
    (HIPAA)

History, 284
  chief complaint, 285
  elements of, 284–288, 289f
  family history, 287–288
  levels of, 288–289
  past history, 287–288
  of present illness, 285
  review of systems, 286–287
  social history, 287–288
HIV infection, 119–120
  in pregnancy, childbirth and the
    puerperium, 119–120, 155
HMOs, 22–23
Hodgkin's Disease, 99
Holter monitor, 498, 498f
Holter report, 499f
Home care plan oversight services,
    327
Home health procedures/services,
    743
Home services, 327
Hormone pellet implantation,
    subcutaneous, 397–398
Hospital inpatient services, 311
  admission services, 313
  attending physician, 313
  critical care services
    see Critical care services
  discharge services, 313–314
  emergency department services,
    320–321
  initial hospital care, 311
  inpatient coding
    see Inpatient coding and
      reporting
  pediatric critical care
    see Pediatric critical care
  subsequent hospital care,
    312–313
Hospital observation services, 309
  initial observation care, 309–310
  observation care discharge
    services, 309
H-reflex studies, 730
Human immunodeficiency virus
  see HIV infection
Hydatidiform, 619f
Hydration services, 732–733
Hypertension, 87, 134–137
  benign hypertension, 135
    congestive heart failure with,
      138
  controlled, 137
  elevated blood pressure, 137
  malignant, 135
  Official Guidelines for Coding
    and Reporting, 136–137
  with renal failure, acute, 138
  secondary, 137, 139, 139f
  transient, 137
  uncontrolled, 137
  unspecified, 135
Hypertension Table, 135f
Hypertensive chronic kidney
    disease, 136
Hypertensive heart disease, 136, 138
Hypertensive renal disease, 136, 137
Hypertensive retinopathy, 137
Hyperthermia, 683
Hypospadias, 585
Hysterectomies, 609–610
Hysterosalpingraphy, 611
Hysteroscopy, 611–612, 612f
Hysterotomy, 618, 621

I
ICD-9-CM manual, 27
  abnormal investigations, 165
  acute conditions, 107–108
  additional code, use of, 56
  Alphabetic Index to Volume 1,
    40–41
    carryover lines, 43, 43f
    conventions used, 43–55
    cross references, 55
    E codes, 170–171, 171f
    eponyms, 59
    etiology, 52
    main terms, 41, 42f
      modifiers following, 42
      notes following, 57–58
    manifestation of disease, 52
    modifiers, 42
    Section 2: Table of Drugs and
      Chemicals, 172–178,
      176f
    Section 3: Alphabetic Index
      to External Causes of
      Injuries, 170–171
    Section 3: Alphabetic Index to
      External Causes of Injuries
      and Poisonings, 171f
    subclassification codes, 458
    subterms, 42–43, 42f
  Alphabetic Index to Volume 3,
    65–70
  "and" and "with," 54
  appendices, Volume 1, 38–40
  blood and blood-forming organs,
    diseases of, 130–131
  bold type, 34
  braces-{ }, 48
  brackets-[ ], 46
    codes in, 52
  burns, 180–182, 184
  categories, 33, 33f
  cerebrovascular disease, late
    effects of, 111
  chapters, 33, 33f
  chronic conditions, 107–108
  circulatory system, diseases of,
    134–140
  Classification of Diseases and
    Injuries, 32–34
    Supplementary Classification.
      E codes, *below*; V codes,
      below
  "code, if applicable, any causal
    condition," 57
  "code first underlying disease,"
    56–57
  coding guidelines. Official
    Guidelines for Coding and
    Reporting, *below*
  colons-:, 48
  combination codes, 109
  congenital anomalies and
    conditions, 161, 163, 164
  conventions used, 43–55
  diabetes/diabetes mellitus,
    128–129
  diagnosis codes, 34–35
  digestive system, diseases of,
    148–149
  diseases
    Alphabetic Index to Volume 1,
      above
    Tabular List, Volume 1, *below*

ICD-9-CM manual (Continued)
  DRG numbers and
    see Medicare program
  E codes
    Alphabetic Index to Volume 1,
        170–171, 171f
    injury/poisoning and
        complications, 166–170,
        177, 185–186
    late effects of external cause
        guidelines, 169
    misadventures and
        complications of care
        guidelines, 170
    multiple cause guidelines,
        167–168
    place-of-occurrence guideline,
        168
    terrorism guidelines, 170
    undetermined cause guidelines,
        169
    unknown or suspected intent
        guidelines, 169
  endocrine diseases, 128–129
  Ethical Coding, Standards of,
      27, 28f
  excludes notes, 49–50
  format of, 29
  fractures, 185–187
  general guidelines, 99–100
  genitourinary system, diseases of,
      150
  good coding habits, 99
  health service contact, factors
      influencing. V codes, below
  health status, factors influencing.
      V codes, below
  HIV infection, 119–120
  ill-defined conditions, 165
    inpatient coding and reporting,
        749
  immunity disorders, 128–129
  impending condition, 113–114
  includes notes, 48–49
  Index(es)
    Alphabetic Index to Volume 1,
        above
    Alphabetic Index to Volume 3,
        above
  infectious diseases, 49, 118–120
  injury/poisoning and
      complications, 166–170, 177,
      185–186
  inpatient coding and reporting
    abnormal findings, 762
    additional diagnoses, 760–761
    comparative or contrasting
        conditions, 753
    complications, 756
    ill-defined conditions, 749
    interrelated conditions, 751
    multiple diagnoses, 752
    observation unit admissions,
        759
    original treatment plan not
        carried out, 755
    outpatient coding,
        distinguished, 748–749
    outpatient surgery admissions,
        760
    Present on Admission (POA),
        763
    principal diagnosis, 748, 749
    signs, 749

ICD-9-CM manual (Continued)
  symptoms, 749
  symptoms following
      contrasting/comparative
      diagnoses, 755
  uncertain diagnoses, 757–758,
      763
  italicized type, 34
  late effects codes, 110–112
  mental disorders, 131–133
  metabolic diseases, 128–129
  multiple coding, 104–106
  musculoskeletal system and
      connective tissue diseases,
      159–160
  NEC ("not elsewhere
      classifiable"), 44, 45
  neoplasms, 120
    coding, 121–123, 122f
    Official Guidelines for Coding
        and Reporting, 123–125
    "unknown site or unspecified,"
        127
    V codes, 125–126
  nervous system, diseases of,
      133–134
  newborn guidelines, 161–163
  NOS ("not otherwise specified"), 4
  nutritional diseases, 128–129
  Official Guidelines for Coding
      and Reporting
    acute conditions, 107–108
    brackets, codes in, 52
    burns, 180–182, 184
    chronic conditions, 107–108
    circulatory system, diseases of,
        136–137
    combination codes, 109
    detail in coding, level of,
        100–101
    elevated blood pressure, 137
    general guidelines, 99–100
    good coding habits, 99
    health service contact, factors
        influencing. V codes, below
    health status, factors
        influencing. V codes, below
    impending condition, 113–114
    injury/poisoning and
        complications, 166–170,
        177, 185–186
    inpatient coding and reporting,
        above
    integral conditions, 102–104
    medical care complications, 188
    multiple coding, 104–106
    neoplasms, 123–125
    newborn guidelines, 161–163
    organization of, 98–100
    "other" codes, 51
    outpatient coding and
        reporting, below
    parasitic diseases, 118–120
    pregnancy, childbirth, and
        puerperium complications,
        153–157
    specificity in coding, 100–101
    subcategories, 51
    surgery complications, 188
    therapeutic substances, adverse
        effects of, 175
    threatened condition, 113–114
    "unspecified" codes, 51
  "other" codes, 51

ICD-9-CM manual (Continued)
  outpatient coding and reporting
    additional diagnoses, 80–91
    chronic diseases, 89–90
    diagnostic services, 90–91
    first-listed diagnoses, 76
    inpatient coding,
        distinguished, 748–749
    observation stays, 79, 86
    prenatal visits, 93
    specificity in, 87
    surgery codes, 78, 79, 92–93
    therapeutic services, 91
    uncertain diagnoses, 88
    unconfirmed diagnoses, 77
    V codes, 81–86
  parasitic diseases, 49, 118–120
  parentheses-( ), 47
  pregnancy, childbirth, and
      puerperium complications,
      151–157
  Procedures, Volume 3, 60
    alphabetic index, 65–70
    format, 61–62
    history, 60–61
    replacement with ICD-10-PCS
        manual, 197–198
    see also ICD-10-PCS manual
    Tabular List, 63–64, 487f
  replacement
    with ICD-10-CM
        see also ICD-10-CM manual
    Procedures, Volume 3, 197–198
        see also ICD-10-PCS manual
  reporting guidelines. Official
      Guidelines for Coding and
      Reporting, above
  respiratory system, diseases of,
      140–141
  sections, 33, 33f
  sense organs, diseases of, 133–134
  signs, 165
    inpatient coding and reporting,
        749
  skin and subcutaneous tissue,
      diseases of, 157–158
  slanted brackets-[ ], 46
  subcategories, 33, 33f
  subclassification codes, 33f, 34
  Supplementary Classification
    E codes, above
    V codes, below
  symptoms, 165
    inpatient coding and reporting,
        749, 755
  systemic inflammatory response
      syndrome, 167
  tables of contents
    Volume 1, 32f
    Volume 3, 63f
  Tabular List, Volume 1, 29
    Appendix A-Morphology of
        Neoplasms, 38–39
    Appendix B-Glossary of Mental
        Disorders (deleted in
        2005), 39
    Appendix C-Classification
        of Drugs by American
        Hospital Formulary Service
        List Number and Their
        ICD-9-CM Equivalents, 39
    Appendix D-Classification
        of Industrial Accidents
        According to Agency, 39–40

ICD-9-CM manual (*Continued*)
　Tabular List (*Continued*)
　　Appendix E-List of Three-Digit
　　　Categories, 40
　　Classification of Diseases and
　　　Injuries, 32–34
　　divisions, 29, 32–34
　　fourth/fifth-digit specificity,
　　　35–36
　　Tabular List, Volume 3, 63–64
　therapeutic substances, adverse
　　effects of, 175
　threatened condition, 113–114
　tumors. Neoplasms, *above*
　"unspecified" codes, 51
　V codes
　　neoplasms, 125–126
　　outpatient services, 81–86
　"with" and "and," 54
　wounds, 187–188
ICD-10-CM manual, 193
　crosswalk, 195–196, 195f
　development of, 193–194
　ICD-9-CM, replacement of,
　　193–194
　improvements in, 194–195
　index, 196, 196f
　mapping, 195–196, 195f
　preface, 194, 194f
　structure of system, 195
　Tabular chapters, 196, 197f
ICD-10-PCS manual
　characters of, 198
　　changing characters, 199, 199f
　　character 1, 198
　　character 2, 199
　　character 3, 199–200, 201t–203t
　　Tabular List, 206–207, 207f
　development of, 197–198
　index, 205–206, 206f
　root operations (medical and
　　surgical), 201t–205t
　Tabular List, 206–207, 207f
Ill-defined conditions, 165
　inpatient coding and reporting,
　　749
Immune globulins, 709–710
Immunity disorders, 128–129
　human immunodeficiency virus
　　see HIV infection
　sarcoidosis, chronic iridocyclitis
　　in, 134
Immunization agents, 709–713
Immunology codes, 698
Implants
　cardioverter-defibrillators, 476–478
　cochlear devices, 655–656, 655f
　contraceptive capsules, 397
　eyeball, 646, 647f
　hormone pellet implantation,
　　subcutaneous, 397–398
　pacemakers, 476–478
　penile, 585
Incarcerated hernia, 558
Incentive spirometry, 726, 726f
Indicator dilution studies, 504
Individual Practice Associations
　(IPAs), 22
Infants
　see Newborns
Infectious diseases, 118–120
　includes/excludes notes, 49
Infertility, female, 48
Influenza immunizations, 712

Influenzae, hemophilus, 141
Infusion services, 732–733
　home infusion procedures
　　services, 743
Ingrown toenail, 396
　removal of, 396f
Injection services, 732–733
　biopsy codes, 433
　bladder procedures, 575
　cardiovascular vascular injection
　　procedures, 491–492, 493f,
　　494f
　nasal turbinate injections, 453,
　　454f
　pneumothorax injection, 465
　sinus tract injection procedure
　　codes, 433
Injury coding, 166–170, 185–186
　burn injuries, 180–182, 184
　traumatic fractures, 186
Inner ear procedures, 655–656
Inpatient coding and reporting
　abnormal findings, 762
　additional diagnoses, 760–761
　comparative or contrasting
　　conditions, 753
　complications, 756
　ill-defined conditions, 749
　interrelated conditions, 751
　multiple diagnoses, 752
　observation unit admissions, 759
　original treatment plan not
　　carried out, 755
　outpatient coding, distinguished,
　　748–749
　outpatient surgery admissions, 760
　Present on Admission (POA), 763
　principal diagnosis, 748, 749
　signs, 749
　symptoms, 749
　symptoms following contrasting/
　　comparative diagnoses, 755
　uncertain diagnoses, 757–758, 763
Inpatient services
　hospital
　　see Hospital inpatient services
　neonatal and pediatric critical
　　care services, 334
Insemination, artificial, 611
Integumentary system
　CPT manual subsection, 382
　　format of, 382
　skin
　　see Skin, subcutaneous, and
　　　accessory structures
　subcutaneous structures
　　see Skin, subcutaneous, and
　　　accessory structures
Intermediate care facility, 324
International Classification of Diseases
　Clinical Modification
　　9th revision
　　　see ICD-9-CM manual
　　10th revision
　　　see ICD-10-CM manual
　Procedure Coding System
　　see ICD-10-PCS manual
Intersex surgery, 600
Interstitial fluid pressure, 438
Intestines, 543–545
Intracapsular cataract extraction, 649
Intracoronary stent placement,
　496–497, 496f
Intrauterine devices, 610–611, 610f

Intravascular ultrasound, 496
Introitus
　see Vulva, perineum, and introitus
In utero surgery, 154–155
In vitro fertilization, 611, 614
IPAs, 22
Iridocyclitis
　in sarcoidosis, chronic, 134
　unspecified, 129
Iris, 649
Ischemia
　coronary arteries, 482
　reversible, 685
Island pedicle flap, 407
IUDs, 610–611, 610f

J

Jaundice, 87, 89

K

Keratoplasty, 648
Kidneys, 564f
　donors, 83
　endoscopy, 571
　end-stage renal disease, 717, 719
　excision, 567
　hypertensive chronic kidney
　　disease, 136
　hypertensive renal disease, 136, 137
　incision, 564–567
　index locations, 571
　introduction codes, 568–569
　laparoscopy, 571
　renal transplantation, 567–568
　repair, 569–570
　structure of, 570f
Knife wounds, 432–433

L

Labia majora, 603f
Labia minora, 603f
Laboratory section
　see Pathology/laboratory section,
　　of the CPT manual
Labyrinth, 655
Labyrinthectomy, 655
Labyrinthotomy, 655
Lacerations
　see Wound(s)
Lacrimal apparatus, 645f
Lacrimal sac, 645f
Laminectomy, 636, 636f
Laparoscopic retropubic
　prostatectomy (LRP), 593
Laparoscopy
　bladder, 577–578
　corpus uteri, 611–612, 612f
　esophagus, 540, 540f
　kidney, 571
　oviduct/ovary, 613
　spermatic cord, 589
Laryngoplasty for a laryngeal web,
　459
Laryngoscopy
　biopsies, 535
　direct, 449, 450
　indirect, 450
Laryngotomy, 459
Larynx, 458
　excision, 459
　intubation, 459
　laryngoplasty for a laryngeal web,
　　459

Laser coagulation of the prostate, 592
Laser transmyocardial revascularization, 476
Laser vaporization of the prostate, 592–593
Lesions
    kidney, ablation of, 567, 568f
    nasal lesions, excision or destruction of, 453
    penile lesions, destruction of, 583
    skin
        see Skin lesions
Ligature strangulation, 390
Limited lymphadenectomy, 519
Lingual frenum, 530
Lip reconstruction, 528
Lip repair, 529
Lipectomy, 410
Lips, 527–529
Liver, 556
    abnormal scan, 165
    biopsy, 556
    cirrhosis of, 104
    transplant, 556
Local anesthesia, 347, 347f
Long-term care facility, 325
Lumbar puncture, 636, 637f
Lund-Browder chart/classification of burns, 183f, 412f
Lungs and pleura, 463
    excision, 463
    incision, 463
    injury to lung, 49–50
    pneumonolysis, 465
    pneumothorax injection, 465
    thoracoplasty, 463
Lymphadenectomies, 519
Lymphatic system
    see Hemic and lymphatic systems

M

Magnetic resonance angiography, 672
Magnetic resonance imaging, 662, 672, 673f
    cardiac MRIs, 511, 512f
    see also Radiology
Magnifying loupes, 651, 656, 656f
Male genital system, 583f
    diseases of, 150
    epididymis, 587–588
    format of subsection, 582
    ICD-9-CM manual, 150
    intersex surgery, 600
    penis
        see Penis
    prostate
        see Prostate
    scrotum, 588
    seminal vesicles, 590–591
    spermatic cord, 589–590
    testis, 586–587
    tunica vaginalis, 588
    vas deferens, 588–589
Malignancies
    see Cancer
Mammography, 674–675
Managed Care Organizations (MCOs), 22
Managed health care, 21–23
Manometric studies, 573
Mapping, 507
Mastectomies, 264, 418–419, 418f, 419f, 420f

Maternity care and delivery, 617
    abortion services
        see Abortion services
    antepartum services, 616, 618
        amniocentesis, 618
        cordocentesis, 618
        excision, 618–619
        introduction codes, 619–620
        repair services, 620
    complications of, 151–157
    congenital anomalies and conditions originating in the perinatal period, 161, 163
    estimated date of delivery, 615
    format of subsection, 615
    HIV-infected persons, 155
    ICD-9-CM manual, 151–157
    normal delivery, 155
    postpartum care, 616
MCOs, 22
Meckel's diverticulum, 545
Mediastinum, 522–523
    biopsy, 463
Medical decision making, 294–295
    complexity levels, 295
    complications or death, risk of, 296–299
    data to be reviewed, 296
    elements of, 297f
    examples, 296, 298–299
Medical examination
    see Examination
Medical necessity, certificates of
    oxygen necessity, 244f
    transcutaneous electrical nerve stimulation, 243f
Medical records
    anesthesia, 356f–357f
    documentation, 282–283
        Guidelines, 338–340
        1995 Guidelines
            see also E/M services
    electronic records, 9
    management options, 295–301
    patient history
        see History
    risk of complications or death, 296–299
Medical team conferences, 330
Medically Unlikely Units, 671
Medicare Administrative Contractors (MACs), 3–4, 3f
Medicare Advantage, 6, 22–23
    nonphysicians' services, 19
Medicare fraud and abuse
    form of fraud, 18
    protecting yourself from, 20
    regulations, 20
    violators, 18
    what constitutes, 17–18
    who determines, 18–19
Medicare program, 2–4
    abuse
        see Medicare fraud and abuse
    accepting assignment, 4
    anesthesia service time, 355
    bypass procedures, 542
    coinsurance payments, 4
    DRGs. Inpatient diagnosis-related groups, below
    Electronic Remittance Advice, 14
    E/M services, 252, 254, 264, 265, 266, 268
    Federal Register, 9–10, 11f

Medicare program (Continued)
    fraud
        see Medicare fraud and abuse
    hospital insurance, 5–6
    Medicare Advantage, 6, 22–23
    outpatient resource-based relative value scale, 11–12
        adjustments, 15
        beneficiary protection, 14
        conversion factor, 13
        Geographic Practice Cost Index, 13
        limiting charge, 14–15
        Medicare Volume Performance Standards, 13–14
        relative value unit, 12–13
        site-of-service limitations, 15
        surgical procedures/supplies, 15–17, 375, 376, 377
        uniformity provision, 15
        wound debridement, 385
    Part A, 5–6
    Part B, 6
    Part C, 6
    Part D, 6
    pneumococcal vaccines, 711
    prescription drugs, 6
    Quality Improvement Organizations, agreements with, 4–5
    RBRVS. Outpatient resource-based relative value scale, above
    skin closures, 401
    Standard Paper Remittance Advice (SPR), 14
    supplementary insurance, 6
    surgical trays, 375
    volume performance standards, 13–14
Medication therapy management services, 742
Medicine codes
    allergen immunotherapy, 728
    allergy testing, 727
    anesthesia
        see Anesthesia
    behavior assessment/intervention, 732
    biofeedback, 716
    cardiovascular system
        see Cardiovascular system
    chemotherapy, 733–736
    chiropractic manipulative treatment, 741
    CNS assessments/tests, 731
    dermatological procedures, special, 737–738
    dialysis, 717–720
    gastroenterology, 720
    glucose monitoring, 728–729
    HCPCS
        see Healthcare Common Procedure Coding System
    home health procedures/services, 743
    hydration services, 732–733
    immune globulins, 709–710
    immunization agents, 709–713
    influenza immunizations, 712
    infusion services, 732–733
        home infusion procedures services, 743
    injection services
        see Injection services

Medicine codes (Continued)
  medication therapy management services, 742
  muscle testing, 729–731
  National Codes
    see National Codes
  neurologic function tests, 729–731
  non-face-to-face nonphysician services, 742
  nutritional therapy, medical, 741
  ophthalmologic services, 721–723
  osteopathic manipulative treatment, 741
  other services and procedures, 743
  otorhinolaryngologic services, special, 724
  photodynamic therapy, 737
  physical medicine and rehabilitation, 738–739
  pneumococcal immunizations, 712
  psychiatric treatments, 714–716, 732
  pulmonary tests/therapies, 726
  range-of-motion measurements, 729, 729f
  sedation
    see Anesthesia
  sleep testing, 729–731
  special services, procedures, and reports, 742
  transfusion medicine, 698–699, 699f
  vaccines, 709–713
    immunization administration for, 710–711
  vascular diagnostic studies, noninvasive, 725
  wound care management, 739, 740f
Medicine section, of the CPT manual, 708
  format of, 708–709
  see also Medicine codes
Meninges, 631
Meningitis, 133
Menstrual period, last, 615
Mental disorders, 131–133
  ICD-9-CM manual: Tabular List, Volume 1, Appendix B, 39
  psychiatric treatments, 714–716, 732
Metabolic diseases, 128–129
Microbiology, 699–700
Miscarriages, 620
Missed abortion, 620
Mohs' micrographic surgery, 416–417
Mouth, 530–531
  candidiasis infection of, 118
  dentoalveolar structures, 531
  floor of, 530–531
  lips
    see Lips
  palate, 533
    cleft, 529, 529f
  salivary gland and ducts, 533–534, 533f, 534f
  vestibule of, 529
MRA, 678
MRI, 662, 672, 673f
  cardiac MRIs, 511, 512f
  see also Radiology
Mullerian ducts, 591
Muscle testing, 729–731

Musculoskeletal system
  arthroscopy, 443
  arthroscopy codes, 443–444
  bone grafts, 438
  casts and strapping codes, 440–442
  coding tips, 424
  connective tissue diseases, 159–160
  diseases of, 159–160
  dislocations, 429, 430f
  electrical stimulation, 438
  endoscopy, 443–444
  excision, 433
  foot repairs, 440
  format of subsection, 424
  fractures
    see Fractures
  free osteocutaneous flaps, 438
  ICD-9-CM manual, 159–160
  incisions, 431
  interstitial fluid pressure, 438
  other procedures codes, 438
  spinal fixation, 438–439
  spinal instrumentation, 439, 439f
  toe repairs, 440
  ultrasound stimulation, 438
  wound exploration, 432–433
Myocardial infarction
  acute, 137
  impending, 114
Myringotomy, 653

N

Nails, 394
  avulsion, 395–396
  debridement, 394
Nasal fractures, 426, 426f
  therapeutic fracture of nasal turbinate, 455
National Codes, 233, 234–235
  colorectal cancer screening, 549–551
  durable medical equipment, 241
  general guidelines, 235–237
  index, 237, 237f, 238f
  national physician fee schedule, 241, 245f
  routes of administration of drugs, 239, 240, 240f
  table of drugs, 238–239, 239f
National Provider Identification (NPI), 9
Nebulizers, 726, 727f
Neck
  lymph nodes, 520, 521f, 522
  radical dissection, 459
  suprahyoid dissection, 520
Negative Pressure Wound Therapy, 739, 740f
Neonatal critical care services, 334
Neoplasms
  bladder tumors, transurethral resection of, 579
  cardiac, 476
  coding, 121–126
  ICD-9-CM manual: Tabular List, Volume 1, Appendix A, 38–39
    see also ICD-9-CM manual
  peritoneum, malignant neoplasm of, 47
  retroperitoneum, malignant neoplasm of, 47

Nephrectomy, 567
Nephrolithotomy, 565, 566f
  percutaneous, 566–567
Nephrolithotripsy, 566–567
Nephrorrhaphy, 298
Nephrostolithotomy, percutaneous, 567
Nephrostomy, 565
Nephrotomy, 565
Nervous system, 630
  autonomic, 638–639
  brain, 639–640
    aneurysm, 633
    arteriovenous malformation, 633
    vascular disease, 633
  cerebrospinal fluid shunts, 633, 634f
  CNS
    see Central nervous system
  code assignments, 631–632
  diseases of, 133–134
  extracranial nerves, 638–639
  meninges, 631
  peripheral, 630, 638–639
  skull surgery, 632–633
  spine/spinal cord
    see Spine and spinal cord
Neurologic function tests, 729–731
Neuroplasty, 639–640
Neurovascular pedicle flap, 407–408
Newborns
  anesthesia for infant less than 4 kg, 270
  care, 333
    see also Maternity care and delivery
  congenital anomalies, 161, 163
  critical care services, 334
  perinatal guidelines, 161–163
  sepsis, 163
  single live born, 84
Non-face-to-face physician services, 332
Nose, 451
  biopsy of skin outside of, 204
  excision, 452–453
  foreign body, removal of, 454
  hemorrhage control
    anterior nasal packing, 455, 456f
    posterior nasal packing, 455, 456f
  incision, 451, 451f
  introduction codes, 453–454
  lesions, excision or destruction of, 453
  nasal button, insertion of, 453–454, 454f
  polyps, excision of, 452, 453f
  sinuses
    see Sinuses
  turbinate injections, 453, 454f
NPI (National Provider Identification), 9
Nuclear cardiology, 472
Nuclear medicine, 684–685
Nursing facilities, 324–325
  discharge services, 325
  initial care, 325
  intermediate care facility, 324
  long-term care facility, 325
  other services, 325–326
  skilled nursing facility, 324
  subsequent care, 325
Nutritional diseases, 128–129
Nutritional therapy, medical, 741

O

Observation codes
  hospital, 309–310
  outpatient reporting, 79, 86
Obstetric care
  see Maternity care and delivery
Occlusion, 100
Ocular adnexa
  see Eye and ocular adnexa
Office/outpatient consultations, 315
Office/outpatient services
  established patient services, 307
  Medicare coverage
    see Medicare program
  new patient services, 305
  outpatient coding
    see Outpatient coding and
      reporting
  unconfirmed diagnoses, 77
Official Guidelines for Coding and
    Reporting
  see ICD-9-CM manual
Omentum, 557
OMT, 741
Oncology
  cancer
    see Cancer
  radiation
    see Radiation oncology
Online medical evaluations, 332
Onychocryptosis, 396
  removal of nail, 396f
Open reduction, 67
Operating microscope, 651, 656,
    656f
Operation, 70
  see also Surgery codes
Ophthalmologic services,
    721–723
Orchiectomy, 58
Orchiopexy, 586
Oscheoplasty, 588
Ossicular chain, 655
Ostectomy, 411
Osteoarthritis, 425
Osteopathic manipulative treatment,
    741
Ostomies, 544–545, 545f
Otoplasty, 653
Otorhinolaryngologic services,
    special, 724
Outpatient coding and reporting
  additional diagnoses, 80–91
  chronic diseases, 89–90
  diagnostic services, 90–91
  first-listed diagnoses, 76
  inpatient coding, distinguished,
    748–749
  observation stays, 79, 86
  prenatal visits, 93
  specificity in, 87
  surgery codes, 78, 79, 92–93
  therapeutic services, 91
  uncertain diagnoses, 88
  unconfirmed diagnoses, 77
  V codes, 81–86
Outpatient resource-based relative
    value scale (RBRVS)
  see Medicare program
Outpatient services
  see Office/outpatient services
Ovary
  see Oviduct/ovary

Oviduct/ovary, 601f, 612
  excision, 613
  incision, 612–613
  laparoscopy, 613
  lysis of adhesions, 613–614
  repair, 613–614
  in vitro fertilization, 614
Oxygen necessity, certificate for, 244f

P

PACE, 23
Pacemaker/cardioverter-defibrillator,
    476–478
Pacing, 506, 507
Palate, 533
  cleft, 529, 529f
Pancreas, 557, 626f, 627
  removal of, 557
Pancreatitis, 107
Panniculectomy, 410, 410f
Paracentesis, 648
Parasitic diseases, 118–120
  includes/excludes notes, 49
Parathyroid glands, 627
  incision and excision, 629
Paraurethral glands
  see Skene's glands
Parotid duct, 534, 534f
Past history, 287–288
Patella fracture, 187
Pathology/laboratory section, of the
    CPT manual, 690
  anatomic pathology, 700–701
  chemistry, 695–696
  clinical pathology, 694–695
  coagulation tests, 696–698
  cytogenic studies, 701
  cytopathology, 701
  drug assays, 692–693
  drug testing, 691–692
  evocative/suppression testing,
    693–694
  format of, 690
  hematology, 696–698
  immunology codes, 698
  microbiology, 699–700
  Organ or Disease Oriented Panels,
    690–691
  other procedures, 703
  surgical pathology, 701–702
  transfusion medicine, 698–699,
    699f
  urinalysis, 695–696
Patient history
  see History
Patient-activated event recorder, 480
Patient-controlled analgesia, 347
Pediatric critical care
  inpatient services, 334
  patient transport, 334
Pedicle flaps, 407–408
Pelvic exenteration, 576
Penicillin
  allergy, personal history of, 84
  urticaria due to, 175
Penile amputation, 584
Penile implant, 585
Penis
  excision, 583–584
  incisions, 582
  introduction codes, 584–585
  lesions, destruction of, 583
  repair, 585

Percutaneous biopsy, 433
Percutaneous skeletal fixation, 427,
    428f
Percutaneous transluminal coronary
    angioplasty, 482, 483f
Pericardiocentesis, 475, 475f
Pericarditis, 108
Pericardium, 475
Perinatal guidelines, 161–163
Perineoplasty, 603
Perineum
  see Vulva, perineum, and introitus
Peripheral arterial disease
    rehabilitation, 508
Peripheral nervous system, 630,
    638–639
Peritoneal dialysis, 717
Peritoneum, 557
  malignant neoplasm of, 47
Pernicious anemia, 91
Peyronie disease, 584, 584f
Pharyngitis, streptococcal, 109
Pharyngoplasty, 536
Pharyngostomy, 536
Pharynx, 535–536
Photodynamic therapy, 737
Physical medicine and
    rehabilitation, 738–739
Physician standby services, 329–330
Pilonidal cysts, 396–398
Pinch graft, 403f
Plethysmography, 508
Pleura
  see Lungs and pleura
Pleurectomy, 463
Pneumococcal meningitis, 133
Pneumococcal vaccines, 711, 712
Pneumonia
  dehydration due to, 103
  from gram-negative bacteria, 45
  Klebsiella pneumoniae, due to, 140
  organism unspecified, 102
Pneumonocentesis, 463
Pneumonolysis, 465
Pneumothorax injection, 465
POA (Present on Admission), 763
Point-of-Service (POS) benefits, 23
Poisoning codes, 166–170, 177
Polio vaccines, 83
Polycythemia vera, 91
Polyps
  endocervical polyps, 606–607, 607f
  nasal polyps, excision of, 452, 453f
Polysomnography, 729–730, 730f
Posterior synechiae, 648
Postoperative evaluations, 92
Postpartum care, 616
Postpartum curettage, 619
Post/preoperative diagnoses
  different diagnoses, 93
  same diagnosis, 93
PPOs, 22
Preferred Provider Organizations
    (PPOs), 22
Pregnancy
  abortions
    see Abortion services
  amniocentesis, 618
  artificial insemination, 611
  birth
    see Maternity care and delivery
  care during
    see Maternity care and delivery
  complications, late effect of, 156

Pregnancy (Continued)
  complications of, 151–157
  diabetes in, 155
  ectopic, 151, 618–619, 619f
  first pregnancy with
      complication, 93
  first pregnancy without
      complication, 93
  HIV infection in, 119–120, 155
  miscarriages, 620
  peripartum and postpartum
      periods, 156
  prenatal visits, 93
  in vitro fertilization, 611, 614
  see also Fetuses
Premature infants, 163
Prenatal visits, 93
Preoperative evaluations, 92
Pre/postoperative diagnoses
  different diagnoses, 93
  same diagnosis, 93
Present on Admission (POA), 763
Presenting problem, nature of,
    302–303
Pressure ulcers, 410–411, 411f
Preventive medicine services,
    331–332
Priapism, 585
Problem focused examination, 290
Proctosigmoidoscopy, 547
Program for All-Inclusive Care for
    the Elderly (PACE), 23
Programmed stimulation, 506
Prolonged physician services,
    328–330
Prostate, 591
  acute prostatitis due to
      streptococcus, 150
  benign prostatic hyperplasia,
      591–593
  biopsies, 593–594
  vesical neck and prostate codes,
      580
Prostate cancer
  biopsies, 593–594
  brachytherapy, 594–595
Prostatectomy, 591–593
Prostatotomy, 594
Proton beam treatment delivery,
    683
Pseudophakia, 648
Psychiatric treatments, 714–716, 732
Psychiatrists, 715
Psychologists, 715
Psychosocial circumstances, 83
Pulmonary tests/therapies, 726
Punch biopsy, 389, 390f
Puncture aspiration, 383
Pyeloplasty, 569–570
Pyelostolithotomy, 567

Q
QIO providers, 4–5
Quality Improvement
    Organizations, 4–5

R
Radiation oncology, 679
  clinical brachytherapy, 683–684,
      684f
  clinical treatment planning, 679
  dosimetry, 680
  hyperthermia, 683

Radiation oncology (Continued)
  medical radiation physics, 680
  proton beam treatment delivery,
      683
  radiation treatment delivery, 681
  radiation treatment management,
      682
  simulation, 679–680
  special services, 680
  treatment devices, 680
Radical lymphadenectomy, 519
Radiofrequency energy, 507
Radiologists, 661
  interventional, 676
Radiology, 661
  anteroposterior body position,
      663, 664f
  axial projection, 667, 667f
  body planes/positioning, 662–667
  cardiovascular codes
      see Cardiovascular system
  component/combination coding,
      669, 670
  decubitus body positions,
      664–665, 666f
  diagnostic, 627–674
  distal body references, 663, 664f
  global radiology service, 509–510
  Guidelines, 668–671
  lateral body positions, 360f,
      663–664, 665, 666f
  Medically Unlikely Units, 671
  nuclear medicine, 684–685
  oblique views, 665, 666f, 667
  posteroanterior body position,
      663, 664f, 666f
  prone body position, 662, 664,
      666f
  proximal body references, 644f,
      663
  recumbent body position, 665,
      666f
  supervision and interpretation,
      669, 670
  supine body position, 664, 666f
  tangential projections, 667, 667f
  terminology, 661–667
  ultrasound
      see Ultrasound
  "with contrast," 671
Radiology section, of the CPT
    manual
  format of, 661
  generally
      see Radiology
Radiotherapy
  brachytherapy
      see Brachytherapy
  oncology
      see Radiation oncology
Range-of-motion measurements,
    729, 729f
RBRVS
    see Medicare program
Rectum, 546–547
Referral, 314
Regional anesthesia, 346–347, 348
Reimbursement
  managed health care, 21–23
  Medicare
      see Medicare program
Relative Value Guide, 352, 354f
Renal cysts, 569
Renal transplantation, 567–568

Reproductive system(s)
  female
      see Female genital system
  male
      see Male genital system
  procedures, 600
Request for consultation, 314
Requesting physician, 314
Respiratory system
  bronchi
      see Trachea and bronchi
  diseases of, 140–141
  endoscopy, 448–449
  format of subsection, 448
  ICD-9-CM manual, 140–141
  larynx
      see Larynx
  lungs
      see Lungs and pleura
  nose
      see Nose
  pleura
      see Lungs and pleura
  sinuses
      see Sinuses
  trachea
      see Trachea and bronchi
Rest home services, 327
Retinopathy
  diabetic retinopathy, with type I
      diabetes, 105
  hypertensive, 137
Retroperitoneal, 564
Retroperitoneum, malignant
    neoplasm of, 47
Review of systems, 286–287
Rhinoplasty, 454–455, 529
Rhytidectomy, 408, 409
RNY gastric bypass, 541, 542f
Robotic assisted prostatectomy
    (RAP), 593
Rotation flaps, 402, 403f
Roux-en-Y gastric bypass, 541, 542f
Rubeosis iridis, 129
Rule of Nines, 183f, 412f

S
Salivary gland and ducts, 533–534,
    533f, 534f
Sarcoidosis, chronic iridocyclitis in,
    134
Scarlet fever and streptococcal
    pharyngitis, 109
Scissors removal, 390, 391f
Scrotoplasty, 588
Scrotum, 588
Sedation
    see Anesthesia
Segmental instrumentation, 439f
Seldinger technique, 502, 503f
Seminal vesicles, 590–591
Sense organs, diseases of, 133–134
Sentinel node biopsy, 520, 522
Sepsis in newborns, 163
Septic abortion, 620
Septoplasty, 455
Seton, 553, 554f
Shoulder relocation, 429, 430f
Shunts, 633
  cerebrospinal fluid, 633, 634f
  ventriculoperitoneal
      see Ventriculoperitoneal shunts
Sigmoidoscopy, 547–548

Signal-averaged electrocardiography, 500
Signs, 165
  inpatient coding and reporting, 749
Sinuses
  accessory, 457–458
  displacement therapy, 453
  tract injection procedure codes, 433
Sinusitis
  acute maxillary, 141
  chronic, 48
Sinusotomies, 458
SIRS (systemic inflammatory response syndrome), 167
Skeletal system
  see Musculoskeletal system
Skeletal traction, 427, 428f
Skene's glands, 5, 581, 601
Skilled nursing facilities, 324
Skin, subcutaneous, and accessory structures
  burn treatment, 412–414, 413f
  burns, 411–412, 412f
  debridement, 383–385
  diseases of, 157–158
  excision-debridement, 384
  grafting procedures
    see Skin grafts
  hormone pellet implantation, 397–398
  ICD-9-CM manual, 157–158
  incision and drainage codes, 384, 384f
  lesions
    see Skin lesions
  nails, 394–396
  nose biopsy, 452
  pilonidal cysts, 396–398
  wound repair
    see Wound repair
Skin flaps, 406–408
  rotation flaps, 402, 403f
Skin grafts
  adjacent tissue transfers, 402–403
  donor site, 401
  for facial nerve paralysis, 410
  recipient site, 401
  skin replacement surgery/skin substitutes, 403–405
Skin lesions, 386
  biopsies, 389–390, 417
    breast procedures, 417–418
  closure of excision sites, 387–388
  cutting, 388–389
  destruction, 386
    other than excision, 415–416
  excision, 386–389
    benign lesions, 392–393
    malignant lesions, 393, 394f
  paring, 388–389
  shaving of, 391–392
  skin tags, 390–391
  types of, 386f
Skin replacement surgery, 403–405
Skin substitutes, 403–405
Skin tags, 390–391
Skin traction, 429, 429f
Skull surgery, 632–633
Sleep testing, 729–731

Slit lamp, 647
Social history, 287–288
Sore throat, streptococcal, 109
Special E/M services, 332
Spermatic cord, 589–590
Spinal anesthesia, 346, 348
Spinal cord
  see Spine and spinal cord
Spinal fixation, 438–439
Spinal instrumentation, 439, 439f
Spinal tap, 636, 637f
Spine and spinal cord, 631
  autonomic nervous system, 638–639
  CNS
    see Central nervous system
  coding procedures, 635–637
  extracranial nerves, 638–639
  peripheral nerves, 638–639
Spine surgery codes, 437
Spirometry, incentive, 726, 726f
Spleen, 518
Splints, 440, 441f
  removal of, 440
Spondylolisthesis, acquired, 50
Spontaneous abortions, 620
Staff Model HMOs, 22
Standard Paper Remittance Advice (SPR), 14
Stem cell harvesting, 519
Stensen's duct, 534, 534f
Stents
  in the biliary tract, 557
  intracoronary placement, 496–497, 496f
  prostatic, 591
  renal, 568
Stimson technique, 429, 430f
Stoma, 544, 544f
Stomach, 541
  ulcers, 103, 149
Strabismus surgery, 649
Strangulated hernia, 558
Strapping, 440
  codes, 440–442
  removal of, 440
  types of, 441f
Streptococcal sore throat, 109
Stress tests, 684
  cardiovascular, 497–500
Stroke, 100
Subcutaneous structures
  see Skin, subcutaneous, and accessory structures
Subungual hematoma, nails, 395
Suppositories, vaginal, 621
Suprahyoid neck dissection, 520
Surfer's ear, 653
Surgery codes
  ambulatory surgery, 92
  birthing
    see Maternity care and delivery
  cardiovascular system
    see Cardiovascular system
  computer-assisted surgical navigation, 438
  deleted codes, 371, 371f
  diaphragm, 523
  fine needle biopsies, 378, 378f
  global surgery period, 375
  integumentary system
    see Integumentary system
  materials and supplies, 375

Surgery codes (Continued)
  maternity care
    see Maternity care and delivery
  mediastinum, 523
  Mohs' micrographic surgery, 416–417
  musculoskeletal system
    see Musculoskeletal system
  outpatient coding and reporting, 78, 79, 92–93
  parathyroid glands, 629
  parenthetical phrases, 370, 370f
  pathology codes, 701–702
  postoperative evaluations, 92
  preoperative evaluations, 92
  respiratory system
    see Respiratory system
  separate procedures, 372–373
  special reports, 372
  surgical packages, 374–377
  thyroid gland, 628–629
  unlisted procedures, 371
  see also specific anatomic/physiological sites
Surgery Guidelines, 368–371
  unlisted procedures, 371
Surgery section, of the CPT manual, 368
  birth deliveries
    see Maternity care and delivery
  codes
    see Surgery codes
  Guidelines
    see Surgery Guidelines
  maternity care
    see Maternity care and delivery
  "New Text" symbols, 368, 369f
  notes, 368, 369f
  "Revised Text" symbols, 369–370
  subsections
    auditory system
      see Auditory system
    diaphragm, 523
    digestive system
      see Digestive system
    ear
      see Ear
    endocrine system, 626–629, 626f
    general subsections, 382
    hemic system
      see Hemic and lymphatic systems
    lymphatic system
      see Hemic and lymphatic systems
    male genital system
      see Male genital system
    mediastinum, 523
    nervous system
      see Nervous system
    ocular adnexa
      see Eye and ocular adnexa
    urinary system
      see Urinary system
Surgical packages, 374–377
Surgical pathology, 701–702
Swan-Ganz catheter, 351f, 352
Symptoms, 165
  inpatient coding and reporting, 749, 755
Systemic inflammatory response syndrome (SIRS), 167

T

Tandem cuff, 581
Tattooing codes, 397
Telephone services, 332
TENS, certificate for, 243f
Terrorism E coding guidelines, 170
Testis, 586–587
Third-party reimbursement
  managed health care, 21–23
  Medicare
    see Medicare program
Thompson operation, 70
Thoracentesis, 464, 464f
Thoracoplasty, 465
Thoracoscopy, 449
Thoracotomy, 449, 463
Thrombectomy, 488–489
Thrombolysis, 495
Thrombus, 488
Thymus gland, 626f, 627
Thyroid gland, 626–627
  incision and excision, 628–629
Thyroiditis, 108
Tibia, areas of, 429, 430f
Tissue grafts
  musculoskeletal system, 437
  skin
    see Skin grafts
Tissue-expander codes, 397
Toe repairs, 440
Toenails, 394
  ingrown, 396, 396f
Tomography, 662
  see also Radiology
Tongue, 530–531
Tonsillectomy, 535–536
Tonsillitis, acute, 50
Tonsils, 535–536
  chronic disease of, 54
Topical anesthesia, 347
Total pelvic exenteration, 576
Toxicity codes, 166–170, 177
Toxoids, 709–713
Trabeculectomy ab externo, 649
Trachea and bronchi, 460
  incision, 460
  introduction codes, 462
  repair procedures, 462
Trachelorrhaphy, 609
Tracheoplasty, 462
Tracheostomy, 460, 461f
Traction, 427, 428f
Transconjunctival approach, 649–650, 649f
Transcutaneous electrical nerve simulation, certificate for, 243f
Transfusion medicine, 698–699, 699f
Transmyocardial revascularization, 476
Transplantation
  bone marrow, 519
  kidney, 567–568
  liver, 556
  pancreas, 557
Transtracheal tracheostomy, 460, 461f
Transurethral incision of the prostate (TUIP), 592
Transurethral microwave heat treatment (TUMT), 591

Transurethral needle ablation (TUNA), 591
Transurethral resection of a bladder tumor, 579
Transurethral resection of the prostate (TURP), 591
Transurethral surgery, 579–580
Transverse wedge excision, 527
Tubal ligation, 612–613
Tube graft, 406, 406f
Tuberculosis, 49
Tumors
  see Neoplasms
Tunica vaginalis, 588
Turbinate injections, 453, 454f
Tympanostomy, 653

U

Ulcers
  gastrointestinal hemorrhage, 148, 149
  lower limbs, 57
  pressure, 410–411, 411f
  sacral, 403f
  stomach, 103, 149
Ultrasound
  A-mode, 677
  B-scan, 677
  coronary vessels, 496
  diagnostic, 675–678
  Doppler, 678
  echocardiography, 501–502, 501f, 725
  examinations, 677
  M-mode, 677
  musculoskeletal system stimulation, 438
  real-time scan, 678
  transrectal, 595
Ultraviolet light therapy, 738
Uncertain diagnoses
  inpatient coding and reporting, 757–758, 763
  outpatient coding and reporting, 88
Undescended testis, 586
Unit/floor time, 302–303
Urachal cyst, 576
Ureter, 564f, 572
  endoscopy, 573–575
  excision, 572–573
  incision, 572
  introduction codes, 573
  laparoscopy, 573
  repair procedures, 573
Ureterolithotomy, 572
Ureterolysis, 573
Ureteroneocystostomy, 573
Ureteroplasty, 573
Ureteropyelostomy, 573
Ureterosigmoidostomy, 573
Urethra, 564f, 581
  excision, 581
  incision, 581
  manipulation codes, 582
  repair procedures, 581
Urethrectomy, 581
Urethromeatoplasty, 581
Urethroplasty, 581
Urinalysis, 695–696
Urinary system, 564f
  bladder
    see Bladder

Urinary system (*Continued*)
  E. coli infection, 118
  format of subsection, 564
  kidneys
    see Kidneys
  ureter
    see Ureter
  urethra
    see Urethra
Urine, aspiration of, 576
Urodynamics, 577
Urticaria due to penicillin, 175
Uvula, 533

V

Vaccines, 709–713
Vagina, 604
  biopsies, 607
  destruction, 604
  endocervical polyps, 606–607, 607f
  endoscopy, 606–607
  excision, 604
  insertion of devices, 605, 605f
  irrigation, 605
  manipulation of, 606
  repair, 606
  suppositories, 621
Valium overdose, coma from, 178
Valvuloplasty, 497
Varicocele, on spermatic cord, 589
Vas deferens, 588–589
Vascular diagnostic studies, noninvasive, 725
Vasectomy, 589
Vasogram, 589
Vasotomy, 589
Vasovasorrhaphy, 589
Vasovasostomy, 589
Veins, 485f
Ventricular puncture, 632
Ventriculoperitoneal shunts, 633, 634f
  laminectomy, 636, 636f
  lumbar puncture, 636, 637f
Vermilionectomy, 527
Vertebrae, 636f
Vertebral column, 635f
Vesiculotomy, 591
Vulva, perineum, and introitus, 601
  destruction, 602
  excision, 602–603
  incision, 602
  repair, 603
Vulvectomy, 602–603
V-Y plasty, 402

W

Wound(s), 187–188
  complicated, 187
  gunshot, 432–433
  knife, 432–433
  repair
    see Wound repair
  types of, 400f
Wound repair
  abrasion codes, 408
  active care management, 739, 740f
  blepharoplasty, 408
  burn treatment, 412–414, 413f
  cervicoplasty, 408
  chemical peels, 408, 409f

Wound repair *(Continued)*
  complex repairs, 399
  components, 401
  debridement, 181, 401, 402f
  dermabrasion, 408, 409f
  exploration, 401
  factors, 398–401
  grafting procedures
    see Skin grafts

Wound repair *(Continued)*
  intermediate repairs, 399
  ligation, 401
  lipectomy, 410
  pressure ulcers, 410–411, 411f
  rhytidectomy, 409
  simple repairs, 399
W-plasty, 402

X
X-ray films, 672
  see also Radiology

Z
Z-plasty, 402, 402f

Trust Carol J. Buck and Elsevier for the
resources you need at *each step* of your coding career!

Track your progress toward complete coding success!

Step 1: Learn

- ❏ Step-by-Step Medical Coding 2010 Edition • ISBN: 978-1-4160-6836-5
- ❏ Workbook for Step-by-Step Medical Coding 2010 Edition • ISBN: 978-1-4377-0218-7
- ❏ Medical Coding Online for Step-by-Step Medical Coding 2010 • ISBN: 978-1-4377-0369-6
- ❏ Virtual Medical Office for Step-by-Step Medical Coding 2010 Edition • ISBN: 978-1-4377-1505-7

Step 2: Practice

- ❏ The Next Step: Advanced Medical Coding 2010 Edition • ISBN: 978-1-4377-0441-9
- ❏ Workbook for The Next Step: Advanced Medical Coding 2010 Edition • ISBN: 978-1-4377-0675-8
- ❏ Advanced Medical Coding Online for The Next Step 2010 Edition • ISBN: 978-1-4377-0442-6
- ❏ Online Internship for Medical Coding 2010 Edition • ISBN: 978-1-4377-0819-6

Step 3: Certify

- ❏ CPC® Coding Exam Review 2010: The Certification Step • ISBN: 978-1-4377-0817-2
- ❏ CCS Coding Exam Review 2010: The Certification Step • ISBN: 978-1-4377-0815-8
- ❏ The Extra Step: Facility-Based Coding Practice 2010 Edition • ISBN: 978-1-4377-1365-7
- ❏ The Extra Step: Physician-Based Coding Practice 2010 Edition • ISBN: 978-1-4377-0767-0

Step 4: Specialize

- ❏ Evaluation and Management Step: An Auditing Tool • ISBN: 978-1-4160-6724-5

Coding References

- ❏ 2010 ICD-9-CM for Physicians, Volumes 1 & 2, Professional Edition • ISBN: 978-1-4377-0208-8
- ❏ 2010 ICD-9-CM for Hospitals, Volumes 1, 2 & 3, Professional Edition • ISBN: 978-1-4377-0207-1
- ❏ 2010 ICD-9-CM for Physicians, Volumes 1 & 2, Standard Edition • ISBN: 978-1-4377-0748-9
- ❏ 2010 ICD-9-CM for Hospitals, Volumes 1, 2 & 3, Standard Edition • ISBN: 978-1-4377-0747-2
- ❏ 2010 ICD-9-CM for Physicians, Volumes 1 & 2, Professional Softcover Edition • ISBN: 978-1-4377-1434-0
- ❏ 2010 ICD-9-CM for Physicians, Volumes 1 & 2, Professional Compact Edition • ISBN: 978-1-4377-1433-3
- ❏ 2010 ICD-9-CM for Hospitals, Volumes 1, 2 & 3, Professional Compact Edition • ISBN: 978-1-4377-1432-6
- ❏ 2010 HCPCS Level II Professional Edition • ISBN: 978-1-4377-0211-8
- ❏ 2010 HCPCS Level II Standard Edition • ISBN: 978-1-4377-0818-9
- ❏ 2010 ICD-10-CM Standard Edition Draft Manual • ISBN: 978-1-4160-2567-2
- ❏ 2010 ICD-10-PCS Standard Edition Draft Manual • ISBN: 978-1-4160-6412-1

Author and
Educator
Carol J. Buck,
MS, CPC-I, CPC,
CPC-H, CCS-P

Get the next resources on your list today!

- Order securely at **www.elsevierhealth.com**
- Call toll-free **1-800-545-2522**
- Visit your local bookstore

PC-10

ELSEVIER